THE PHYSIOLOGICAL BASES OF COGNITIVE AND BEHAVIORAL DISORDERS

THE PHYSIOLOGICAL BASES OF COGNITIVE AND BEHAVIORAL DISORDERS

Lisa L. Weyandt

LEA LAWRENCE ERLBAUM ASSOCIATES, PUBLISHERS
2006 Mahwah, New Jersey   London

Senior Editor: Steve Rutter
Editorial Assistant: Victoria Forsythe
Cover Design: Kathryn Houghtaling Lacey
Textbook Production Manager: Paul Smolenski
Full-Service Compositor: TechBooks
Text and Cover Printer: Hamilton Printing Company

This book was typeset in 10/12 pt. Times New Roman, Bold, and Italic.
The heads were typeset in Sabon Bold and Bold Italic.

Lawrence Erlbaum Associates, Inc., Publishers
10 Industrial Avenue
Mahwah, New Jersey 07430
www.erlbaum.com

Library of Congress Cataloging-in-Publication Data

Weyandt, Lisa L.
    The physiological bases of cognitive and behavioral disorders /
Lisa L. Weyandt.
        p.   cm.
    Includes bibliographical references and index.
    ISBN 0-8058-4718-9 (case : alk. paper) — ISBN 0-8058-4719-7
(pbk. : alk. paper)
    1. Psychology, Pathological—Physiological aspects.   2. Cognition
disorders—Physiological aspects.   3. Neuropsychiatry.   I. Title.
    [DNLM: 1. Mental Disorders—physiopathology.   2. Brain Diseases
—physiopathology.   3. Brain Diseases—complications.   4. Brain
Injuries—complications.   WM 140 W546p 2005]
    RC455.4.B5W49   2005
    616.89—dc22   2005014272

Printed in the United States of America
10 9 8 7 6 5 4 3 2 1

To Bruce

Contents

Foreword

In his seminal historical work, *The Structure of Scientific Revolutions*, Thomas Kuhn taught us that science occurs in one of two modes: incremental step-by-step "puzzle-solving," and revolutionary changes in perspective and fundamental assumptions, which he first termed "paradigm shifts." Kuhn had noticed that all sciences, like all other human endeavors, require a trellis of shared and largely unspoken assumptions that include tenaciously held consensus on what questions can be asked, the methods that can be used to address those questions, and the criteria by which answers are judged valid or not. This implicit yet essential framework within which knowledge is organized and accumulated is the "paradigm." Working within a given paradigm provides the basis for the alchemy of science: the results are greater than the sum of the small individual findings because of the overall mosaic that emerges. Inevitably, as Kuhn observed, knowledge accumulates within a given paradigm until a tipping point is reached, beyond which the newly acquired data tiles no longer fit the previously agreed on framework/mosaic. This conflict between data and theory is first resolved by rejecting the data, which in isolation, are always flawed and subject to multiple interpretations. Eventually, as data that conflict with the dominant paradigm continue to accrue, the theory is altered ad hoc. Such improvised patches can continue indefinitely, but their progressive esthetic and predictive deficiencies make the improvised paradigm vulnerable. Following a period of fertile but disturbing confusion, a new paradigm emerges, which encompasses the old and provides a new "higher" plateau for continued scientific exploration. And so on.

Exactly one hundred years ago, Albert Einstein published three papers that ultimately led to the paradigm shifts that became known as the theory of relativity and quantum mechanics. Although it took several decades for these fundamental ideas to take firm hold within the community of physicists, now it is difficult to take seriously the previous perseverative attempts to measure the ether through which the earth was supposedly moving or the Euclidian definitions of space and time that prevailed at the time. Despite those undoubted achievements, even physics continues to struggle with incipient paradigm shifts, whether in the form of a "superstring theory" of the universe or in the continuing attempts to build a grand unified theory of gravity and electromagnetism.

However, the most challenging, fascinating, and necessary task before the community of 21st century scientists is the attempt to understand the physiological bases of cognitive and behavioral disorders. This unimaginably vast task stretches to the 19th century, but it truly began to accelerate only in the past two decades or so, as the necessary tools to allow study of the living brain have become available. The human brain is the most complex object in the universe, having over 100 billion neurons, each of which is continuously integrating inputs from 10,000 to 500,000 other neurons. Fortunately, the pace of discovery in brain sciences is now accelerating exponentially, so that we can be nearly certain that new paradigms will soon emerge that will dramatically alter the way in which we understand brain function and dysfunction. The elements of this vast mosaic are emerging from clinics in which the suffering of individual patients is systematically cataloged, thus improving our diagnostic systems. Other elements are increasingly provided by the panoply of emerging neuroimaging technologies, including positron emission tomography, magnetic resonance imaging, electroencephalography, magnetoencephalography, or near-infrared spectroscopic imaging. The fruits of molecular genetic studies are also beginning to illuminate unsuspected links and relationships as well as some of the usual suspects, such as the serotonin transporter promoter. Perhaps the most important part of this process is the Herculean effort to understand brain function in model organisms, including humans (cognitive neuroscience), non-human primates, rodents, fruit flies, and even flatworms. It is through the interplay of these multiple ways of knowing that the new paradigms of brain function that we so badly need will emerge. Ironically and wonderfully, it is much more likely that such new paradigms will be conceived by members of the generation of students who will be introduced to these topics by this comprehensive text, rather than by one of the authors cited in its list of references. And that is as it should be.

> —F. Xavier Castellanos, M.D.
> Brooke and Daniel Neidich Professor of Child
>   and Adolescent Psychiatry
> Director, Institute for Pediatric Neuroscience
> NYU Child Study Center
> New York, NY

Preface

It has been estimated that one in five adults and 15–20% of children and adolescents in the United States suffer from a diagnosable mental disorder (Costello & Angold, 1995; US Surgeon General, 1999). Cross-national studies have also reported alarmingly high prevalence rates of psychiatric disorders such as major depression (Simon, Fleck, Lucas, Bushnell, & LIDO Group, 2004); however, prevalence rates vary across countries due to classification systems and methods of defining and assessing mental illness. Both national and cross-national studies consistently indicate that despite the high prevalence of psychiatric disorders, only a minority of children and adults receive timely, appropriate, and consistent treatment. Many individuals suffer from more than one mental illness, and psychiatric disturbances are commonly found in patients with other medical conditions. For example, a variety of psychiatric symptoms have been found in patients with Parkinson's or Alzheimer's disease, most frequently depression, anxiety, and hallucinations (Aarsland et al., 1999; Menza, Robertson-Hoffman, & Bonapace, 1993; Paulsen et al., 2003). In 2003, neurologists Fink and colleagues assessed the prevalence of psychiatric disorders among newly referred, neurological inpatients and outpatients and discovered 46% of the men and 63% of the women had a psychiatric disorder (Fink, Hansen, Sondergaard, & Frydenberg, 2003). As studies by others had suggested, Fink and his colleagues found that more than two thirds had not received treatment. Freeman, Freeman, and McElroy (2002) reported that bipolar disorder, panic disorder, obsessive compulsive disorder, social phobia, and posttraumatic stress disorder frequently co-occur and that psychobiological mechanisms likely account for these high comorbidity rates. Bankier, Januzzi, and Littman (2004) recently reported a high prevalence of comorbid psychiatric disorders in patients with coronary heart disease including major depression, posttraumatic stress disorder, eating disorders, and alcohol abuse. Massagli and colleagues (2004) found that children were at significant increased risk for psychiatric disorders following mild traumatic brain injury, and Burns et al. (2004) reported nearly half of children aged 2 to 14 years with completed child welfare investigations suffered from emotional and behavioral problems. Vega, Sribney, Aguilar-Gaxiola, and Kolody (2004) recently completed a 12-month prevalence study of psychiatric disorders among Mexican Americans and reported that 14.2% of immigrant women and 12.6% of immigrant men suffered from mood, anxiety, and substance disorders. Rates were significantly higher for U.S.-born Mexican-American women and men. Following the events of September

11, 2001, Fullerton, Ursano, and Wang (2004) studied rates of psychiatric disorders in rescue and disaster workers and found 40.5% of disaster workers had developed acute stress disorder, posttraumatic stress disorder, or major depression. These studies underscore the extent of mental illness in the general population, the need to better understand the biological underpinnings of these disorders, and the necessity for developing effective treatment approaches.

Numerous psychological and psychiatric theories exist about the origin, continuity–discontinuity, and treatment of mental illness. These theories differ in many respects including the degree to which biological (e.g., genetics, neurochemistry) and/or environmental factors (e.g., stimulation, deprivation, learning) contribute to pathology. Theoretical perspectives and explanations of behavior typically influence choice of treatment such as therapy, skills training, medication, or a combination of approaches. Although many argue that clinical conditions such as depression are the result of both biological and environmental influences, others disagree. Peter Breggin, for example, argues that depression is a common human experience and that environmental factors and life circumstances are the cause, not genetics or biochemistry (Breggin & Breggin, 1994). In contrast, LeDoux, (2002) recently described mental illness as abnormal patterns of synaptic transmission, neural circuits, and neurotransmitters. Similarly, Kendall and Jablensky (2003) argue that biological factors contribute significantly to mental illness and recently noted that "psychiatry is in a state of flux, and advances in neuroscience and genetics are soon likely to challenge many of its current theoretical underpinnings, particularly those related to the causation and definition of mental disorders" (p. 4). The common-sense approach to explaining mental illness is to acknowledge that both biological factors and environmental factors contribute to aberrant brain functioning and the expression of disorders. The question then becomes to what extent do biological and environmental factors contribute to the expression of pathology, and which of these factors precipitates the other? Unfortunately, many of the studies described in this text are based on correlational findings and, therefore, preclude causal inference. Scientists from disciplines as varied as molecular genetics, neuroscience, neuropsychology, neuroimaging, neurophysiology, and neurology have all contributed to the understanding of brain functioning, although current knowledge is rudimentary relative to that which is yet to be discovered. Part of the difficulty in uncovering the nature of brain functioning is a result of the enormous complexity of neuronal circuitry. Each cognitive or behavioral function is dependent on the interactions of millions of neurons and glial cells and, according to Skinner and colleagues (2000), these interactions are "both dynamically variable and mathematically nonlinear." Nevertheless, researchers have gained considerable progress in understanding the functions associated with brain regions, fundamental neural networks, and the neurochemistry involved in memory, movement, and emotion, as well as numerous clinical disorders.

This is a revolutionary era for neuroscience, particularly in the areas of genetics, pharmacology, brain stimulation techniques, and neuroimaging of the brain. The implications of recent neuroscience findings are staggering. For example, scientists a the Highland Psychiatric Research Foundation in Inverness, Scotland, have developed breath and skin patch tests that may one day be useful in the early diagnosis of schizophrenia. With regard to brain cells, one of the more recent discoveries is that, contrary to dogma, certain areas of the human brain can generate new neurons (a process known as neurogenesis) and that medications used to treat depression may foster neurogenesis in at least one area of the brain, the hippocampus. This knowledge has critical ramifications for drug development and treatment of clinical disorders that are characterized by neuronal death, such as Parkinson's and Alzheimer's diseases. It is conceivable that drugs may be developed to stimulate neurogenesis and thus slow the progression or even ameliorate brain disease. Research has also demonstrated that the brain is mutable, although little is known about the parameters of the brain's ability to revise itself. The most convincing evidence is based on studies of patients who have sustained brain injuries and have recovered varying degrees of behavioral and cognitive function. Controversially, some researchers have argued that cognitive disorders such as reading and language disabilities may be modified at a physiological level through nonpharmacological, environmental stimulation, a view supported by only a preliminary study thus far (e.g., Merzenich et al., 1999; Temple et al., 2003).

In addition to improving pathological conditions, neuroscientific research—and, in particular, pharmacological research—has produced drugs that may actually enhance normal functioning. For example, it has been well established that pharmacological interventions, such as Ritalin, can drastically improve the cognitive and behavioral functioning of children, adolescents, and adults with ADHD. There is also a large body of research that substantiates the ability of antidepressants and anti-anxiety medications to drastically improve the symptoms of depression and anxiety disorders. With regard to self-improvement, psychiatrist and author Peter Kramer (1997) has described patients who achieve an enhanced brain (i.e., a brain that is "better than well" (p. xvii)) while taking Prozac. "Cosmetic psychopharmacology" (Kramer, 1997, p. 7) may indeed be a futuristic method to improve cognitive and behavioral functioning in healthy people. Pharmaceutical companies have invested billions of dollars in an effort to develop memory-enhancing drugs to slow memory loss and restore memory functions for patients with dementia, such as Alzheimer's disease. Perhaps, these drugs will also enhance the memory skills of healthy individuals. Robert Langreth (2002), a reporter for Forbes, aptly referred to such memory-enhancing drugs as "Viagra for the brain" and, based on interviews with various scientists, reported that these drugs will soon be available.

Altering brain functioning through genetic engineering, implants, transplants, psychosurgery, or medication poses a plethora of ethical questions. In May 2002, the Dana Alliance for Brain Initiatives, in collaboration with Stanford University Center for Biomedical Ethics and the University of California, San Francisco, held a conference that delineated a new field, "neuroethics," to address the social, legal, and ethical implications of modern brain research. Adina Roskies (2002) from the MIT Department of Linguistics and Philosophy identified two main divisions of neuroethics: the ethics of neuroscience and the neuroscience of ethics. Clearly, with the rapid advancement of technology, and as researchers continue to unravel the complexities of the human brain and better understand normal as well as abnormal brain functioning, the ethical discussions and debates will only continue.

Given the recent advances in clinical neuroscience, the purpose of this book is to summarize the literature concerning the physiological bases of various cognitive and behavioral disorders. Along the same lines, physiologically based (e.g., ECT) and pharmacological interventions are also discussed throughout the text. Although research clearly supports the use of nonpharmacological therapy based interventions for various disorders, coverage of these approaches is beyond the scope of this book. It should be noted that the disorders covered in this book are described according to the Diagnostic and Statistical Manual of the American Psychiatric Association, now on its fourth edition, partially updated in 2000. (DSM IV-TR, APA, 2000). The DSM will undergo future revisions as our knowledge of mental illness advances. Critics such as Kendell and Jalbensky (2003) argue that although the DSM classification system is invaluable and extremely useful, it does not necessarily represent independent, valid disorders. Indeed, there are often overlapping symptoms among disorders, and conditions such as depression and anxiety may exist as a continuous distribution of symptoms rather than a distinct dichotomy between abnormality and normalcy. Furthermore, that line is often arbitrary, as noted by Johns and van Os (2001), who have found that psychotic experiences exist on a continuum and even "normal" individuals experience hallucinations and delusions. As technology advances, particularly with regard to genetics and neuroimaging, psychiatric disorders may one day be conceptualized in a pathophysiologically classification system. But, at present, most psychiatric diagnoses are based on a number of cognitive and behavioral indicators in conjunction with factors such as frequency and duration of behavior, level of impairment, age, gender, and sociocultural factors. As Steven Hyman, Provost of Harvard University and former head of the National Institute of Mental Health, recently noted, "defining a rational nosology for disorders of the brain, the body's most complex organ, is clearly one of the greatest challenges for modern medical science" (Hyman, 2002).

The intention of this book is to provide the reader with a greater understanding of what is known and what is still not fully understood about the physiological bases of cognitive and behavioral disorders. We begin with a review of basic principles of neuroscience—neuroanatomy, cellular function, and neurotransmission. Also included is information on physiological techniques and neuroimaging, neuroplasticity, and research regarding physiologically based interventions. The remaining chapters review research findings, their limitations, and the unanswered questions concerning the physiological basis of specific cognitive and behavioral disorders.

Acknowledgments

I would like to express my gratitude to Central Washington University and the Department of Psychology for supporting my professional leave so that I could devote my time to writing *The Physiological Bases of Cognitive and Behavioral Disorders*. I would also like to acknowledge the following students who served as my research assistants during the formation and writing stages: Meghan Alderson, Katie Fulton, Deborah Gaidos, Meredith Miller, Nif Obeid, Amy Shoaf, and Bilyana Yakova. Sarah Dunkin and Michelle Lillard provided valuable assistance in the preparation of the index. The staff at the CWU Interlibrary loan office—Rebecca Smith, Carol Peterson, and Jennifer Jaques—deserves special acknowledgment for the tireless tracking down and ordering of thousands of articles cited in this book. I would also like to acknowledge Estelle Mathews, and Donna Miglino Secretaries, Department of Psychology, for their practical assistance. I thank my friend and colleague, Dr. Terry Devietti, for his encouragement to pursue this project and for reading sample chapters along the way.

I am particularly grateful for the illustrations provided by Blausen Medical Communications and would like to acknowledge and thank Bruce Blausen, the CEO and president, for his willingness to participate in this project. Blausen Medical Communications is a specialty scientific medical and animation and illustration company that has an international reputation for excellence in scientific precision and product development. I would also like to offer special recognition to Grant Peterson, the creator of the illustrations, whose attention to design, detail, and accuracy resulted in extraordinary images.

Special thanks go to my 4-year-old son, Sebastian, for his unwavering love and patience, especially during the times when my mind was distracted by the development of this book. Finally, I would like to thank my editor, Steve Rutter, for his support and encouragement throughout this process.

THE PHYSIOLOGICAL BASES
OF COGNITIVE AND
BEHAVIORAL DISORDERS

1

Neuroanatomy, Brain Development, and Plasticity

This chapter reviews the anatomy of the brain: the structures and associated functions of the forebrain, midbrain, and hindbrain. It also explains the role of glial cells and neurons and addresses the processes involved in prenatal and postnatal brain development including neurulation, dendritic arborization, and myelination. Finally, it presents research on the brain's capacity to change in response to environmental stimulation, stroke, developmental anomalies, or deprivation.

OVERVIEW OF THE NERVOUS SYSTEM

The nervous system has two main divisions: the peripheral nervous system (PNS) and the central nervous system (CNS). The PNS is located outside the skull and spine and detects environmental information via sensory receptors. It then transmits this information to the CNS by way of sensory nerves known as *afferent* nerves (from the Latin for carry information *to* the CNS). The PNS also transmits information from the CNS to muscles, glands, and internal organs by way of motor nerves known as *efferent* nerves (from the Latin for carry information *away* from the CNS). The PNS is subdivided into the somatic and autonomic nervous systems. The somatic division controls skeletal movement, and the autonomic division controls glands and muscles of internal organs. The autonomic division regulates internal bodily processes and consists of the sympathetic (arousal) and parasympathetic (restoration) nervous systems. The CNS is located in the skull and spine and consists of the brain and the spinal cord. Twelve pairs of cranial nerves and 31 pairs of spinal nerves connect the brain and spinal cord to the PNS. As shown in Fig. 1.1, the cranial nerves are located on the ventral surface of the brain and involve numerous functions of the head, neck, and face. The cranial nerves found on the brain stem involve vital functions.

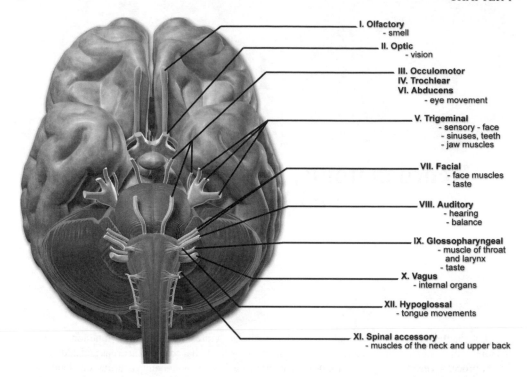

FIG. 1.1.   Location and function of cranial nerves.
Copyright Blausen Medical Communications. Reproduced by permission.

BRAIN REGIONS, STRUCTURES, AND FUNCTIONS

Directionality and Terminology

The brain can be viewed from various anatomical directions based on three axes: anterior–posterior, dorsal–ventral, and medial–lateral. *Anterior* refers to the front (also known as rostral) and *posterior* the rear or tail (also known as caudal). *Dorsal* means toward the back or top and *ventral* toward the belly or ground. *Lateral* refers to the side and *medial* the midline (Fig. 1.2). Ipsilateral refers to the same side of the body and contralateral to the opposite side of the body. The structures of the brain can also be viewed from several perspectives: horizontal, saggittal, and coronal planes. A *horizontal* plane runs parallel to the top of the brain, a *saggittal* plane runs parallel to the side of the brain, and a *coronal* plane runs parallel to the front of the brain. This directional terminology will be important for understanding the information to follow as well as interpreting the scientific literature.

BRAIN DIVISIONS

The brain consists of five major divisions: telencephalon, diencephalon, mesencephalon, metencephalon, and myelencephalon. The telencephalon and diencephalon comprise the forebrain. The mesencephalon refers to the midbrain, and the metencephalon and myelencephalon comprise the hindbrain (Fig. 1.3).

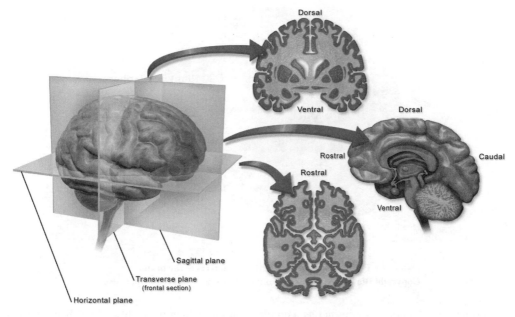

FIG. 1.2.   Directionality and planes.
Copyright Blausen Medical Communications. Reproduced by permission.

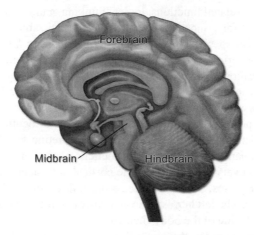

FIG. 1.3.   Sagittal section depicting three primary divisions
of the brain. Copyright Blausen Medical Communications. Reproduced by permission.

Forebrain

The *telencephalon* is the largest division of the human brain and is involved in developing complex cognitive and behavioral processes such as initiating movement, interpreting sensory stimulation, and higher-level cognition such as planning, problem solving, and language. The telencephalon is made up of two cerebral hemispheres—the right and the left (Fig. 1.4), which are connected by a number of bundles of nerve fibers (i.e., commissures) including the corpus callosum, anterior and posterior commissures, hippocampal commissure, and habenular

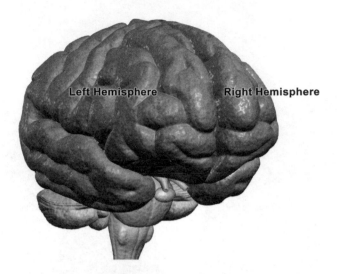

FIG. 1.4.   Left and right hemispheres of the brain.
Copyright Blausen Medical Communications. Reproduced by permission.

commissure. The commissures act as a conduit through which the right and left hemispheres exchange information and function interdependently (Springer & Deutsch, 1993). The hemispheres are asymmetrical and vary in size depending on specific structures or regions (e.g., left frontal is larger in size than right frontal; Watkins et al., 2001). In general, the left hemisphere is specialized for language-related functions, logical thinking, and writing; the right hemisphere is specialized in function for visuospatial, musical, and artistic abilities (Springer & Deutsch, 1993). This asymmetrical specialization of function is known as *lateralization*. Evidence of these processing hemispheric differences derives largely from individuals with brain damage, surgically cut corpus callosum ("split-brain patients"), and neuropsychological studies. For example, damage to the left frontal lobe (Broca's area) or left temporal lobe (Wernicke's area) can result in difficulties with language production and comprehension (Damasio, 1991). Damage to the right hemisphere can result in spatial reasoning difficulties such as judging line orientation (Benton, Hannay, & Varney, 1975) and interpreting facial expressions (Bowers, Bauer, Coslett, & Heilman, 1985). Many other deficits have been ascribed to left and right hemisphere damage and vary depending on the cortical and subcortical regions involved as well as factors such as age, sex, intelligence, location, and severity of the damage (Kolb, 1989; Kolb & Whishaw, 1996). The left hemisphere generally controls the right side of the body, the right hemisphere the left side of the body (i.e., contralateral control).

The hemispheres are covered by the cerebral cortex and separated by the longitudinal fissure (Fig. 1.5). The cerebral cortex is approximately 3 mm thick and consists of six layers of cells (of varying thickness) running parallel to its surface. Because the cortex consists mainly of cell bodies, it has a grayish appearance and is commonly referred to as "gray matter." Extentions of the cell body (*axons*) project to other areas of the cortex and to subcortical regions. According to Martini (1998), the total surface area of the cortex is roughly equivalent to 2.5 square feet of flat surface. The size and shape of the skull cause the cortical structure of the brain to fold inward. Hence much of the brain is hidden within the grooves. These folds or bumps are called gyri, and the grooves are known as sulci (smaller grooves) and fissures (major grooves). During evolution the human brain increased in size, in particular the volume of the cerebral cortex. Rakic (1995) has suggested that a genetic alteration may have played a significant role in the large surface size of the cortex in humans relative to other animals.

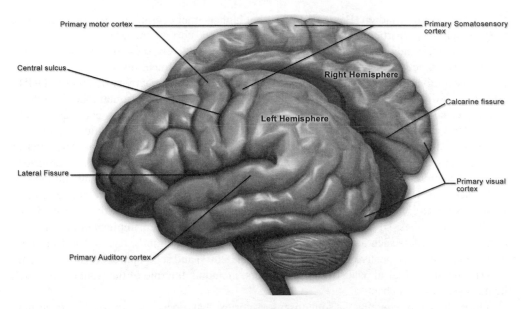

FIG. 1.5. Left and right hemispheres, corti, fissures, and central sulcus. Copyright Blausen Medical Communications. Reproduced by permission.

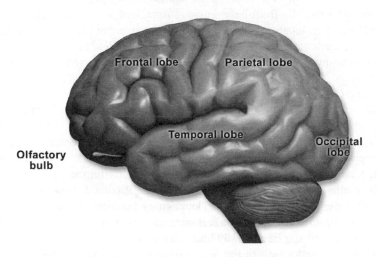

FIG. 1.6. Olfactory bulb and four lobes of the brain. Copyright Blausen Medical Communications. Reproduced by permission.

The telencephalon also includes the frontal, parietal, temporal, and occipital lobes (Fig. 1.6). The frontal lobe is the most anterior, and the parietal lobe is posterior and dorsal to the frontal lobe. Located on the lateral surface, the temporal lobe is separated from the frontal and parietal lobes by the lateral sulcus. The occipital lobe is the most posterior of the four lobes. Although each lobe has primary functions, all four are highly interconnected. The frontal lobe, the largest of the four lobes, contains the motor cortex that is involved in voluntary movement. A specialized region important in language production, known as Broca's area, is found in the frontal lobe of the left hemisphere. The right frontal lobe has also been found to play a role in language functions in young children (Basser, 1962). Other higher-order cognitive processes ascribed to the frontal lobes, in particular the anterior region (prefrontal cortex), include strategic planning, impulse control, and flexibility of thought and action. Collectively, these processes are known as executive functions retain (Fletcher, 1996). A number of clinical disorders are characterized by executive function deficits including attention-deficit/hyperactivity disorder (ADHD), Alzheimer's disease, schizophrenia, and others (Weyandt, 2004). The frontal lobes have three primary circuits: dorsolateral, orbitofrontal, and anterior cingulate (Burruss et al., 2000). The dorsolateral circuit is postulated to be specifically involved in executive functions and the orbitofrontal circuit in regulation of emotions and socially appropriate behavior. The anterior cingulate circuit is thought to mediate motivation and wakefulness and arousal. As described by Burruss and colleagues, damage to this circuit can result in profound apathy, immobility, and absence of behavior. Christ, White, Mandernach, and Keys (2001) have suggested that inhibitory control, that develops early in childhood and declines in late adulthood, is mediated by the frontal lobes. Dysfunction of frontal lobe circuitry has been implicated in a number of clinical disorders such as ADHD (Ernst et al., 2003), Alzheimer's disease (Sultzer et al., 2003), obsessive compulsive disorder (Saxena et al., 2003) and schizophrenia (Callicott et al., 2003). The physiological basis of these disorders, including the role of the frontal lobes, will be discussed in later chapters.

The parietal lobe contains the somatosensory cortex, that processes information concerning the body's position in space and sensory information from the skin such as touch, pressure, and pain (see Fig. 1.5). Stimulating any part of the skin—for example, on the nose, finger, or foot—leads to activation of neurons in the somatosensory cortex that represent that area. Damage to the parietal lobe from head injury, stroke, and so on can result in a number of effects depending on the location and severity of the damage. For example, damage to the right parietal lobe can result in contralateral neglect, that is, complete lack of awareness of visual, auditory, and somatosensory stimulation on the left side of the body (McFie & Zangwill, 1960). Disorders of tactile function, spatial ability, and drawing are also associated with damage to the parietal lobe (Kolb & Whishaw, 1996). Like the other lobes, the temporal lobes are rich in afferent and efferent pathways that connect to cortical and subcortical regions of the brain. The primary auditory cortex located in the temporal lobe plays a critical role in hearing and the processing of sounds. The left hemisphere of the temporal lobe contains a region known as Wernicke's area that is critical to understanding spoken language. Damage to the temporal lobe can result in a variety of disturbances affecting auditory sensation and perception, long-term memory, personality, and language comprehension (e.g., Blumer & Benson, 1975; Samson & Zatorre, 1988; Scoville & Milner, 1957). The primary function of the occipital lobes is the analysis of visual information, and damage therein can result in a number of visual perception disturbances (*agnosias*) (see Banich, 1997 for a review).

Additional structures located in the telencephalon include the limbic system and basal ganglia. The limbic system is actually a set of interconnected structures that form a ring around the thalamus and include the limbic cortex, hippocampus, amygdala, and fornix. The limbic system regulates motivated behaviors such as sexual behavior, eating, and aggressive behavior as well as learning, memory, and recognition and expression of emotion. Recent research has implicated part of the limbic cortex, the anterior cingulate cortex, in a variety of cognitive and emotional functions. Bush, Luu, and Posner (2000), for example, described two main subdivisions of the anterior cingulate cortex: the cognitive and affective subdivisions. They suggested that connections with the lateral prefrontal cortex, parietal, and motor corti are tied to cognitive processing such as the modulation of attention, motor control, pain aversiveness, and higher-order cognitive processes. Alternatively, the affective subdivision is connected to structures such as the hippocampus, hypothalamus, amygdala, and nucleus accumbens and is

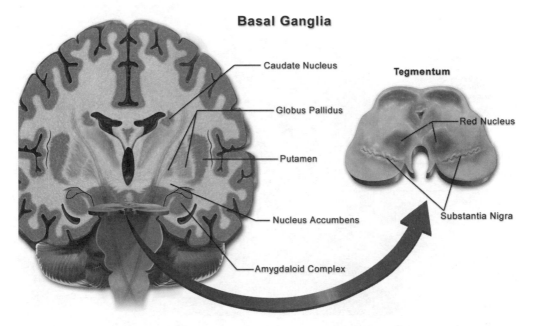

FIG. 1.7. Basal ganglia. Copyright Blausen Medical Communications. Reproduced by permission.

involved in the interpretation and regulation of emotional responses. Bush and colleagues also suggested that the cingulate cortex undergoes a long developmental process and the volume of the cingulate cortex is related to regulation of emotional and behavioral responses. Heimer (2003) recently noted that the interconnections among these structures are so complex that it is a misconception to regard the limbic system as a separate system from the basal ganglia. He described additional circuits within the limbic region and explained how these pathways project from the cerebral cortex, hippocampus, amygdala, and other structures to the basal ganglia. Quirk and Gehlert (2003) suggested that the amygdala plays an important role in the development of anxiety disorders and drug-seeking behaviors. Specifically, they hypothesized that the neuronal pathways that extend from the amygdala to the prefrontal cortex are deficient in inhibitory tone (i.e., overactivity) and thus drugs targeting these pathways could prevent addiction relapse and anxiety disorders.

The basal ganglia are a complex group of subcortical cell bodies that play a critical role in movement. They consist of the caudate nucleus, putamen, and the globus pallidus (Fig. 1.7). The caudate nucleus and putamen together are known as the striatum. The striatum receives input from the cortex and other structures (e.g., thalamus and amygdala) and projects information to widespread regions such as the brain stem and the prefrontal cortex (van Dongen & Groenewegen, 2002). The nucleus accumbens is a group of cell bodies located adjacent to the striatum. One pathway known as the nigrostriatal system extends from the substantia nigra (located in the midbrain) to the striatum. Parkinson's disease is associated with degeneration of cell bodies of the substantia nigra that affect functioning of the nigrostriatal system and, consequently, movement. A second pathway, the mesolimbic system, extends from the tegmentum (midbrain cell bodies) to the nucleus accumbens, amygdala, and hippocampus. This pathway has been implicated in rewarding brain stimulation and clinical disorders such as schizophrenia and addictive behavior (Koob & Nestler, 1997; Soares & Innis, 1999). Heimer (2003) discussed additional pathways that connect the cerebral cortex, limbic system, and basal ganglia, arguing that "all major telencephalic disorders are, to some extent at least, disorders

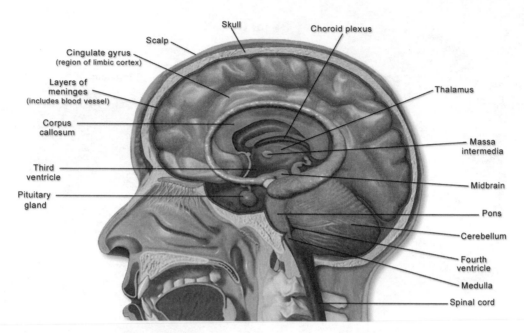

Skull

Scalp

Cingulate gyrus
(region of limbic cortex)

Layers of
meninges
(includes blood vessel)

Corpus
callosum

Third
ventricle

Pituitary
gland

Choroid plexus

Thalamus

Massa
intermedia

Midbrain

Pons

Cerebellum

Fourth
ventricle

Medulla

Spinal cord

FIG. 1.8.   Sagittal section showing the pituitary gland, ventricle system, corpus callosum, and additional brain structures. Copyright Blausen Medical Communications. Reproduced by permission.

of the basal ganglia" (p. 1737). These topics and pathways will be examined in greater detail in subsequent chapters (see Nicholson & Faull, 2002 for additional information about the basal ganglia).

The *diencephalon*, also part of the forebrain, is comprised of the thalamus and the hypothalamus. The thalamus consists of cell bodies that receive, process, and transmit sensory input to appropriate areas of the cortex. For this reason, it is often referred to as a "relay station" for visual, auditory, and somatosensory information. The hypothalamus also consists of a group of cell bodies and is located below the anterior portion of the thalamus. It plays a critical role in regulating the autonomic nervous system as well as numerous survival behaviors such as eating, drinking, emotional regulation, and mating. The hypothalamus is also involved in functioning of the endocrine system and releasing hormones that stimulate the pituitary gland, which in turn controls other endocrine glands. The pituitary gland is located on the ventral surface of the hypothalamus near the optic chiasm and mamillary bodies (Fig. 1.8).

The *optic chiasm* is the point at which the nerves extending from each eye come together. The *mamillary bodies* are a collection of cell bodies located posterior to the pituitary gland and are part of the hypothalamus. Chugani (1998) recently reported that the sensorimotor cortex, thalamus, amygdala, basal ganglia, and areas of the brain stem were more active in newborn infants compared to other areas of the cortex where cellular activity was relatively low. Chugani's study supports other brain development studies which have suggested that different regions of the brain mature at different rates and that this level of brain maturation is related to behavioral competencies.

Midbrain

The *mesencephalon*, also known as the *midbrain*, contains numerous ascending and descending pathways that project from the subcortical to cortical regions. The midbrain is involved in maintaining alertness as well as many basic behavioral reactions. It is comprised of two subdivisions: the tectum and the tegmentum. The tectum is composed of two pairs of bumps: the superior and the inferior colliculi. The superior colliculi are involved in vision and the inferior colliculi are involved in hearing. The tegmentum lies ventrally to the tectum and contains a number of structures that play an important role in attention, arousal, sleep, sensitivity to pain, and movement. These structures include the reticular formation, periaqueductal gray matter, red nucleus, and substantia nigra (Fig. 1.7; see Henricus, Domburg, & Donklaar, 1991 for additional information).

Hindbrain

The *metencephalon* and *myelencephalon* comprise the *hindbrain* (Fig. 1.3). The metencephalon consists of the pons and the cerebellum. The myelencephalon contains one structure, the medulla oblongata. The pons lies between the midbrain and the medulla oblongata, ventrally to the cerebellum. The pons also serves as a relay station from the cortex to the cerebellum and is important in regulating sleep (Jones, 1993). The cerebellum is attached to the pons by bundles of axons called cerebellar peduncles. The cerebellum receives information from other parts of the brain and projects information throughout regions of the brain. It plays a critical role in movement, and damage to the cerebellum impairs coordinated movements as well as standing and walking. Recent research suggests that the cerebellum is involved in additional functions such as language, memory, and emotions and may play a role in psychiatric disorders such as schizophrenia (Caplan, Gomez Beldarrain, Bier, Vokaer, Bartholme, & Pandolfo, 2002; Herb & Thyen, 1992; Leroi et al., 2002; Martin & Albers, 1995; Vokaer et al., 2002).

The myelencephalon consists of the medulla oblongata and structures therein. Contained within the medulla is a complex network of cell bodies that project to the midbrain. This network is known as the *reticular formation* (or activating system) and is important in a variety of functions such as attention, arousal, sleep, and certain reflexes that are necessary for survival.

BRAIN DEVELOPMENT

There is no universally accepted theory of brain functioning, although as Hynd and Willis (1988) have indicated, it is generally understood that the brain works as a functional system. Specifically, Hynd and Willis extrapolated on Luria's (1970) theory of functional brain units and postulated that various regions and structures of the brain are specialized in function yet function interdependently. Research clearly indicates that a relationship exists between brain development and behavior and that the brain develops in a hierarchical fashion (Huttenlocher, 2002). For example, Luria (1980) suggested that posterior and subcortical regions of the brain that are associated with early survival behaviors (e.g., sucking, swallowing) are more developed at birth than cortical regions that are involved in higher-order cognitive processes (e.g., executive functions, problem solving). Indeed, structural and functional imaging studies of the brain have found a consistent pattern of evolving changes with greater cellular activity in the brain stem and subcortical structures shortly after birth and gradual increase in cortical activity during the first 2 years (Tokumaru et al., 1999). In addition, neuroimaging studies have found that as development progresses, activity at the level of the cerebral cortex changes from more diffuse involvement to greater localization of brain activity. Just et al. (1996), for example, studied adults using fMRI and found that more regions of the brain were activated during a complex sentence comprehension task and fewer regions were activated as the task decreased in complexity. Studies with children have found similar findings, supporting the view that different regions of the brain are specialized in function and these functions are related to stages of brain development. Recent neuroimaging studies also suggest that higher-level cognitive functions such as abstract reasoning, problem solving, and planning are processed at the level of the cortex and the pattern of activation for these tasks may vary greatly among individuals (e.g., Derbyshire, Vogt, & Jones, 1998). Brain development begins shortly after conception with the onset of neurulation.

PRENATAL BRAIN GROWTH

Neurulation

The first prenatal period of development is the *germinal period* and is characterized by the union of egg and sperm, division of cells, and implantation of this group of cells in the uterine wall. The second prenatal period begins around the 14th day of gestation and is known as the *embryonic period*. At approximately 2 weeks gestation, a portion of the embryonic tissue (*ectoderm*) begins to thicken and forms the neural plate. In the middle of the neural plate is a fissure that continues to deepen and fold inward, forming the neural groove. The folds of the neural groove eventually fuse and form the neural tube. A portion of the tube later becomes the brain's ventricles and spinal canal. At approximately 3 weeks gestation, the ectoderm separates from the neural tube, and cells from the ectoderm migrate laterally and eventually form the spinal and cranial nerves. Between the 3rd and 4th weeks of gestation, the anterior and posterior ends of the neural tube fuse, and the posterior end develops into the spinal cord. The anterior end of the neural tube gives rise to brain vesicles that later develop into the structures that form the major subdivisions of the brain (forebrain, midbrain, hindbrain; see Swanson, 2003 for more information). During the fetal period, which lasts from the beginning of the 3rd month gestation until birth, the brain continues to develop at a rapid pace, at a rate of 250,000 neurons per minute (Cowan, 1979). This growth is associated with functional abilities in the fetus (e.g., somatosensory, hearing, movement) as well as noticeable morphological changes (e.g., gyri and sulci form around the 7th month (Kolb & Whishaw, 2001, p. 242). By 5 months gestation, most nerve cells (neurons) have formed. By the end of the fetal period, all of the brain's structures have formed and become functional. A number of cellular events contribute to brain maturation including cell birth, migration, differentiation, synaptogenesis, mylenization, synaptic pruning, and cellular death.

BRAIN CELLS AND BRAIN MATURATION

Neurons and Glial Cells

The brain consists of two main types of cells: neurons and glial cells (Figs. 1.9 and 1.10). In general, neurons communicate messages and glial cells were thought to serve ancillary functions such as providing structure and support to neurons. Recent research, however, suggests that glial cells play a role in a number of cellular processes such as facilitating communication among neurons, plasticity, and production of substances that nourish neurons and enhance their survival (*neurotrophins*; Otten et al., 2001). Glial cells are subdivided into several types; the two main types found in the CNS are the *astrocytes* and *oligodendrocytes*. Astrocytes are the largest type of glial cell and provide structural support for neurons. In addition, they are in physical contact with blood vessels and form a protective barrier so toxic substances do not penetrate the brain. Astrocytes also transport substances from the blood to and from

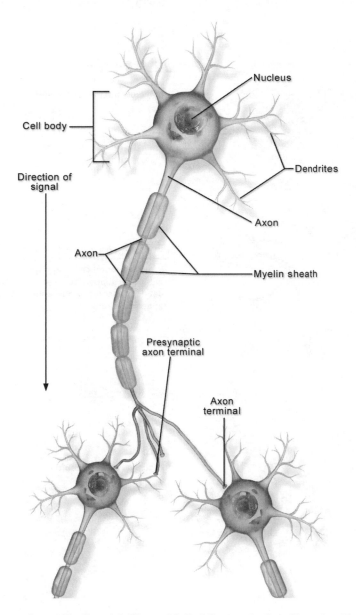

FIG. 1.9.   Image of a neuron. Copyright Blausen Medical Communications. Reproduced by permission.

neurons. Recent evidence suggests that astrocytes are involved in the production of chemicals that neurons use to communicate with each other and that the interaction between astrocytes and neurons may be impaired during degenerative brain diseases such as dementia (Hertz, Yu, Kala, & Schousboe, 2000). Recent research also suggests that astrocytes may strengthen signaling among neurons by releasing substances that amplify the effects of neurotransmitters (Do, Benz, Binns, Eaton, & Salt, 2004).

Oligodendrocytes form a protective sheath, known as *myelin*, around part of the neuron, the axon. Myelin consists of lipids and proteins and helps to insulate and facilitate the transduction of messages sent from one neuron to another. Many, but not all, axons are myelinated in the CNS.

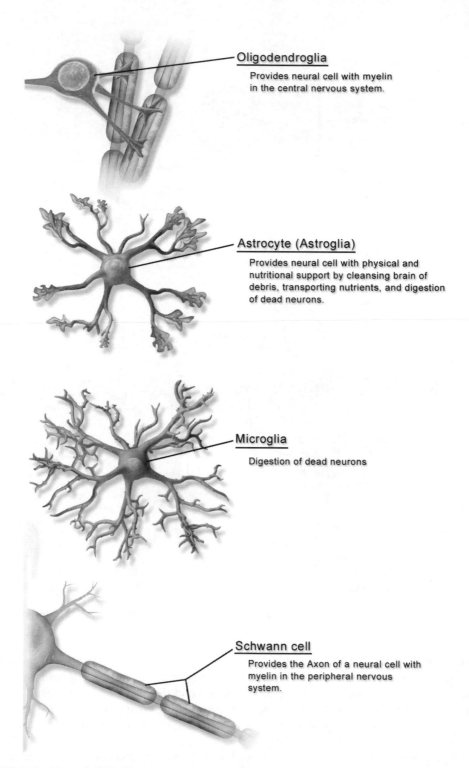

Oligodendroglia

Provides neural cell with myelin in the central nervous system.

Astrocyte (Astroglia)

Provides neural cell with physical and nutritional support by cleansing brain of debris, transporting nutrients, and digestion of dead neurons.

Microglia

Digestion of dead neurons

Schwann cell

Provides the Axon of a neural cell with myelin in the peripheral nervous system.

FIG. 1.10. Types of glial cells. Copyright Blausen Medical Communications. Reproduced by permission.

According to Levitan and Kaczmarek (1997, p. 25), glial cells are also thought to (a) participate in the uptake and breakdown of chemicals that neurons use for communication, (b) act as scavengers and remove debris including dead neurons, (c) take up ions from the extracellular environment, (d) provide proteins and other substances to neurons, (e) segregate groups of neurons from one another, and (f) alter neuronal signaling by changing ion concentrations in the extracellular fluid. Piet, Vargova, Sykova, Poulain, and Oliet (2004) recently reported that glia cells (*astrocytes*) help to regulate communication among neurons and enhance or hinder neurotransmission by facilitating or impeding diffusion of neurotransmitters in the brain.

Neurons come in different shapes, sizes, and types. As reviewed by Thompson (2000), there are four main classifications of neurons: motor, sensory, principal, and interneurons. *Motor* neurons have axons that project to the spinal cord where they communicate with other motor neurons that innervate muscles and glands. *Sensory* neurons convey information from the peripheral nervous system to the CNS. Within the brain are principal and interneurons. *Principal* neurons have long axons that extend to other locations in the brain whereas *interneurons* have shorter axons that communicate messages to nearby cells. The basic components of a neuron include a cell body (*soma*), dendrites, and an axon. The cell body contains the nucleus and other structures that help a neuron process and transmit information. Dendrites are very thin structures that emerge from the cell body of the neuron and are formed in a variety of shapes and sizes. They receive messages from other neurons while axons transmit messages to other cells. Dendrites continue to develop and mature postnatally and are believed to play an integral role in plasticity (Kennedy, 2000). Axons of neurons extend from the cell body and transmit information from the cell body to other neurons, a process known as *neurotransmission*. Neurotransmission is covered in detail in the chapter 2.

Cell Migration

Neurons and glial cells originate prenatally from stem cells. Stem cells line the cerebral ventricles and give rise to progenitor cells that in turn produce neuroblasts and glioblasts. *Neuroblasts* are immature neurons and *glioblasts* are immature glial cells; the formation of these cells is known as *neurogenesis* and *gliogenesis*, respectively. Factors that regulate the processes of neurogenesis and gliogenesis are not well understood, but neuroscientists are studying the role of genes and various proteins that may trigger cellular change and maturation. For example, Conti et al. (2001) proposed that the presence of certain proteins (i.e., ShcA and ShcC) in progenitor cells is involved in the division of neural stem cells and appear to critically affect the survival and maturation of these cells. They also suggested that these proteins may affect the neuroblast's responsiveness to extracellular factors (i.e., neurotropic substances) that may further enhance their survival. Sun and colleagues (2001) reported that the presence of an intracellular substance (i.e., neurogenin) can activate certain genes in neurons that facilitate neurogenesis and at the same time suppress glial genes. This is an active area of research, in which future studies will likely reveal the complexities involved in the formation of neurons and glial cells.

Once neuroblasts and glial cells have been created, they migrate from the ventricular zone to other brain locations. Researchers have discovered that one type of glial cell, known as a radial glial, extends from the ventricular zone to various parts of the brain including the cortex. Cells apparently migrate by crawling along the radial glial fibers until they reach their destination. The mechanisms that govern the migration process are under investigation but appear to involve an interaction between genetic and environmental factors. For example, Rakic (1995) hypothesized that in addition to building scaffolds, glial cells offer chemical trails for neurons to follow to their destinations. Indeed, several types of extracellular molecules have been identified in other animals and insects that either attract or repel migrating neurons including netrins, ephirins, semiphorins, and slit molecules (Halim, 1999; Mueller, 1999). Recently, Shen and Bargmann (2003) discovered a protein molecule known as SYG-1 in roundworms that directs neurons to form connections with other neurons. They speculated that the discovery of similar proteins in humans may help treat human disorders such as epilepsy and chronic pain in which synapse formation goes awry.

Migrating neurons are not fully formed and have a structure that extends from the tip of the axon called a *growth cone*. The cones are believed to contain proteins (i.e., receptors) that are attracted to and repelled by other proteins in the migration path (Terman & Kolodkin, 1999). Thus, the developing neuron crawls along a pathway, led by the growth cone that moves forward and turns in response to molecules that attract or repel the cell. Once the cell's destination is reached, the growth cone is replaced by an axon terminal that forms connections (*synapses*) with other cells (Mueller, 1999). Substances on the surface of cells have been found to facilitate synaptic connections among neurons, and these substances are known as *cell adhesion molecules*. According to Levitan and Kaczmarek (1997), a variety of cell adhesion molecules exist, and many more will likely be discovered. The process of formation of synapses with nearby or distant neurons is known as *synaptogenesis*.

Synaptogenesis

When the developing neurons have migrated, they differentiate into different sizes and shapes and align themselves with other neurons in the same vicinity to form networks (*aggregation*). The initial process of aggregation is believed to be under genetic control, but chemicals surrounding neurons appear to be involved in the maturation and functional role of neurons. For example, research has found that if predifferentiated cells are removed from one brain region and placed in another, they will serve the same functions as those in their new vicinity (Schlaggar & O'Leary, 1991). After developing neurons reach their destinations, they begin to sprout axons that eventually form synapses with nearby or distant neurons, that is, synaptogenesis. By 5 months gestation, most neurons have migrated to their correct location but are morphologically immature, that is, they lack axons, dendrites, and connections with other neurons. Synaptogenesis begins prenatally after neurons have reached their destination and continues after birth. Subcortical structures such as the hippocampus undergo synaptogenesis much earlier than cortical regions (Kostovic et al., 1989). During the first 1 to 2 years of post-natal life, synaptogenesis increases dramatically and is followed by a substantial reduction, or pruning phase. Different regions of the cortex increase in synaptic density and experience pruning at different times. The visual cortex, for example, increases in synaptic connections after birth during months 2–4, while other areas of cortex increase in synaptic connections during the first 12 months.

Huttenlocher (1979) explored synaptic density in the frontal cortex of 21 postmortem normal human brains ranging from newborn to 90 years. Results indicated that synaptic density in newborns was similar to the density level in adults. The morphology of the connections was immature, however, and did not resemble adult appearance until approximately 24 months. Synaptic density continued to increase from birth until 1–2 years, at which time the level was about 50% above the adult mean. The synaptic and neuronal density levels slowly declined from ages 2–16, but then remained constant throughout adulthood. These data suggest that neurons establish their synapses during the first 1–2 years of life, followed by loss of connections until late adolescence. Abnormalities in synaptic density found in individuals with mental retardation and schizophrenia suggest that the synaptic elimination process is crucial to normal brain development (Armstrong, Dunn, Antalffi, & Trivetti, 1995; Cragg, 1975; Feinberg, 1982). This pruning process likely depends on genetic and nongenetic factors, but it has been argued that those synaptic connections that are used and reinforced will evolve, while other idle synapses will not survive (Edelman, 1987). For example, Pallier, Dehaene, Poline, and LeBihan (2003) used fMRI to find that adults who had been exposed to a native language during childhood but were adopted and subsequently reared with a second language, did not show specific cortical activation when exposed to their native language. They interpreted these findings as supporting the notion that brain plasticity for language progressively closes as networks for language stabilize. In other words, the plasticity for language is available during childhood, but if the language is not used the brain does not appear to show evidence of exposure to the language over time. Similar assertions have been made with regard to the ability to play a musical instrument. The Suzuki method, for example, stresses the importance of training in early childhood. Elbert et al. (1995) compared the size of the area of the right hemisphere somatosensory cortex that controls finger movements on the left hand and found that this region was significantly larger in adults who had begun playing the violin in childhood. These studies suggest that there is a relationship between size and function of a given area of the cortex and that early childhood experiences can facilitate the synaptic connections among neurons. A direct relationship does not exist, however, between brain anatomy size and function. On average, male brains tend to be 10% larger than female brains, but larger brains are not predictive of higher cognitive capabilities such as intelligence. Albert Einstein's brain was in the low average range for weight (Diamond, Scheibel, Murphy, & Harvey, 1985), and some individuals who have had an entire hemisphere removed remain of average to superior intelligence (Smith & Sugar, 1975; St. James-Roberts, 1981).

Apoptosis

In addition to an excessive production of synapses followed by synaptic pruning, neurons are overproduced prenatally and subsequently die off before and after birth (*apoptosis*). Neuronal cell death takes place both cortically and subcortically athough the specific loss of neurons in each region is not well understood. It has been estimated that approximately 50% of neurons follow a programmed cell death, and this process continues during childhood and puberty (Pinel, 2000, p. 408; Durston et al., 2001). Eriksson and colleagues (1998), however, recently discovered that neurons in the hippocampus of adult humans reproduce after birth. Prior to this discovery, neurogenesis was believed to be complete before birth. It is possible that scientists will discover neurogenesis in other brain regions, which would have obvious implications for treatment of brain diseases ranging from Alzheimer's disease to depression. The relevance and extent of apoptosis in the human brain remain somewhat a mystery.

Circuity

Research has identified a number of factors that appear to contribute to cellular death. For example, one reason that neurons die is that they must compete with other neurons to establish synapses. If synapses are not established, neurons will be deprived of neurotropic factors, that is, substances that nourish and promote the survival of neurons. Neurotrophins are released by target neurons, taken up by part of the axon, and transported back to the cell body where they are believed to alter gene expression and protein synthesis (Pettmann & Henderson, 1998). Several types of neurotropic factors has been identified, and the absence of these substances has been found to trigger genetic processes that result in cell death (Nishi, 1994). The purpose of programmed cell death and synaptic pruning is not fully understood. Scientists have hypothesized that an overproduction of neurons and subsequent competition for synapses increase the likelihood that an appropriate number and degree of complexity among synapses will be achieved (Gordon, 1995). Huttenlocher (2002, p. 80) has also suggested that apoptosis removes unnecessary cell populations, resulting in more efficient connections among neurons.

Eventually neurons form systems and circuits of synapses that are thought to be similar across individuals, such as those found in the visual or auditory systems. Individuals vary tremendously in their environmental experiences, however, which likely shapes and develops the brain in unique ways. Psychologist Donald Hebb (1949) proposed that neurons that fire repeatedly and are located in close proximity will undergo growth and metabolic changes that ultimately strengthen the connections between them. Recent research has supported Hebb's original hypothesis. For example, studies have found that active neurons sprout and form new connections and those that are active are nourished by chemical substances (i.e., neurotrophins) that further contribute to growth of the cell (Martin & Kandel, 1996; Schuman, 1999). Studies have also demonstrated that the sensory system of the fetus is functional and that the fetus responds to sounds such as music or a familiar voice. Some researchers have speculated that stimulation of the fetus during prenatal development may help to foster brain development and consequently enhance cognitive functions later in life (e.g., Kolata, 1984; Shelter, 1985), leading to an explosion of so-called prenatal educational programs. These programs typically recommend activities such as playing classical music, speaking, singing, and reading to the fetus. Huttenlocher (2002), however, stated that "to date there is no convincing evidence that such stimulation will enhance cognitive functions later in life" (p. 16). Most research on the physiological effects of environmental stimulation has focused on postnatal brain growth.

POSTNATAL BRAIN GROWTH AND PLASTICITY

As noted previously, prenatally the brain produces approximately 250,000 neurons per minute (Cowan, 1979), and at birth the brain has billions of neurons and glial cells. Neurons in general do not reproduce postnatally, but glial cells continue to reproduce throughout childhood and adulthood. The newborn's brain is nearly two thirds the adult size but only 25% of the adult weight. After age 5, however, total brain size does not increase significantly. The brain's weight, however, increases fourfold from birth to 10 years (Webb, Monk, & Nelson, 2001). The postnatal increase in the brain's volume and weight is due to a number of factors including proliferation and maturation of glial cells, synaptogenesis, myelination of axons, and maturation of neurons characterized by axonal development and dendritic expansion. As noted by Huttenlocher (1979), the morphology of neurons and the connections among neurons, especially at the level of the cortex, are immature at birth and these connections increase dramatically shortly after birth. For example, Webb, Monk, and Nelson (2001) reported that the length of dendrites in the prefrontal cortex increases five to ten times during the first 6 months (postnatal). Buell and Coleman (1981) found that dendrites continue to grow and elongate throughout adulthood, even late adulthood. Growth of axons and increased complexity of synaptic connections also characterize cell maturation. Different regions of the cortex mature at different rates and, based on anatomical and neuroimaging studies, the prefrontal cortex is the last region to mature (Huttenlocher, 1979). Synaptogenesis is also associated with brain function. For example, during the first and second years of life, synaptogenesis occurs in areas of the brain associated with language comprehension and language production, during the time that children begin to understand spoken language and subsequently begin to use language to communicate.

Developmental changes also occur with respect to the ratio of white matter (*myelinated axons*) to gray matter (*cell bodies*). Webb, Monk, and Nelson (2001), for example, reported that whereas at birth 50% of the total brain volume is composed of gray matter, gray matter decreases substantially with age due to neuronal death and pruning of synapses. During early childhood and into adolescence, there is a steady decrease in the percentage of gray matter (Rapoport et al., 1999). Conversely, white matter increases with age at the level of the cortex, and according to Huppi et al. (1998) there is a fivefold increase in prenatal white matter between 29 and 41 weeks. Postnatally, myelination of axons increases in the cortex throughout childhood and adolescence and levels off during late adolescence, but continues throughout life (Klingberg et al., 1999; Sowell et al., 1999; Tokumaru et al., 1999). MRI studies have shown that several areas of the cortex are myelinated at birth and myelinate rapidly within a few months after birth (e.g., visual system, somatosensory cortex). Other regions such as the prefrontal cortex myelinate more slowly, a process that continues into at least late adolescence and perhaps young adulthood (Kinney, Brody, Kloman, & Gilles, 1998). With regard to subcortical structures, research suggests that substantial myelination is present at birth and growth occurs at a rapid pace between birth and 6 months. Additional white matter growth occurs in subcortical areas during adolescence and young adulthood but at a slower rate (Kinney, Brody, Kloman, & Gilles, 1998; Nomura et al., 1994). These studies demonstrate that myelination of the brain is clearly related to brain function in infancy and childhood. Myelination may also be associated with cognitive capabilities later in life. Green, Kaye, and Ball (2000), for example, recently examined the postmortem brains of 19 men and women ages 85–104 years and reported that those who remained cognitively unimpaired showed very few changes in white matter, neuronal, and glial cell density.

It is generally accepted that prenatal brain development is initiated as a result of genetic factors but postnatally environmental factors play a significant role (Huttenlocher, 1994). The relative contributions of genetic and environmental influences on brain development remain unclear. For example, the appearance and functional organization of the brain from the cortex to subcortical structures are similar across individuals. Humans vary tremendously, however, with respect to their personalities as well as their cognitive and behavioral capabilities. As Joseph LeDoux (2002) recently suggested, "the key to individuality, therefore, is not to be found in the overall organization of the brain, but rather in the fine-tuning of the underlying networks" (p. 36). In other words, the connections between neurons appear to define individuality, and these connections are influenced greatly by environmental experiences, particularly after birth. Research has demonstrated that environmental experiences can have profound negative or positive effects on the structure of the brain. For example, it has been well established that toxic substances such as alcohol can have deleterious effects on a developing embryo or fetus, interrupt normal brain functioning, and perhaps permanently damage the corpus callosum as is seen in fetal alcohol syndrome (Bookstein, Sampson, Connor, & Streissguth, 2002). McEwen and Sapolsky (1995) have postulated that children who are abused may have elevated levels of stress hormones (e.g., cortisol) that are toxic to the hippocampus due to the large number of cortisol receptors located on this structure. Higher levels of cortisol may interfere with the normal development and functioning of the cells of the hippocampus. On the other hand, environmental experiences can have a positive effect on brain development. Research with other animals, for example, has shown that rats reared in enriched, complex environments show increased complexity of neuronal connections as well as superior task performance compared to rats reared in less stimulating environments (Greenough & Black, 1992). With regard to humans, Elbert and colleagues (1995) found that the area of the cortex that subserves the fingers is larger in musicians who play string instruments than in nonmusicians. Certainly the concept of rehabilitation following brain injury is based on the notion that environmental stimulation can affect brain functioning. The process of the brain's ability to change in response to environmental experience is called *plasticity* (Konorski, 1948). During periods of brain development, the brain is believed to be more plastic as more synapses are available to support developing functions. Plasticity declines in adulthood, but the brain remains capable of responding to environmental experiences throughout the life span (Stiles, 2000).

PLASTICITY

Kennard (1936) was among the first to systematically study plasticity with regard to the behavioral effects of brain injury in monkeys. Based on her studies, she concluded that the earlier in life brain damage occurs, the less severe the behavioral effects. Subsequent research challenged the Kennard doctrine and demonstrated that although in some cases brain injury in early childhood is associated with better outcome, usually the outcome depends on a variety of modulating factors other than age. Kolb (1989) identified and studied factors such as intelligence, handedness, sex, location and severity of the damage, environmental experiences, and type of assessment techniques and concluded that all of these factors could influence the behavioral effects of the brain damage. In other words, two individuals can suffer the same type of brain damage but the effects resulting from the damage may vary significantly due to mediating variables.

For decades, the bulk of information on brain plasticity derived from studies of other animals. These studies were and continue to be conducted with monkeys, chimpanzees, rats, cats, dogs, rabbits, and other animals. Although a variety of methods are used, most studies involve damaging part or parts of the brain, altering the environment, and observing the subsequent physiological and behavioral effects. In general, results from these studies have demonstrated that the brain has the ability to reorganize its connections depending on a large number of factors such as the age of the animal, location and severity of the damage, and environmental conditions. The problem with this body of literature is that the brains of other animals are not morphologically or functionally the same as the human brain. As Huttenlocher (2002, p. 113) stated, "the newborn monkey brain is not a good model in which to study the likely effects of cortical lesions in human neonates," and further added, "the results obtained in lesions made in a 2 or 3 month old monkey therefore have limited relevance to the study of plasticity related to perinatal brain lesions in humans." Therefore, although there is voluminous information available on plasticity in other animals, the following section focuses primarily on the human literature to date.

TRAUMATIC BRAIN INJURY

According to the Brain Injury Association of America, every 21 seconds a person in the United States sustains a traumatic brain injury (TBI), that is, approximately 1.5 million people each year. A traumatic brain injury is an insult to the brain caused by an external force that results in temporary or sustained impairments in cognitive, emotional, behavioral, or physical functioning. The risk of TBI is highest among adolescents (ages 15–17) and those older than 75 years. Overall, accidents involving vehicles are the leading cause of TBI, followed by falls (Thurman, Alverson, Dunn, Guerreor, & Sniezek, 1999). The leading cause of TBI in infants is abuse (i.e., shaken baby sydrome). During TBI, the internal brain tissue and blood vessels become bruised and the jarring of the brain can cause tearing of the tissues and blood vessels. This bruising and jarring can result in internal bleeding and swelling. In addition, cells that are damaged and die release their contents (e.g., ions, proteins) into the extracellular space, which can be toxic and ultimately fatal to other neurons and glial cells (Stein, Brailowsky, & Will, 1995). The effects of the injury vary depending on the location and severity of the injury as well as other factors such as age and timing of treatment interventions (Watanabe, Miller, &

McElligott, 2003). Taylor et al. (2002) recently reported that the behavioral and academic outcomes were poorer for children with moderate to severe TBI. They also found that family factors moderated the long-term effects of TBI, and unfavorable family circumstances (high stress, economically disadvantaged) were associated with a poorer prognosis.

Research indicates that participation in a rehabilitation program enhances the rapidity and extent of recovery following TBI (Cope, 1995). As with plasticity in general, the precise mechanisms responsible for recovery are not well understood, and there is tremendous variability in methods used in rehabilitation programs to treat TBI. One method, constraint induced movement therapy (CIMT), has been found to improve the functional capabilities of brain injury victims (Taub et al., 1993). CIMT involves constraining the unaffected extremity and gradually inducing patients to use the affected limb. Kunkel et al. (1999), for example, investigated cortical activity of stroke patients following CIMT. Results indicated substantial reorganization of motor areas in the hemisphere that controlled the unaffected limb, and this was correlated to recovery of movement in the affected limbs. Presumably motor systems in the intact hemisphere became involved in motor function of the affected limb. Bilateral training has also been used with stroke victims to avoid loss of strength and range of motion in the unaffected limb. Results by Whitall et al. (2000) have supported the use of this rehabilitation technique at improving strength and range of motion in both the affected and unaffected limbs. Regardless of the intervention method, research indicates that rehabilitation should begin shortly after the injury to increase the likelihood of greater recovery (Gonzalez-Rothi, 2001). The neurophysiological basis of rehabilitation is uncertain, but as Gonzalez-Rothi described, recovery of behavioral and cognitive function is likely the result of focusing on specific, desired behaviors and providing a stimulating, enriched environment that leads to synaptic and neuronal changes (see Dobkin, 2003 for a review). Taub, Uswatte, and Elbert (2002) recently noted that although historically the field of rehabilitation has been disconnected from neuroscience, recent discoveries in behavioral neuroscience—particularly with regard to plasticity—will likely lead to more effective intervention techniques to enhance recovery following brain injury.

BRAIN INJURY—STROKE

Strokes are sudden disruptions to the blood supply to the brain that cause damage to brain cells. The loss of blood to the brain tissue restricts the supply of oxygen and glucose and consequently results in damage and death of brain cells. In addition, neurons in damaged areas tend to fire excessively, releasing the neurotransmitter glutamate. This excessive release of glutamate is toxic to neurons and results in further cellular death. Dying cells spill their contents into the affected region, causing additional damage. A medication, tissue plasminogen activator (t-PA), has been developed that blocks glutamate receptors and helps to diminish the subsequent degree of brain damage. In order to be effective, the medication needs to be administered within 3 hours of the onset of the stroke (Katzan et al., 2000).

The specific effects of a stroke vary depending on the region of the brain affected and the severity of the stroke. Compared to adults who suffer a stroke, children tend to have fewer long-lasting behavioral effects such as facial weakness and difficulties with walking (Lenn & Freinkel, 1989). Approximately 50% of children experience chronic problems with speech, movement, and learning, but the effects tend to be mild relative to adult impairment (Walsh & Garg, 1997). The cognitive and behavioral effects of the stroke appear to be vary significantly among individuals, however, as Delsing, Catsman-Berrevoets, and Appel (2001) were unable to identify a relationship between etiology, age, or gender and stroke outcome. According to Thirumala, Hier, and Patel (2002), the most powerful predictor of recovery is the severity of the stroke. The mechanisms responsible for varying levels of recovery are uncertain but likely include reorganization of neuronal pathways at the cortical and subcortical levels, use of pathways in the undamaged hemisphere, and possibly the development of new motor networks (Azari & Seitz, 2000; Thirumala, Hier, & Patel, 2002). Using neuroimaging, Blasi and colleagues (2002) recently discovered that the right hemisphere can take over and learn how to perform language tasks when the language-related areas of the left hemisphere in adults are damaged by stroke. They also found that similarly to healthy patients, individuals who had suffered a stroke in the left hemisphere became more efficient with language tasks over time and this was reflected in decreased activity in the right hemisphere. Overall, research with stroke victims suggests that depending on the severity of the stroke, recovery is possible and the physiological factors associated with recovery of function differ in children and adults. In general, children are less likely to suffer from chronic behavioral and cognitive effects of stroke and their symptoms are usually milder than adults. Presumably the child and adolescent brain is still developing and is therefore more plastic than the mature, adult brain.

DEVELOPMENTAL ANOMALIES

Lesions are injury-related changes in brain tissue that may affect functioning at various levels of development. A large number of factors may produce lesions early or later in life, and the timing of the lesions may have different behavioral effects. Brain injury that severely damages language-related regions results in permanent or transient language deficits in adults, but the prognosis is more positive in young children. Research indicates brain lesions that occur in infancy, prior to the onset of language, are associated with normal development of receptive language. Productive language (i.e., speaking) is usually delayed but subsequently progresses normally (Bates, 1999b).

Children who have had a hemisphere completely or partially removed (known as *anatomical* and *functional hemispherectomy*, respectively) due to drug-resistant epilepsy or brain diseases have been found to develop language in the intact hemisphere (Sperry, 1974). The degree of recovery and nature of impairment are variable, however (Curtiss & Schaeffer, 1997; de Bode & Curtiss, 2000). Research also indicates that children who have had the left hemisphere removed tend to have more problems acquiring and restoring their language and the course is more prolonged than children who have had the right hemisphere removed (de Bode & Curtiss, 2000). In adults, hemispherectomy leads to more severe language-related deficits (Ogden, 1996; St. James-Roberts, 1981). The physiological reasons for the disparity between child and adult outcomes of hemispherectomy are unclear although several hypotheses have been advanced. Several studies have found, for example, that children tend to process language more diffusely and language is not yet localized in the left hemisphere as is characteristic of adults (e.g., Mills, Coffey-Corina, & Neville, 1993; Ojemann & Schoenfield-McNeill, 1999). In addition, the child brain, relative to the adult brain, has more synaptic connections available for plasticity, that is, reorganization (Huttenlocher, 1979). Holloway et al. (2000) used fMRI to investigate sensorimotor functions of 17 children and adolescents (1 to 19 years) who had either part or all of the left or right hemisphere removed due to congenital or acquired brain disease. Results indicated that the somatosensory cortex of the remaining hemisphere was activated with both hands in all children regardless of the onset of the brain damage. These findings demonstrated that ipsilateral pathways had become activated but the source of these pathways was unknown. Holloway et al. speculated that the ipsilateral pathways may have been present since early childhood but silent. After the hemispherectomy, however, the silent pathways may have become activated and strengthened due to demand. Alternatively, intact neurons may have sprouted projections from intact axons and created new pathways.

Other evidence of plasticity comes from studies of individuals who were born deaf or blind and those with reading disabilities. Neville and colleagues (1983) examined cortical activity among adults who were congenitally deaf and of normal hearing and results indicated that areas that were normally devoted to hearing were now devoted to vision in these individuals. Sterr, Elbert, and Rockstroh (2002) reported that the area of the somatosensory cortex that controlled the fingers was significantly larger in blind adults who were experienced Braille readers than a group of sighted adults who did not read Braille. They also compared the somatosensory arrangement in one-finger versus multfinger Braille readers and found that the cortical arrangements were different in these groups. In a related study, Sadato and colleagues (1998) used PET to study the areas of the cortex that were activated during Braille reading in blind and sighted subjects. As predicted, findings indicated that different areas were activated in the two groups. Specifically, areas of the occipital cortex (primary visual cortex) were activated in the blind subjects during Braille reading, whereas areas of the somatosensory cortex were activated in sighted subjects. Sadato et al. (2002) later discovered that the age at which sight was lost was associated with areas of cortical activation in blind subjects during a tactile task. Specifically, an area of the visual cortex was activated in blind subjects who lost their sight prior to age 16, but this same area was suppressed in blind subjects who lost their sight past that age.

The results of these studies support Ramachandran's (1993) hypothesis that reorganization of synapses at the level of the cortex is characteristic of the adult brain, and that these changes can occur in response to environmental demands but may be mediated by other variables such as age. For example, Temple et al. (2003) investigated brain activation in children with reading disability before and after a remediation program that focused on auditory training and oral language training. Using fMRI, Temple and colleagues found increased activity in brain regions associated with reading following the remediation program. In fact, the investigators reported that the level of brain activation approximated that of normal-reading children and these changes were correlated with improvement on oral language and phonological awareness tasks. No significant correlation was found, however, between increased brain activity and reading improvement.

BRAIN INJURY—AMPUTATION

Ramachandran (1993) reported that adults who had a limb amputated often had sensory experiences as if the limb were still present when part of their face was touched. He hypothesized that areas of the cortex devoted to the face invaded and took over the area of the cortex that had previously been devoted to the limb. Ramachandran and Rogers-Ramachandran (2000) later discussed neuroimaging studies that documented changes at the level of the somatosensory cortex in phantom limb patients. The physiological substrates that are responsible for these cortical changes are unclear, but one hypothesis is that silent synapses are present in the surrounding region of the cortex and these synapses become activated or "unmasked" (Ramachandran, 1993). Another factor that may contribute to the reorganization is axonal sprouting and increased complexity of connections of neighboring neurons, known as collateral sprouting.

DEPRIVATION STUDIES

Relative to other animals, few studies are available on the physiological effects of sensory deprivation. Heron (1957) was among the first to study the behavioral effects of depriving young adults of nearly all sensory input. In this study, college students were paid to remain in an isolated, soundproofed room, lying on a bed with their eyes, ears, and extremities covered. Most participants became distressed after a few hours and very few could remain for the duration of the study. Several of the students who participated the longest (not more than 24 hours) reported having visual hallucinations. Grassian (1983) has written about the pathological effects of prisoners held in solitary confinement—perceptual distortions; hallucinations; delusions; generalized anxiety; and impulsive, violent behavior. Research on the physiological effects of deprivation in children is limited, but the available studies suggest that there are brain changes in response to reduced environmental stimulation. White and Held (1966), for example, studied reaching behavior and attentiveness in institutionalized infants reared in nonstimulating environments. By simply introducing a visual stimulus at 1 month of age, the infant's reach and visual attentiveness nearly doubled relative to infants not exposed to the stimulus. Recently, Chugani et al. (2001) used PET to study brain activity in human infants who had been reared in deprived conditions. Specifically, Chugani and colleagues studied ten children (average age of 8) who had been placed in Romanian orphanages 4–6 weeks after birth and had resided in the orphanage for a mean of 38 months before being adopted. PET scans taken during an awake, resting state found that these children had decreased metabolism in several areas of the cortex, particularly the prefrontal cortex, relative to 7 children with epilepsy and 17 healthy adults. In addition, the Romanian children demonstrated mild neuropsychological, attention, impulsivity, and social skill deficits. The researchers hypothesized that these deficits may be a result of early and pervasive sensory deprivation that altered the development of the limbic system and the circuits that project to and from limbic structures.

Glaser (2000) recently reviewed the literature on child abuse and neglect and concluded that child maltreatment induces stress in victims which may result in permanent dysregulation of brain structures and systems. Specifically, he suggested that child maltreatment can disrupt normal brain development in the region of the hypothalamic–pituitary–adrenal axis and the parasympathetic system. Impairments in these systems are associated with increased levels of stress hormones (e.g., cortisol, adrenaline) and over time may be toxic to hippocampal and other neurons. Carlson and Earls (1997) and Davies (2002), for example, found that children who were reared in Romanian orphanages showed abnormal cortisol levels and these levels were associated with poorer performance on developmental screening tests. De Bellis (2001) argued that child maltreatment should be regarded as "an environmentally induced complex developmental disorder" (p. 558) that is often characterized by profound and long-lasting physiological as well as emotional effects. Recently, Bugental, Martorell, and Barraza (2003) reported that "subtle" forms of maltreatment (e.g., frequent spanking or emotional maternal withdrawal) during infancy may alter the hypothalamic–pituitary–adrenal axis in ways that foster social–emotional problems, immune disorders, cognitive deficits, and sensitization to later stress. Balbernie (2001) suggested that childhood maltreatment interferes with normal development of the limbic system and connections with the prefrontal cortex, which in turn results in an impaired ability to regulate emotion and behavior. He hypothesized that early prevention and intervention programs, for infants and children who are at risk for abuse or who have been abused, can capitalize on the brain's plasticity and decrease the likelihood of abnormal brain development.

ENRICHMENT STUDIES

The effect of enriched environments has been investigated in other animals for decades. Overall, the results indicate that complex environments, relative to simple environments, are associated with increased connections among synapses as well as dendritic and axonal expansion (e.g., Greenough, Withers, & Anderson, 1992). These physiological changes are also associated with improved behavioral performance on learning and memory tasks. Kolb and Elliott (1987), for example, demonstrated that rats who had sustained brain damage and were then reared in complex environments performed significantly better on behavioral tasks than brain-damaged rats who were reared in standard, nonstimulating laboratory cages.

With regard to humans, Diamond and Hopson (1998) have suggested that an enriched environment is one that is characterized by consistent and positive emotional support, stimulation that is multisensory, relatively stress-free, promotes exploration and active learning, is reasonably challenging, encourages social interactions, and practices good health care. Although these suggestions make intuitive sense, very little empirical information is available about the relative contribution of enriching experiences to physiological changes in the human brain. For example, it is well established that the brain develops in a hierarchal fashion and that substantial growth occurs during early childhood and slower growth continues during adolescence and to a lesser extent during adulthood. The types and nature of experiences that would facilitate optimal brain development at different stages of brain development are speculative, however. In other words, a gap exists between neuroscience research and pedagogy. A few studies have, however, found a relationship between environmental–educational stimulation and behavioral gains. Campbell and Ramey (1994), for example, studied the effects of enrichment programs on the intellectual and academic achievement of at-risk children and found substantial positive behavioral effects. Huttenlocher and colleagues (1998) compared the language growth of children when school was in session versus summer vacation periods. Results indicated that there was a significant difference in language growth with greater performance during the school session (i.e., enrichment period). Although one may hypothesize that the enriched environment had physiological effects that corresponded with behavioral effects, physiological measures were not included in these studies. As a result of the recent discoveries in neuroscience on brain development and plasticity, numerous popular books have become available touting educational methods to enhance children's learning in the classroom (e.g., Wolfe, 2001). Although these stragtegies are well-intended, research studies are needed to explore the effectiveness of these methods.

MECHANISMS OF PLASTICITY

Glial Cells, Dendritic Arborization, Axonal Sprouting, and Synaptogenesis

As mentioned previously, the majority of physiological studies on plasticity have been conducted with other animals or postmortem human brain tissue. Recent advances in neuroimaging have provided insight into anatomical and functional brain changes in human children and adults. The mechanisms responsible for plasticity are not well understood but are believed to involve a number of events such as proliferation of glial cells, dendritic arborization, axonal sprouting, synaptogenesis, and perhaps neurogenesis and involvement of neurotrophins. Collectively, these factors result in the modification of existing synaptic connections and/or create new synaptic connections and circuits. Unlike neurons, glial cells continue to reproduce postnatally and serve a number of functions that promote the development, maturation, and sustenance of neurons. Dendritic arborization is characterized by increases in dendritic length, branching, and dendritic spine density. Axonal sprouting occurs when neighboring neurons send off-shoots to the damaged region and form synapses with remaining neurons that no longer have synaptic connections. This process is also known as *collateral sprouting*, and evidence of this process has been substantiated in humans and other animals (e.g., Ramachandran, 1993; Fritschy & Grzanna, 1992).

The cellular mechanisms responsible for learning and behavioral adaptation are poorly understood. Research does suggest that stimulation of synaptic pathways facilitates the maturation and strength of these pathways. The process by which this strengthening occurs is unknown but has been linked to *long-term potentiation* (LTP). LTP has been studied primarily in the hippocampus of other animals and refers to the increased excitability of a neuron in response to repeated stimulation. Increased excitability of cells over time is thought to result in more efficient communication among neurons. More efficient communication among neurons is associated with enhanced learning and memory (see Levitan & Kaczmarek, 1997 for a review) and has been described as a major factor in neural plasticity during childhood as well as adulthood (Huttenlocher, 2002). McEachern and Shaw (2001) have argued that the case for LTP and plasticity is weak; however, LTP may also be involved in neuronal pathology. As an example, they suggested that LTP in the adult brain may arise in response to injury or gene dysfunction and produce pathological changes in neuron numbers or connections. McEachern and Shaw also proposed that plasticity is the result of interactions across multiple levels of neural organization; however, these relationships and dynamics are poorly understood. With respect to human pathology, Duman (2002) has suggested that mood disorders are likely characterized by atrophy and loss of neurons, especially in the hippocampus, and that antidepressants may actually reverse this process by promoting cell proliferation. This information will be covered in more detail in chapter 6.

Medication, Neurotrophins, and Neurogenesis

Researchers have begun to explore the role of medication in facilitating plasticity with regard to recovery from brain injury (TBI). These medications include stimulants, antihypertensives, and, more recently, medications that are used to treat memory problems of Alzheimer's disease (e.g., Rao, Dogan, Todd, Bowen, & Dempsey, 2001). In general, stimulants appear to have the most robust effects on improving attention and memory in patients with TBI. Ritalin, for example, is a central nervous system stimulant that has been found to augment activity of injured neuronal tissue in comatose patients and facilitate consciousness, and improve attention of children with pediatric brain injury (Kajs-Wyllie, 2002; Williams, Ris, & Ayangar, 1998). Studies are currently underway at several locations across the country to further investigate the effects of stimulants and other medications in children and adults with moderate to severe TBI who are in the early stages of recovery.

In the future, other medications may be useful in facilitating plasticity in the human brain. For example, following injury or damage, regrowth of axons and tracts does not occur in the brain and spinal cord. Z'Graggen et al.'s (1998) study of rats suggests that substances in the extracellular fluid may inhibit regrowth of axons and nerve tracts and it may be possible prevent the action of these substances. One such axon outgrowth inhibitor is known as Nogo. GrandPre, Li, and Strittmatter (2002) recently reported that a drug that inhibits the actions of Nogo can result in regrowth of axons in the spinal cord of rats. Consequently, they suggested that Nogo antagonists may be an effective form of treatment for spinal cord injuries as well as brain injuries. Medications may also be useful in promoting birth of new neurons, a process known as *neurogenesis*. Eriksson and colleagues (1998), for example, discovered that contrary to what was believed previously, neurons in the hippocampus of adult humans actually reproduced. Studies with other animals suggest that neurogenesis may occur in other areas of the brain, which has obvious implications for treatment of brain diseases (e.g., Barnea & Nottebohm, 1996). In the meantime, several drugs have been associated with synaptogenesis and neurogenesis. Zhang and colleagues (2002) at the Henry Ford Health Science Center in Detroit, for example, recently discovered that rats that were treated with Viagra for 6 days following an induced stroke showed new blood vessel growth and an increase in dendritic arborization as well as synaptic connections. Compared to rats that had not received the drug, Viagra-treated rats performed significantly better on behavioral and health measures.

Banasr, Hery, Brezun, and Daszuta (2001) have studied the role of serotonin and estrogen in neurogenesis in the hippocampus of rats and have suggested that these substances may play a critical role in the birth or death of neurons in the hippocampus. For example, according to Banasr and colleagues, increasing brain levels of serotonin has been associated with an increase in neurogenesis but studies with estrogen have been less consistent. Other studies have suggested that increased levels of serotonin may facilitate neurogenesis in humans as well. Duman (2002) postulated that human mood disorders may be characterized by cellular atrophy and loss and that antidepressants may reverse this process. Indeed, a number of studies with other animals have found that administration of antidepressants can influence the production of neurons in the hippocampus and depletion of serotonin reduces neurogenesis (e.g., Fuchs et al., 2002). Interestingly, van Praag, Kempermann, and Gage (1999) found that running on an exercise wheel significantly increased the number of new neurons in the hippocampus of mice, and Gomez-Pinilla and colleagues (2002) found that running increased levels of substances that nourish brain cells (BDNF) in rats. Research with humans has found that exercise is associated with improved mood in subjects with mild to moderate depression (Dimeo, Bauer, Varahram, Proest, & Halter, 2001), and it is plausible that the findings of van Pragg et al. (1999) may also apply to humans.

Neurotrophins

Neurotrophins are substances that are thought to play a role in plasticity by promoting the growth of surviving neurons. Several types of neurotrophins have been identified such as nerve growth factor (NGF), brain-derived neurotrophin factor (BDNF), neurotrophin 3 (NT-3), transforming growth factor (TGF), and epidermal growth factor (EGF). Neurotrophins are produced by neurons and glial cells, but little is known about the dynamics of neurotrophins or the factors that regulate the production and release of neurotrophins because they cannot yet be visualized in intact tissue (Schuman, 1999). Altar and colleagues (1997) demonstrated that at least one neurotrophin, BDNF, is widely distributed in the rat brain and in nerve terminals. They also showed that BDNF is produced in the cell body and transported to the nerve terminals where it is released. Thoenen, Zafra, Hengerer, and Lindholm (1991) found that drugs that increased the amount of a certain neurotransmitter (GABA) reduced basic levels of NGF and BDNF, suggesting that the regulation of neurotrophins is at least partially mediated by the brain's neurotransmitter systems. Neurotrophins have been found to facilitate the development of immature neurons and to enhance functioning of mature synapses. For example, research with other animals and insects has found that neurotrophins help to regulate ongoing neurogenesis in young and adult rats (Wagner, Black, & DiCicco-Bloom, 1999) and speed up the neurotransmission process in hippocampal neurons (Messaoudi, Bardsen, Srebro, & Bramham, 1998). Mice that have been genetically altered so that BDNF is reduced demonstrate learning deficits (Linnarsson, Bjorklund, & Ernfors, 1997), implicating neurotrophins in learning and memory. King, Heaton, and Walker (2002) recently found that chronic ethanol intake led to learning and memory deficits in rats, and these deficits were correlated with a significant reduction of neurotrophins in the forebrain and hippocampus. King and colleagues argued that compromised levels of neurotrophins interfered with synaptic connections in the hippocampus and other regions of the forebrain, resulting in memory and learning deficits.

With regard to humans, a number of studies have found reduced levels of neurotrophins in postmortem brains of individuals with various disorders such as Alzheimer's disease, Parkinson's disease, and depression (D'Sa & Duman, 2002; Fahnestock, Garzon, Holsinger, & Michalski, 2002; Momose et al., 2002). Indeed, D'Sa and Duman (2002) have suggested that medications used to treat depression may increase neurogenesis and modulate processes associated with the production and release of neurotrophins. Garzon and colleagues (2002) have suggested that decreasing levels of neurotrophins (BDNF) is an early symptom of Alzheimer's disease. Studies are currently underway to determine whether raising levels of neurotrophins improves the symptoms associated with brain-based diseases such as Parkinson's disease and Alzheimer's disease and brain injury resulting from stroke (Ovbiagele, Kindwell, Starkman, & Saver, 2003). In general, these studies are based on the premise that neurotrophins can facilitate plasticity even in diseased or injured brains.

In addition to brain development and plasticity, researchers have investigated other aspects of brain function and anatomy such as the metabolic needs of the brain and gender differences. The results of these studies suggest that the body prioritizes the needs of the brain and the metabolism of the brain changes with age. Studies concerning anatomical and functional brain differences between males and females have been equivocal.

METABOLIC NEEDS OF THE BRAIN

The adult brain weighs approximately 3 pounds and comprises about 2% of the body's weight. Due to its high metabolic activity, it uses 20% of the body's oxygen consumption in an adult (Sokoloff, 1989). Most of the brain's metabolism is used for cellular processes involved in neuronal communication. This high level of oxygen consumption continues 24 hours a day with very little decrease during sleep. If the cerebral blood flow delivering the oxygen is interrupted, loss of consciousness occurs within seconds, and cessation of blood flow for a few minutes can result in irreversible damage to the brain. According to Sokoloff, blood flow rates vary throughout the brain, with four to five times greater blood flow to gray matter compared to white matter regions. Cerebral oxygen consumption changes with development, characterized by low levels at birth and unusually high levels during childhood. For example, Sokoloff reported that the brain's oxygen consumption at age 5 is greater than that of an adult brain. Specifically, the cerebral oxygen consumption of a child of 5 or 6 equals more than 50% of his or her total body basal oxygen consumption. This high level of oxygen consumption steadily declines during childhood and levels off during adolescence. Cerebral oxygen consumption corresponds to cellular activity, and the brain's primary fuel is glucose. Consistent with the high demand for oxygen during childhood, Chugani and Phelps (1991), using neuroimaging (PET), reported that glucose consumption nearly triples during the first few years of life. Between the ages of 3 and 8, the consumption levels off and is reduced to approximately 30% above the initial high levels. This high rate of glucose metabolism has been correlated with regions of brain development and behavior. Specifically, at birth the sensorimotor cortex is highly active corresponding to survival behaviors such as sucking and mobility of limbs. The prefrontal cortex is the last to mature and is associated with higher-order cognitive skills such as hypothetical thinking, abstract reasoning, planning, and problem solving (Hemmingsen et al., 1999).

The role of brain metabolism indices has been studied in drug abuse (Volkow, Fowler, Wolf, & Gillespi, 1991) and more recently as a predictor of outcome after moderate or severe head injury. Glenn and colleagues (2003) compared the cerebral metabolic rate of oxygen and glucose consumption as well as mean cerebral blood flow in 49 patients with traumatic brain injury. Results indicated that during the first 6 days following the injury, cerebral metabolic rate of oxygen consumption was one of the best predictors of neurologic outcome. These results support an earlier study by Kelly et al. (1997), who reported that an acute elevation in cerebral blood flow after TBI is necessary for recovery of cognitive and behavioral functions. Research has also attempted to predict factors that lead to successful outcomes for individuals with TBI, with differences found between males and females in terms of cognitive, emotional, and vocational outcomes (Bounds, Schopp, Johnstone, Unger, & Goldman, 2003). Studies have also found differences between males and females with respect to brain anatomy and processing.

SEX DIFFERENCES IN BRAIN MORPHOLOGY

According to a review by Durston et al. (2001), on the average the male brain is 10% larger than the female brain, although there are numerous size differences between males and females with regard to specific brain structures. Boys tend to have larger total brain size than girls beginning prenatally and continuing postnatally (Giedd et al., 1996). Females, however, have been found to have a larger caudate, hippocampus, globus pallidus, and parts of the corpus callosum. Males have been found to have larger total brain volume, amygdala, and greater gray matter percentage in certain cortical regions than females. Females have been found to have a larger corpus callosum and greater gray matter percentages in several cortical regions relative to males (Dekaban, 1978; Schlaepfer et al., 1995). Some researchers have speculated that these structural differences between the brains of males and females are related to the cognitive differences (i.e., language and spatial reasoning) that have been found between the sexes. For example, girls on average learn to read earlier than boys, which may be related to language-related processing differences or environmental factors. Shaywitz et al. (1995) investigated regions of the brain that were activated in males and females during a language task (rhyming). Results indicated that compared to males, females had greater bilateral activation of areas of the frontal lobe. Harasty, Double, Halliday, Kril, and McRitchie (1997) also found that the language-associated areas of the cortex were larger in females compared to males. Although these findings may be due to a number of factors, they do suggest that males and females may process language differently, at least on some types of language tasks.

Frederikse et al. (1999) found that males had larger gray matter volumes of a particular area in the left parietal lobe (inferior parietal lobule). In females, however, this same area was larger in the right hemisphere relative to the left hemisphere. The meaning of this anatomical difference is unclear, but researchers have speculated that this region of the parietal lobe plays a role in spatial and mathematical abilities. Interestingly, Frederikse et al. (2000) found that males with schizophrenia had a reversed pattern of asymmetry in this area. Not all studies have found morphological differences between males and females, however. Witelson (1989) examined 50 postmortem brains of males and females and found that females did not have an overall larger corpus callosum than males. Size differences were found between males and females, however, in specific areas of the corpus callosum (males had larger genu and females had larger isthmus). Frost et al. (1999) have suggested that processing of higher-order cognitive functions such as language is actually similar in males and females, and argued that studies investigating morphological differences between the brains of males and females are fraught with methodological problems. Indeed, many of the studies are conducted with small samples, include only one sex, and differ radically in the types of tasks and measures used to assess brain anatomy and functioning. In addition, anatomical differences do not reflect functional differences and the origin of the anatomical differences is uncertain. Given the previous discussion of plasticity, daily living experiences can affect the developing brain in ways that remain obscure. Clearly, more research is needed to explore potential brain differences between males and females and the relevance of these findings (see Hines, 2003 for a review).

SUMMARY

The brain can be divided into three main regions: the forebrain, midbrain and hindbrain. Brain development begins prenatally with the onset of neurulation and continues postnatally. During the first 2 years of life, the brain has an overabundant number of connections among neurons, and these connections rapidly decrease in number during early childhood. Environmental factors are believed to contribute to postnatal brain growth that is characterized by reproduction of glial cells, increased complexity of connections among neurons, dendritic arborization, and myelination of axons. The brain has the capacity to change in response to environmental stimulation or deprivation, a process known as plasticity. Plasticity occurs throughout the life span but, in general, the brain is more plastic during childhood. Morphological brain differences have been found between males and females, but the meaning of these differences is unclear. Although there is no universally accepted theory of how the brain functions, it is generally understood that the brain works as an interdependent system. The basis of this system is cellular communication, the details of which will be explained in the next chapter.

2

Cellular Function, Neurotransmission, and Pharmacology

This chapter reviews the principles of cellular function and explains the process of neurotransmission. Information is also presented on the specific types of neurotransmitters and the general functions associated with each. The chapter concludes with an overview of psychopharmacology, including pharmokinetics, and its use in the treatment of mental disorders.

INTRACELLULAR COMPONENTS AND FUNCTIONS

As depicted in Fig. 2.1 (see also Color Plate 1), the numerous internal components of a cell each serve a particular function. These structures include the cell membrane, nucleus, ribosomes, endoplasmic reticulum, mitochondria, golgi complex, microtubules, and synaptic vesicles as well as other structures. The cell body is encased in a semipermeable membrane consisting of a double layer of lipid molecules. Embedded in the membrane are proteins that have a number of functions and serve an essential role in communication between neurons. The intracellular space of the cell is filled with cytoplasm; within the cytoplasm is the nucleus of the cell containing the chromosomes and nucleolus. Chromosomes consist of strands of DNA, and portions of the DNA—the genes—initiate production of messenger ribonucleic acid (mRNA). The nucleolus produces ribosomes, and ribosomes interact with the mRNA to synthesize proteins for the cell. The endoplasmic reticulum is of two forms, rough and smooth. Rough endoplasmic reticulum contains ribosomes that produce proteins to be transported within and out of the cell. The smooth endoplasmic reticulum plays an important role in the production of lipids. The cell's energy supply is produced by mitochondria. Mitochondria produce adenosine triphosphate (ATP), which the cell uses as an energy source. The main function of the golgi complex (or apparatus) is to assemble proteins and package molecules in vesicles such as neurotransmitters.

The structure of the cell is maintained by strands of proteins (known as the *cytoskeleton*), some thin and others large. The large strands of proteins, or microtubules, extend from the cell body through the axon to the terminal button. Various substances and organelles are transported from the cell body by specialized molecules down the microtubules to the terminal button, a

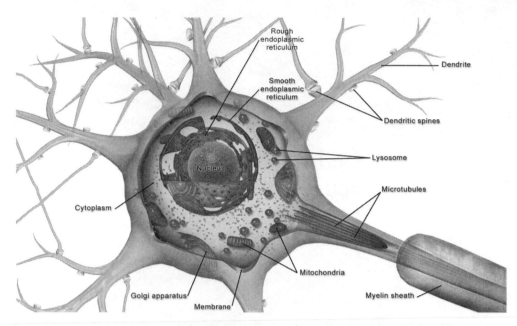

Rough
endoplasmic
reticulum

Dendrite

Smooth
endoplasmic
reticulum

Dendritic spines

Lysosome

Nucleus

Microtubules

Cytoplasm

Mitochondria

Golgi apparatus

Myelin sheath

Membrane

**FIG. 2.1.   Internal components of a cell. Copyright Blausen
Medical Communications. Reproduced by permission. (See Color Plate 1.)**

process called *anterograde transport*. Substances are also transported from the terminal button
to the cell body along these same microtubules (*retrograde transport*). For example, mitochondria, lysosomes, and vesicles filled with neurotransmitter substances are all transported down
the microtubules to the terminal button, and this movement is achieved by motor proteins (e.g,
kinesin; Morris & Hollenbeck, 1995). According to a recent review by De Camilli, Haucke,
Takei, and Mugnaini (2001), the movement of substances within a neuron via anterograde and
retrograde transport can take anywhere from hours to several weeks depending on a variety of
factors.

    Proteins have also been found to stabilize the microtubules within the cytoplasm of the cell.
One such stabilizing protein is tau protein. Research by Ebneth et al. (1998) found overexpression of tau protein interfered with the internal trafficking processes of cells and significantly
slowed the transport of substances down the microtubules. They speculated that elevated levels
of tau protein and mislocated, tangled filaments of tau protein cause a gradual degeneration
of neurons followed by cognitive impairment. Patients with Alzheimer's disease, for example,
have been found to have neurofibrillary tangles of tau protein and elevated levels of tau protein
compared to adults without the disease (Kahle et al., 2000). Felipo and colleagues (1993) also
studied the role of microtubules in neuronal degeneration and found that toxic substances (e.g.,
ammonia) can interfere with the integrity and functioning of microtubules and the transport
process.

    The terminal button, located at the end of the axon, contains many of the structures found
in the cell body (Fig. 2.2; see also Color Plate 2). The terminal button contains vesicles filled
with substances that are released by the cell and cause a reaction in nearby and, in some cases,
distant cells. This process, known as exocytosis, will be covered in detail later in the chapter.
At the other end of the cell body are dendrites. *Dendrites* are very thin, treelike structures of
various shapes and sizes that emerge from the cell body of the neuron and receive messages
from other neurons.

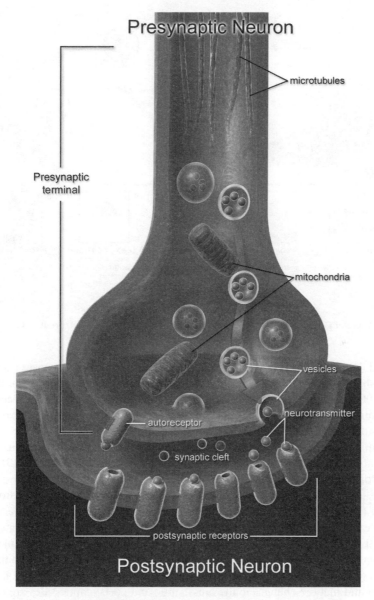

FIG. 2.2.   Terminal button of presynaptic neuron and cell membrane depicting receptors of postsynaptic neuron. Copyright Blausen Medical Communications. Reproduced by permission. (See Color Plate 2.)

Dendrites and Synapses

As mentioned in the previous chapter, dendrites continue to develop and expand throughout the life span and help to establish connections among neurons. As the principal reception sites for information from other neurons, each dendrite receives thousands of inputs from other neurons via synapses. The term *synapse*, first identified by Sherrington in 1897, refers to the site at which axons make functional contact with their target cells (Cowan, Sudhof, & Stevens, 2001, p. vii). Specifically, a synapse is the space between the terminal button of a neuron sending a

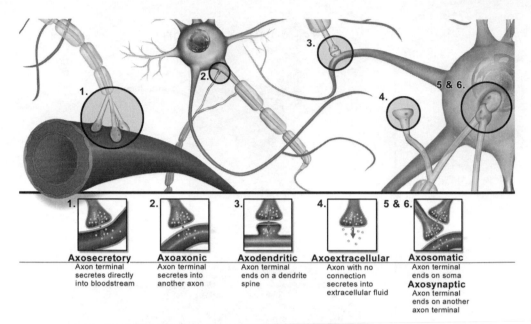

FIG. 2.3.   Types of synapses. Copyright Blausen Medical Communications. Reproduced by permission.

message and the area of a neuron that is receiving the message. Most synapses occur on small mushroom-shaped structures, or dendritic spines, that protrude from the shaft of the dendrite (Kennedy, 2000). Synapses can also occur on the dendrites soma, axon, or nonspecifically into the extracellular fluid; these synapses are known as axodendritic, axosomatic, axoaxonic, and axoextracellular, respectively. Other types of synapses are also possible, for example, when an axon terminal forms a synapse with a small blood vessel and releases chemicals such as hormones into the bloodstream (i.e., axosecretory synapse; Cowan & Kandel, 2001) (Fig. 2.3).

Features of the synapse include the terminal button of the neuron ("presynaptic") that is sending a message, vesicles filled with neurotransmitter, the membrane of the neuron receiving the message ("postsynaptic") that contains receptors for the neurotransmitter, and the space ("synaptic cleft") between the presynaptic and postsynaptic neurons (refer to Color Plate 2). The synaptic cleft is small, with an average width of 20 nm, and contains protein filaments that are thought to stabilize the synaptic connections (Südof, 2001). Studies have found that synaptic connections change in size and appearance during certain cellular events (e.g., long-term potentiation) and that the changes in the presynaptic and postsynaptic sides are coordinated, that is, they enlarge and contract together (Toni et al., 1999). As Südof (2001) noted, the factors that mediate these synchronized changes are not understood but may involve cell adhesion molecules.

Located on the dendritic spines are receptors that consist of protein channels that can change shape (i.e., open and close) to allow the exchange of substances across the cell membrane (Fig. 2.4). The pattern and distribution of these channels are diverse. For example, in some neurons, channels that respond to particles in the extracellular fluid such as ions (particles that have a positive or negative charge, e.g., Na+, K+, Ca_2+) are evenly distributed along the dendrites. In other neurons, however, these channels may be present along the cell body but occur in very low density along the dendrites (Häusser, Spruston, & Stuart, 2000). Historically, dendrites have been recognized for their structural role in synaptic connections, but recently researchers have reported that dendrites play an active role in processing the thousands of

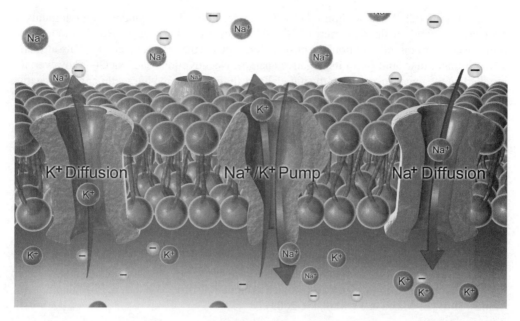

FIG. 2.4.   Exchange of ions across cell membrane.
Copyright Blausen Medical Communications. Reproduced by permission.

inputs they receive from other neurons (Häusser, Spruston, & Stuart, 2000). For example, the distribution and density of dendritic spines and ion channels likely affect neuronal signaling although the mechanisms are not well understood. In a recent review article, Matus (2000) reported that the production of dendritic spines is influenced by environmental experiences and that increased numbers of dendritic spines are associated with brain development, plasticity, and learning. Robinson and Kolb (2004) recently reported that exposure to drugs such as cocaine, nicotine, and morphine alters the functioning of neurons and neuronal systems by inducing changes in the structure of dendrites and dendritic spines. Although many questions remain about the role of dendrites in neuronal processing of information, it is well established that dendrites receive messages from other neurons and that these messages affect the distribution of energy across the cell's membrane. If the sum total of all of the synaptic inputs changes the cell membrane to a degree that an action potential develops, the recipient neuron will send a message to other neurons.

DEVELOPMENT OF THE ACTION POTENTIAL

Electrostatic Pressure and Diffusion

A neuron that is not actively communicating with other neurons is said to be at rest. When a neuron is at rest, particles called ions, which have either a negative (*anion*) or positive (*cation*) charge, are unevenly distributed in the intracellular and extracellular fluid (refer to Fig. 2.4). Specifically, ions are distributed in such a way that the inside of the cell has a negative charge (-70 mv) relative to the outside of the cell. This is because the intracellular fluid contains organic anions not found in the extracelluar fluid ($A-$), which largely accounts for the negative charge inside the cell relative to the outside of the cell. The intracellular fluid also contains more potassium ions ($K+$) than the extracellular fluid and smaller amounts of cloride ions (Cl−) and sodium (Na+). The extracellular fluid contains larger amounts of Na+ and Cl− and smaller amounts of K+ and has a positive charge relative to the intracellular fluid. Because of this distribution, the positive ions outside the cell (Na+ and K+) are attracted to the intracellular fluid (with its negative charge). Negative ions such as Cl−, however, are repelled by the negative charge of the intracellular fluid. Within the intracellular fluid, negative ions (A−) are attracted to the positive charge of the extracellular fluid but cannot leave the cell because of their large size. Positive ions (K+) are repelled by the positive charge of the extracellular fluid. This attraction between positive and negative ions and the repulsion between like-charged ions produce energy in the form of electrostatic pressure. In addition, because ions are unevenly distributed inside and outside the cell, they try to diffuse. The only ion that is more abundant in the extracellular fluid and is also attracted to the intracellular fluid is Na+. Because of electrostatic pressure and diffusion, Na+ enters the intracellular fluid. However, it is pushed back out by the sodium potassium pump. The sodium potassium pump consists of proteins located in the cell membrane that actively and efficiently pump out the extra Na+ that has entered the cell and retrieve K+ ions that have leaked out of the intracellular fluid. To function, the sodium potassium pump uses a considerable amount of the cell's energy supply. Abnormalities of the sodium potassium pump as well as elevated levels of extracellular sodium have been implicated in clinical disorders such as bipolar disorder (Looney & El-Mallakh, 1997; Valdes, Huff, El-Masri, & El-Mallakh, 2003).

Depolarization and Hyperpolarization

An action potential develops as a result of stimulation to the cell that changes the permeability of the membrane to sodium and potassium ions. Specifically, a single neuron receives thousands of messages from other neurons. If these messages selectively open the Na+ channels on one or many parts of the cell membrane, sodium enters the intracellular fluid and the intracellular fluid becomes less negative, that is, it becomes more positive (*depolarization*). This reduction in the negative charge of the intracellular fluid is known as excitatory postsynaptic potential because it increases the likelihood that an action potential will develop. On the other hand, if K+ channels are selectively opened and K+ exits the inside of the cell, the intracellular fluid becomes even more negative. This increase in the negative charge of the inside of the cell— inhibitory postsynaptic potential—hyperpolarizes the cell because it decreases the likelihood that the neuron will develop an action potential. These excitatory and inhibitory potentials occur at thousands of places on the cell. Their net effect is integrated at the junction between the cell body and the axon—the axon hillock. If the sum of the total depolarizations and hyperpolarizations is sufficient to depolarize the cell membrane to a certain point called the threshold of excitation, an action potential will develop. An action potential is a rapid and complete reversal of the neuron's membrane potential from −70 mv to approximately +50 mv, meaning that the inside becomes positive relative to the extracellular fluid, mainly because of the influx of Na+ (Fig. 2.5).

An action potential lasts less than 1 millisecond until neurons are quickly restored to the resting potential. This is achieved by the outflow of K+ ions to the extracellular fluid after the threshold of excitation is reached. In fact, the outflow of K+ ions results in the membrane over-shooting the −70 mv resting potential for a brief period during which another action potential cannot develop (*absolute refractory period*). Within a millisecond or two, the sodium potassium pump removes the extra Na+ ions from the intracellular fluid and retrieves the K+ ions from the extracellular fluid. The resting potential is restored. In summary, an action potential is the result of a neuron receiving inputs from many presynaptic cells within milliseconds. The likelihood of a neuron developing an action potential is the net result of excitatory and

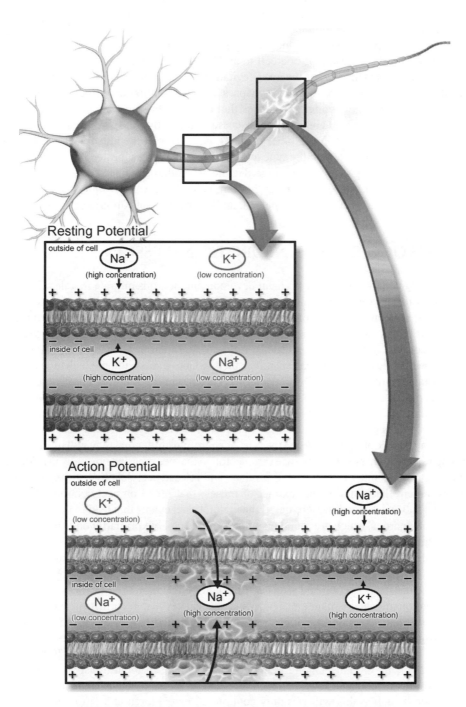

FIG. 2.5. Distribution of ions during resting and action potentials.
Copyright Blausen Medical Communications. Reproduced by permission.

inhibitory inputs to that cell. Once the action potential develops, the role of the neuron as a recipient of information changes to one of a transmitter of information.

Transmission of information between cells occurs by two general methods: electrical synapses and chemical synapses. Electrical synapses involve the rapid movement of ions or molecules from the cytoplasm of one cell to another via gap junctions, such as are found in tissues of the liver and the lens of the eye (Levitan and Kaczmarek, 1997). More prominent in the central nervous system are chemical synapses, the focus of this chapter. Chemical synapses involve the release of transmitter substances that result in the depolarization or hyperpolarization of the postsynaptic membrane, as discussed. In addition to their variable location on the neuron, synapses also differ in other respects. For example, the number of synapses on a neuron varies among cells, as do the type and number of receptors located on a neuron. There is also variability among neurons with regard to the biosynthesis of neurotransmitters, the type of neurotransmitter that is released from the terminal button, whether more than one type of transmitter substance is found within the cell, and reuptake/deactivation processes.

PROCESS OF CHEMICAL NEUROTRANSMISSION

As discussed in chapter 1, during prenatal development, neurons migrate to a destination and immediately form synapses with other neurons. Within the axons of these immature neurons are synaptic vesicles containing neurotransmitter fluid. These vesicles coalesce in areas of the axon that will later form the presynaptic terminal button (De Camilli, Haucke, Takei, & Mugnaini, 2001). According to Huttenlocher (2002), a developing neuron releases a neurotransmitter from a growth cone and this neurotransmitter then induces a morphological change on part of the dendritic membrane of neighboring neurons. This part of the dendritic membrane develops into a receptor and, according to Huttenlocher the receptor will continue to respond to the neurotransmitter in the future. According to De Camilli, Haucke, Takei, and Mugnaini (2001), clusters of vesicles will not remain in areas of the axon that do not form synapses. Interestingly, neurons may be flexible with regard to the type of neurotransmitter that they will ultimately produce and release. Patterson (1978), for example, found that neurons that normally use dopamine as their neurotransmitter could instead produce and release acetylcholine if they matured in an environment that contained an extract of muscle that relied on acetylcholine. Craig and Lichtman (2001) described in more detail the maturational events that lead to the formation of receptors on neurons, which are found on all parts of the cell but primarily on dendritic spines.

Although the general process of neurotransmission is fairly well understood, many of the specifics processes remain theoretical. For example, unanswered questions remain concerning (a) the details by which vesicles fuse and release a neurotransmitter, (b) methods by which transmitter substances may interact and affect cellular communication, (c) the process by which the terminal button membrane maintains it size and shape, (d) synapse formation and maturation, (e) the role of neurotrophins in cellular communication, and (f) the relevance of lesser-known neurotransmitters to cellular communication and brain function. Questions also remain about the role of genes in neurotransmission. For example, Cravchik and Goldman (2000) recently argued that genetic diversity among human dopamine and serotonin transporters and receptors leads to neurochemical individuality, which can be seen in behavioral differences among humans. Ideas such as this will certainly continue to be explored and unfold as technology advances our understanding of the interactions between genetics, environmental experiences, and cellular communication.

The following section provides an overview of the processes involved in neurotransmission, followed by a discussion of transmitter substances and the effects of several classes of drugs at the level of the synapse.

Exocytosis

Traditional explanations concerning communication among neurons usually describe the release of neurotransmitters from the ends of the axon at the terminal button. Some neurotransmitters (i.e., catecholamines), however, are released from areas on branched axons called axonal varicosities. From these axonal varicosities, described as beadlike in appearance, neurotransmitters such as norepinephrine are released (Cooper, Bloom, & Roth, 2003). According to von Bohlen und Halbach and Dermietzel (2002), a single dopamine-releasing neuron can form up to 100,000 varicosities that synapse with other neurons.

When an action potential reaches the terminal button, a number of events occur that facilitate the release of a neurotransmitter (*exocytosis*). First, the membrane of the terminal button depolarizes with the arrival of the action potential and calcium (Ca+) enters the intracellular fluid. The entry of calcium triggers a process that results in neurotransmitter release from vesicles contained within the terminal button. Large and small vesicles filled with transmitter substances (i.e., peptides and neurotransmitters) are located throughout the terminal button but are most abundant near the membrane. According to Betz et al. (1992), synaptic vesicles are adaptable and can merge to form large clusters. Vesicles filled with larger transmitter substances (*peptides*) are packaged in the soma and transported to the axon terminal, while vesicles that contain smaller substances (e.g., catecholamines) are packaged in the terminal button. Their containment in the vesicles protects neurotransmitters from enzymes in the intracellular fluid that could metabolize the substances.

Although there is disagreement in the literature concerning the specifics of the neurotransmitter release process, some vesicles are believed to be "docked" at the membrane and ready for release. This area of the membrane is referred to as an *active zone*. Entry of Ca+ and subsequent protein reactions are believed to cause the docked vesicles to fuse completely with the membrane and for at least one vesicle to spill its contents into the synaptic cleft (von Bohlen und Halbach & Dermietzel, 2002). Proteins (e.g., synaptotagmin) are believed to be important in facilitating fusion of a synaptic vesicle with the cell membrane (Wang et al., 2001). Meanwhile, other vesicles migrate to the active zone area in preparation for release (Greengard et al., 1993). Although the details of this process are not well understood, it has been hypothesized that proteins play a critical role in providing structural support and serve as scaffolding for the "docked" and reserve vesicles (Pieribone et al., 1995). Recently, Murphy, Rueter, Trojanowski, and Lee (2000) reported that a particular family of proteins (synuclein proteins) are involved in maintaining reserve pools of synaptic vesicles in the terminal button of neurons. They suggested that pathologies in the synuclein proteins could lead to impaired synaptic function and degeneration of neurons. These findings may be particularly relevant to understanding neural degeneration in Parkinson's and Alzheimer's diseases as studies have found synuclein proteins in plaque deposits in the brains of individuals with these diseases (Baba et al., 1998).

Neurotransmitter Regulation

Factors that help regulate the amount of neurotransmitter produced and released by a cell include rate-limiting enzymes autoreceptors, heteroreceptors, and vesicular transporters. *Rate-limiting enzymes* are enzymes that essentially control the amount of neurotransmitter that can be produced. For example, when dopamine is biosynthesized by the cell, tyrosine is converted to dopamine by tyrosine hydroxylase. Tyrosine hydroxylase is found in all catecholamine neurons and is essential for the synthesis of dopamine. Increasing the level of tyrosine itself does not result in increased levels of dopamine. Manipulation of tyrosine hydroxylase by drugs, however, can affect the levels of dopamine that is produced. Thus, tyrosine hydroxylase is a rate-limiting enzyme. More detailed information concerning the biosynthesis of dopamine is presented later in this chapter.

Autoreceptors are located on the presynaptic terminal membrane, cell body, and dendrites and respond to neurotransmitter released by that neuron. They moderate the amount of neurotransmitter released and generally decrease the synthesis and release of neurotransmitter (Hunt, 2000). For example, when autoreceptors that are located on the terminal button are stimulated, they trigger feedback mechanisms to the cell (i.e., second messenger systems) and transmitter release is reduced. Drugs have been developed, for example, that target the dopamine system and stimulate autoreceptors. The result is that dopamine synthesis and release is inhibited. Drugs that block these autoreceptors increase dopamine synthesis and release (Cooper, Bloom, & Roth, 2003). The role of autoreceptors located on the soma and dendrites is less well understood and their effect on neurotransmitter release is dependent on a variety of factors (von Bohlen und Halbach et al., 2002; Webster, 2001a).

Heteroreceptors on the presynaptic membrane respond to different neurotransmitters than the one released by the neuron on which they are located. According to Carvey (1998), heteroreceptors modulate the activity of neurons by influencing the increased or decreased release of neurotransmitters. Most research with autoreceptors and heteroreceptors has been conducted in other animals; their role in human brain functioning is not well understood. Schlicker and Gothert (1998), for example, suggested that autoreceptors and heteroreceptors may have complex interactive effects on neurons. Raiteri (2001) recently noted that "due to the multiplicity of the proteins that seem to be involved in the exocytotic process, understanding their interactions with presynaptic receptors will be a formidable task" (p. 674). What can be concluded is that the regulation of neurotransmitter release is influenced by a number of factors including presynaptic and postsynaptic receptors. Neuroimaging methods are currently available that make it possible to study receptor distributions in the brain of living individuals by using substances that are tagged with tracers. These studies have provided valuable information concerning normal distribution of receptors as well as target sites for drugs and areas of neuronal degeneration (Sedvall, Farde, Persson, & Wiesel, 1986).

Small molecule transmitters are synthesized in the cytoplasm and then transported into the synaptic vesicles via vesicular transporters that are specific for each neurotransmitter substance (McIntire, Reimer, Schuske, Edwards, & Jorgensen, 1997). Compared with transporter proteins that assist in the reuptake of neurotransmitters into the terminal button, less is known about vesicular transporters. *Vesicular transporters* are proteins that move neurotransmitters from the cytoplasm to the vesicle by way of a pump located on vesicular plasma membrane. Studies that have genetically altered the expression of these transporter proteins have found significant reductions in the amount of neurotransmitter stored in vesicles and released with exocytosis (Reimer, Fon, & Edwards, 1998). Recent findings by Sandoval and colleagues (2003) indicate drugs such as methamphetamine rapidly decrease dopamine uptake into the vesicles and contribute to abnormal levels of dopamine within the cytoplasm. However, the precise mechanisms involved in vesicular reuptake are poorly understood. Chen, Wei, Fowler, and Wu (2003) have suggested that newly synthesized neurotransmitters (e.g., dopamine) are preferentially taken up into vesicles rather than preexisting neurotransmitters in the cytoplasm. They also suggest that vesicular reuptake involves a multistage process.

POSTSYNAPTIC RECEPTORS

After a neurotransmitter is released, it diffuses across the cleft and attaches to postsynaptic receptors. Postsynaptic receptors can be classified into two types: ionotropic and metabotropic. Activation of ionotropic receptors results in rapid, short-lasting effects, whereas activation of

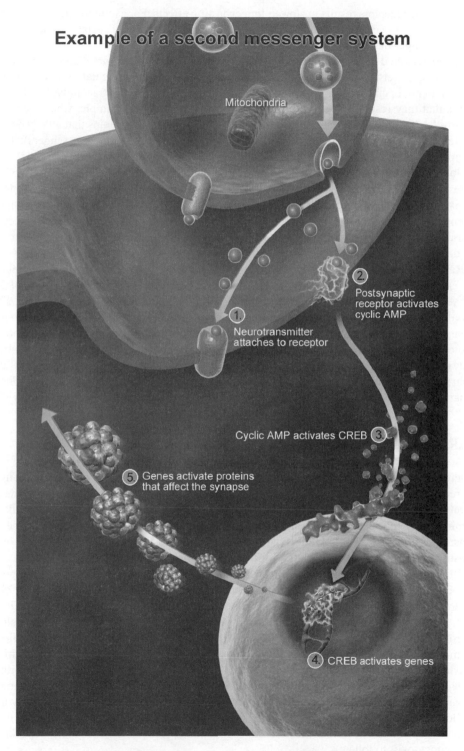

FIG. 2.6.   Second messenger system. Copyright Blausen
Medical Communications. Reproduced by permission. (See Color Plate 3.)

metabotropic receptors results in slower, longer-lasting effects. For example, the opening of an ion channel can occur in less than 5 milliseconds while activation of metabotropic receptors may take longer than 30 milliseconds (Hunt, 2000).

When activated by a neurotransmitter substance, ionotropic receptors directly open membrane ion channels, resulting in a rapid change in the membrane potential. Metabotropic receptors do not open channels directly but instead activate a series of intracellular biochemical events that may result in opening or closing of ion channels. For example, when the neurotransmitter (the first messenger) attaches to the receptor, it causes proteins that attached to the inside of the receptor to activate other chemicals in the cell (the second messengers). These chemicals can then send additional messages causing ion channels on the membrane to open or close or to initiate changes in the cell's DNA or metabolic acitivity (Fig. 2.6; see also Color Plate 3). Examples of second messengers include G-proteins, cAMP, and cGMP. The end result is that the cell membrane either becomes slightly depolarized (i.e., excitatory postsynaptic potential) or hyperpolarized (i.e., inhibitory postsynaptic potential). Depending on effects of neural integration—that is, temporal and spatial summation—an action potential may or may not develop and the neuron may or may not fire.

Research has found that postsynaptic receptors are adaptive and can increase ("upregulation") in number if a substance such as a drug blocks the receptor for an extended period of time (e.g., a dopamine antagonist such as an antipsychotic) (Cooper, Bloom, & Roth, 2003). They can also decrease ("downregulation") in number if a stimulus is chronically present (e.g., a dopamine agonist such as cocaine; Volkow et al., 2001). Rao and colleagues (1998) reported that serotonin receptors were upregulated in a acutely suicidal patients relative to healthy controls. They hypothesized that a reduction in the availability of serotonin resulted in an increase of serotonin receptors. Some antidepressant medications (SSRIs) increase the amount of serotonin that remains in the synaptic cleft, resulting in a downregulation of serotonin receptors (Stahl, 1998).

TERMINATION OF NEUROTRANSMISSION

If neurotransmitters were to remain in the cleft, these substances would continue to activate the receptors resulting in prolonged effects. Hence, mechanisms are needed to terminate the effects of neurotransmitters. Specifically, excitatory and inhibitory postsynaptic potentials are terminated by four main processes: reuptake, enzymatic deactivation, diffusion of the neurotransmitter into the extracellular fluid, and reuptake by glia cells. *Reuptake* is the removal of the transmitter substance from the cleft by the protein pumps that are located on the presynaptic membrane. These proteins are specific to the neurotransmitter and are known as transporter proteins. For example, SERT is the transporter protein that removes serotonin from the cleft; the transporter proteins that remove dopamine and norepinephrine are known as DAT and NET, respectively. In other animals, different types of transporters have been found for a single neurotransmitter. For example, four types of GABA transporter proteins have been identified in the mouse (von Bohlen und Halback & Dermietzel, 2002). Although the precise mechanisms by which the transporter proteins function in humans are not well understood, various drugs developed to inhibit these proteins are associated with certain behavioral effects. For example, Prozac inhibits the tranporter protein for serotonin and thus is frequently and effectively used to alleviate depression (Schloss & Williams, 1998). Once the neurotransmitter is taken up by the presynaptic neuron, various theories exist concerning the method by which it is repackaged (see pinocytosis, to follow).

Enzymatic deactivation occurs when an enzyme breaks down the neurotransmitter while it remains in the cleft. For example, acetylcholinesterase (AchE) breaks down Ach into choline and acetate. Diffusion occurs when neurotransmitters drift away from the receptor sites and are no longer capable of activating the receptors. Finally, research suggests that glia cells take up neurotransmitters (or their metabolites) and assist in the recycling process of neurotransmitters (Kettenmann & Ransom, 1995).

Endocytosis and Pinocytosis

The process of release of a neurotransmitter is known as exocytosis, while the process of reuptake, recycling, and repackaging of a neurotransmitter is known as endocytosis. Once the neurotransmitter has been released, there are several theories about the process by which the vesicle is recycled and the membrane maintains its shape (*pinocytosis*). Two main theories are the "kiss-and-tell" and "budding" theories (De Camilli, Slepnev, Shupliakov, & Brodin, 2001). The kiss-and-tell theory suggests that after a vesicle fuses with the presynaptic membrane and releases its neurotransmitter, it reseals, remains intact, and is released back into the terminal button to be recycled after various staging processes. In contrast, the budding theory suggests that after the vesicle fuses with the membrane and releases its contents, pieces of the membrane break off, a number of proteins attach to the pieces (e.g., clathrin), and the pieces are formed into vesicles by the cisternae located in the terminal button.

Harris, Hartwieg, Orvitz, and Jorgensen (2000) recently reported that a protein, snyapto-janin, facilitates vesicle recycling and that mutuations in the gene which produces this protein can significantly interfere with the recycling process. Bloom et al. (2003) have identified a role for the proteins synapsin and actin in the vesicle recycling process. These studies suggest that multiple proteins are involved in the recycling of synaptic vesicles, but the interactive effects of these proteins are not understood. After the vesicles are recycled, they are filled with neuro-transmitter and transported to the appropriate areas in the terminal button, where they will once again fuse with the membrane and release their contents. According to De Camilli, Slepnev, Shupliakov, and Brodin (2001), precursor membranes for synaptic vesicles are transported from the cell body to the terminal button, and recycling of synaptic vesicles may occur only in the terminal button. Koenig and Ikeda (1996) suggested that at least two vesicle recycling pathways may exist within a terminal button; one near the active zone and rapid in function, another away from the active zone and more slow. The entire process of release, recycle, and repackaging is hypothesized to occur within 60 seconds (De Camilli, Slepnev, Shupliakov, & Brodin, 2001; Levitan & Kaczmarek, 1997).

NEUROTRANSMITTER SUBSTANCES

Neuroscientists estimate that the brain contains hundreds of different neurotransmitters; the majority have yet to be identified. According to Werman (1966), chemicals found in the brain are considered to be a neurotransmitter if:

- They are synthesized in the neuron;
- They are released, occupy a receptor, and result in an effect in another cell;
- They are cleared from the synaptic cleft following release; and
- Their effects can be replicated by an experimental substance.

Neurotransmitters can be classified in a number of ways (Webster, 2001b), but the simplest is a breakdown by size into three categories: transmitter gases, large molecule transmitters, and small molecule transmitters. Small molecule transmitters have molecular weights less than 200 while large molecule transmitters have molecular weights ranging from 200–5,000 (Beart, 2000). Different types of transmitter substances can coexist in neurons and may be co-released and have interactive effects (von Bohlen und Halbach & Dermietzel, 2002). Transmitter substances are not equally distributed throughout the brain and, depending on the specific substance, are found in higher and lower concentrations. For example, large molecule transmitters are most concentrated in the nuclei of the hypothalamus; glycine, a small molecule transmitter, is the most abundant inhibitory neurotransmitter in the spinal cord; and dopamine, a small molecule transmitter, is heavily concentrated in the substantia nigra and surrounding systems (Ashwell, Tancred, & Paxinos, 2000). In addition, neurotransmitter substances are unequally distributed within the cell depending on processes such as biosynthesis and axoplasmatic transport (von Bohlen und Halbach & Dermietzel, 2002).

Transmitter Gases

Unlike large and small molecule transmitters, once transmitter gases are synthesized in various locations by the cell, they cross the cell membrane, diffuse across the cleft, and enter other cell membranes. After they enter the cells of neighboring neurons, transmitter gases are short-lived and are believed to exert their effects by activating internal processes within the cell, that is, second messenger systems. Relative to what is known about large and small molecule transmitters, the role of transmitter gases in brain function is poorly understood. Examples of transmitter gases include carbon monoxide (CO) and nitric oxide (NO). Nitric oxide is involved in the dilation of the brain's blood vessels and has been hypothesized to play a mediating role in learning and memory (Levitan & Kaczmarek, 1997). The role of carbon monoxide is unclear but may be involved in regulating functions in olfactory neurons and stimulating neurons in the hypothalamus (Kim & Rivier, 2000; Snyder, Jaffrey, & Zakhary, 1998). Recently, Wang (2002) hypothesized that hydrogen sulfide (H_2S) is the third endogenous gaseous transmitter and that it is implicated in brain development and long-term potentiation in the hippocampus. Kimura (2002) reported that H_2S is produced in response to neuronal firing and that it plays a role in the release of hormones from the hypothalamus. More empirical information is available, however, on large and small molecule transmitters.

Large Molecule Transmitters

Large molecule transmitters include a variety of peptides that consist of two or more amino acids connected by peptide bonds. Peptides are synthesized by neurons and released from the terminal button. Some peptides attach to receptors and influence changes on the postsynaptic membrane while others exert indirect effects on cells by diffusing throughout the extracellular fluid and are referred to as neurohormones (e.g., follicle-stimulating hormone). As reviewed by von Bohlen und Halbach and Dermietzel (2002), peptides, unlike small molecule neurotransmitters, are involved in a number of processes such as immune responses and physiological growth and development.

Examples of peptides include angiotensin, cholecystokinin, somastostatin, and vasopressin (see Hökfelt, 1991 for a review). Vrontakis (2002) reviewed the role of a lesser-known peptide, galanin, and indicated that this peptide alters the release of several neurotransmitters and has multiple biological effects. He suggested that drugs that interfere with the effects of galanin may be beneficial in the treatment of eating disorders, depression, and Alzheimer's disease, among others. The most well-studied peptides are probably the endogenous opiates (e.g., endorphins). Opiate drugs such as morphine and heroin bind to these naturally occurring opioid receptors that both activate pain suppression (i.e., analgesia) and are involved in reinforcement or "pleasure" systems. Quirk and Gehlert (2003) recently suggested that as peptides can excite or inhibit certain behavioral responses such as anxiety in the pathways extending from the limbic region to the prefrontal cortex, medications that target these peptides may prove useful in treating anxiety disorders as well as cue-induced cravings in humans.

Relative to small molecule transmitters, peptides have slower, longer-lasting effects. They can augment or reduce the effect of small molecule transmitters when they are released. Peptides can be present in the same terminal button as small molecule transmitters but are located in separate vesicles. Peptides differ from small molecules in a number of ways (see Cooper, Bloom, & Roth, 2003 for a review):

- Synthesis and packaging of peptides occurs in the soma, and the vesicles containing the peptides are delivered via microtubules to the terminal button.
- Once released, peptides are deactivated by enzymes and are not taken up by the terminal button and recycled.
- Peptides are released in larger amounts from various regions of the terminal button.
- Peptides diffuse throughout the extracellular fluid and are capable of modulating the activity of neurons in a wider region.
- Peptides can increase the sensitivity of postsynaptic receptors to neurotransmitters.

Small Molecule Transmitters

The three classes of small molecule transmitters are amino acids, monoamines, and acetylcholine. The amino acids include aspartic acid, gamma-aminobutyric acid (GABA), glutamate, and glycine. The monoamines include catecholamines—for example, dopamine (DA), epinephrine (EP), and norepinephrine (NE)—and indolamines (serotonin [5HT]). Amino acids are the building blocks of proteins and are widely distributed throughout the brain. They contain both a carboxyl group and an amino group attached to the same carbon. According to Cooper, Bloom, and Roth (2003), the amino acids are likely the major transmitters in the brain while the remaining neurotransmitters account for a relatively small percentage of synapses.

Aspartate

Although abundant in the brain, relatively little is known about aspartate (aspartic acid). Both aspartate and glutamate serve as building blocks for proteins and peptide synthesis and are involved in intracellular metabolism (Cooper, Bloom, & Roth, 2003). Aspartate produces an excitatory effect (depolarizes) on the membrane and is closely related to glutamate. According to von Bohlen und Halbach and Dermietzel (2002), aspartate and glutamate are synthesized in the terminal button, attach to similar postsynaptic receptors (N-methyl-D-aspartate, NMDA), and produce comparable effects. Consequently, it is often difficult to distinguish between the metabolic and neurotransmitter functions of aspartate and glutamate. Receptor dysfunction for both amino acids has been implicated in schizophrenia (Olney & Farber, 1995). Recently, Morgan, Mofeez, Brandner, Bromley, and Curran (2003) found that a drug that blocks NMDA receptors—ketamine—impaired learning and memory but not attention or executive functioning in healthy adult subjects. In addition, ketamine produced schizophrenia-like symptoms in these healthy adults, further evidence that glutamate is involved in learning and memory as well as psychotic symptoms. The NMDA receptor has also been implicated in bipolar disorder. For example, Mundo et al. (2003) investigated a subunit of the NMDA receptor and the gene (GRIN1) that codes this subunit. Results indicating that a variant in this gene was associated with bipolar disorder suggest that the gene may be involved in its pathogenesis.

Glutamate

Glutamate is the principal excitatory neurotransmitter in the brain, accounting for approximately 50% of synapses (Snyder & Ferris, 2001). Glutamatergic neurons are widely distributed—in subcortical structures, throughout the cortex, and in other areas of the brain. Like aspartate, glutamate is synthesized in the axon terminal by a series of enzymatic changes and stored in synaptic vesicles. Several types of glutamate receptors have been identified including NMDA, AMPA, and the Kainate ionotrophic receptors as well as several metabotrophic receptors specific to glutamate (Sheng, 2001). These receptors consist of complex subunits that interact with intracellular proteins, but the specific functions of the subunits are not fully understood. For example, the NMDA receptor has been found to have at least six different binding sites that have varying effects when occupied (Dickenson, 2001). For the ion channels to open (e.g., calcium), glutamate must bind to one of the sites and glycine must bind to another site. Opening of the ion channels results in the influx of sodium, which depolarizes the cell membrane, and the influx of calcium triggers complex second messenger systems. The AMPA and kainate receptors are thought to control sodium channels. When glutamate binds to these receptors, depolarization results (i.e., EPSPs). Glutamate receptors are usually located on parts of the dendrite and less commonly near or on the cell body (see von Bohlen und Halbach & Dermietzel, 2002 for a review).

Glutamate is cleared from the cleft primarily by glia cells via reuptake transporter proteins found on the glial cell membrane. Glutamate is also taken up by transporter proteins on the presynaptic terminal button, soma, and dendrites as well as glia cells, a process that is less well understood (Cooper, Bloom, & Roth, 2003). Several subtypes of glutamate transporters have been identified. After glutamate is cleared from the cleft by glial cells, it is converted by enzymes into glutamine. Glutamine is then transported to neuronal terminal buttons, where it serves as a precursor for glutamate. The reuptake process is particularly important as high levels of extracellular glutamate can be toxic to other neurons and glia cells, as discussed in chapter 1.

Glutamate has been implicated in learning and memory (e.g., Riedel, Platt, & Micheau, 2003) as well as a number of psychiatric illnesses. For example, Michael and colleagues (2003) recently reported that adults suffering from bipolar disorder and mania had significantly elevated levels of glutamate in the region of the prefrontal cortex. Schiffer (2002) reviewed the molecular genetics literature and concluded that mutations in glutamate receptor genes might increase the risk of developing schizophrenia, bipolar disorder, or depression. Levine and colleagues (2000) compared cerebral spinal fluid glutamate metabolites in adults with depression (unipolar and bipolar) relative to control subjects and found that those suffering from depression had higher metabolite concentrations. Meador-Woodruff, Hogg, and Smith (2001) investigated the density of glutamate receptors in postmortem samples of adults with schizophrenia, biolar disorder, depression, and a control group and reported similar findings across samples. Recently, Friedman and colleagues (2004) found significant decreases in glutamate metabolites in patients with bipolar disorder treated with lithium relative to control subjects. Glutamate has also been found to influence the release and inhibition of other neurotransmitters such as serotonin. Marek (2002), for example, reported that drugs that stimulate glutamate autoreceptors suppress the release of glutamate, which in turn reduces the release of serotonin in the prefrontal cortex. Given the hypothesis that glutamate dysfunction is involved in schizophrenia, Marek suggested drugs that target glutamate autoreceptors may be warranted in the treatment of the disorder. One of the difficulties in determining the role of glutamate or other neurotransmitters in pathological conditions is that the complexities of these systems in the normal brain are not yet understood.

y-Amino Butyric Acid (GABA)

GABA is the principal inhibitory neurotransmitter in the brain, expressed in approximately 30% of all synapses (Synder & Ferris, 2001). Widely distributed throughout the brain, it is found in high concentrations in the basal ganglia, thalamus, and cortex. It is synthesized in the terminal button from glutamate by GAD (glutamic acid decarboxylase), an enzyme that removes a carboxyl group (Cooper, Bloom, & Roth, 2003). At least three types of GABA postsynpatic receptors have been identified: GABAa, GABAb, and GABAc receptors. GABAa and GABAc are ionotropic receptors and when occupied by GABA, the chloride channel opens. GABAb is a metabotropic receptor and when occupied activates a cascade of intracellular events that ultimately results in a reduction of neurotransmitter release. GABA receptors are mainly located on dendrites close to the cell body or on the cell body. In addition, GABA autoreceptors have been identified on the membrane of the terminal button, where they help inhibit the release of GABA (Sarup, Larsson, & Schousboe, 2003).

GABA is cleared from the cleft by reuptake via GABA transporters (GAT) found on the presynaptic membrane of the terminal button and the glia cell membrane. Several types of GABA transporters have been identified. The reason for multiple types of transporter proteins is unknown. Cooper, Bloom, and Roth (2003) suggested that different types of transporter proteins may serve as cotransporters for other types of amino acids or that they may have the capacity to function in an outward direction, "serving as a paradoxical mechanism for release, rather than the removal of GABA" (p. 114). Like most neurotransmitters, GABA has been implicated in psychiatric disorders, including epilepsy, Tourette's Disorder, stress, and a variety of anxiety disorders. Sepkuty and colleagues (2002), for example, reported that a specific glutamate transporter protein (EAAC1) found on the soma and dendrites of many neurons plays a critical role in GABA synthesis. Specifically, they found excessive neuronal activity and seizures were induced in rats treated with a drug that blocked the EAAC1 transporters. In addition, a 50% loss of GABA in the hippocampus demonstrated that GABA synthesis is partially dependent on glutamate transporter proteins (i.e., glutamate is a GABA precursor). Sepkuty et al. hypothesized that epilepsy can result from a disruption in the process of EAAC1 reuptake and GABA metabolism. Drake et al. (2003) reported that a drug (Baclofen) that activates GABA postsynaptic receptors was effective at decreasing symptoms of posttraumatic stress disorder (PTSD) in patients with PTSD due to combat. Ketter and Wang (2003) and Maubach (2003) recently suggested that drugs that enhance GABA inhibitory effects may be useful in treating bipolar disorder as well as the memory deficits characteristic of Alzheimer's disease. Additional studies have implicated the GABA system in psychiatric disorders and are discussed in subsequent chapters.

Monoamine Neurotransmitters

The monoamine neurotransmitters fall into two groups, catecholamines and indolamines, based on their chemical structure. The catecholamines include dopamine (DA), epinephrine (EP), and norepinephrine (NE). Neurons that release epinephrine are referred to as *adrenergic* while neurons that release norepinephrine are referred to as *noradrenergic*.

Dopamine

Dopamine is widely distributed throughout the brain and several complex dopaminergic systems have been identified. These systems originate in the midbrain and forebrain and include the nigrostriatal, mesolimbic, and mesocortical systems (Fig. 2.7). Each systems is associated

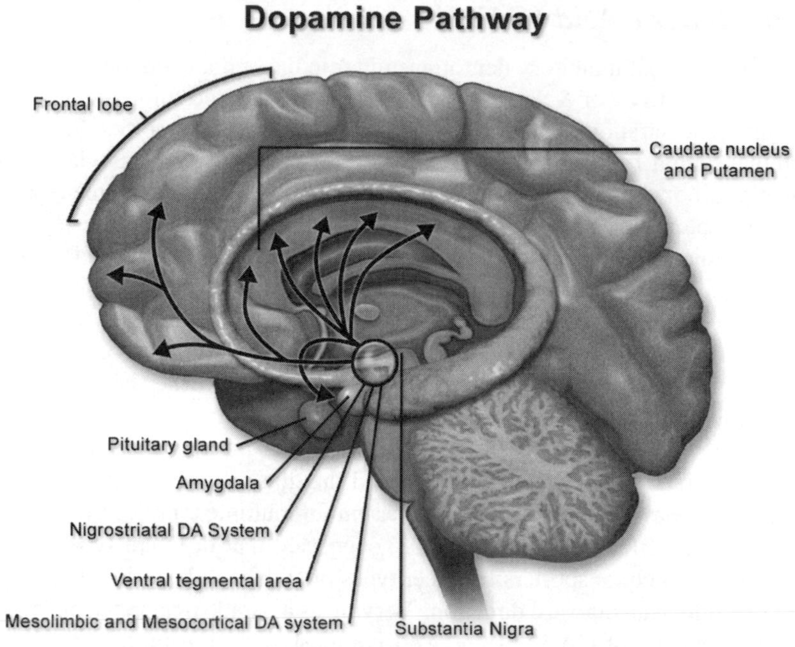

Dopamine Pathway

FIG. 2.7. Dopaminergic pathways and projections.
Copyright Blausen Medical Communications. Reproduced by permission.

with specific functions, and the morphology and density of the neurons vary among the systems (Cooper, Bloom, & Roth, 2003). Dopamine is involved in numerous functions (e.g., movement, attention, motivation, learning) and has been implicated in a variety of disorders such as schizophrenia, obsessive compulsive disorder, Tourette's disorder, and Parkinson's disease. These disorders and the role of the dopaminerigic systems, as well as other neurotransmitter systems, are addressed in subsequent chapters.

Dopamine is synthesized in the terminal button from the precursor amino acid tyrosine. Found in certain foods, tyrosine is converted into L-DOPA by the enzyme tyrosine hydroxylase (which adds a hydroxyl group to the tyrosine). The enzyme DOPA decarboxlyase then removes a carboxyl group from the L-DOPA, which results in dopamine. Dopamine is stored in synaptic vesicles to prevent breakdown by the enzyme monoamine oxidase (MAO). Five families of dopamine receptors have been identified, all metabotropic. According to Greengard (2001), the second messenger pathways involved in these metabotropic receptors are enormously complicated. In addition, dopamine receptors vary in their distribution throughout the brain and, depending on the receptor, dopamine can have an excitatory, inhibitory, or modulating effect on the cell (Cooper, Bloom, & Roth, 2003). This variance in distribution of receptors is consistent with the large number of brain functions in which dopamine appears to be involved. The synthesis and release of dopamine are also regulated by presynaptic autoreceptors. In general, drugs that stimulate autoreceptors inhibit dopamine release; drugs that block autoreceptors elicit its release.

Dopamine is cleared primarily by transporter proteins, known as DAT, found on the dendrites, terminal button, soma, and in the *extrasynaptic* region of the terminal button of dopamine-releasing neurons (Kuhar, 1998). Unlike GABA, which has several types of transporter proteins, DAT appears to be the only transporter protein for dopamine. According to Cooper, Bloom, and Roth (2003), 80% of dopamine is retrieved from the extracellular fluid by reuptake. Different levels of DAT are found in different dopamine neurons, however, which suggests that diffusion is also involved in removing dopamine from the synaptic cleft (Kuhar, 1998). Drugs such as cocaine and methylphenidate selectively target and block DAT, thereby prolonging dopamine's effects in the synaptic cleft (Volkow et al., 1999). Drugs with a high affinity for DAT have also been used by neuroimaging researchers to measure the density of DAT in patients who suffer from Parkinson's disease. Neuroimaging studies revealed that the disease is characterized by a loss of DAT in the striatum (Varrone, Marek, Jennings, Innis, & Seibyl, 2001). Conversely, obsessive compulsive disorder may be characterized by an increased density of DAT (Kim et al., 2003), while the density of DAT appears to be normal in schizophrenia (Laruelle et al., 2000). Mozley, Gur, Mozley, and Gur (2001) measured DAT levels in 30 men and 36 women and reported age as well as sex differences, with women and younger subjects having higher DAT availability in the striatum (caudate and putamen). For women and younger participants, increased DAT availability was associated with better neuropsychological task performance.

After reuptake, dopamine is broken down by monoamine oxidase (MAO) or catechol-O-methyltransferase (COMT) into homovanillic acid (HVA). HVA levels in the cerebral spinal fluid have been used as an index of dopamine activity in the brain. For example, levels of HVA have been reduced in Parkinson's and alzheimer's diseases (Gibson, Logue, & Growdon, 1985) as well as epilepsy (Laxer et al., 1979). Increased levels of HVA have been found with patients with Tourette's syndrome (Cohen, Shaywitz, Caparulo, Young, & Bowers, 1978) and bipolar disorder (Swann et al., 1983). Developmentally, children have been found to have higher levels of cerebral spinal fluid HVA and other neurotransmitter metabolites compared to adults (Leckman et al., 1980). Harper Mozley and colleagues (2001) recently investigated dopamine transporter levels and density of dopamine postsynaptic receptors in healthy college students of various ages. Results indicated that dopamine receptor availability declined with age and that the rate of dopamine reuptake differed between males and females. Specifically, better fine-motor coordination and faster performance on a verbal inhibition task were linked to higher levels of dopamine uptake in females but not in males. The authors suggested that cognitive and motor functions may be differentially regulated by dopamine in males and females, possibly by the hormonal system.

Norepinephrine and Epinephrine

Norepinephrine is differentially distributed in the brain, with most cell bodies contained in the brain stem in the locus coeruleus (Fig. 2.8). These neurons form tracts and project to many areas such as the hypothalamus, thalamus, and the cortex. Norepincphrine is synthesized in the terminal vesicles from dopamine by the enzyme dopamine B-hyroxylase. In some cells, norepinephrine is not released but instead is further metabolized to create epinephrine. Norepinephrine is released both from the terminal button and from swellings located along branches of the axon known as varicosities (von Bohlen und Halbach & Dermietzel, 2002). Epinephrine is released by the adrenal glands located above the kidneys. The adrenergic receptors in the brain respond to epinephrine as well as norepinephrine. Like dopamine and other neurotransmitters, norepinephrine release is partially regulated by autoreceptors. According to Cooper, Bloom, and Roth (2003), other substances (e.g., prostaglandins) may also affect (increase) the release of norepinephrine. Several types of norepinephrine postsynaptic receptors (i.e., adrenergic receptors) have been identified and all are metabotropic. Norepinephrine is cleared from the extracellular fluid by norepinephrine transporters (NET). Densities of NET vary in the brain, with the highest concentrations found in the locus coeruleus and the lowest in the caudate and putamen (Charnay et al., 1995). Interestingly, the norepinephrine transporter may

Norepinephrine Pathway

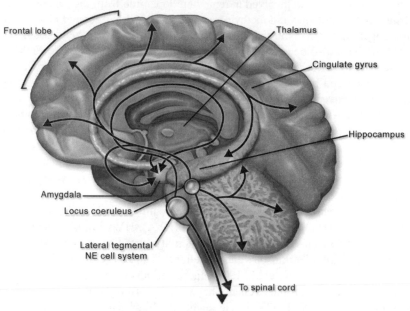

Frontal lobe

Thalamus

Cingulate gyrus

Hippocampus

Amygdala

Locus coeruleus

Lateral tegmental
NE cell system

To spinal cord

FIG. 2.8. Norepinephrine pathways and projections.
Copyright Blausen Medical Communications. Reproduced by permission.

have a greater affinity for dopamine and, according to Cooper, Bloom, and Roth (2003), can thus influence dopamine transmission. Norepinephrine that is taken back into the cell is either repackaged into synaptic vesicles or broken down by MAO or COMT and recycled.

Norepinephrine has been implicated in a number of psychiatric disorders, in particular anxiety and mood disorders (Charney, 2003). For example, some, but not all, studies have reported lower urinary metabolites of norepinephrine in patients with bipolar disorder relative to control participants (Wehr, Muscettola, & Goodwin, 1980). Recently, Bhanji, Margolese, Saint-Laurent, and Chouinard (2002) suggested that mania is likely due to hyperactivity of norepinephrine systems. They based this hypothesis on the fact that mirtazapine, a drug that increases levels of norepinephrine in the brain, was found to induce mania in adults. Norepinephrine has also been implicated in panic disorder (Sand et al., 2002), ADHD (Biederman & Spencer, 1999; Biederman & Faraone, 2002), and other psychiatric conditions.

Serotonin

Serotonin (5-hydroxytryptamine; 5HT) is categorized as an indolamine. It is also differentially distributed throughout the brain, with higher concentrations located in the brain stem (i.e., raphe nuclei) and midbrain. Similar to dopamine, the projection systems for serotonin are complex and widespread (Fig. 2.9). Although serotonin's role in the brain is not fully understood, studies suggest it helps regulates arousal, wakefulness, appetite and eating behavior, stress response, mood, and motor behavior (Stanford, 2001b). Developmentally, serotonin synthesis is substantially higher in children than adults, and during ages 5–15 there is a gradual decline in synthesis values toward adult levels (Chugani et al., 1999). According to Sodhi and Sanders-Bush (2004), serotonin interacts with other growth factors and neurotransmitter systems to facilitate prenatal and postnatal brain growth.

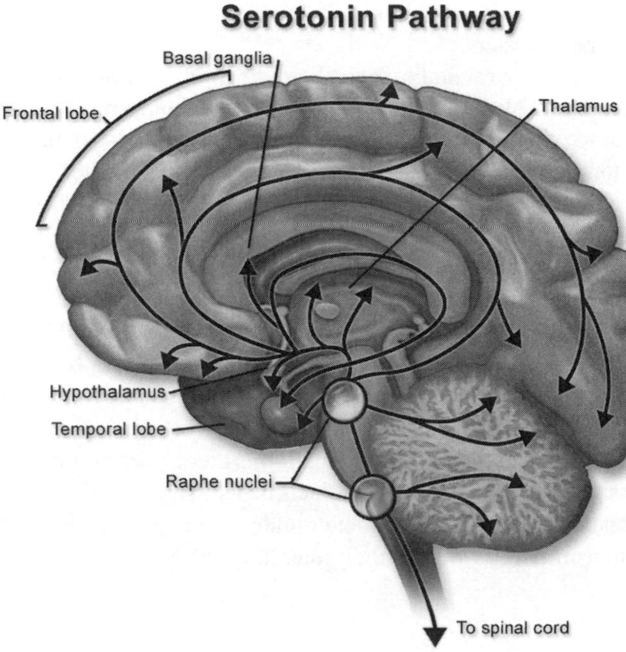

Serotonin Pathway

Basal ganglia

Frontal lobe

Thalamus

Hypothalamus

Temporal lobe

Raphe nuclei

To spinal cord

**FIG. 2.9. Serotonergic pathways and projections.
Copyright Blausen Medical Communications. Reproduced by permission.**

Serotonin is synthesized from a precursor—amino acid tryptophan. Tryptophan is found in various foods and converted into serotonin by several enzymatic events in the terminal button. Stanford (2001b) reported that serotonin is synthesized in glial cells as well, but very little information is available concerning this process. The first step of serotonin synthesis in neurons is that the enzyme tryptophan hydroxylase adds a hydroxyl group to the tryptophan, resulting in 5-hydroxytryptophan (5-HTP). Next, the enzyme 5-HTP decarboxylase removes a carboxyl group from the 5-HTP, producing serotonin. Serotonin is stored in synaptic vesicles, and its synthesis and release are regulated by autoreceptors and heteroreceptors. Serotonin autoreceptors are found on the terminal button as well as the cell body of neurons. Like other neurotransmitter autoreceptors, their function is primarily inhibitory. The role of heteroreceptors in serotonin synthesis and release is poorly understood. Harsing and colleagues (2004) recently speculated that glutamate-releasing neurons may possess serotonin heteroreceptors that inhibit glutamate release. Inhibition of glutamate release ultimately leads to decreased activity of serotonin-releasing neurons, suggesting that serotonin synthesis and release are partially mediated by a glutamaterigic–serotonergic interaction.

With regard to postsynaptic receptors, Cooper, Bloom, and Roth (2003) reported that at least eight types of serotonin postsynaptic receptors have been identified, all but one metabotropic. The reason for such a large number of receptors is unclear. Stanford (2001b) hypothesized that the variety of receptors allows for greater flexibility and refinement of response to serotonin. Schott et al. (2003) recently investigated antibodies to serotonin in blood serum of patients with depression, schizophrenia, Alzheimer's disease, alcoholism, rheumatoid arthritis, and multiple sclerosis as well as healthy volunteers. Results indicated that patients with depression and multiple sclerosis had decreased antibody reactivity to serotonin, while increased reactivity was found in those with arthritis and alcoholism. The authors speculated that serotonin antibodies could influence receptor function and thus produce cognitive and behavioral symptoms associated with the disorders.

Serotonin is deactivated by reuptake from the cleft by the serotonin transporter (SERT) and further degraded by MAO. The final metabolite of serotonin—5-hydroxyindolic acid (5-HIAA)—is similar to other neurotransmitter metabolites in that it can be detected and measured in the urine. However, as Potter, Hsiao, and Goldman (1989) noted, this is an unreliable measure of brain levels of neurotransmitters. Abnormalities of the serotonin transporter (SERT) have been implicated in a number of psychiatric conditions. Ozaki et al. (2003), for example, linked a mutation on the SERT gene (I425V) to obsessive compulsive disorder, Asperger's syndrome, social phobia, anorexia nervosa, tic disorder, and substance abuse. The authors speculated that the mutation could result in different neuropsychiatric phenotypes depending on a number of factors. General dysfunction of the serotonin system has been implicated in numerous disorders. Petty et al. (1996) hypothesized that a balance of neurotransmitters is necessary for the brain to achieve a healthy state of homeostasis and an imbalance among neurotransmitters results in pathology. According to this theory, serotonin is a stabilizing neurotransmitter that assists in returning the brain's neurochemistry to a homeostatic set point. At present, this idea remains theoretical and a better understanding is needed of the specific role of individual neurotransmitters as well as their interactive effects.

Acetylcholine

Acetylcholine (Ach) was the first neurotransmitter discovered and is in its own class. Acetylcholine is widespread throughout the central (Fig. 2.10) and peripheral nervous systems. Neurons that release Ach are referred to as *cholinergic*. Ach is synthesized from choline found in

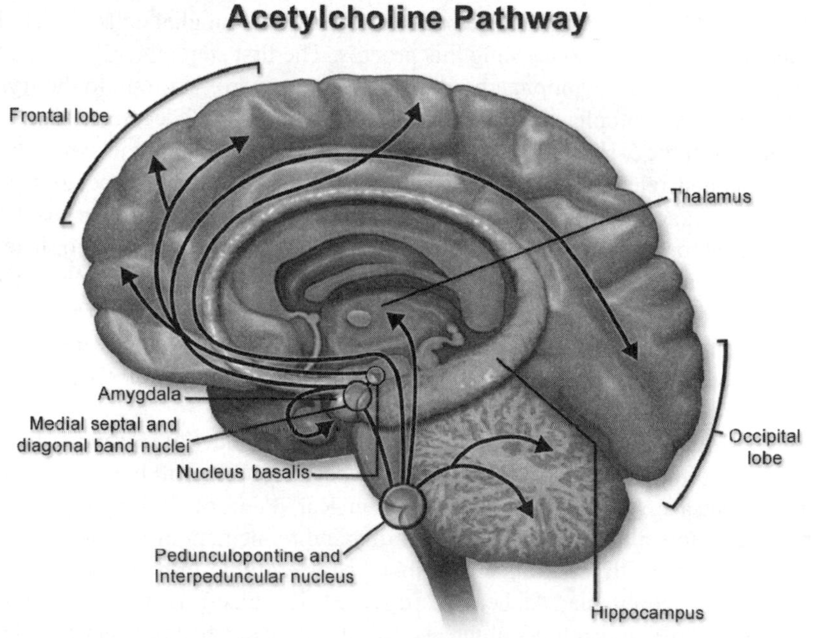

FIG. 2.10. Acetylcholine pathways and projections.
Copyright Blausen Medical Communications. Reproduced by permission.

various foods and is a by-product when fats are broken down. As the enzyme acetylcholine-transferase transfers an acetate ion to choline, this process results in Ach. Ach is then stored in synaptic vesicles in the terminal button. Similar to other neurotransmitters, the synthesis and release of Ach are partially regulated by autoreceptors. Two main types of postsynaptic receptors have been identified for Ach: nicotinic (ionotropic) and muscarinic (metabotropic) receptors. They were so named after the drugs that were found to stimulate or inhibit the receptors—namely nicotine, found in cigarettes, and muscarine, found in certain types of mushrooms.

The nicotonic receptor is complex, consisting of at least eight subunits. Binding Ach to one of the subunits alters the conformation of the receptor, a change that opens the $Na+$ channels and depolarizes the membrane. The roles of each of the subunits of the nicotinic receptor are not fully understood (Webster, 2001b). Nicotonic receptors (i.e., heteroreceptors) are found on GABA, dopamine, and glutamate-releasing neurons and, according to von Bohlen und Halbach and Dermietzel (2003), activation of these receptors by Ach can increase the synthesis and release of these neurotransmitters. The muscarinic receptor functions quite differently than the nicotonic receptor and is coupled to second messenger systems. Different classes and subtypes of the muscarinic receptor have been identified; they differ in their distribution in the brain as well as their second messenger pathways. After release from the terminal button, Ach is not terminated by reuptake but instead is degraded by acetylcholineesterase, and next choline is cleared from the cleft by a choline transporter (von Bohlen und Halbach & Dermietzel, 2003).

Acetylcholine has been implicated in complex cognitive functions such as attention, memory, and learning as well as a variety of psychiatric disorders. For example, Mihailescu and Drucker-Colin (2000) suggested that Ach, and specifically the nicotonic receptor, may be involved in the pathogenesis of schizophrenia, depression, Tourette's disorder, Alzheimer's disease, and Parkinson's disease. McEvoy and Allen (2002) noted that many patients with schizophrenia and half of their first-degree relatives have abnormalities in smooth pursuit eye movements that can be corrected by nicotine. They also noted that nicotine can temporarily reduce the frequency of tics associated with Tourette's disorder. McEvoy and Allen hypothesized that smooth eye pursuit movements and perhaps involuntary tics are due to genetic variations in Ach nicotonic receptor number and function. The role of Ach in dementia has been studied extensively and is covered in chapter 4. Blennow and Vanmechelen (2003) recently reviewed the therapeutic benefits of acetylcholineesterase inhibitors in the treatment of Alzheimer's disease and suggested that several proteins detected in cerebral spinal fluid may serve as reliable markers for early dementia and other psychiatric disorders. Kaufer, Friedman, Seidman, and Soreq (1998) suggested that drugs that inhibit acetylcholineesterase can induce a pathological state similar to posttraumatic stress disorder. They hypothesized that acute stress stimulates excessive Ach activity that in turn triggers long-lasting genetic changes that affect acetylcholine metabolism in the brain. The role of acetylcholine in psychiatric disorders is explored further in subsequent chapters.

PSYCHOPHARMACOLOGY

Drugs have been used to treat psychiatric conditions since the early 1900s, but the first major breakthrough in psychopharmacology occurred during the 1950s with the release of the antipsychotic drug Thorazine (chlorpromazine). Thorazine was used to reduce psychotic symptoms and to calm patients with schizophrenia and mania. Tofranil (imipramine), the first tricyclic antidepressant, was released during the mid-1950's. Librium, a benzodiazepine, was made available during the late 1950s and the mood stabilizer lithium during the early 1960s

(Stanford, 2001c). Drugs prescribed to treat the symptoms of mental illness are known as *psychotropic* medications. Psychotropic drugs are commonly prescribed to treat a wide range of disorders such as anxiety disorders, mood disorders, and behavioral disorders. It is critical to note that psychotropic medications are palliative in nature, not curative, that is, although they can improve symptoms these drugs do not cure the underlying cause of disorders.

Studies indicate that the use of psychotropic medications has increased among children of all ages as well as adults (e.g., DeBar, Lynch, Powell, & Gale, 2003; Herman et al., 2002). For example, Zito and colleagues (2003) reported a two- to threefold increase in psychotropic medication use in children and adolescents from 1987 to 1996, with stimulants and antidepressants prescribed most frequently followed by mood stabilizers. DeBar, Lynch, Powell, and Gale (2003) investigated psychotropic use in 743 preschool children identified as having behavioral or emotional problems. They found that 16% received such medication and 48% were prescribed a stimulant medication only. Safer, Zito, and dosReis (2003) found that over 20% of outpatient youths treated in community mental health centers and over 40% of youth treated in inpatient facilities were given more than one psychotropic medication. Ryan et al. (2002) reported that 51% to 94% of individuals living in nursing homes have psychiatric symptoms and thus psychotropic medications are widely prescribed within this population.

Despite the increase use of psychotropic medications among children, adolescents, and adults, the precise mode action of most drugs used to treat psychiatric disorders is unknown. Cooper, Bloom, and Roth (2003) stated that "at the molecular level an explanation of the action of a drug is often possible; at the cellular level, an explanation is sometimes possible; but at the behavioral level, our ignorance is abysmal" (p. 2). Part of the difficulty in understanding the precise effects of drugs is that it is likely that many unknown factors influence neuronal signaling. In addition, research suggests significant variation among individuals in drug sensitivity that may correlate with behavioral variation (Iwata et al., 1999). The field of neuropharmacology is actively seeking to understand (a) the role of genes in drug response; (b) how genes are activated or suppressed by exposure to drugs; (c) the structure and function of postsynaptic receptors, autoreceptors, and heteroreceptors and the effects of drugs on these receptors; (d) trophic factors involved in neuronal regulation and the effects of drugs on these trophic factors; and (e) the role of glial cells in neuronal signaling and the effects of drugs on glial cell functioning.

Although a plethora of questions remain concerning the mode of action of psychotropic drugs and factors that may influence these mechanisms, information is available about the pharmacology of medications used to treat mental illness. The following section reviews the basic principles of pharmacology and describes generally the purported mode of action of commonly prescribed psychotropic medications. Additional details on the use, effectiveness, and side effects of these medications are discussed in subsequent chapters.

Pharmacokinetics

The process of drugs being absorbed, distributed, metabolized, and excreted is known as pharmacokinetics. The most common means of administering psychotropic medications is orally. Most drugs are absorbed in the gastrointestinal system, and a number of factors can determine the degree of absorption (e.g., food in digestive system, drug concentration, effects of other drugs). After a drug is absorbed into the bloodstream, it is distributed to various sites throughout the body such as the kidneys, liver, heart, brain, fat tissue, and muscle. Distribution of a psychotropic drug is influenced by blood flow, diffusion of the drug from the blood to the target area, and the degree to which the drug can pass through membranes (i.e., lipid soluble;

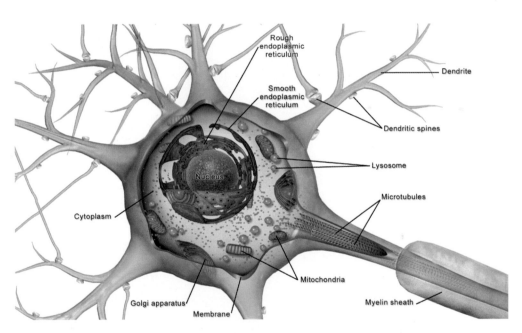

Color Plate 1. Internal components of a cell.
Copyright Blausen Medical Communications. Reproduced by permission.

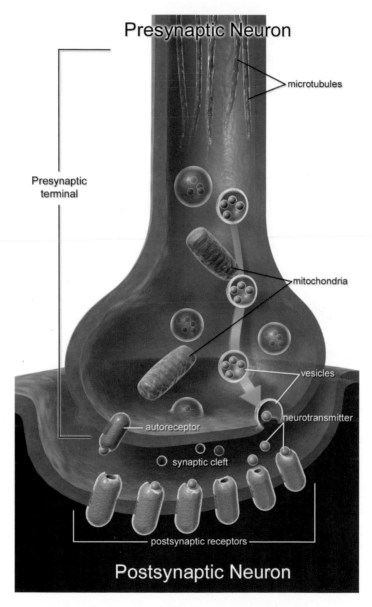

Presynaptic Neuron

microtubules

Presynaptic
terminal

mitochondria

vesicles

neurotransmitter

autoreceptor

synaptic cleft

postsynaptic receptors

Postsynaptic Neuron

Color Plate 2. Terminal button of presynaptic neuron
and cell membrane depicting receptors of postsynaptic neuron.
Copyright Blausen Medical Communications. Reproduced by permission.

Example of a second messenger system

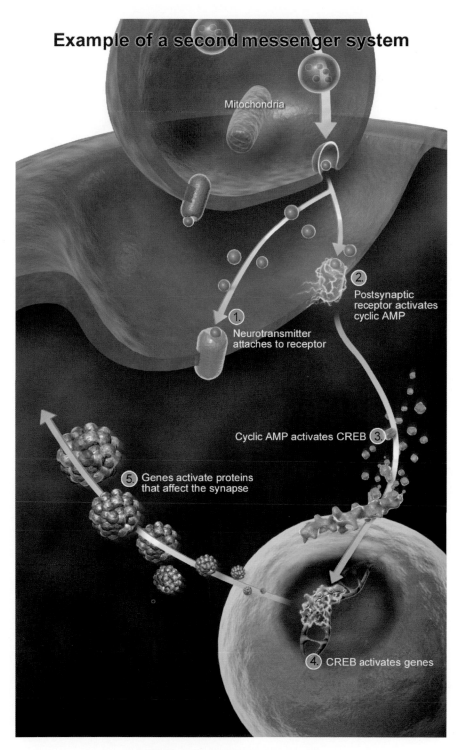

Mitochondria

1. Neurotransmitter attaches to receptor

2. Postsynaptic receptor activates cyclic AMP

Cyclic AMP activates CREB 3.

5 Genes activate proteins that affect the synapse

4. CREB activates genes

Color Plate 3.   Second messenger system.
Copyright Blausen Medical Communications. Reproduced by permission.

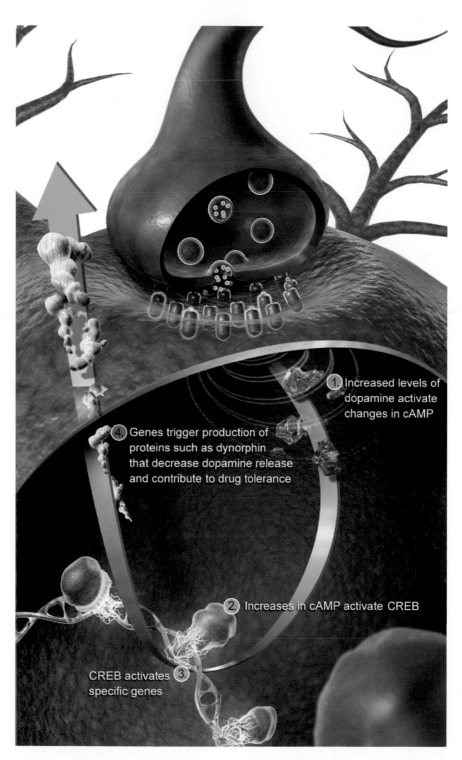

Color Plate 4. Physiological changes associated with drug tolerance.
Copyright Blausen Medical Communications. Reproduced by permission.

Carvey, 1998). Some psychotropic drugs such as antipsychotic and tricyclic antidepressant medications collect in muscle and fat tissue and are slowly released into the bloodstream. This storage and slow release process helps to explain why individuals with schizophrenia or depression who stop taking their medications sometimes remain symptom-free for several weeks (Perrine, 1996).

Metabolism (or biotransformation) of psychotropic medications occurs primarily in the liver, but also in the brain and blood, through a complex system of enzymatic processes. The by-products of drug metabolism are known as *metabolites*, the actions of which can have therapeutic effects. For example, the main metabolites of some antipsychotic drugs (e.g., risperidone, zotepine) have been found to contribute to the therapeutic effects of the drug (Caccia, 2000a). During metabolism, metabolites can interact and produce a range of effects from toxicity to canceling out desired drug effects. Trenton, Currier, and Zwemer (2003) recently reported that toxic doses of psychotropic drugs such as antipsychotics are highly variable and may be increased by coingestion of other drugs. For example, some prescription drugs can inhibit the enzymes that metabolize antipsychotic drugs and consequently may increase the probability of toxic effects of these antipsychotic medications. Unfortunately, as noted by Caccia (2000a), information is scarce concerning the effects of drug metabolites as well as the interactive effects of these metabolites with other drugs.

The process by which drugs are eliminated from the body is called *excretion*. Excretion occurs primarily in the kidneys, and the by-products are passed in urine. According to Carvey (1998), the bowel, sweat glands, skin, lungs, and saliva can also participate in drug excretion. Some studies have found that the substantial differences among individuals in their ability to metabolize psychotropic medications may be related in part to their genetic makeup. Dahl (2002) suggested that genotyping and phenotyping may one day be used to determine optimal dosages for individuals, especially for poor or ultrarapid metabolizers of psychotropic medications.

Medication Effects

The amount of psychotropic drug needed to attain a therapeutic effect can vary widely among individuals, as can the undesirable effects of psychotropic drugs (Iwata et al., 1999; Trenton, Currier, & Zwemer, 2003). Undesirable effects of psychotropic drugs (i.e., *side effects*) vary among individuals and types of drugs. Most side effects of psychotropic medications have been well documented, both common and uncommon. For example, common side effects associated with antidepressant medications (SSRIs) include constipation, dry mouth, headache, sweating, and reduced libido; rare effects could include seizures and severe allergic reactions (Physician's Desk Reference [PDR], 2003). Edwards and Anderson (1999) completed a meta-analysis of five SSRIs and reported that although there was no difference in efficacy among the antidepressant medications, the degree of side effects varied widely. Recent findings also suggest that polymorphisms of the norepinephrine neurotransporter gene (NET) are associated with patients' response to the antidepressant milnacipran (Yoshida et al., 2004). Specifically, Yoshida and colleagues treated 96 Japanese patients who suffered from major depression with milnacipran, a dual serotonin and norepinephrine reuptake inhibitor, and correlated their response to the medication with the presence of polymorphisms of the serotonin and norepinephrine transporter genes. Results revealed that the presence of a specific polymorphism of the norepinephrine gene was associated with a greater therapeutic response. Additional studies are needed to substantiate this finding and explore the role of genetic variations in the therapeutic response to other types of medications.

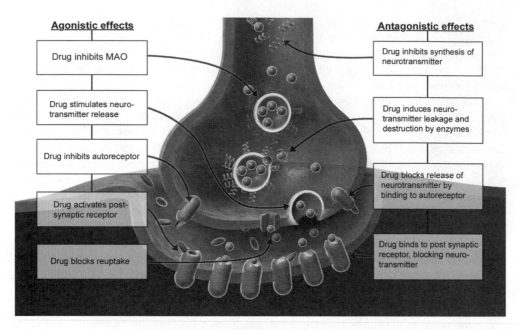

FIG. 2.11. Agonistic and antagonistic drug effects.
Copyright Blausen Medical Communications. Reproduced by permission.

Agonists and Antagonists

Drugs can be classified into two main categories: Those that facilitate the effects of neurotransmitters are known as *agonists* whereas drugs that interfere with the effects of neurotransmitters are known as *antagonists*. Agonists may facilitate neurotransmission by (a) serving as a precursor, (b) stimulating the release of neurotransmitter, (c) occupying and activating the postsynaptic receptors, (d) blocking the autoreceptors, (e) blocking reuptake by inhibiting the transporter proteins, (f) inhibiting deactivating enzymes, or (g) facilitating postsynaptic affinity. Conversely, antagonists may interfere with transmission by (a) preventing storage of neurotransmitter in the vesicles, (b) preventing the release of neurotransmitter, (c) occupying and blocking postsynaptic receptors, (d) activating autoreceptors, (e) preventing synthesis of the neurotransmitter, or (f) deactivating enzymes that naturally inhibit the synthesis of neurotransmitters (Fig. 2.11).

Neurotoxins are a good example of substances that can produce either antagonistic or agonistic effects. For instance, curare, which is derived from a plant berry, occupies acetylcholine receptors and blocks acetylcholine from attaching to the receptor. By blocking the receptor, curare prevents release of acetylcholine from the cell. Curare is therefore an acetylcholine antagonist and large doses can prevent movement and respiration. In contrast, black widow spider venom increases the amount of acetylcholine released by the terminal button and is therefore an acetylcholine agonist. Other neurotoxins inhibit the breakdown, prevent their release, and/or stimulate the production of neurotransmitters (Webster, 2001b). Many analgesics are considered antagonists because they block receptor sites involved in pain regulation. Antipsychotic medications often target and block dopamine receptors and hence are considered dopamine antagonists. More recently, drugs have been developed that have both antagonistic and agonistic effects.

Hundreds of drugs have been developed to treat cognitive and behavioral disorders and various systems exist to classify these medications. The five main classes of psychotropic drugs are antianxiety, antidepressants, antipsychotic, mood stabilizers, and stimulants. The next section provides an overview of the mode of action of each these classes. Drugs also will be discussed in subsequent chapters as they pertain to the disorders covered therein.

AN OVERVIEW OF PSYCHOTROPIC DRUGS AND MODE OF ACTION

As mentioned previously, drugs either facilitate or interfere with the process of neurotransmission. By pharmacologically altering the process of neurotransmission, behavior and cognition are affected. For example, drugs have been developed that decrease anxiety, improve or stabilize mood, enhance attention and concentration levels, and decrease symptoms that interfere with daily living such as compulsions, hallucinations, and delusions.

Antianxiety Medications

Anxiety disorders, a heterogeneous group of conditions that have been categorized by the DSM IV-TR as 12 separate disorders, include generalized anxiety disorder, obsessive compulsive disorder (OCD), panic disorder phobias, and posttraumatic stress disorder (APA, 2000). According to Lepine (2002), even though anxiety disorders are the most prevalent psychiatric disorders, nearly two thirds of individuals who suffer from them do not seek treatment. Anxiety disorders affect children as well as adults, and it has been estimated that 30 million people in the United States will experience an anxiety disorder at some point in their lives (Lepine, 2002). Anxiety disorders frequently co-occur with depression, adding to the level of disability experienced by individuals with these disorders (Lecrubier, 2001). The most commonly prescribed medication to treat anxiety disorders are benzodiazepines although other medications such as antidepressants are also used (Wittchen, 2002). Examples of benzodiazepines include Xanax, Valium, and Klonipin (see Table 2.1).

Benzodiazepines

Benzodiazepines attach to part of the GABAa receptor (Fig. 2.12). When a benzodiazepine occupies this site, GABA attaches to a different part of the receptor more frequently. When GABA attaches to the receptor, chloride (Cl−) channels open and the cell membrane hyperpolarizes (Stanford, 2001a). As the principal inhibitory neurotransmitter, GABA is widely distributed throughout the brain. The end result is that neural inhibition is increased throughout the brain and behavioral relaxation is increased. In other words, drugs such as Valium enhance GABA's ability to decrease neuronal excitation by increasing neuronal inhibition. The GABA receptor is complex and consists of multiple subunits. Other drugs such as barbituates and alcohol attach to a different part of the GABAa receptor. When a barbituate occupies the site, it mimics the effects of GABA. Specifically, the Cl− channels remain open significantly longer, even in the absence of GABA. The end result of these drugs (e.g., Seconal) is similar to the benzodiazepines in that neural inhibition is increased throughout the brain. Additional information concerning the physiological effects of antianxiety medications in included in chapter 7.

Antidepressant Medications

Antidepressants are used most often to treat individuals suffering from mood disorders, specifically depressive disorders. The DSM IV-TR categorizes mood disorders as depressive disorders

TABLE 2.1

Psychotropic Medications: Brand and Drug Names

Antidepressants: (SSRIs)
- Celexa (citalopram)
- Lexapro (escitalopram)
- Luvox (fluoxamine)
- Paxil (paroxetine)
- Prozac (fluoxetine)
- Zoloft (sertraline)

Miscellaneous Antidepressants
- Effexor (venlafaxine)
- Remeron (mirtazapine)
- Serzone (nefazodone)
- Wellbutrin (Bupropion)

MAO Inhibitors
- Deprenyl (selegilene)
- Manerix (moclobemide)
- Marplan (isocarboxazid)
- Nardil (phenylzine)
- Parnate (tranylcypromine)

Tricyclic Antidepressants
- Anafranil (clomipramine)
- Asendin (amoxapine)
- Aventyl (nortriptyline)
- Desyrel (trazodone)
- Elavil (amitriptyline)
- Ludiomil (maprotiline)
- Norpramin (desipramine)
- Sinequan (doxepin)
- Surmontil (trimipramine)
- Trofranil (imipramine)
- Vivactil (protriptyline)

Antianxiety
Benzodiazepines
- Atarax (vistaril)
- Ativan (lorazepam)
- Centrax (prazepam)
- Klonipin (clonazepam)
- Serax (oxazepam)
- Tranxene (clorazepate)
- Valium (diazepam)
- Xanax (alprazolam)

Anxiolytic
- BuSpar (buspirone)
- Catapress (clonidine)
- Librium (chlordiazepoxide)

Antipsychotic
- Abilify (aripiprazole)
- Chlorpromazine (thorazine)
- Clozapine (clozaril)
- Geodon (ziprasidone)
- Haldol (haloperidol)
- Loxapa (loxapine)
- Mellaril (thioridazine)
- Moban (molindone)
- Navane (thioxthixene)
- Orap (pimozide)
- Permitil (fluphenazine)
- Quide (piperacetazine)
- Risperdal (risperidone)
- Serentil (mesoridazine)
- Stelazine (trifluoperazine)
- Seroquel (quetiapine)
- Taractan (chlorprothixene)
- Tindal (acetophenazine)
- Trilafon (perphenazine)
- Zyprexa (olanzapine)

Mood Stabilizers
- Depakote (divalproex)
- Eskalith (lithobid)
- Lamactil (lamotrigine)
- Neurontin (gabapentin)
- Tegretol (carbamazepine)
- Topamaz (topiramate)
- Lithium

Anticonvulsants
- Depakene (valproate)
- Tegretol (carbamazepine)
- Lamotrigine (lamictal)
- Gabapentin (neurontin)
- Topiramate (topamax)
- Oxcarbazepine (trileptal)
- Zonisamide (zonegran)

Stimulants
- Adderall (adderall)
- Dexedrine (dextroamphetamine)
- Methylphenidate (Ritalin, Concerta, Metadate, Methylin)
- Cylert (pemoline)

Nonstimulant
- Strattera (atomoxetine)

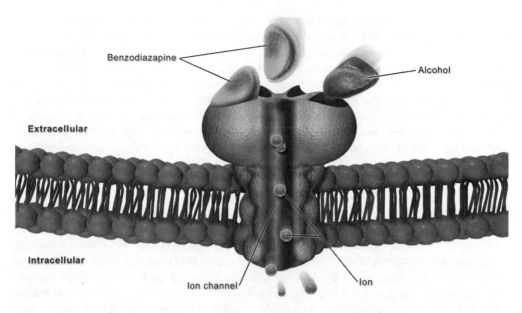

**FIG. 2.12.   GABA receptor depicting attachment of benzodiazepine
and alcohol. Copyright Blausen Medical Communications. Reproduced by permission.**

and bipolar disorders. Depressive disorders include major depressive disorder, dysthymic disorder, and depressive disorder not otherwise specified. Major depressive disorder is the most common of the depressive disorders: The lifetime risk is estimated to be 10% to 25% for women and 5% to 15% for men (APA, 2000). Those suffering from major depression have been found to experience impairment in physical and role functioning, lost work days, and high use of health services (Lecrubier, 2001). According to the American Psychiatric Association, up to 80% of individuals with a mood disorder respond to treatment that typically involves antidepressants and some form of psychotherapy. Stahl (2000) reported that the majority of patients respond to an antidepressant and 90% or more show improvement with combinations of antidepressants. In addition, antidepressants significantly reduce relapse rates of depression, especially if they are continued for at least a 12-month period. Antidepressants have a number of side effects; recently some researchers have suggested a possible link between antidepressant use and cancer. When Sternbach (2003) conducted a review of the literature concerning the connection between antidepressant use and cancer for articles published from 1966 to 2002, however, he concluded that the link was questionable and additional studies were warranted. With regard to increased risk of suicidal thoughts or committing suicide, Khan and colleagues (2003) reported that of 48,277 depressed individuals treated with antidepressants, 77 committed suicide. Similar rates were found among those who received an SSRI—another type of antidepressant—or a placebo. They concluded that the findings did not support an increased risk between antidepressants and suicide. But in 2003, the United Kingdom banned the use of the antidepressant paroxetine with children, stating that the drug was ineffective in treating children and carried too many risks (Abbott, 2003). In 2004, the U.S. Food and Drug Administration (FDA) reviewed 24 trials involving over 4,400 children and adolescents treated with 9 antidepressant drugs (or placebo) for OCD, major depression, or other psychiatric disorders. Results revealed an average suicide risk of 4% compared to 2% for placebo (no suicides actually occurred during the trials). As a result of these findings, the FDA directed manufacturers of all antidepressant drugs to include a boxed warning statement about the increased risk of suicidal thinking or behavior among children and adolescents treated with these medications.

Studies have documented that some of the improvement in behavioral symptoms can be attributed to a placebo effect. A *placebo* is a treatment that is devoid of specific actions on the individual's symptoms yet somehow causes a beneficial effect. Mayberg and colleagues (2002) were the first to use neuroimaging techniques to investigate areas of brain activation in depressed patients who took a placebo or an antidepressant. Results revealed that a similar pattern of brain activation occurred in both those taking the drug and those taking a placebo. Additional areas were activated in those taking the antidepressant, however, and the authors speculated that these regions may be particularly important in the therapeutic effects of antidepressant medications. Three broad classes of antidepressants are used to treat depression: monoamine oxidase inhibitors, tricyclic, and atypical antidepressants. The mode of action differs with each type.

Monoamine Oxidase Inhibitors (MAOIs)

Monoamine oxidases are enzymes (MAO-A and MAO-B) that metabolize serotonin, dopamine, and norepinephrine. Research has found that MAO activity varies greatly in the normal population (Brunner et al., 1993). Monoamine oxidase inhibitors are drugs that prevent monoamine oxidase from breaking down neurotransmitters within the terminal button. The first MAOIs produced inhibited both MAO-A and MAO-B, but newer MAOIs target one or the other of these enzymes. Some MAOIs have a weak affinity for blocking serotonin and norepinephrine presynaptic transporter proteins and inhibit reuptake to some degree (e.g., Nardil, Iproniazid; Stanford, 2001a, b, c). The end result of both cases is that more neurotransmitter is available for release and for activating postsynaptic receptors. Use of MAOIs is associated with improvement of depression symptoms although the precise cellular mechanisms that result in behavioral improvement are not well understood. Brunner and colleagues (1993) identified a genetic mutation that resulted in complete MAO deficiency of one type of MAO (MAOA). This deficiency was associated with aggressive, impulsive behavior in male subjects. Monoamine oxidase inhibitors are prescribed less frequently than other depressants due to their negative interaction with the amino acide tyramine, commonly found in foods such as cheese, coffee, chocolate, and other items. Specifically, when MAO is inhibited, tyramine is not broken down and consequently accumulates in the intracellular and extracellular fluid. This accumulation elevates blood pressure and can cause hypertension and stroke (PDR, 2003).

Tricyclic and Atypical Antidepressants

Tricyclic antidepressants (e.g., imipramine, desipramine) block the reuptake of norepinephrine and, to a lesser degree, serotonin, by binding to the presynaptic transporter proteins. The major limitation of tricyclic antidepressants is their adverse side effects. Singhal et al. (2002) recently reported that, in rare instances, antidepressants can produce sudden-onset headaches, seizures, and stroke, a condition known as Call-Fleming syndrome. In addition to blocking reuptake of norepinephrine and serotonin, tricyclic antidepressants attach to acetylcholine and histamine receptors. The consequence of attaching to these receptors is sedation, dry mouth, blurred vision, and dizziness, among other symptoms (PDR, 2003).

The atypical antidepressants, selective serotonin reuptake inhibitors (SSRIs; e.g., fluoxetine, Paxil), are the most commonly prescribed antidepressant medications and account for half or more antidepressant prescriptions (Stahl, 1998). Relative to tricyclic antidepressants, SSRIs produce fewer side effects, have a greater compliance rate, and can be used to treat a large number of disorders. According to Stahl, the mode of action of SSRIs is not completely understood but appears to involve a four-step process: (a) SSRIs immediately attach to the serotonin transporter (SERT) and prevent the reuptake of serotonin; (b) this blockage causes a rapid increase of serotonin in the soma; (c) autoreceptors become desensitized to the increased levels of serotonin and more serotonin is released from the terminal button; and (d) after several weeks, the postsynaptic receptors also desensitize and symptoms are alleviated. In summary, SSRIs are hypothesized to disinhibit the serotonergic process at the level of the presynaptic and postsynaptic neurons.

The mode of action of SSRIs implicates the serotonergic system in the physiological basis of depression although dysfunction of the serotonergic system has been associated with several conditions including suicidal behavior and impulsive–aggressive behavior (Coccaro et al., 1989). Interestingly, as Petty, Davis, Kabel, and Kramer (1996) noted, no psychiatric disorder appears to worsen with SSRIs. Indeed, SSRIs are used to treat a variety of psychiatric conditions including anxiety, eating, and mood disorders. In addition, Donnelly (2003) recommended that SSRIs be the first approach to treating PTSD in children, and recommended use of medications such as mood stabilizers and adrenergic medications if problems of dyscontrol or impulsivity coexist in children suffering from PTSD. Silver (2003) suggested that SSRIs, particularly fluoxetine and fluvoxamine, are useful in ameliorating the negative symptoms associated with schizophrenia and noted that they can be used safely with antipsychotic medications. Johnson (2003) recently suggested that SSRIs are useful in treating late-onset alcoholism, especially in alcoholics with comorbid major depression. Wittchen (2002) has suggested that antidepressants may play a role in *preventing* the development of major depression in individuals who suffer from generalized anxiety disorder. Although SSRIs may indeed improve the symptoms of a variety of psychiatric disorders, the way in which SSRIs produce these improvements is largely speculative.

With regard to efficacy among SSRIs, Edwards and Anderson (1999) conducted a meta-analysis of 20 SSRI studies and found that they appeared to be equally efficacious. Fluoxetine (Prozac) was associated with more side effects such as weight loss, agitation, and skin reactions compared to the other four SSRIs included in the meta-analysis. Learned-Coughlin and colleagues (2003) recently discovered that the antidepressant Bupropion (Wellbutrin) blocked the dopamine transporter rather than the serotonin transporter, suggesting that changes in the dopaminergic system may be responsible in part for the therapeutic effects of the drug. Additional information concerning the physiological effects of antidepressants is provided in chapter 6.

Antipsychotic Medications

Antipsychotic medications are primarily used to treat psychotic disorders although they are sometimes used to treat nonpsychotic disorders such as Tourette's disorder (Gaffney et al., 2002). The DSM IV-TR identifies nine psychotic disorders including schizophrenia, and the specific constellation of symptoms varies among these disorders. Several definitions exist for "psychotic" ranging from the presence of hallucinations and delusions to the presence of disorganized speech and behavior or catatonic behavior (APA, 2000). Schizophrenia occurs in .5 to 1.5% of adults and is described in detail in chapter 8 of this text. Schizophrenia is characterized by positive (e.g., hallucinations) and negative (e.g., flat affect, absence of behavior) symptoms. Antipsychotic medications such as chlorpromazine, clozapine, and haloperidol primarily lessen the psychotic symptoms but have a minimal effect on negative symptoms. Silver (2003) suggested that SSRIs, particularly fluoxetine and fluvoxamine, be used to treat the negative symptoms associated with schizophrenia. One of the most disturbing side effects of antipsychotic medications is tardive dyskinesia, characterized by involuntary muscle movements, primarily in the facial region. The risk of tardive dyskinesia differs among the antipsychotic medications; overall, 20 to 40% of patients will develop the condition (Jest et al., 1999). According to Webster (2001c), tardive dyskinesia can take months or years to develop and the symptoms may continue or even worsen after the medication is ceased.

With regard to mode of action, antipsychotic medications primarily block the dopamine (D2) receptors. Depending on the drug, however, one or several types of dopamine receptors may be blocked. For example, cholorpromazine blocks D2 receptors while clozapine is believed to block D4 and serotonin receptors (Strange, 2001). Recently, Grunder et al. (2003) reported that in addition to blocking dopamine postsynaptic receptors, antipsychotic medications reduce the level of dopamine that is synthesized by neurons.

Mood Stabilizers

Mood stabilizers are primarily used to treat a mood disorder—bipolar disorder. Recently, mood stabilizers have been used to augment antidepressants or antipsychotics in patients who do not respond to standard medication treatment for major depressive disorder or schizophrenia (Bertschy et al., 2003; Conley & Kelly, 2001). For example, Birkenhager and colleagues (2004) reported that a combination of imipramine and lithium was superior to treatment with an antidepressant (fluvoxamine) in individuals with severe depression. Mood stabilizers are also used with children and adults with explosive, aggressive behavior (Fava, 1997) as well as with aggressive adults with OCD (Hollander, 1999). According to the DSM IV-TR, there are actually four types of bipolar disorder: bipolar I, bipolar II, cyclothymia, and bipolar disorder not otherwise specified. These disorders differ with respect to the presence and frequency of manic symptoms and depressive symptoms. The prevalence and associated features differ with each disorder, but the overall lifetime prevalence is significantly lower for bipolar disorders than depressive disorders.

Two main types of mood stabilizers are used in the treatment of bipolar disorders—lithium and anticonvulsants (e.g., Carbamazepine, Divalproex). The precise mode of action of lithium is poorly understood, but current research suggests that it inhibits second messenger systems in glial cells (astrocytes) and neurons (Pardo, Andreolotti, Ramos, Picatoste, & Claro, 2003). Bown, Wang, and Young (2003) recently suggested that lithium may inhibit cellular processes that result in neurotoxicity and death of neurons and glial cells in the hippocampus and frontal cortex with individuals with bipolar disorder. Lenox and Hahn (2000) reviewed the progress in understanding the mode of action of lithium during the past 50 years and concluded that "we are currently still at the stage of identifying the pieces of the lithium puzzle; within the next 50 years, we will be putting the puzzle together" (p. 12). The mode of action of anticonvulsants is also unclear, but studies suggest they inhibit norepinephrine reuptake, block sodium channels, and enhance the action of GABA (Perrine, 1996). Additional information concerning the physiological effects of mood stabilizers is provided in chapter 5.

Stimulants

Stimulants are used primarily for the treatment of behavior disorders, particularly ADHD. ADHD affects 3 to 7% of the school-age population and the majority of individuals experience significant symptoms throughout adolescence and adulthood (Weyandt, 2001). Although several types of stimulants are available (e.g., Dexedrine, Adderall), methylphenidate (Ritalin) is the most commonly prescribed stimulant for ADHD. It is used in over 80% of childhood cases (Safer & Zito, 2000). Like most medications, the precise mode of action of stimulants is unclear. According to Grace (2001), methylphenidate disrupts the reuptake process by blocking the transporter protein for dopamine (DAT) and, to a lesser extent, norepinephrine.

This blockade results in more dopamine available in the synaptic cleft and helps to regulate dopaminergic systems, particularly in the regions of the prefrontal cortex and basal ganglia. Volkow et al. (2001) used neuroimaging and found significant increases in the extracellular fluid after methylphenidate was administered orally to adults. They suggested that individuals with ADHD have increased dopamine transporters and by blocking the transporters, dopamine levels increase. Additional information concerning the effects of methylphenidate is provided in chapter 9.

SUMMARY

This chapter reviewed the processes involved in neurotransmission including exocytosis, endocytosis, and pinocytosis. Neurotransmitter classifications and neurotransmitter systems were also reviewed including acetylcholine, aspartate, dopamine, GABA, glutamate, and serotonin. An overview of psychopharmacology was provided as well as a general description of the purpose and mode of action for various classes of psychotropic drugs. Although medications can often improve behavioral symptoms of various disorders, it is important to note that they do not remedy the underlying physiological condition that contributes to the expression of the disorder.

3

Techniques of Brain Imaging

During the past decade, understanding of human brain functioning has increased exponentially. This chapter reviews techniques that are commonly used to study brain functioning. Physiological techniques measure or reflect brain activity or structure and include computed tomography (CT), electroencephalogram (EEG), magnetic resonance imaging (MRI), functional magnetic resonance imaging (fMRI), and positron emission tomography (PET). These techniques vary with respect to their ability to measure (a) cellular activity, (b) brain structure, and (c) brain function. Additional techniques are available such as event-related optical signal (EROS), magnetoencephalography (MEG), magnetic resonance spectroscopic imaging (MRSI), near-infrared imagining (nIR), and single photon emission tomography (SPECT). However, because these latter methods are used more infrequently in the study of psychiatric disorders, they will not be discussed here. Background information regarding basic principles of brain activation is reviewed followed by specific neurophysiological and neuroimaging techniques. The final section of the chapter examines brain stimulation techniques, some of which are now being used in the treatment of psychiatric disorders.

BASIC PRINCIPLES OF BRAIN ACTIVATION AND MEASUREMENT

Brain activation includes many events but all can be grouped into two basic physiological processes: neuronal signaling and brain metabolism. Neuronal signaling refers to the movement of ions across the cell membrane, and brain metabolism refers to changes in oxygen and glucose consumption. These processes of metabolism and neuronal signaling occur continually, but their rate of activity varies across brain regions and during different states (e.g., sleeping, awake, cognitive demands). Some of these cellular changes, such as movement of oxygen molecules, produce patterns of electromagnetic signals that radiate to the outside of the brain and can be detected by measurement devices. Other cellular changes, such as increased glucose consumption, can be tracked and measured with radioactive substances that are attached to glucose molecules and taken up by active neurons. Thus, neuroimaging techniques measure either metabolism (glucose, oxygen consumption, or changes in blood volume) or neural signaling (flow of ions, release of neurotransmitters, or density of receptors). Other techniques, such as CT and MRI measure brain structure, not function, and provide information about the morphology of the brain. Physiological techniques such as EEG measure the summed postsynaptic activity of many individual neurons at the level of the cortex.

In general, there are two main purposes of brain imaging techniques. The first is to compare *structural* images of a normal brain to those of a diseased brain in order to determine whether certain structural changes are characteristic of various diseases. These types of images are useful for diagnostic purposes such as brain tumors, ventricle enlargement, or tissue loss. A second purpose is to determine whether *functional* changes are associated with brain disease or with cognitive processes. For example, epilepsy is characterized by excessive neuronal firing and Parkinson's disease is characterized by chronic activation in the area of the globus pallidus (Dostrovsky et al., 2000). Studies have also reported, albeit inconsistently, that schizophrenia and major depression are characterized by hypoactivity of the frontal lobes (Ingvar & Franzen, 1974; Ito et al., 1996). More recently, researchers have begun to explore whether certain regions of the brain become more or less activated during various task demands. Cabeza and Nyberg (1997), for example, reviewed PET studies of higher-order cognitive processes in normal subjects and identified different patterns of activation depending on the cognitive task.

Measurement Design

It is important to note that the structural and functional images of the brain produced by CT, MRI, fMRI, PET, and SPECT are actually reconstructed computerized images. Each method varies with respect to the mathematical formulas used for the reconstruction. Depending on the purpose of the imaging technique, different procedures are used to produce and interpret the brain image. For example, for structural questions, images of a brain suspected of disease can be compared to a normal brain. For questions of brain function, brain activity measurements of an individual who is suspected of having a brain disease such as schizophrenia, Parkinson's disease, or Alzheimer's disease can be compared to those taken while a healthy individual is at rest. Alternatively, measurement of brain activity can be taken while an individual is at rest and these measurements can be used as a baseline for comparison to brain activity measurements of the same individual while they are engaged in a task. These comparisons can therefore be used to target brain regions that are likely involved in various cognitive tasks. This same comparison method can be repeated across numerous subjects, and the data can be collapsed to identify general areas of increased activation among subjects during specific tasks.

In addition to whether the techniques provide structural or functional information about the brain, the techniques also differ with regard to (a) time required to complete the image(s), (b) use of radioactive substances, (c) degree of resolution, and (d) expense.

BRAIN IMAGING TECHNIQUES, STRUCTURAL IMAGING

Computed Tomography (CT)

The two most common techniques for gathering information about brain structure are computed tomography (CT) and magnetic resonance imaging (MRI). A CT scan is achieved by an X-ray tube and detector that is placed around a individual's head. The Tube moves in a circular process passes beams through the head at all angles. The X-ray tube and detector are located opposite each other and, after the X-ray beam passes through an individual's head, the detector records the amount of radioactivity that passes through. A computer translates the information from the detector into pictures of the brain and skull. Based on a mathematical formula incorporating density and corresponding voxels, various shades of black, gray, or white can then be assigned to the image. Cerebral spinal fluid appears nearly black on the image, and bone appears white. Compared to MRI, the resolution of the CT images is low and consequently it is difficult to differentiate between gray (tissues rich in cell bodies) and white matter (myelinated axons).

Computed tomography has been used to research a number of psychiatric disorders, but primarily schizophrenia. Johnstone and colleagues (1976), who were among the first to use CT with patients with schizophrenia and healthy controls, found that patients with schizophrenia had enlarged ventricles and smaller cortical gyri than individuals without the disorder. Since that time, hundreds of CT studies have been conducted with numerous disorders ranging from dementia to anxiety disorders. O'Brien et al. (2000) investigated CT images in two groups of patients with two types of dementia and a group with major depression. Results indicated that CT scans did not differentiate between types of dementia but did distinguish between individuals with major depression and dementia. According to Colohan, O'Callaghan, Larkin, and Waddington (1989), brain morphology as examined by CT can vary depending on the age of the subject, and occasionally CT scans appear falsely abnormal. Furthermore, they reported a poor correlation between CT scan findings, laboratory testing, EEG, physical exam, and psychiatric status. Similarly, Ghaziuddin and colleagues (1993) reported that the widespread use of CT in child and adolescent psychiatry was unfounded because not only do very few of these patients have abnormal CT scans, but also changes in diagnoses or treatment are rarely the result of such scans. Collectively, these studies suggest that the use of CT in psychiatric studies and practice is of limited use. Techniques with greater resolution such as MRI and those that provide information about brain functioning are more suitable for understanding and diagnosing clinical disorders.

Magnetic Resonance Imaging (MRI)

Magnetic resonance imaging provides more detailed images than CT scans with clear contrasts between gray and white matter and cerebral spinal fluid. MRI does not use X-rays; instead, a strong magnetic field is passed through an individual's head and the MRI scanner detects the movement of hydrogen molecules in response to the magnetic field. The details of this process are complex, but, essentially, the nuclei of hydrogen molecules are protons and act as tiny magnets. When the MRI scanner sends a magnetic field through the head, the protons align in one direction. When a pulse of radio waves is delivered by the scanner, the protons move to a different orientation and this movement is detected by the scanner. These protons are present in different concentrations in the brain (e.g., cerebral spinal fluid versus myelinated axons), and the scanner uses this information to produce the MRI image (see Papanicolaou, 1998 for additional information).

A plethora of studies has been published concerning the use of MRI in dementia, Parkinson's disease, and psychiatric disorders. It is important to emphasize that MRI produces structural images and not information concerning cellular functioning. Nevertheless, comparisons of brain MRI have found morphological deviations in individuals with schizophrenia (e.g., enlarged lateral and third ventricles, reduction of total brain volume, reduction of size of prefrontal and temporal lobes) (Lawrie & Abukmeil, 1998). Recently, Milev and colleagues (2003) found that MRI scans taken at the onset of schizophrenia were predictive of continued hallucinations 5 years later. Differences between MRI scans in patients with major depression, bipolar disorder, and healthy control subjects have also been found (e.g., Shioiri, 1996). Castellanos et al. (1996) found that the caudate nucleus was significantly smaller in boys with ADHD than boys without the disorder. These results are not consistently found, however, as some studies have reported no MRI differences between individuals with and without psychiatric disorders. MRI has been exceedingly useful in providing information about the normally developing brain in childhood and adolescence. Overall, these developmental studies indicate both changes in regional brain volume with increasing age and specific sex differences. For example, in both boys and girls white and gray matter volume increased during childhood, and on average boys have larger brains than girls. After correcting for brain volume, the caudate nucleus is larger in girls than boys and the amygdala is larger in boys than girls (Durston et al., 2001).

BRAIN IMAGING TECHNIQUES, FUNCTIONAL IMAGING

Functional Magnetic Resonance Imaging (fMRI)

Functional magnetic resonance imaging (fMRI) indirectly assesses changes in brain metabolism by measuring the level of oxygenated to deoxygenated blood in the bloodstream near the area of increased neuronal activity. According to Papanicolaou (1998), the amount of oxygenated blood that is delivered to brain tissue depends on the rate of metabolism in that area. For example, following increased metabolic activity the amount of oxygenated blood delivered to the area increases, although this relationship is not necessarily linear. Instead, the amount of oxygenated blood that is delivered to an active area exceeds that of the amount that was actually used and this can take up to several seconds. fMRI detects this increase in oxygenated blood. fMRI can detect metabolic activity at a good resolution but does not measure actual quantitative changes in blood flow or metabolism. In other words, fMRI has good spatial resolution but poor temporal resolution. An advantage of fMRI is that it does not require the use of radiation and is considered safe for both adults and children. Although previously MRI and fMRI were exceedingly difficult to use with infants, particularly neonates, Erberich, Fiedlich, Seri, Nelson, and Bluml (2003) recently developed MRI equipment that can be used for MRI and fMRI with newborns.

Use of fMRI with normal and psychiatric populations has increased dramatically during the past decade. With regard to normal brain functioning, fMRI studies have found anatomical correlates of various aspects of attention and memory as well as possible circuitry between temporal regions and prefrontal regions on episodic memory tasks (Mandzia & Black, 2001). According to Grady (1998), older adults tend to use different areas of the brain—and perhaps functional networks—than younger individuals when performing the same cognitive task. Maestu et al. (2003) recently reviewed the current status of neuroimaging studies of cognition and noted that most studies attempt to locate brain regions associated with particular cognitive functions when, in fact, most cognitive processes are widely distributed. They recommended that future studies focus on the role of neural networks and attempt to identify the spatial and temporal patterns of brain activity that support cognition.

With regard to clinical disorders, fMRI studies are plentiful and usually involve a comparison between individuals with and without a specific disorder. Schizophrenia has received the most attention, and a summary of findings appears in chapter 5. In general, fMRI studies suggest that patients with schizophrenia exhibit reduced activation in several brain regions relative to individuals without the disorder (e.g., Menon, Anagnoson, Glover, & Pfefferbaum, 2001). Other disorders that have been investigated with fMRI include anxiety disorders, eating disorders, OCD, posttraumatic stress disorder, and others. For example, Shapira and colleagues (2003) compared fMRI scans of eight individuals with OCD and control participants taken during a picture-viewing, disgust-inducing task. Results indicated that different brain regions were activated in OCD subjects compared to control subjects. Lanius, Hopper, and Menon (2003) compared fMRI scans of a husband and wife with acute PTSD during a script-driven traumatic imagery task and found significant differences in areas of activation despite exposure to the same traumatic event. Lanius and colleagues emphasized that patients with PTSD—and most likely other disorders—can have very different subject and biological responses to traumatic events and that different neuronal mechanisms may underlie these different responses.

A major concern in interpreting the fMRI literature is that most studies focus on changes in brain activity but relatively little information is available regarding baseline activity of the brain. Gusnard and Raichle (2001) have suggested there may be a baseline or normal resting state of brain function that involves consistent activity in some areas and less activity in others. For example, even at rest, the brain is involved in a continuous process of monitoring the environment (e.g., for potential predators), and this monitoring is correlated with neuronal activity in certain brain regions (posterior cingulate cortex). Gusnard and Raichle also suggest that processes such as daydreaming may represent another type of continuous brain activity; such "stimulus-independent" activity has been associated with areas of the prefrontal cortex (McGuire, Paulesu, Frackowiak, & Frith, 1996). The bottom line is, there is currently no validated model of baseline brain activity and it is plausible that it varies among individuals and is affected by factors such as age, health, gender, and genetics. Kosslyn (1999) has argued that simply observing which brain regions are activated during task performance is unlikely to lead to a better understanding of brain functioning. Instead, Kusslyn proposed that scientists should first develop a taxonomy of questions concerning the manner in which cognitive processes occur in the brain, design tasks that capitalize on the strengths of neuroimaging techniques, and then offer specific hypotheses based on the research questions. To increase interpretation accuracy of fMRI images, Cox and Savoy (2003) have suggested that multivariate statistical procedures be used rather than multiple univariate analyses. Relative to other neuroimaging techniques (i.e., PET), fMRI is less expensive, does not require radiation exposure, and can be used safely with children as well as adults.

Positron Emission Tomography (PET)

As mentioned in chapter 2, neurons use a variety of organic molecules to function that are delivered via blood (e.g., glucose, water) or manufactured within the cell. Their concentration varies depending on the activity of the neurons. The constituents of these substances (e.g., hydrogen, oxygen, nitrogen) do not emit electromagnetic signals and therefore cannot be tracked or measured with neuroimaging devices. Organic substances such as oxygen and glucose, however, can be bombarded with radioactive isotopes and combined with other substances to create compounds such as glucose or water. These compounds can then be inhaled injected into a person's bloodstream, they then pass the blood–brain barrier and enter the brain. These compounds are "radioactive" and shed positively charged particles *(positrons)* that can be traced in the brain. Two methods are used to measures neuronal activity: glucose metabolism and blood flow. Glucose is the primary source of energy for neurons and, as neuronal activity increases, increased amounts of radioactive glucose are taken up by neurons. Alternatively, as discussed with fMRI, blood flow is correlated with increased metabolic activity of neurons and organic molecules such as oxygen or carbon can be tagged and traced in the blood. The time required for the positrons to shed varies among isotopes; the amount of time it takes for half of the positrons to be shed is known as the *half-life*. As positrons are shed, they collide with electrons, which results in photons. These photons pass through the skull and are detected by the PET scanner. The exit location of the photos reflects the distribution of the radioactive compound in the brain and represents the level of brain activity in various regions. The PET scanner records the photon signals and a mathematical algorithm is applied to the data. A computerized image is then projected in shades of gray or color *representing* the neuronal activity changes in the brain. PET images can also be superimposed on a MRI scan. The MRI scan shows the brain anatomy in detail whereas the PET reveals the blood flow or glucose metabolism in various areas.

Recently, researchers have begun using radioactive drugs ("ligands") that attach to specific neurotransmitter receptors (e.g., dopamine, opiate, muscarinic receptors) to determine the concentration of various neurotransmitter sites (Frost, 1992). For example, dopamine antagonists tagged with a radioactive tracer (e.g., [11C]raclopride) can identify areas high in a specific class of dopamine receptor (D2). This information is important as it helps to identify sites of drug action as well as degree of binding to these receptors with various drugs (e.g., antipsychotics, cocaine, antidepressants). For example, Drevets et al. (1997) used PET and a radioactive ligand that binds to serotonin receptors ([11C]WAY-100635) to determine the extent of binding in individuals with bipolar disorder and major depression. Results indicated that binding was significantly reduced in individuals with both types of depression, but the magnitude of the reduction was greater in those with bipolar disorder. Sedvall, Farde, Persson, and Wiesel (1986) suggested that quantitative neuroreceptor measurements may one day be used as a biochemical diagnostic tool for neuropsychiatric disorders. Recently, Volkow, Fowler, and Wang (2003) stressed the importance of PET in substance abuse research and Van Heertum and Tikofsky (2003) suggested that PET is a cost-effective method of establishing an earlier diagnosis of Alzheimer's disease.

PET has been used in hundreds of studies of individuals with aberrant behavior and psychiatric disorders. Raine and colleagues (1994), for example, reported less activation in the prefrontal cortex in a group of men who committed murders relative to a control group, and Das, Barkataki, Kumari, and Sharma (2002) suggested that PET and other neuroimaging techniques may actually help to predict violent behavior. Recently, Tauscher and colleagues (2001) reported an inverse relationship between serotonin receptor binding (5-HT1A) and anxiety symptoms. Numerous PET glucose metabolism and blood flow studies have been conducted with schizophrenia, mood disorders, OCD, and other anxiety disorders. These findings—as well as the limitations of the studies—are discussed in subsequent chapters.

PET has also been used to investigate cognitive processes in individuals without psychiatric disorders. For example, Borg, Andree, Soderstrom, and Farde (2003) examined the relationship between serotonin receptor density and spiritual experiences. In 15 healthy males between the ages of 20 and 45, they found a significant negative correlation between spiritual acceptance and self-transcendence and density of serotonin receptors. The authors speculated that low serotonin activity may increase sensory perception and decrease cognitive inhibition and therefore increase the likelihood of transcendent, spiritual experiences. Corbetta and colleagues (1991) used PET to investigate normal cognitive processes, specifically, the neural systems involved in discriminating shape, color, and speed of a visual stimulus. Results indicated that distinct areas of the cortex appear to be involved in processing visual information and that different neural systems become activated depending on whether a task requires selective or divided attention. Similarly, Haxby et al. (1994) investigated areas of brain activation in healthy adult males who performed a face identity and matching task. Results indicated that depending on the task, different brain regions were activated. Cantor-Graae and colleagues (1993) also used PET to measure regional blood flow in normal subjects while they performed two executive function tasks (Wisconsin Card Sorting Test and verbal fluency). Results revealed differential activation patterns with these neuropsychological tasks.

Cabeza and Nyberg (1997) reviewed PET studies of higher-order cognitive processes such as attention, memory, and language with normal subjects. Based on their review of over 100 such studies, they concluded that different brain regions are consistently activated with different types of cognitive tasks. For example, attention studies found that selective attention activates the anterior cingulate whereas generalized attention engages regions of the frontal and parietal cortex. Auditory language comprehension tasks generally activate the left superior temporal gyrus, comprehension of written material (reading) the occipital lobes. According to Cabeza and Nyberg, different types of memory tasks (e.g., working memory versus semantic memory) activate different brain regions and most studies do not report activation of subcortical structures in higher-order cognitive tasks. Paus and colleagues (1998) also reviewed a large number of PET studies and cautioned that task difficulty, nature of the response, and memory demands can modulate regional cerebral blood flow and should therefore be accounted for in future studies.

Methodological Limitations

Additional methodological issues need to be considered when interpreting the results of fMRI and PET neuroimaging studies. A major concern involves the validity and reliability of the images. For example, a critical assumption is that the particular brain activity observed actually represents the cognitive or behavioral function that the study was intended to measure—which may not be the case. As noted by Papanicolaou (1998), a study's intent may be to measure glucose metabolism, but the resultant brain activity representing oxygen use and increased blood flow does not necessarily covary with the pattern of metabolism. Furthermore, subjects may approach tasks differently and various memories may be triggered while a subject is performing a task. Consequently, the results may not reflect a specific cognitive process (e.g., semantic memory) but instead additional brain functions. This is one reason why PET and fMRI are of questionable use with complex constructs such as measuring "personality" or "emotion." When attempting to measure constructs with PET or fMRI, simplification of concepts and use of operational definitions are crucial. Replication of studies and findings would help support the validity of results but are rare in the literature.

In addition, the use of tasks during neuroimaging techniques such as PET and fMIR to identify brain regions involved in cognitive processes can be problematic, as noted by Humphreys and Price (2001). For example, if an area of the brain that is known to be damaged shows reduced activation and areas distant from the damaged area show reduced activation, one may leap to the conclusion that these distant regions are functionally linked to the damaged region. As Humphreys and Price pointed out, however, there are many other plausible interpretations of this finding. For example, it is possible that a task cannot be performed correctly due to the brain damage itself, and hence distant areas that are normally activated are not needed.

A related methodological issue is whether the same image results would be found over time (i.e., reliability). Standardized measures for administering neuroimaging techniques and tasks could improve validity and reliability, as currently there is great variability across studies in terms of tasks, design, ages of subjects, clinical disorders, and techniques employed. Furthermore, as Cantor-Graae, Warkentin, Franzen, and Risberg (1993) noted, relatively few normative studies have been conducted. Those that have typically include a small sample size and report significant variability among subjects with respect to areas and degree of brain activation. Additionally, many studies do not include information on intelligence or ethnicity, study only one gender, and/or include subjects within a restricted age range. Thus, it remains unknown whether the results of studies with limited sample characteristics would apply to both sexes as well as individuals of different ages and ethnicity. In addition, the frequent inclusion in psychiatric samples of individuals with two or more disorders *(comorbidity)* makes it difficult to determine whether the findings of the study are related to one disorder or a combination of disorders. It is also important to emphasize that PET—like fMRI—is an indirect measure of cellular function and does not directly measure synaptic functioning. Finally, it is critical that neuroimaging findings be considered in a broader context to help determine the clinical relevance of the findings. For example, hypoperfusion of the frontal lobes, and in particular the prefrontal cortex, has been found in individuals with schizoprenia, ADHD, Alzheimer's disease, Parkinson's disease, and borderline personality disorder, as well as violent criminals (Soloff et al., 2003). It would be a mistake to conclude that decreased activity in the frontal lobes causes any of these disorders or that hypoperfusion is unique to a specific disorder.

Electroencephalogram (EEG)

An EEG is a recording of the postsynaptic cortical activity of groups of neurons while an individual is at rest, sleeping, or during a specific sensory stimulation task (e.g., a flash of light). EEGs are recorded by electrodes that are placed on the scalp over different regions of the brain such as the occipital, parietal, temporal, and frontal lobes. Specific systems exist for the placement of electrodes (Nuwer et al., 1994), and the number of electrodes placed on the scalp can vary from approximately 15 to 125 (Gevins, 1998). In conditions in which a stimulus is presented, the recording is called a sensory-evoked potential or an event-related potential. For example, Molfese (1984) was among the first to use an auditory stimulus to demonstrate that the left hemisphere in adults, but not the right, responds to consonant sounds. Molfese, Molfese, Key, and Kelly (2003) later reported that the brain of infants reliably discriminates between familiar and unfamiliar words, based on auditory-evoked reponses.

According to Martin (1991), EEGs are based on frequency and amplitude domains; frequencies of the potentials vary from 1–30 Hz and amplitudes from 20–100 MV. Several dominant frequency and amplitude bands characterize EEG recordings: alpha (8–13 Hz), beta (13–30 Hz), delta (0.5–4 Hz), and theta (4–7 Hz). Alpha waves are associated with relaxed wakefulness, beta waves with alter wakefulness, and delta and theta waves are associated with sleeping states. Several studies, however, suggest that all of these EEG bands may be involved in various physiological brain states, and thus their usefulness for understanding brain activity is questionable (Klimesch, 1999). Given that visual inspections of EEG recordings have limited value except in pathological conditions such as epilepsy, quantitative methods have been developed (qEEG) that analyze frequency, amplitude, and spatial changes of potentials (see Martin, 1991 for additional information concerning EEG).

Among the recent quantitative methods developed is qEEG mapping. The technique involves the creation of a multidimensional matrix that provides a topgraphic representation of qEEG parameters, enabling dynamic changes to be observed as they take place during the EEG. Statistical methods are then used to analyze the data to help identify areas of normal and abnormal brain activity (e.g., Bosch-Bayard et al., 2001). As Raichle (2000) noted, qEEG is not an imaging tool like PET and fMRI, and the source of the cortical activity recorded by EEG is difficult to determine. In addition, artifacts and errors in measurement can influence the results and interpretation of qEEG (Lawson et al., 2003). Raichle (2000) advocated the combined use of EEG and neuroimaging techniques such as PET and fMRI to gain a truer picture of brain functioning. Patterns of cortical activation have been found, however, in individuals with various disorders relative to individuals without the disorders. For example, several studies using qEEG have found that individuals with schizophrenia show an increase in delta and theta waves (slow waves) as well as beta (fast) waves (e.g., Itil, 1977). This pattern has not been found in all studies, however, and these findings are not necessarily unique to schizophrenia. In addition, not all patients with schizophrenia have abnormal qEEG findings (Kirino & Inoue, 1999). More recently, Harris et al. (2001) investigated qEEG in a group of 40 individuals with different types of schizophrenia. According to the results of this study, distinct patterns of qEEG emerged that differentiated between three types of schizophrenia. These findings were similar to those reported by Sponheim et al. (2000), who compared EEG patterns in 112 patients with schizophrenia relative to smaller samples of individuals with bipolar disorder and major depression as well as control subjects. Specifically, they found a significant correlation between EEG results and morphological characteristics (e.g., enlarged ventricles) in the patients with schizophrenia, an association not found in the patients with bipolar disorder or depression. (For a review of EEG studies in mood and anxiety disorders, see Gruzelier, Galderisi, & Strik, 2002.)

Studies have also used EEG and qEEG to investigate a wide range of clinical and cognitive disorders such as anxiety disorders, mood disorders, ADHD, autism, dementia, and learning disorders. Tot and colleagues (2002), for example, found that adults with OCD had higher qEEG frequencies of slow-wave bands and lower frequencies of alpha waves (mainly in the left frontotemporal region) relative to control subjects. Other studies have found EEG pattern differences between individuals with OCD and controls in the anterior regions of the cortex (Molina et al., 1995). Blair Simpson, Tenke, Towey, Liebowitz, and Bruder (2000) reported significant qEEG changes in the anterior region of the cortex when patients with OCD were exposed to feared contaminants. Studies have also explored EEG and qEEG patterns in individuals with other types of anxiety disorders such as social phobia, panic disorder, and PTSD. Jokic-Begic and Begic (2003), for example, recently reported that combat veterans with PTSD had decreased qEEG alpha activity and increased beta activity relative to veterans without PTSD. In 2001, Begic, Hotujac, and Jokic-Begic compared veterans with PTSD and control subjects using qEEG and found increased beta and theta activity in several regions of the cortex.

Numerous EEG studies have been conducted with individuals with mood disorders. Increased alpha and beta activity has been found in individuals with depression relative to control subjects in several studies (e.g., Nystrom, Matousek, & Hallstrom, 1986). Fewer studies have investigated bipolar disorder, but preliminary findings suggest that bipolar disorder is characterized by different qEEG patterns relative to control subjects and at least one clinical disorder—schizophrenia (Oluboka, Stewart, Sharma, Mazmanian, & Persad, 2002; Shagass, Roemer, Straumanis, & Josiassen, 1984). Cook et al. (2002) studied qEEG changes in 51 adults with major depression during baseline, 48 hours, and 1 week, during which time participants were treated with either a placebo or antidepressant. Results indicated that medication responders relative to nonresponders and placebo showed significant qEEG differences over time, particularly in the prefrontal region. Interestingly, Leuchter and colleagues (2002) investigated depressed individuals who were classified as medication or placebo responders. Over a 9-week period, several qEEG recordings were performed and results revealed no pretreatment qEEG differences between subjects. During treatment, however, placebo responders showed an increase in prefrontal cordance, which was not observed in those who responded to medication. The authors concluded that placebo effects can induce changes in brain function that are different from those associated with antidepressant medication.

With regard to childhood-related disorders, Gasser, Rousson, and Schreiter Gasser (2003) recently reported that children with learning disabilities and mental retardation showed an increase in slow qEEG waves relative to children without these disorders. Harrison, Demaree, Shenal, and Everhart (1998) suggested that autism is characterized by different qEEG patterns in the left anterior and right frontal regions of the cortex. In study by Dawson and colleagues (1995) using EEG, children with autism exhibited reduced cortical activity in the frontal and temporal regions but not in the parietal region relative to normal children. Willis and Weiler (2005) recently reviewed the EEG literature concerning children with ADHD and concluded that, in general, EEG patterns of activity differ between children with and without ADHD. Furthermore, boys and girls with ADHD tend to have different EEG profiles and different patterns sometimes also emerge for different subtypes of ADHD. In a rare longitudinal study, Otero and colleagues (2003) explored whether psychosocial risk was associated with alteration of the CNS based on EEG findings. Forty–two preschool-age children living in a socially, economically, and culturally disadvantaged environment in a developing country were evaluated several times over a 6-period and compared to a group of low-risk children. The EEG patterns of the at-risk group showed higher delta and theta values in the frontal regions and less alpha activity in the posterior regions of the cortex. The authors interpreted these results as supporting the hypothesis that insufficient environmental stimulation is associated with developmental lag in children.

Despite the multitude of studies that have found EEG differences between groups of individuals with a specific type of disorder relative to control subjects, EEG and qEEG studies are limited in several ways. First, as Gruzelier, Galderisi, and Strik (2002) noted, measures such as EEG have good temporal resolution but suffer from poor spatial resolution compared to neuroimaging techniques such as PET and fMRI. Second, EEG measures only cortical activity and cannot reveal the subcortical changes that may have affected or produced the cortical activation patterns. Finally, EEG and qEEG have limited diagnostic utility with psychiatric disorders as distinct profiles are not unique to the many different types of disorders. Coutin-Churman et al. (2003) recently evaluated the incidence, sensitivity, and specificity of abnormal quantitative EEG measures in individuals with and without psychiatric conditions. Results revealed abnormal qEEG findings in 83% of patients and 12% of control participants. The most frequent abnormality was a decrease in delta and/or theta bands, a finding not evident in the control group. However, no qEEG pattern was uniquely characteristic of a disorder and, in many cases, patients with the same disorder had different qEEG profiles.

BRAIN STIMULATION TECHNIQUES

A number of brain stimulation techniques have been developed to stimulate neuronal functioning and influence behavior, including deep brain stimulation (DBS), electroconvulsive therapy (ECT), magnetic seizure therapy (MST), transcranial magnetic stimulation (TMS), and vagus nerve stimulation (VNS). Information concerning the use of ECT with psychiatric disorders is plentiful, but relatively few studies are available concerning the remaining techniques and their application in psychiatric treatment.

Electroconvulsive Therapy (ECT)

According to the most recent Task Force Report of the American Psychiatric Association, since its development in 1938 ECT has evolved into a complex procedure "about which much has been learned but many questions remain" (APA Task Force Report, 2001, p. 3). ECT involves the placement of electrodes on the scalp to deliver electricity to the brain, inducing a grand mal seizure. Tremendous variability exists among individuals with respect to the amount of stimulus intensity necessary to produce a seizure. For example, according to Abrams (2000), some individuals have such a high seizure threshold that delivery of maximal stimulus intensity may not be sufficient to achieve a therapeutic response. Children, typically have a much lower threshold (Fink & Coffey, 1998). ECT is used primarily with adults but more recently has been used with both children and adolescents (e.g., Fink & Coffey, 1998). Bolwig (2003) recently reported that seizure activity of at least 20 seconds is a prerequisite for therapeutic efficacy, and the number of ECT sessions required for improvement of symptoms ranges from 6 to 12. According to the APA Task Force Report (2001), the mortality rate of ECT is approximately the same as that of minor surgery. The most common side effect of ECT is headache, occurring in 45% of individuals. Nausea, muscle soreness, and temporary memory loss are also commonly reported following ECT. Less common side effects include mania, delirium, prolonged amnesia, and, rarely, cardiovascular complications and prolonged seizures (APA Task Force Report, 2001). Zink and colleagues (2002) recently suggested that the drug rivastigmine, an acetylcholinesterase inhibitor, could protect against unfavorable cognitive side effects associated with ECT. The efficacy of ECT depends on a number of patient factors (e.g., age, severity of illness) as well as technical factors such as stimulus dosage and electrode placement (Sackheim, 1997). Breakey and Dunn (2004) recently reported that Caucasians were more likely than African Americans to be treated with ECT based on a review of hospital records over the period 1993–2002.

First used as a treatment for schizophrenia, ECT shortly thereafter became the main form of treatment for patients with major depression and mania (APA Task Force Report, 2001). Since the 1940s, ECT has been found to improve symptoms associated with a host of disorders—major depression, bipolar disorder, and schizophrenia (Hoffman, Linkowski, Kerkhofs, Desmedt, & Mendlewicz, 1985; Uesugi, Toyoda, & Iio, 1995) as well as bulimia, Parkinson's disease, and various medical conditions. Bolwig (2003) described ECT as the most effective and most controversial treatment for severe depression. Gorman (2003) noted that although the majority of patients suffering from depression respond favorably to ECT, the effects are short-lived and relapse rates are high. Antidepressant medication begun immediately after a course of ECT has been found to help maintain remission of symptoms (Gorman, 2003). According to the APA Task Force Report, a substantial body of literature supports the use and effectiveness of ECT in the treatment of major depression, mania, and schizophrenia. Less information is available on the use of ECT in treating other psychiatric disorders although several studies have been published concerning the use of ECT in the treatment of OCD, Tourette's disorder, and anorexia nervosa. For example, Maletzky, McFarland, and Burt (1994) and Thomas and Kellner (2003) reported that ECT was effective at improving symptom of OCD, while Rapoport, Feder, and Sandor (1998) and Trivedi, Mendelowitz, and Fink (2003) found that ECT improved symptoms characteristic of Tourette's disorder. In a study by Ferguson (1993), two females with anorexia nervosa responded favorably to ECT while a third patient did not.

Relatively recently, ECT has been used to treat physical symptoms (e.g., motor tremor) in addition to psychiatric symptoms. For example, Fall, Ekman, Granerus, Thorell, and Walinder (1995) reported that ECT improved motor symptoms associated with advanced Parkinson's disease. The period of symptom improvement varied greatly among patients, however, from a few days to over a year. In 2003, Kennedy, Mittal, and O'Jile reviewed the literature from 1990–2000 regarding ECT and movement disorders. Most of the studies investigated the use of ECT with patients with Parkinson's disease, although a few studies included patients with progressive supranuclear palsy (PSP), multiple system atrophy (MSA), Wilson's disease, Huntington's disease, tic disorder, and Meige's syndrome. Many of the patients in the studies also suffered from major depression. The authors concluded that ECT is an effective treatment for depression that co-occurs with movement disorders and may also improve the motor manifestations of movement disorders.

The mechanism by which ECT alleviates depression and in some cases improves motor symptoms is uncertain. Several hypotheses have been presented in the literature. For example, ECT has been found to effect dopaminergic, noradrenergic, and serotonergic transmission

(Fall, Granerus, & Granerus, 2000; Kapur & Mann, 1993) and, according to Kennedy, Mittal, and O'Jile (2003), enhancement of noradrenergic and serontonergic transmission is likely associated with improvement of depression. Improvement in motor functioning following ECT, however, may be due to enhanced dopaminergic transmisssion. Support for this hypothesis was provided by Fall et al. (1995), who found an increase in cerebral spinal fluid dopamine metabolites after ECT that correlated with improvement of motor symptoms. In addition, Hoffmann, Linkowski, Kerkhofs, Desmedt, and Mendlewicz (1985) studied a group of male adults suffering from major depressive disorders and reported that following ECT, cerebral spinal fluid serotonin metabolites increased but no significant changes were found in dopamine metabolites. The increase in serotonin metabolites was associated with improved behavioral symptoms, total sleep time, and sleep efficiency. These findings support the hypothesis that ECT helps to alleviate depression symptoms by enhancing serotonergic transmission and changes in the dopaminergic system are related to improvement in motor symptoms.

Not all studies investigating the effects of ECT on movement disorders (e.g., Parkinson's disease) have found changes in dopamine metabolites, however, and the specific effects of ECT on the dopaminergic system are not well understood. Andersen et al. (1987), for example, found that although ECT improved the severity of Parkinsonian symptoms in 11 patients with severe Parkinson's disease, this improvement was generally short-lived and the concentrations of dopamine metabolites in the cerebral spinal fluid were not affected by the ECT. Kennedy, Mittal, and O'Jile (2003) suggested that ECT may facilitate dopamine binding to postsynaptic receptors. Indeed, Fall, Ekberg, Granerus, and Granerus (2000) used neuroimaging (SPECT) to investigate dopamine reuptake in patients with Parkinson's disease before and after ECT, and results indicated no significant change in reuptake following ECT. Patients with less advanced Parkinson's disease and therefore greater degree of reuptake responded significantly better to ECT than those with more advanced Parkinson's disease. Balldin and colleagues (1982) found ECT enhanced the effects of a dopamine postsynaptic receptor agonist, further suggesting a critical role for dopamine receptors in ECT treatment.

Andrade et al. (2002) reported that the density of dopamine postsynaptic receptors increased following ECT, with the degree of increase dependent on the intensity of the electrical stim-ulus. Bolwig (2003) reported that ECT likely enhances transmission among GABA-releasing neurons, and alterations of this system are correlated with an increase in seizure threshold. When Kronofol, Hamdan-Allen, Goel, and Hill (1991) studied the effects of ECT on hormone release at 2-, 5-, 15-, and 30-minute intervals following ECT, they found an increase in the con-centration of several hormones compared to pre-ECT levels. The magnitude of this hormonal "surge" decreased over time and with repeated treatments. The researchers concluded that the hormonal changes induced by ECT are likely related to changes at the neurotransmitter level (i.e., dopamine). Recently, Henry, Schmidt, Matochik, Stoddard, and Potter (2001) used PET to measure the effect of glucose metabolism in a number of brain regions following ECT in four female and two male patients with major depression. Results indicated a widespread decrease in glucose metabolism (17 regions) but a concurrent increase in glucose metabolism in the basal ganglia, upper brain stem, and occipital lobe. Although some researchers (e.g., Nobler et al., 2001) have suggested that changes in glucose metabolism underlie the therapeutic ef-fects of ECT, Yatham, Clark, and Zis (2000) found that glucose metabolism changes were not persistent 1 week following ECT and not correlated with self-report ratings on the Hamilton Depression Rating Scale. Interestingly, chronic electroconvulsive shock in mice has been as-sociated with increased levels of neurotropic factors and neurogenesis in the hippocampus (Madsen et al., 2000). Bolwig (2003) speculated that ECT in humans might initiate a series of molecular changes that trigger genetic expression of nerve growth factor production as well as neurogenesis in subcortical regions such as the hippocampus. Presumably, changes in this subcortical region impact neural circuitry in the immediate vicinity and thus, given the widespread projections that stem from this region, many areas of the brain are likely affected by these cellular changes.

In summary, ECT historically has been used to treat mood disorders and schizophrenia. More recently, ECT has been used to treat a variety of psychiatric disorders as well as motor symptoms characteristic of Parkinson's disease. Although critics claim that ECT causes brain damage, Gorman (2003) recently noted that "an affluent person in the United States is much more likely to receive ECT for depression than a poor person, quite unusual for something that is truly harmful" (p. 475). Breakey and Dunn (2004) found that Caucasians suffering from major depression are significantly more likely than African Americans to be treated with ECT. Recent evidence also suggests that the memory impairments that are often induced by ECT are temporary and ECT may actually contribute to neuronal plasticity. The mechanisms responsible for the effectiveness of ECT are not well understood but are thought to primarily involve several neurotransmitter systems and possibly morphological changes in subcortical structures.

Transcranial Magnetic Stimulation (TMS)

TMS is a noninvasive brain stimulation technique that can be used to stimulate specific areas of the brain while an individual is awake. TMS uses head-mounted wire coils that deliver strong magnetic impulses to specific areas of the cortex. These magnetic pulses are generated by electricity but, unlike ECT, the magnetic field can be highly focused on specific areas. The pulses last for less than a millisecond and induce changes in the ion distribution across the cell's membrane. Specifically, the magnetic field produces electrical currents in the brain by depolarizing neurons at the level of the cortex and possibly subcortical structures (George et al., 2003). Repetitive TMS (rTMS) involves the delivery of magnetic impulses in rhythmic succession, at an adjustable rate. Stimulation frequencies higher than 25–30 Hz increase the risk of seizures, however, and so are rarely used (George et al., 2003). Padberg and colleagues (1999) explored whether there was an antidepressant difference with fast versus slow repetitive TMS. TMS was found to be safe at both frequencies and neither was superior in terms of improvement of symptoms of depression. TMS is painless and can be applied safely for single or multiple sessions over a period of several weeks (Loo et al., 2001).

According to one of the pioneers in TMS research, Mark George (2003), TMS does not have a single mechanism of action but instead induces different effects depending on several factors: the activity an individual is engaged in while receiving TMS, the region stimulated by TMS, and parameters of the TMS device (e.g., intensity, frequency, coil angles) as well as individual subject differences. Unlike other brain stimulation techniques, TMS can produce immediate effects such as limb movement or cessation of speech. For example, Epstein et al. (1996) demonstrated that TMS applied directly over Broca's area (left frontal lobe) resulted in the immediate cessation of fluid speech, for which the physiological reason is unknown.

TMS is believed to affect neurotransmitter systems but the details of this process are poorly understood. It is plausible that TMS and rTMS have multiple effects: at the level of the synapse and on neural networks, neurotransmitters, gene expression, and glia cell functioning. To help unravel the physiological effects of TMS, researchers have begun to study TMS in combination with fMRI and PET to measure blood flow changes and extracellular neurtransmitter changes in the brain after TMS is applied. For example, Strafella, Paus, Fraraccio, and Dagher (2003) and Strafella, Paus, Barrett, and Dagher (2001) used PET to measure changes in extracellular dopamine concentration after repetitive TMS of the dorsolateral left prefrontal cortex in healthy human participants. Results revealed that TMS induced the release of dopamine in the caudate nucleus in the ipsilateral hemisphere only. The reason for this finding was unclear, but the authors speculated that descending pathways (corticostriatal) extend from the prefrontal cortex and project predominantly to the ipsilateral striatum. By stimulating neurons at the level of the cortex with TMS, other neurons within this pathway are likely activated, including glutamate-releasing neurons, which in turn activate dopamine-releasing neurons in the caudate. Dopamine released into the extracellular fluid in the caudate region is not rapidly taken up by nerve terminals, and therefore measurable changes in dopamine concentration can be detected. Strafella and colleagues reported similar TMS and dopamine-related findings in 2003.

According to George et al. (2003), TMS is a promising technique for treating depression and has been approved in Canada and Israel as a treatment method for this disorder. Several studies have found that TMS applied to the prefrontal cortex improves symptoms of depression short-term and may possibly improve depression long-term (e.g., Janicak et al., 2002; Martis et al., 2003). Trivedi (2003) suggested that TMS, along with other brain stimulation devices, may be especially effective with patients suffering from treatment-resistant depression. Hasey (2001) recently compared the effectiveness of TMS and ECT at improving depression in adults and concluded that they were equally efficacious. Findings from meta-analyses concerning the effectiveness of TMS have been mixed, suggesting that TMS has short-term antidepressant effects but questionable long-term effects (Burt, Lisanby, & Sackeim, 2002; Martin et al., 2003). Martin et al. (2003) harshly criticized the quality of the TMS studies and suggested that there was insufficient evidence to support the use of TMS in the treatment of depression. McNamara and colleagues (2001) also questioned the use of TMS for psychiatric disorders and emphasized the need for studies with more rigorous methods and adequate experimental control.

Exploratory uses of TMS include treatment of movement disorders, seizures, depression, bipolar disorder, Tourette's disorder, schizophrenia, and enhancement of memory and learning (George & Belmaker, 2000). For example, Greenberg et al. (1997) were among the first to investigate the use of TMS in the treatment of OCD. Twelve adults with OCD were given repetitive TMS for 2 seconds a minute for 20 minutes and then rated on compulsive urges for 8 hours following treatment. The results indicated that compulsive urges decreased significantly during the 8 hours of observation, and the authors interpreted these findings as supporting an underlying prefrontal mechanism for OCD. Subsequently, Sachdev and colleagues (2001) reported that TMS was effective at improving OCD symptoms even in patients with treatment-resistant OCD. George, Sallee, Nahas, Oliver, and Wasserman (2001) suggested that TMS may improve motor tics associated with Tourette's disorder but also emphasized that basic research is needed to empirically explore its usefulness. Finally, following a review of the literature on the use of TMS in treating schizophrenia, Nahas, Molloy, Risch, and George (2000) advocated its use in exploring the circuitry implicated in schizophrenia but acknowledged that, given the chronicity of schizophrenia, the therapeutic applications of TMS are limited with this population.

Pascual-Leone and colleagues (1999) recommended that TMS be used to study and perhaps enhance neuroplasticity. For example, following a head injury or amputation TMS can be applied to different positions over the motor cortex while recording evoked potentials. This method allows researchers to generate a cortical map that can be correlated with functional movements, and therefore reorganization of motor outputs can be measured over time. TMS can also be used to stimulate different brain regions to facilitate cellular changes associated with neuroplasticity. Ziemann, Corwell, and Cohen (1998), for example, used a tourniquet around the elbow to stop blood supply to the forearm and nerve signals to the brain (simulating an amputation). This loss of input to the brain caused the cells to reorganize at the cortical level. When TMS was applied to the area undergoing reorganization, plasticity was enhanced. However, when TMS was applied to the same region in the opposite hemisphere, the brain's responsiveness to the TMS decreased. The authors speculated that use of TMS to nonimpaired regions of the brain may actually inhibit plasticity in other brain regions. An important implication of this study is that TMS could potentially be used to increase brain reorganization following brain injury (e.g., stroke) and hence speed up recovery and rehabilitation. The authors also speculated that TMS could be used to promote learning in children and adults, but empirical studies are needed to explore this hypothesis.

Vagus Nerve Stimulation and Deep Brain Stimulation

Newer brain stimulation methods that allow for more precise delivery of electricity include vagus nerve stimulation (VNS) and deep brain stimulation (DBS). According to Henry (2003), VNS is the most widely used nonpharmacological treatment for severe cases of epilepsy. In VNS, an electrode is wrapped around the left vagus nerve located in the neck. The vagus nerve is one of the 12 pairs of cranial nerves and extends from the brain stem through the neck. The vagus nerve lies between the jugular vein and the carotid artery in the neck. It contains both ascending sensory (afferent) and descending motor (efferent) pathways, but according to Bolwig (2003) nearly 80% of the nerves are sensory in nature. The antiseizure effects of VNS are mediated through the afferent fibers of the vagus nerve that project extensively to many parts of the brain (Henry, 2003). The lead and electrode are connected to a battery-operated pulse generator (i.e., pacemaker) implanted in the left side of the chest. The generator is programmed to deliver electrical pulses to the brain via the vagus nerve in order to suppress seizures in both children and adults. According to Henry (2003), patients can be given a magnet that can be swiped across the generator to increase the amount of electrical current released. By doing so, a patient can abort a seizure that is about to occur or turn off the generator for a period of time. The known side effects of VNS are minimal. Due to the location of the nerve, vocalization is usually altered by VNS but, according to Kemeny (2003), this is reversible by altering the electrical output. Other possible, but less likely complications include infection, nerve lesions, blood clots, and lead breakage.

With regard to efficacy, VNS has been found to reduce seizure reduction in patients with epilepsy, reduce the severity of seizures, improve mood, and abort impending seizures when a supplemental magnet is used correctly (Henry, 2003). Rush (2003) reported that VNS can be an effective treatment for patients with moderately to severely resistant depression, although it has not yet been approved by the FDA for such use in the United States. Roslin and Kurian (2003) suggested that it may be useful in the treatment of morbid obesity. Park (2003) reported that VNS reduced seizure frequency in patients with epilepsy and autism and also improved cognitive functioning such as alertness. As Kosel and Schlaepfer (2003) recently noted, one of its major disadvantage is its invasiveness. Nevertheless, application of VNS in the treatment of numerous psychiatric conditions is underway.

As mentioned previously, the precise mechanisms responsible for these effects are unknown. Henry and colleagues (1998) used PET to explore changes in regional cerebral blood flow prior to and during VNS treatment in patients with epilepsy. Results indicated that VNS induced significant increases in blood flow in the medulla and thalamus as well as many other regions. Significant decreases in blood flow in the amygdala and hippocampus were also associated with VNS. Although the relevance of these areas of increased and decreased blood flow was uncertain, the authors speculated that blood flow increases in the thalamus may be particularly important in decreasing seizure activity. Indeed, Henry et al. (1999) reported that bilateral blood flow increases to the thalamus was most predictive of an individual's responsiveness to VNS.

A few studies have compared the blood flow effects of VNS administered acutely versus chronically. In general, the results have been mixed, with some studies reporting similar areas and degree of CBF changes while other studies have reported differences between acute and chronic VNS activation (Henry, 2003). It remains unclear if the brain adapts to chronic stimulation of the left vagus nerve and, if so, what the ramifications of this adaptation might entail. Hammond et al. (1992) and Ben-Menachem et al. (1995) reported that chronic VNS was associated with changes in neurotransmitters as measured by cerebral spinal fluid content. For example, GABA levels reportedly increased as did serotonin metabolite levels. Significant decreases were found in CSF concentration levels of glutamate and aspartate (Ben-Menachem et al., 1995). As Henry (2003) noted, however, the relationship between VNS and neurotransmitters and antiseizure effects is unclear. Henry has suggested that the antiseizure actions of VNS may be due to several factors: (a) an increase in neural transmission in the thalamus and associated projection areas, (b) a decrease in neural transmission in the limbic system, and (c) an increase in the release of norepinephrine and serotonin in widespread regions of the brain. Additional research is needed, however, to determine the cellular mechanisms responsible for the therapeutic effects of VNS.

Deep Brain Stimulation

DBS involves the insertion of a small lead with an electrode in specific target areas of the brain (i.e., globus pallidus, thalamus). The lead and electrode remain in the brain and are connected to a programmed, battery-operated pulse generator (i.e., pacemaker) implanted in the chest. Similar to VNS, the generator sends electrical impulses, but in this case the impulses are sent directly to the target region of the brain. A large number of studies have substantiated that DBS improve tremors characteristic of movement disorders such as Parkinson's disease (Vingerhoets et al., 2002). Similar physiological pathways have been implicated in Parkison's disease and OCD (i.e., cortico–striato–pallido–thalamo–cortical neuronal circuits), and preliminary findings suggest that DBS may be effective as well at decreasing obsessive compulsive behavior in humans (Mallet et al., 2002; Nuttin et al., 1999). Tass et al. (2003) recently suggested that the nucleus accumbens is a promising target for DBS in patients with severe OCD and argued that DBS can desynchronize the chronic overactivity of neurons in the region of the nucleus accumbens. According to Greenberg and Rezai (2003), the effectiveness of DBS is also being investigated for epilepsy, brain injury, chronic pain, and other conditions. Moscarillo and Annunziata (2000) described a case of a patient with an implanted DBS electrode who also received ECT for depression. The DBS generator was turned off during the eight ECT treatments and the patient's mood improved following ECT. Similar to VNS, the side effects and potential complication of DBS resemble those associated with surgery (e.g., infection, hemorrhage) and actual stimulation. Many of the stimulation-related side effects are temporary and/or can be reduced by varying the electrical output of the generator.

The mode of action of DBS is unknown. Greenberg (2002) suggested that DBS may interfere with ("jam") neural circuits or block synaptic transmission. According to Greenberg and Rezai (2003), DBS may impose a meaningless pattern of neuronal activity in the target region that produces a "functional" but not morphological lesion. Alternatively, DBS might enhance rather than inhibit communication among neurons that ultimately results in improved motor function. Greenberg and Rezai identified a number of variables that could affect the outcome of DBS including orientation of the electrode, the morphology of the brain structure receiving stimulation, and DBS technical factors such as duration and frequency of stimulation.

SUMMARY

A number of physiological techniques have been developed to assess brain structure and brain function. This chapter reviewed CT, EED, MCI, fMRI, and PET. Recently the usefulness of brain stimulation techniques such as ECT and DBS have been studied in clinical populations. TMS is a noninvasive brain stimulation technique that may be effective at improving symptoms of several psychiatric conditions. Additional, well-controlled studies are needed to further substantiate the short-term and long-term usefulness of this technique in the treatment of various disorders. The efficacy of DBS for intractable movement disorders is well established. Given the significant number of individuals who do not respond to medication interventions, there is a rapidly growing interest in the use of DBS for treatment of severe psychiatric disorders (Greenberg & Rezai, 2003). The mechanisms of action of DBS are poorly understood. A major advantage of DBS is that it can stimulate areas of the brain implicated in neuropathology with greater precision than ECT, TMS, or VNS. Additional research is needed to better understand the underlying mechanisms of DBS as well as the usefulness of this technique in the treatment of clinical disorders.

4

Dementia of Alzheimer's Type
and Parkinson's Disease

This chapter summarizes background information on diagnostic criteria, prevalence, gender, ethnicity, and other findings relevant to dementia of Alzheimer's type and Parkinson's disease and discusses research findings concerning the etiology and treatment of both diseases. Dementia of Alzheimer's type is addressed first, including information pertaining to genetic, anatomical, neurochemical, and neuroimaging findings. Medications used to treat Alzheimer's disease are also discussed. Genetic, physiological, and anatomical findings concerning Parkinson's disease are then reviewed along with treatment approaches including medication, ablative procedures, ECT, and brain stimulation.

BACKGROUND INFORMATION

According to DSM IV-TR criteria (2000), disorders of dementia are characterized by memory and multiple cognitive deficits but are classified as different disorders based on etiology (e.g., general medical condition, cerebrovascular disease, substance inducement). Prevalence estimates of dementia vary depending on the subjects sampled, type of dementia, severity of impairment, and regions or countries studied, but according to the DSM IV-TR, 3% of the adult population suffers from severe cognitive impairment. In clinical and hospital-based studies, nearly half of all dementia cases are of Alzheimer's type; population-based studies report even higher rates (e.g., Edland, Rocca, Petersen, Cha, & Kokemen, 2002). Prevalence rates of dementia in nursing home residents from other countries such as Durango City, Mexico, were reported as 16.1% with the majority (11.6%) suffering from Alzheimer's disease. Based on a random sample of 1,062 residents age 70 or older in southeastern France, dementia was found in 9.2% of the cases; 5.5% were of Alzheimer's type (Obadia et al., 1997). Baiyewu, Adeyemi, and Ogunniyi (1997) reported that the majority of psychiatric disorders in Nigerian nursing home residents were dementia cases, and Snowdon and Lane (2001) reported that the prevalence of dementia among elderly people living at home in Botany, Australia, was 11%. Recently, Meguro et al. (2002) reported that the overall prevalence rate in adults 65 and older living in Tajiri, Japan, was 8.5%. Collectively, these studies substantiate that dementia occurs in a significant portion of adults worldwide, especially dementia of Alzheimer's type.

DEMENTIA OF ALZHEIMER'S TYPE

Dementia of Alzheimer's type is characterized by multiple cognitive deficits manifested by both memory impairment and cognitive disturbances that cause significant impairment in occupational or social functioning (see Table 4.1).

These impairments, which have a gradual onset and continuing decline, are not due to medical or substance-induced conditions. Dementia of Alzheimer's type usually occurs after age 65 (late-onset subtype), and prevalence rates increase markedly with increasing age. For example, .6% of males and .8% of females are estimated to have Alzheimer's at age 65, numbers that rise to 11% and 14%, respectively, by age 85. By age 95, 36% of all males and 41% of females have dementia of Alzheimer's type, with 40 to 60% marked by moderate to severe impairment (DSM IV-TR, 2000). Early-onset Alzheimer's type (age 65 or younger) is significantly less common than late-onset. Devi et al. (2004) found a higher prevalence of psychiatric disorders (e.g., schizophrenia, bipolar disorder, depression) among parents and siblings of patients with early-onset Alzheimer's disease (26% versus 15%). They speculated that some forms of early-onset Alzheimer's disease may share underlying genetic etiologies, a hypothesis in need of further empirical investigation. The most common cause of dementia is Alzheimer's disease, and some studies have reported a higher incidence of Alzheimer's in African Americans and Hispanics than whites (Tang et al., 2001) and others that the incidence of dementia is comparable among whites and African Americans (Fillenbaum et al., 1998).

According to the DSM IV-TR (2000), Alzheimer's disease is slightly more common in females than males. However, a large population based-study conducted by Ruitenberg and colleagues (2001) found no such gender differences until after 90 years of age. In a recent longitudinal study of Catholic priests, nuns, and brothers, Barnes et al. (2003) reported that the incidence of Alzheimer's disease did not differ between men and women. In addition to cognitive decline, behavioral and psychological symptoms also commonly occur in patients with Alzheimer's disease. Hart et al. (2003), for example, investigated the prevalence of noncognitive symptomology in patients with a 3-year or greater diagnosis of Alzheimer's disease and found that apathy occurred in 88% of the patients, aggression in 66%, sleep disturbances in 54%, irritability and appetite changes in 60%, 56% suffered from depression, 55% had delusions, and 52% experiences significant anxiety symptoms. McCurry and colleagues (2004) found that 56% percent of patients with Alzheimer's disease suffered from anxiety symptoms that positively correlated with nighttime behavioral disturbances such as awakenings. Marder et al. (1999) found that siblings of individuals who had Parkinson's disease and dementia were three times more likely to develop Alzheimer's disease than control subjects. Perl, Olanow, and Calne (1998) noted that many patients with Parkinson's disease develop Alzheimer's disease and, conversely, many patients with Alzheimer's disease develop extrapyramidal symptoms characteristic of Parkinson's disease. Consistent with previous studies (e.g., Nobler, Pleton, & Sackeim, 1999), Hargrave, Reed, and Mungas (2000) found depression was common in patients with Alzheimer's disease—especially women—with the level of functional impairment associated with the severity of depression. Cross-sectional studies have found that the frequency of major depression decreases in severe Alzheimer's disease but aggression, agitation, and psychosis increase (Lopez et al., 2003). Sultzer (2004) reported that psychotic symptoms are common in Alzheimer's disease, and Tran and colleagues (2003) found a significant relationship between frequency of psychotic symptoms and dependency in daily living in patients with Alzheimer's disease. Increased dependency in daily living often leads to greater demands for care such as nursing homes and assisted living programs. Research by Leon, Cheng, and Neumann (1998) indicates that the cost of caring for patients with Alzheimer's disease is increasing yearly and assisted living facilities are significantly less costly than nursing homes.

TABLE 4.1

Diagnostic Criteria for 294.1x Dementia of the Alzheimer's Type (DSM IV-TR, 2000)

A. The development of multiple cognitive deficits manifested by both
   (1) memory impairment (impaired ability to learn new information or to recall previously learned information)
   (2) one (or more) of the following cognitive disturbances:
      (a) aphasia (language disturbance)
      (b) apraxia (impaired ability to carry out motor activities despite intact motor function)
      (c) agnosia (failure to recognize or identify objects despite intact sensory function)
      (d) disturbance in executive functioning (i.e., planning, organizing, sequencing, abstracting)
B. The cognitive deficits in Criteria A1 and A2 each cause significant impairment in social or occupational functioning and represent a significant decline from a previous level of functioning.
C. The course is characterized by gradual onset and continuing cognitive decline.
D. The cognitive deficits in Criteria A1 and A2 are not due to any of the following:
   (1) other central nervous system conditions that cause progressive deficits in memory and cognition (e.g., cerebrovascular disease, Parkinson's disease, Huntington's disease, subdural hematoma, normal-pressure hydrocephalus, brain tumor)
   (2) systemic conditions that are known to cause dementia (e.g., hypothyroidism, vitamin B12 or folic acid deficiency, niacin deficiency, hypercalcemia, neurosyphilis, HIV infection)
   (3) substance-induced conditions
E. The deficits do not occur exclusively during the course of a delirium.
F. The disturbance is not better accounted for by another Axis I disorder (e.g., Major Depressive Disorder, Schizophrenia).

Code based on presence or absence of a clinically significant behavioral disturbance:

294.10 Without Behavioral Disturbance: if the cognitive disturbance is not accompanied by any clinically significant behavioral disturbance

294.11 With Behavioral Disturbance: if the cognitive disturbance is accompanied by a clinically significant behavioral disturbance (e.g., wandering, agitations)

Specify subtype:

With Early Onset: if onset is at age 65 years or below
With Late Onset: if onset is after age 65 years

Coding note: Also code 331.0 Alzheimer's disease on Axis III. Indicate other clinical features related to the Alzheimer's disease on Axis I (e.g., 293.83 Mood Disorder due to Alzheimer's Disease, With Depressive Features, and 310.1 Personality Change due to Alzheimer's Disease, Aggressive Type).

Diagnostic Criteria for 294.1x Dementia Due to Other General Medical Conditions
A. The development of multiple cognitive deficits manifested by both
   (1) memory impairment (impaired ability to learn new information or to recall previously learned information)
   (2) one (or more) of the following cognitive disturbances:
      (a) aphasia (language disturbance)
      (b) apraxia (impaired ability to carry out motor activities despite intact motor function)
      (c) agnosia (failure to recognize or identify objects despite intact sensory function)
      (d) disturbance in executive functioning (i.e., planning, organizing, sequencing, abstracting)
B. The cognitive deficits in Criteria A1 and A2 each cause significant impairment in social or occupational functioning and represent a significant decline from a previous level of functioning.
C. There is evidence from the history, physical examination, or laboratory findings that the disturbance is the direct physiological consequence of a general medical condition other than Alzheimer's disease or cerebrovascular disease (e.g., HIV infection, traumatic brain injury, Parkinson's disease,

(Continued)

TABLE 4.1

(Continued)

Huntington's disease, Pick's disease, Creutzfeldt-Jakob disease, normal-pressure hydrocephalus, hypothyroidism, brain tumor, or vitamin B12 deficiency).

D. The deficits do not occur exclusively during the course of a delirium.

Code based on presence or absence of a clinically significant behavioral disturbance:

294.10 Without Behavioral Disturbance: if the cognitive disturbance is not accompanied by any clinically significant behavioral disturbance

294.11 With Behavioral Disturbance: if the cognitive disturbance is accompanied by a clinically significant behavioral disturbance (e.g., wandering, agitations)

Coding note: Also code the general medical condition on Axis III (e.g., 042 HIV infection, 854.00 head injury, 332.0 Parkinson's disease, 333.4 Huntington's disease, 331.1 Pick's disease, 046.1 Creutzfeldt-Jakob disease; see Appendix G for additional codes).

Paulsen et al. (2000) found the incidence of hallucinations and delusions increased with the progression of the disease and was associated with accelerated cognitive decline. Given that psychotic symptoms occur in 40 to 60% of individuals with Alzheimer's disease, some researchers have suggested that the coexistence of psychotic symptoms may represent a distinct phenotype of Alzheimer's disease (Sweet, Nimgaonkar, Devlin, & Jeste, 2003).

In addition to behavioral and psychological symptoms, individuals with Alzheimer's disease also experience a number of neuropsychological impairments depending on the disease's, severity, including deficits in executive functions (Cahn-Weiner, Ready, & Malloy, 2003). According to a recent study by Swanberg, Tractenberg, Mohs, Thal, and Cummings (2004), 64% of patients with Alzheimer's disease had significant executive function deficits. Compared to patients with mild cognitive impairment, patients with Alzheimer's disease have more pronounced memory impairments, particularly episodic memory impairments (Lambon, Patterson, Graham, Dawson, & Hodges, 2003). A number of studies have found that performance on specific types of neuropsychological tests such as episodic and semantic memory tasks may predict preclinical Alzheimer's disease with considerable accuracy, perhaps as high as 95 to 97% (e.g., Blackwell et al., 2004; Kluger et al., 1999). Boyle (2004) and others have attributed the neuropsychological deficits associated with Alzheimer's disease to dysfunction of the frontal systems. The etiology and physiological underpinnings of Alzheimer's disease are complex, however, and research supports a role for genetic, anatomical, and functional abnormalities in the disorder.

Genetic Studies

Familial studies consistently indicate that Alzheimer's disease aggregates in families (e.g., Farrer et al., 1990; Klünemann et al., 2002). For example, Devi et al. (2000) compared the familial aggregation and lifetime risk of Alzheimer's disease in first-degree relatives of 435 individuals with the disease and unrelated control subjects among whites, African Americans, and Caribbean Hispanics. Results indicated the lifetime risk for Alzheimer's disease was 25.9% in relatives of individuals with the disease compared to 19.1% in control relatives, and the risk was higher than controls in all three ethnic groups. In addition, risk of Alzheimer's disease was greater among relatives of women than men. Silverman and colleagues (2003) reported relatives of individuals who develop Alzheimer's disease very late in life (i.e., age 85 or older) have a substantially lower risk for the disease than relatives of early-onset Alzheimer's disease.

Based on these results, they speculated that very late-onset Alzheimer's may be associated with environmental factors while early-onset Alzheimer's disease has a more prominent genetic basis. Van Duijn, Farrer, Cupples, and Hofman (1993) reported similar results in Dutch families of 198 individuals who developed Alzheimer's disease before the age of 65 (i.e., early onset). The mode of inheritance of Alzheimer's disease is unclear, but many studies suggest an autosomal dominant inheritance model for early-onset Alzheimer's disease (e.g., Farrer et al., 1990). In addition, some studies have suggested maternal transmission of the disease (e.g., Edland et al., 1996) while other studies have found evidence of increased paternal transmission (e.g., Ehrenkrantz et al., 1999).

Twin studies also support a genetic basis for Alzheimer's disease. For example, Bergem, Engedal, and Kringlen (1997) reported a concordance rate of 78% among monozytotic twins and 39% for dizygotic twin pairs for Alzheimer's disease in Norway, and Gatz et al. (1997) reported Alzheimer disease concordance rates of 67% and 22% for monozygotic and dizygotic twins in Sweden. In a Finnish study, Raiha and colleagues also reported that the incidence of Alzheimer's disease was significantly higher in monozygotic twins than dizygotic twins. Rapoport, Pettigrew, and Schapiro (1991) reported that monozygotic twins concordant for Alzheimer's disease are significantly more likely to have a family history for the disease than discordant monozygotic twins, further supporting a heritability component of the disease. Recently, Pedersen, Gatz, Berg, and Johansson (2004) examined 662 Swedish twins ages 52 to 98 and followed them up at 2- to 3-year intervals. Results revealed that 5.8% of the sample was diagnosed with Alzheimer's disease and the average onset was late in life (83.9 years). In 26 monozygotic pairs, at least one twin developed the disease and the concordance rate was 32.2%. The concordance rate was 8.7% for dizygotic twins. Overall, twin studies clearly indicate that Alzheimer's disease is more common in monozygotic than dizygotic twins, but questions remain about the mode of inheritance.

Candidate Genes

One of the first genetic breakthroughs concerning Alzheimer's disease was the recognition that individuals with Down syndrome inevitably develop neuropathological changes that are also characteristic of Alzheimer's disease, namely, the accumulation of amyloid plaques and neurofibrillary tangles in the brain. Given that Down syndrome is due to trisomy 21, scientists focused on chromosome 21 and specifically the amyloid precursor protein gene (APP) to study Alzheimer's disease. The APP gene codes the production of the precursor protein amyloid beta-peptide that accumulates in the plaques of patients with Alzheimer's disease. According to Kowalska (2003), early-onset Alzheimer's disease has been linked to over 20 mutations of the APP gene, all of which lead to overproduction of the amyloid protein. In 2000, another mutation of the APP gene was identified and linked to early-onset Alzheimer's disease based on a five-member family, three of whom were found to have the mutation and two developed Alzheimer's disease before age 40 (Murrell, Hake, Quaid, Farlow, & Ghetti, 2000). As Lannfelt et al. (1995) noted, DNA analysis can reveal whether family members have inherited APP mutations, but these gene variants account for only a small percentage of total Alzheimer cases (Kowalska et al., 2004).

In addition to mutations on chromosome 21, researchers have linked chromosomes 14, 1, and 19 to early-onset Alzheimer's disease. For example, a variety of mutations of the presenilin 1 gene (PS1) on chromosome 14 and presenilin 2 gene (PS2) found on chromosome 1 have also been associated with increased production and deposits of amyloid protein plaques in patients with Alzheimer's disease (e.g., Ezquerra et al., 2003; Heckmann et al., 2004). Chromosome 19 is also a focus of study as the APOE gene on this chromosome has been linked to a majority of cases of Alzheimer's disease (Ashford & Mortimer, 2002). Specifically, the APOE gene has several alleles (E2, E3, E4) and not all of these alleles are found in all persons. The E4 allele is associated with increased risk of Alzheimer's disease because of its effect on the production of apolipoprotein, which binds with tau protein. The tau protein is found in the neurofibrillary tangles of individuals with Alzheimer's disease. Not everyone with the APOE gene variant (i.e., E4 allele) develops Alzheimer's disease, but even carriers of the gene tend to have lower glucose metabolism rates in various brain regions, suggesting functional abnormalities are associated with the APOE gene (Reiman et al., 2001). Tolar et al. (1999) hypothesized that apolipoprotein may interfere with cellular functioning at the level of the cellular membrane and lead to neurotoxicity and cellular death. Interestingly, Bergem and Lannfelt (1997) did not find a difference in the frequency of this gene variant in monozygotic and dizygotic twins concordant or discordant for Alzheimer's disease. Graves et al. (1999) found that presence of the APOE-E4 allele in conjunction with impaired olfaction was associated with a 4.9 times increased risk of cognitive decline compared to individuals without the E4 allele and without olfactory impairment. They noted that as plaques and tangles are commonly found throughout the olfactory pathways in patients with Alzheimer's disease, these measures of olfaction could serve as preclinical markers of the disease, especially in individuals with the APOE-E4 allele.

The relationship of the APOE-E4 allele to Alzheimer's disease varies by ethnic group. For example, Tang et al. (1998) found when the APOE-E4 allele was present, the risks for Alzheimer's disease were similar for whites, African Americans, and Hispanics; but in the absence of the APOE-E4 allele, the cumulative risks for Alzheimer's were four times higher for African Americans and two times higher for Hispanics compared to whites. Tang et al. suggested that other genes may contribute to the increased risk of Alzheimer's disease in Hispanics and African Americans. Among Koreans, Kim et al. (1999) found the APOE-E4 allele was more prevalent in patients with Alzheimer's disease than controls, and that the presence of this allele was associated with both early-onset and late-onset Alzheimer's. Ganguli et al. (2000) studied the prevalence of Alzheimer's disease in Ballabgarh, India, and the United States (specifically, southwestern Pennsylvania). The prevalence was significantly lower in India, but the association of the disease with the APOE-E4 allele in the Indian sample was similar to that found in the U.S. sample. Senanarong et al. (2001) found that 59% of individuals with Alzheimer's disease in a sample from Thailand carried the EPOE-E4 allele.

Lauderback and colleagues (2002) suggested that APOE alleles 2 and 3 have antioxidant effects that offer some protection against Alzheimer's disease, whereas allele 4 is associated with oxidative damage in Alzheimer's patients. Silverman et al. (1999) noted that some families' demonstrably low risk of Alzheimer's disease may be due to the fact that they are not carriers of the APOE-E4 allele, or the presence of the E2 allele, or because of some protective gene or genes yet to be identified. Some researchers have suggested that behavioral factors may interact with genetic factors to decrease or increase the risk of Alzheimer's disease. For example, Asada and colleagues (2000) found napping for less than 60 minutes 3 or more days a week was associated with reduced risk of Alzheimer's disease, especially in individuals who were carriers of the APOE-E4 allele. Napping for greater than 60 minutes, however, was associated with increased risk, perhaps because it interferes with normal circadian functions.

One of the most consistently documented neurotransmitter findings in Alzheimer's disease is early and continued loss of cholinergic neurons and downregulation of both nicotinic and NMDA acetylcholine receptors. To decrease turnover of acetylcholine, cholinesterase inhibitors are widely used in the treatment of Alzheimer's disease and are often effective at reducing symptoms of the disease (Lopez et al., 2002). Consequently, polymorphisms of nicotinic and NMDA receptor genes have been investigated. Some studies have found a relationship between Alzheimer's disease and variants of these receptor genes (e.g., Cook et al., 2004; Kawamata & Shimohama, 2002) while others have found no link between polymorphism of cholinergic receptor genes and reduction of receptors (Steinlein et al., 1999). Given the number of chromosomal regions and genes that have been linked to Alzheimer's disease thus far, it is apparent that multiple genes are involved in the disorder and it is highly probable that additional genes and gene variants will be identified in the future.

Anatomical Findings

As mentioned previously, dementia of Alzheimer's type is characterized by plaques and neurofibrillary tangles (Fig. 4.1). The plaques consist of amyloid beta-peptide deposits. Although associated with dementia and Alzheimer's disease, amyloid β deposits alone do not result in Alzheimer's disease (Iqbal et al., 1998; Näslund et al., 2000). Lorenzo and colleagues (2000) noted that the way in which amyloid β becomes toxic is not fully understood, but suggested that an interaction occurs between amyloid β and its precursor protein (amyloid precursor protein, APP) that leads to neurodegeneration. Haroutunian et al. (1998) reported evidence of plaque formation in elderly subjects without dementia, although in general, density of plaque formation was associated with dementia severity. In the brains of individuals with Alzheimer's disease, amyloid plaques are surrounded by neurofibrillary tangles that are composed of tau protein. In healthy neurons, tau helps to stabilize microtubules found in axons but when hyperphosphorylated, tau inhibits the normal functioning and assembly of microtubles and instead forms neurofibrillary tangles (Kahle et al., 2000). Evidence also suggests that the formation and pattern of these tangles may increase rapidly with increasing age and severity of Alzheimer's disease (Uboga and Price, 2000). According to Iqbal et al. (1998), the disassembly of microtubules leads to retrograde neuronal degeneration. Ebneth et al. (1998) also found that an overexpression of tau is toxic to healthy neurons as it retards cell growth, causes changes in the shape of cells, and leads to the disappearance of mitochondria. Neurons that are in the process of neurofibrillary degeneration release the tau protein, which can be detected in the cerebral spinal fluid (CSF) of individuals with Alzheimer's disease. Kahle et al. (2000), for example, measured CSF levels of tau and a second protein (AD7C-neuronal thread protein, or AD7C-NTP) that increases during the early stages of neurofibrillary degeneration in patients with Alzheimer's disease, patients with Parkinson's disease, and healthy control subjects. Results revealed that tau and AD7C-NTP were elevated in patients with Alzheimer's relative to control subjects, but significant differences were not found between control subjects and patients with Parkinson's disease. Studies have also found higher levels of tau protein in patients with a family history of Alzheimer's disease and the APOE geneotype compared to patients without a family history of Alzheimer's disease (Thaker et al., 2003). Ishihara et al. (1999) argued that mutations of the tau gene may cause abnormal functioning of the tau protein in individuals with Alzheimer's disease. Indeed, several studies have reported a relationship between polymorphisms of the tau gene and Alzheimer's disease (e.g., Bullido et al., 2000; Tanahashi, Asada, & Tabira, 2004), although other studies have failed to substantiate these findings (e.g., Crawford et al., 1999; Roks et al., 1999; Russ et al., 2001).

In addition to plaques and tangles, individuals with dementia of Alzheimer's type often have other neuritic pathology such as Lewy bodies. Lewy bodies are inclusions that are comprised of the synaptic protein alpha-synuclein which characterize a specific type of dementia—Lewy body dementia. Arai et al. (2001) found that 48% of patients with Alzheimer's disease had Lewy bodies in addition to plaques and tangles, leading them to speculate that Lewy body formation may be promoted by increased levels of tau aggregation. Kotzbauer, Trojanowsk, and Lee (2001) reported that Lewy bodies occur in approximately 60% of Alzheimer cases

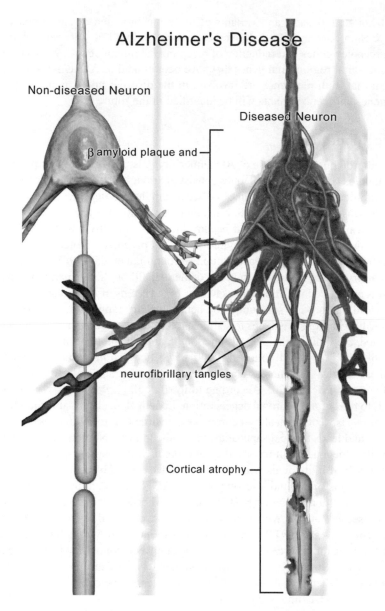

Alzheimer's Disease

**FIG. 4.1. Neurons depicting plaques and neurofibrillary
tangles commonly found in brains of individuals with Alzheimer's
disease. Copyright Blausen Medical Communications. Reproduced by permission.**

and are most commonly found in the amygdala. Ballard et al. (2004) compared postmortem
brains of individuals with Alzheimer's disease and Lewy body dementia and concluded that
persistent visual hallucinations and psychiatric features were more frequent in Lewy body
dementia than Alzheimer's disease. As tangle pathology increased in patients with Lewy body
dementia, however, clinical symptoms prior to death were similar to Alzheimer's patients.

Weiner et al. (2003) also compared postmortem tissue of Alzheimer's patients and patients
with Lewy body dementia and reported that hallucinations, delusions, and extrapyramidal
symptoms were more frequent in the latter. Gilman and colleagues (2004) used PET to measure

striatal presynaptic binding potential in patients with Lewy body dementia and patients with Alzheimer's disease and found substantial decreased binding in patients with Lewy body dementia but not in Alzheimer's patients. Tiraboschi et al. (2002) recently examined postmortem tissue of patients with Alzheimer's disease and patients with Lewy body dementia and found that acetylcholinetransferase activity was substantially reduced in the latter even at early stages of the disease, whereas reductions were less severe in Alzheimer's disease and occurred later in the course of the illness. Collectively, these studies suggest that although Lewy bodies may be present in some cases of Alzheimer's disease, these two types of dementia can be differentiated based on anatomical, physiological, and clinical pathology (Iseki, 2004). In addition to Lewy bodies, the presence of "cotton wool" plaques, consisting of two subtypes of amyloid beta proteins (Abeta42 and Abeta40), have been documented in some cases of Alzheimer's disease and are associated with specific mutations of the presenilin1 gene (e.g., Mann et al., 2001).

Josephs et al. (2003) found evidence of a novel protein pathology in the brains of four individuals with dementia and described the inclusions as neurofilament inclusion bodies. Additional studies are needed to determine whether these neurofilament inclusion bodies are present in Alzheimer's disease as well. Hatanpää et al. (1999) reported that during the normal aging process, synaptic proteins involved in structural plasticity of axons and dendrites decrease significantly. Once such protein is drebrin that is abundant in neurons during development. Their in the adult brain, however, debrin is mainly localized to dendritic spines. Hatanpää et al. found an 81% reduction in drebrin in postmortem brains of patients with Alzheimer's disease relative to similarly aged control subjects, and hypothesized that abnormalities of synaptic proteins may contribute to the cognitive symptoms of Alzheimer's disease. Several studies have reported significant reductions in neurotrophic factors in patients with Alzheimer's disease, particularly in the hippocampus and parietal cortex, which is likely related to the vulnerability of neurons in these regions even at early stages of the disease (e.g., Fahnestock, Garzon, Holsinger, & Michalski, 2002; Michalski & Fahnestock, 2003).

MRI Findings

Brain volume changes are associated with Alzheimer's disease pathology, and hence recent studies have found that MRI measurements taken over time can predict the extent of disease progression. For example, Silbert et al. (2003) followed 24 patients with cognitive impairment and 15 nondemented patients until their deaths, and at regular intervals measured brain volume and ventricular CSF volume. These findings were compared to postmortem measurements of plaques and neurofibrillary tangles and revealed that the accumulation of cortical tangles was strongly associated with total brain volume loss, and the rate of increase of ventricular CSF volume was related to both plaques and tangles. Chan and colleagues (2003) followed 12 patients who were presymptomatic for Alzheimer's disease through to moderate and severe stages using MRI. Results revealed a 2.8% mean yearly loss of brain volume during the mild stage, figure that increased by .32% each year thereafter. Lopez et al. (2003) recently reported that severity of Alzheimer's disease was associated with a progressive deterioration of frontal–temporal structures, evidenced by psychiatric symptoms such as uncooperativeness, wandering, emotional lability, and psychotic symptoms.

Järvenpää et al. (2004) used MRI to compare hippocampal volume in seven pairs of monozygotic twins discordant for Alzheimer's disease compared to control twins and found that the hippocampus was significantly smaller in twins with Alzheimer's disease compared to controls and to nondemented twins. Earlier MRI studies substantiated that atrophy of the hippocampal formation was associated with mild to severe Alzheimer's disease; with more severe dementia, neuronal atrophy was observed in the parahippocampal gyrus and the cortex of the temporal lobe (Detoledo-Morrell et al., 1997). Numerous studies have found a relationship between hippocampal volume reduction and memory loss on behavioral measures (e.g., Convit et al., 2000; Peterson et al., 2000). Killiany et al. (2000) reported that MRI scans of structures of the medial temporal lobe (entorhinal cortex, temporal sulcus, anterior cingulate) could differentiate patients with mild Alzheimer's disease from control subjects with 100% accuracy. Laakso et al. (2000) reported that atrophy of the hippocampus was diffuse in patients with Alzheimer's disease compared to other types of dementia (frontotemporal dementia) in which hippocampal atrophy tended to be more localized to the anterior portion of the hippocampus. Recent studies have found that changes in the shape of the hippocampus over time as well as the rate of change can distinguish even very mild dementia of Alzheimer's type from the normal aging process in healthy individuals (Wang et al., 2003). Head et al. (2004) also found differential age effects in the white matter of the corpus callosum, frontal, temporal, parietal, and occipital lobes in patients with Alzheimer's disease relative to healthy aging control subjects. These finding suggest that the underlying physiology of normal aging and that of Alzheimer's disease likely involve distinctly different mechanisms.

PET, fMRI, SPECT Findings

Functional imaging studies have consistently found reductions in rCBF and glucose metabolism in brains of patients with Alzheimer's disease relative to control subjects. For example, when Friedland et al. (1989) examined glucose metabolism in individuals with probable Alzheimer's disease and healthy age-matched control subjects, despite normal blood–brain–barrier transport of glucose, reduced metabolism in the temporal and parietal cortices was found in individuals with Alzheimer's disease. Rapoport et al. (1991) and Ogawa et al. (1996) reported that resting rates of global glucose metabolism were lower in subjects with Alzheimer's disorder relative to control subjects, even early in the disease. Kumar and colleagues (1991) also found early and widespread metabolic disturbances in subjects with probable Alzheimer's disease and reported that these disturbances increase as the disease progresses.

Rapoport (2003) recently suggested that the early reductions in glucose metabolism observed in Alzheimer's disease are due to changes in synaptic structure and cellular function, such as changes in mitochodria functioning that eventually lead to cellular death. Indeed, glucose metabolism studies that have statistically controlled for degree of brain atrophy in subjects with Alzheimer's disease have found that reductions in glucose metabolism persist, indicating that abnormalities in cellular function are genuine and not simply an artifact of brain atrophy. Mielke and colleagues (1998) found a relationship between reduced glucose metabolism, severity of dementia, and the APOE genotype in patients with Alzheimer's disease. Kessler and colleagues (2000) and Eustache et al. (2004) also reported a relationship between reduced glucose metabolism in the frontal, temporal, and parietal regions and performance on neuropsychological tasks. Sultzer et al. (2003) recently studied the relationship between delusional thoughts and glucose metabolism in patients with Alzheimer's disease and, based on PET scans, reported a significant relationship between metabolic rates in three right frontal regions and severity of delusional thoughts. Collectively, these studies indicate that Alzheimer's disease is characterized by widespread reductions in glucose metabolism, particularly in the right frontal, temporal, and parietal regions.

Studies that have investigated rCBF have also found functional differences between subjects with and without Alzheimer's disease (DeCarli et al., 1996). For example, Warkentin and colleagues (2004) recently reported reduced blood flow in the temporoparietal regions of both hemispheres in patients with Alzheimer's relative to control subjects. Rodriguez et al. (1998) studied 42 patients with probable Alzheimer's disease relative to control subjects and found that rCBF measures of the temporoparietal regions were able to identify subjects with Alzheimer's disease with 75% accuracy. Kogure et al. (2000) found a longitudinal pattern of decline with respect to rCBF in subjects with mild cognitive impairment who developed Alzheimer's within a subsequent 2-year period, using SPECT. Specifically, at baseline, subjects with mild cognitive impairment had significant rCBF reductions in the posterior cingulate gyri (bilaterally) and in the left hippocampus, and parahippocampal gyrus at 2- or-more-year follow-ups relative to control subjects. Recently, Kanetaka et al. (2004) reported similar findings as rCBF was substantially reduced in the posterior cingulate gyrus in patients with very early Alzheimer's disease relative to healthy control subjects. Tonini, Shanks, and Venneri (2003) also measured rCBF longitudinally in patients with Alzheimer's disease (over a period of 6 months) and found significant reductions in blood flow in numerous brain regions. These studies clearly indicate that Alzheimer's disease is characterized by functional blood flow changes which progressively worsen over time. Furthermore, Grady et al. (2001) found that individuals with Alzheimer's disease show a different pattern of rCBF compared to control subjects while performing a short-term visual recognition task. Control subjects showed increased activity in the bilateral prefrontal cortices, right hippocampus, and bilateral parietal areas. Patients with Alzheimer's disease, however, showed increased activation primarily in the prefrontal cortex, and according to Grady et al. these findings support a functional disconnection between prefrontal regions and subcortical structures important in memory in patients with Alzheimer's disease.

Several rCBF studies suggest that PET and rCBF measures can be used to discriminate medication responders from nonresponders. For example, given the evidence that Alzheimer's disease is associated with a loss of presynaptic cholinergic functioning, donepezil (a cholinergic inhibitor) is used to treat some of the symptoms of the disease. Hanyu et al. (2003) compared rCBF in the lateral and medial frontal lobes in responders and nonresponders to donepezil and discovered significantly lower rCBF in the lateral and medial frontal lobes of nonresponders. Interestingly, Staff and colleagues (2000) found that donepezil treatment increased global as well as regional (frontal lobes) blood flow in patients with Alzheimer's disease, who showed symptomatic improvement after taking the medication. Several studies investigating the potential long-term effects of donepezil on rCBF in patients with Alzheimer's disease, revealed that after a year or more of treatment, rCBF did not decline in several regions of the brain (e.g., anterior cingulate, temporal gyrus, prefrontal cortex, temporal lobes) (e.g., Nakano, Asada, Matsuda, Uno, & Takasaki, 2001; Nobili et al., 2002). These studies suggest that donepezil may help to maintain functional brain activity in patients with Alzheimer's disease.

In summary, glucose metabolism and rCBF studies have found global and regional reductions in functional activity in patients with Alzheimer's disease relative to control subjects, and these functional abnormalities worsen with time. Neural circuitry between subcortical structures such as the hippocampus and the prefrontal cortex as well as the parietal and temporal cortices appear to be particularly impaired in patients with Alzheimer's disease (Nobler, Pelton, & Sackeim, 1999). Whereas many early-onset cases of Alzheimer's disease are associated with specific genotypes, late-onset cases are often of unknown etiology.

Risk and Protective Factors Implicated in Dementia of Alzheimer's Type

In addition to gene variants, a variety of factors have been associated with increased risk of Alzheimer's disease. For example, Moceri et al. (2000) predicted that early childhood environment is associated with risk of Alzheimer's disease. Their study of 393 patients with the disease and 377 control families indicated that growing up in a family of five or more siblings increased the risk of developing Alzheimer's by 39%; the risk increased by 8% with each additional family member. Growing up in an urban area (versus a suburb) was also associated with increased risk. Hall and colleagues (2000) also found that growing up in a rural residence combined with less than 6 years of schooling was associated with increased risk of Alzheimer's disease in a sample of 2,212 African Americans. Moceri et al. (2000) suggested that number of siblings and area of residence are related to socioeconomic level and may reflect a poorer quality of living environment. In turn, a poor-quality environment could interfere with normal brain development and maturation and therefore increase the risk of Alzheimer's disease later in life. This study was based on retrospective reports, however, and longitudinal studies that document quality of living and cognitive outcome in later life are needed to adequately explore this hypothesis. Gatz et al. (2001) examined the relationship between years of schooling and Alzheimer's disease in twins discordant for the disease. Contrary to expectations, demented twins and their nondemented twin pair did not differ significantly with respect to education. A number of studies have reported, however, that fewer years of education are associated with greater Alzheimer's risk (e.g., Garre-Olmo et al., 2004; Tyas, Manfreda, Strain, & Montgomery, 2001; Ravaglia et al., 2002), and Harmanci et al. (2003) suggested that having a college degree had a protective effect on the risk of Alzheimer's disease.

Numerous studies have also found a relationship between moderate and severe head injuries and increased risk of Alzheimer's disease as well as other dementias later in life (e.g., Plassman et al., 2000). Findings have been mixed as to whether the magnitude of Alzheimer's risk is greater among persons with carriers of a certain APOE genotype (APOE-E4) who sustain head injury relative to those head injury victims who are noncarriers (e.g., Guo et al., 2000). Wilson and colleagues recently reported that individuals who are prone to psychological distress have a significantly greater risk of developing Alzheimer's disease compared to those who are low in distress proneness. Others have reported a greater risk of Alzheimer's disease among individuals who have a history of migraines (e.g., Tyas, Manfreda, Strain, & Montgomery, 2001). Studies have conflicted with respect to occupational hazards and Alzheimer's risk. For example, Palmer and colleagues (1998) reported a strong relationship between Alzheimer's risk and extreme exposure to solvents but concluded overall there was a small influence of exposure to solvents to the development of dementia in the general population. Kukull et al. (1995) reported that exposure to solvents (e.g., ketones, benzene, phenols) was likely associated with the onset of Alzheimer's disease while Graves et al. (1998) concluded that it is unlikely to be an important risk factor. The relationship between occupational exposure to electromagnetic fields and Alzheimer's risk has also been investigated and, again, the findings have been mixed (e.g., Feychting, Pedersen, Svedberg, Floderus, & Gatz, 1998; Graves, Rosner, Echeverria, Yost, & Larson, 1999; Li, Sung, & Wu, 2002). Li, Sung, and Wu (2002) recently reported that blue-collar workers had the highest risk of dementia compared to other types of occupations. Cigarette smoking, in particular moderate and heavy smoking, is also associated with increased risk of Alzheimer's disease (Juan et al., 2004). Luchsinger, Tang, Shea, and Mayeux (2002) reported individuals with a high caloric and fat intake were at greater risk for Alzheimer's disease (compared to those in the lowest quartiles of caloric intake); carriers of the APOE-E4 allele in conjunction with high caloric and fat intake were at greatest risk for the disease. Several studies have found a relationship between cholesterol levels and Alzheimer's disease although other studies have not substantiated these findings (e.g., Austen, Christodoulou, & Terry, 2002; Evans et al., 2000; Zaldy et al., 2003). Petanceska et al. (2003) noted that the APOE gene mediates cholesterol levels in the brain via the APOE-E4 allele and apolipoprotein, which transports cholesterol in the brain. According to their work, disruptions in cholesterol metabolism may lead to increased production of apolipoprotein and ultimately the plaques and tangles characteristic of Alzheimer's disease. Evans et al. (2000) suggested that modifying cholesterol levels may decrease the risk of Alzheimer's disease.

Butterfield and colleagues (1999) have proposed that free radicals are associated with increased production of amyloid β, and these free radicals alter cell membrane structure and function and ultimately result in cellular death. According to Bickford et al. (2000), diets rich in antioxidants, such as those found in fresh fruits and vegetables, have been shown to improve learning and memory performance in aged rats. Numerous human studies have reported that diets rich in antioxidants (e.g., vitamins C and E) are associated with a lower risk of Alzheimer's diease (e.g., Engelhart et al., 2002; Morris et al., 2002). Zandi et al. (2004) recently found that use of vitamin E and C supplements in combination were associated with a reduced risk of Alzheimer's disease, but use of either vitamin alone was not associated with reduced risk. Luchsinger, Tang, Shea, and Mayeux (2003) did not find a relationship, however, between dietary or supplemental intake of vitamins E and C and Alzheimer's risk. Similarly, Laurin and colleagues (2003) did not find that the dietary intake of omega-3 polyunsaturated fatty acids served a protective role in cognitive impairment and dementia. Other studies, however, have reported that weekly intake of fish and omega-3 fatty acids may reduce the risk of Alzheimer's disease (e.g., Morris et al., 2003). Interestingly, a number of studies have reported that light to moderate alcohol consumption may reduce the risk of dementia and Alzheimer's (e.g., Huang, Qiu, Winblad, & Fratiglioni, 2002; Ruitenberg et al., 2002). Recent findings, however, suggest that this reduced risk may be limited to individuals without the APOE-E4 allele (Luchsinger, Tang, Siddiqui, Shea, & Mayeux, 2004).

Crowe and colleagues (2003) found that participation in leisure activities was negatively correlated with risk of Alzheimer's disease and dementia in general. They also found that greater participation in intellectual activities was associated with a lower risk of Alzheimer's disease—but in women only. Wilson and colleagues (2002) conducted a 7-year longitudinal study of nearly 800 catholic nuns, priests, and brothers from 40 Catholic organizations across the United States. The researchers measured degree of participation in cognitively stimulating activities (e.g., reading books, magazines, or newspapers; doing crossword puzzles; playing cards or checkers) and incidence of Alzheimer's disease. Results indicated that frequent participation in cognitively stimulating activities was associated with a reduced risk of Alzheimer's disease in both males and females. Other studies have found that regular exercise improves the physical health as well as depression levels of patients with Alzheimer's disease (Mahendra & Arkin, 2003; Teri et al., 2003).

Although some studies have reported that hormone replacement therapy (HRT) reduces a woman's risk of Alzheimer's disease, other studies have not supported this finding (Zandi et al., 2002). Estrogen treatment has, however, been found to increase receptor binding of serotonin in regions associated with Alzheimer's disease including the prefrontal cortex, anterior cingulate cortex, and inferior frontal gyrus in postmenopausal women (Kugaya ct al., 2003). Maki, Zonderman, and Resnick (2001) compared memory performance of nondemented women who received HRT to those who had not and found that specific aspects of memory performance were superior in those receiving the therapy. Maki and Resnick (2000) compared rCBF changes over a 2-year period in 12 nondemented women who received hormone replacement therapy to 16 women who did not, and found increased rCBF in several memory-related areas (e.g., hippocampus, parahippocampal gyrus, temporal lobe) in those who received the therapy. Given the encouraging results of studies with individuals without dementia, Wang et al. (2000) explored the effects of 12 weeks of estrogen therapy on cognitive performance, dementia severity, mood, and cerebral perfusion using SPECT and concluded that no meaningful effects were found. Other HRT studies have reported similar conclusions based on samples of women with mild to moderate Alzheimer's disease (e.g., Henderson et al., 2000; Mulnard et al., 2000).

Pharmacological Treatment

Medications that have been approved by the FDA to treat symptoms of Alzheimer's disease during its early stages include donepezil (aricept) rivastigmine (exelon), galantamine (reminyl), and cognex (tacrine). All these drugs are cholinesterase inhibitors and prevent the enzyme acetylcholinesterase from breaking down acetylcholine; thus, more of the neurotransmitter is available at the level of the synapse. As mentioned previously, Alzheimer's disease is characterized by degeneration of the cholinergic system, which projects from nuclei in the basal forebrain to areas of the limbic system as well as the cortex. Degeneration of these neurons is associated with disturbance of attention processes and gradual cognitive decline. Although cholinesterase inhibitors improve memory and cognitive abilities in many, but not all, patients with Alzheimer's disease, they do not slow the progression of the disease at a physiological level. Lopez et al. (2002) reported that the effectiveness of these medications appears to wane as the disease progresses. A number of short-term side effects are associated with cholinesterase inhibitors including nausea, diarrhea, vomiting, suppression of appetite, weight loss, and indigestion. Cognex has been associated with liver toxicity and is therefore rarely used in the treatment of Alzheimer's disease (Ibach & Haen, 2004; Watkins et al., 1994). Rees and Brimijoin (2003) recently reported that cholinesterase may actually facilitate amyloid β plaque formation and suggested that cholinesterase inhibitors may help to protect neurons from degeneration.

In addition to acetylcholine, the neurotransmitter glutamate has been implicated in Alzheimer's disease. Specifically, overstimulation of glutamate receptors is thought to characterize the disease, leading to neurotoxicity and cellular death (e.g., Mishizen-Eberz et al., 2004). A drug that blocks glutamate receptors (NMDA) was recently approved by the FDA in 2003 for late-stage Alzheimer's disease. Memantine (namenda) is a glutamate receptor (NMDA) antagonist that studies have found reduces clinical deterioration in individuals with moderate to severe Alzheimer's (e.g., Reisberg et al., 2003; Tariot et al., 2004). Rive and colleagues (2004) recently reported that memantine also enhances autonomy in Alzheimer's patients. Side effects are similar to cholinesterase inhibitors and include diarrhea, insomnia, dizziness, headache, and, less commonly, hallucinations (Jarvis & Figgitt, 2003).

A drug approved for the treatment of Parkinson's disease is also being used to treat Alzheimer's—selegiline (deprenyl), a MAO-B inhibitor. Studies have produced mixed findings concerning the drug's effectiveness with Alzheimer's patients. For example, Sano et al. (1997) reported that selegiline slowed the progression of Alzheimer's disease, and Knoll (1992) reported chronic treatment with selegiline improves cognitive skills of patients with the disease. Other studies have reported short- but not long-term improvement in cognitive skills of patients with Alzheimer's disease (Wilcock, Birks, Whitehead, & Evans, 2002). In a recent review of the literature, Birks and Flicker (2003) concluded the scientific evidence does not support the use of selegiline in the treatment of Alzheimer's disease. The use of vitamin E in the treatment of Alzheimer's disease is also controversial. In general, studies suggest that antioxidants such as vitamin E may reduce the risk of Alzheimer's disease but do not appear to improve cognitive performance in individuals with moderate or severe Alzheimer's (e.g., Laurin et al., 2004; Tabet, Birks, and Evans, 2000; Zandi et al., 2004). Based on other animal studies, Sung and colleagues (2004) suggested that antioxidants may be beneficial only in the early stages of Alzheimer's disease when oxidative stress is likely to contribute to the development of the disease. Anti-inflammatory medications have also been investigated in the treatment of Alzheimer's disease based on evidence that a chronic inflammatory response may contribute to the disease's pathology (Hoozemans, Rozemuller, Veerhuis, & Eikelenboom, 2001). Aisen and Davis (1994) suggested that low doses of corticosteroids (e.g. prednisone), anti-inflammatories (e.g., indomethacin, ibruprofen), and perhaps colchicine may be effective in slowing the progression of the disease. In a later study, however, Aisen et al. (2000) found that a low-dose regimen of prednisone was not effective in the treatment of Alzheimer's disease and, in a recent review of the anti-inflammatory literature, Eikelenboom and van Gool (2004) concluded that anti-inflammatory medications may be useful in lowering the risk but not in the treatment of the disease.

In addition to medications designed to improve cognitive skills, patients with Alzheimer's disease are sometimes prescribed antipsychotic (e.g., seroquel, zyprexa) and anticonvulsant (e.g., tegretol, depakene) medications to help improve behavioral symptoms such as hallucinations, agitation, and violent outbursts. De Deyn et al. (2004), for example, recently reported that the antipsychotic medication olanzapine significantly decreased psychosis and behavioral disturbances in Alzheimer's patients. Lagnaoui et al. (2003) found that 20% of patients with Alzheimer's disease had been prescribed antianxiety medications within a 3-month period and noted that these medications often have a greater risk of adverse side effects (e.g., increased confusion, dependency) in such patients.

Future Treatments

In a recent review, Samuels and Grossman (2003) suggested that future approaches to the treatment of Alzheimer's disease may include antioxidants, neurotrophic factors, glutamate modulators, tau protein modulators, and heavy metal chelators. Recent research suggests that Alzheimer's disease may be characterized by increased levels of metals such as copper and iron and these metals may interact with amyloid β and result in substances such as hydrogen peroxide, which is toxic to brain cells (Maynard et al., 2002). A chelator is a substance that binds to and removes a particular metal, which, in the case of Alzheimer's disease, conceivably could be used to target amyloid β plaques. Vaccines that target amyloid protein buildup or tau overexpression may also prove successful in the treatment of Alzheimer's disease. Tohda, Tamura, and Komatsu (2003) reported that Zokumei-to, a formula composed of traditional Chinese and Japanese herbal drugs, increased synaptophysin levels in mice that had previously been injected with amyloid β. They speculated that Zokumei-to may also be able to reconstruct synaptic connections in patients with Alzheimer's disease. Given that amyloid β plaques can trigger an immune response that leads to inflammation, neuronal loss, and further plaque formation, scientists developed a vaccination that induced an anti-amyloid β immune response. Results indicated that the vaccination slowed the progression of Alzheimer's disease, but after some patients experienced severe negative reactions including meningoencephalitis, the trials were terminated (Broytman & Malter, 2004; Ferrer et al., 2004). Experimental studies with other animals such as rats have found that chronic nasal administration of amyloid β peptide can decrease amyloid β deposits in the brain (Weiner et al., 2000). Webster and colleagues (2000) have suggested that inhibition of proteins that bind to amyloid β may help to prevent the formation of plaques, and Sigurdsson et al. (2000) have demonstrated that amyloid β lesions can be reversed in the brains of mice with injections of certain peptides. Atwood et al. (2003), however, cautioned that amyloid-beta protein also has trophic properties and excessive removal or inhibition of this protein may increase—rather than decrease—oxidative stress to neurons. Other studies with mice have found that calorie-restricted diets can protect neurons in the hippocampus against death, even when the mice are carriers of genetic mutations (e.g., presenilin 1) associated with Alzheimer's disease (Zhu, Guo, & Mattson, 1999). Preliminary research also suggests that the saliva from Gila monsters contains a chemical ("gilatide") that may enhance memory function in humans, including those with Alzheimer's disease (Beck, in press; Haile et al., 2001).

Summary

Dementia of Alzheimer's type is the most common type of dementia, estimated to affect 11% of males and 14% of females by age 85. Alzheimer's disease is characterized by multiple cognitive impairments including memory loss and cognitive disturbances that cause significant problems in social and occupational functioning. Familial and twin studies support a genetic component of Alzheimer's disease in both late- and early-onset cases. Although no specific gene has been identified for late-onset Alzheimer's disease, cases of early-onset Alzheimer's disease (<65 years) are associated with a variety of genetic mutations, most frequently involving the APP gene. A number of risk and protective factors are associated with the disease. Neuroanatomically, Alzheimer's disease is characterized by plaques and tangles made up of amyloid beta and tau proteins. The disease is also associated with degeneration of acetylcholine-releasing neurons—particularly in the basal forebrain—accompanied by cognitive decline. Collectively, these findings support a physiological basis for Alzheimer's disease. The precise mechanisms that contribute to the disease and the ways in which these mechanisms may interact to contribute to the progression of Alzheimer's disease, however, are not yet understood. Acetylcholinesterase inhibitors are the most effective treatment to date, but these medications treat only the symptoms and do not slow the progress of the disease.

PARKINSON'S DISEASE

Parkinson's disease was first defined in 1871 by James Parkinson, who referred to it as "shaking palsy" (Parkinson, 1871). Parkinson's disease is a progressive neurological disorder characterized by resting tremor, rigidity, postural instability, and slowed ability to start and continue movements (*bradykinesia*; Guttman, Kish, & Furukawa, 2003). Research indicates that men are at 1.5 times greater risk for Parkinson's disease than women (Wooten, Currie, Bovbjerg, Lee, & Patrie, 2004). It is estimated that 1 in 100 people over 65 years of age and 1 in 10 people over age 80 have Parkinson's disease although cross-cultural studies have reported differences in prevalence rates (Strickland and Bertoni, 2004). For example, Sanchez and colleagues (2004) reported a prevalence rate of 176 cases per 100,000 in people over age 50 in Antioquia; Columbia; Caradoc-Davies and colleagues (1992) reported a prevalence rate of 76 per 100,000 in New Zealand; while Woo, Lau, Ziea, and Chan (2004) reported a .5% prevalence among those age 55 and older in Hong Kong. Claveria et al. (2002) found 9 cases per 1,000 in individuals age 40 and over in Cantalejo, Spain, a figure that is substantially higher than other studies. Schrag, Ben-Shlomo, and Quinn (2002) assessed the prevalence of Parkinson's disease in London and found that 20% of patients who had received medical attention had not been diagnosed with the disease when the diagnosis was warranted, and approximately 15% had been inaccurately diagnosed with the disease. Twelves, Perkins, and Counsell (2003) noted that the methods used in epidemiological studies vary considerably and recommended that minimal scientific criteria be developed to help establish more accurate prevalence rates for Parkinson's disease. Interestingly, Ebersbach and colleagues (2000) found sociocultural differences in gait among patients with Parkinson's disease in Berlin, Germany, and Innsbruck, Austria. Specifically, patients with Parkinson's disease from Berlin had significantly faster walking speeds than patients and control subjects from Austria.

Individuals with Parkinson's disease often have neuropsychological deficits such as impairments in executive functioning and language processing (Grossman, 1999). Dementia occurs in approximately 20 to 60% of individuals with Parkinson's disease (DSM IV-TR, 2000). Studies also suggest that patients' awareness of their body in space may diminish with the progression of the disease. Maschke, Gomez, Tuite, and Konczak (2003), for example, found only 55% of patients with Parkinson's disease were able to correctly identify forearm displacement compared to 75% of control subjects. Individuals with Parkinson's disease are at high risk for psychiatric problems: Studies indicate that at least one psychiatric symptom is reported in approximately 61% of Parkinson's patients (Aarsland et al., 1999). It has been estimated that 30 to 40% of patients with the disease suffer from depression (Cummings, 1992; Slaughter et al., 2001), for which most do not receive treatment (Weintraub, Moberg, Duda, Katz, & Stern, 2003). According to Schrag, Jahanshahi, and Quinn (2001), depression is associated with advancing severity of Parkinson's disease, occurrence of falls, recent disease deterioration, and the patient's negative perceptions of the disease. Patients with Parkinson's disease and depression are believed to have greater deficits in frontal lobe functioning as well as dopaminergic and noradrenergic systems relative to Parkinson's disease patients without depression (Cummings, 1992). Glosser (2001) suggested that depression in patients with Parkinson's disease results from multiple factors including reduced levels of serotonin and disruptions in dopamine-rich reward-oriented pathways extending to and from the midbrain to the frontal regions. Changes in dopamine pathways are also associated with deficits in processing emotionally laden facial expressions in Parkinson's patients (Dujardin et al., 2004).

Anxiety disorders such as generalized anxiety disorder and panic disorder are common in Parkinson's disease (Lauterbach, Freeman, & Vogel, 2003). Maia, Pinto, Barbosa, Menezes, and Miguel (2003) reported the incidence of OCD was not higher in patients with Parkinson's disease relative to control subjects, but Kurlan (2004) reported on six patients who developed pathological gambling as well as cleaning, rearranging, and ordering rituals. Sleep problems such as difficulty falling asleep, frequent waking, and excessive daytime fatigue and sleepiness are also common with the disease (Lai & Siegel, 2003; Pal et al., 2004). Nomura et al. (2003) found a relationship between the presence of visual hallucinations and a higher amount of stage 1 REM sleep in patients with Parkinson's disease. Approximately 30% of Parkinson's patients develop psychotic symptoms, most frequently visual hallucinations (D'Souza, Gupta, Alldrick, & Sastry, 2003; Holroyd, Currie, & Wooten, 2001). Patients who take antipsychotic medications have a better prognosis compared to patients with Parkinson's disease with untreated psychotic symptoms (Factor et al., 2003). Menza, Robertson-Hoffman, and Bonapace (1993) suggested that depression and anxiety are related to the underlying neurophysiological changes of Parkinson's disease and are unlikely to be due to psychological reactions to the disease. Late-stage Parkinson's disease is associated with loss of autonomy and self-esteem, social isolation, and substantial deterioration in both physical and mental health (Calne, 2003). Recent studies have found that vascular disease such as hypertension and stroke tends to aggravate the severity of Parkinson's disease (Papapetropoulos et al., 2004). In a recent review, Menza (2000) noted that individuals with specific personality traits (e.g., inflexibility, industriousness, lack of novelty seeking) may be at increased risk for Parkinson's disease although these findings are only correlational in nature.

Genetic Findings

Family and twin studies support the existence of genetic risk factors in the development of Parkinson's disease, particularly in cases of rare, early-onset Parkinsonism (Gaser, 2001). For example, the parkin gene on chromosome 6 and the SPR gene on chromosome 2 have been linked to the development of the disease in individuals younger than 40 years (Karamohamed et al., 2003; Scott et al., 2001), and regions on chromosomes 5, 8, and 17 have been linked to late-onset Parkinson's disease (Scott et al., 2001). Toft and Aasly (2004) recently noted a region of chromosome 1 was linked to late-onset Parkinson's disease in an Icelandic population, and

Valente et al. (2004) also linked a rare form of familial Parkinson's disease to chromosome 1 in patients from Italy. As West and Maidment (2004) noted, however, genetic mutations that result in Parkinson's disease exist in only a small number of individuals; in most cases, genetic factors have not been identified. Twin studies have produced mixed findings, with some studies reporting higher concordance rates in monozygotic than dizygotic twins. Laihinen et al. (2000) used PET to study dopaminergic functioning in controls and four monozygotic and four dizygotic pairs of twins. Each pair consisted of a symptomatic and asymptomatic twin. Results indicated reduced activity in the putamen of the twin pairs, even in the asymptomatic twins relative to control subjects. The researchers speculated that a preclinical stage of Parkinson's disease may exist even when individuals are symptom-free. Interestingly, Tanner et al. (2002) found risk of Parkinson's disease was inversely related to cigarette smoking in monozygotic and dizygotic twins, suggesting that it may have a protective effect.

Other studies have focused on specific genetic mutations that may be linked to Parkinson's disease such as polymorphisms of the parkin gene on chromosome 6, the a-synuclein gene on chromosome 4, and others such as the ACE, Tau, monoamine oxidase, COMT, and Saitohin genes (e.g., Costa et al., 1997; Lee, Kim, Cho, Lim, & Rinne, 2002; Levecque et al., 2004; Lin, Yueh, Chang, & Lin, 2002; Pastor et al., 2000; Zarranz et al., 2004). These mutations are believed to interfere with normal protein functioning and therefore contribute to the degeneration of dopaminergic neurons in the striatum. Xu and colleagues (2002) recently found that a polymorphism of the Nurr1 gene, a gene important in the development and sustenance of dopamine neurons, was significantly higher in patients with Parkinson's disease relative to control subjects. Le Couteur, Leighton, McCann, and Pond (1997) and Kim, Kim, Kim, and Cha (2000) found a rare polymorphism of the dopamine transporter gene was associated with Parkinson's disease, while Oliveri et al. (2000) reported that polymorphisms of the dopamine D2 receptor increased the risk of the disease. It is important to note that not all studies have found an association between genetic mutations and Parkinson's disease (e.g., de Silva et al., 2002; Spadafora et al., 2003). More research is needed to investigate and replicate these genetic findings. In fact, Healy et al. (2004) reported that polymorphisms may actually *decrease* susceptibility of developing Parkinson's disease. Lin et al. (2003) suggested that a specific polymorphism of the dopamine transporter gene may reduce the risk of Parkinson's disease in males but not females. Olson (2000) as well as Warner and Schapira (2003) and others stress that for most cases there is a complex interaction between genetic and environmental factors that leads to the disease.

Anatomical Findings

Parkinson's disease is a progressive neurological disorder characterized by resting tremor, rigidity, postural instability, and slowed ability to start and continue movements (bradykinesia; Guttman, Kish, & Furukawa, 2003). It is important to note that movement is a complex process that involves coordination among numerous brain regions and motor pathways. For example, several descending pathways including the ventromedial pathway originate at the level of the midbrain or motor cortex and traverse through the brain and brain stem to innervate specific body parts (Figs. 4.2 and 4.3). The lateral corticospinal tract, for example, begins at the motor cortex and terminates in the spinal cord and is responsible for movement of fingers, hands, and arms (Fig. 4.3). Other ascending and descending pathways are involved in movement of the face and tongue (Fig. 4.4). Anatomically, Parkinson's disease is characterized by degeneration of dopaminergic neurons in the substantia nigra and to some degree in the ventral tegmental area (Fig. 4.5). Depending on the severity of the disease, most motor pathways are affected. The cause of the degeneration of neurons is not completely understood but is believed to be due to

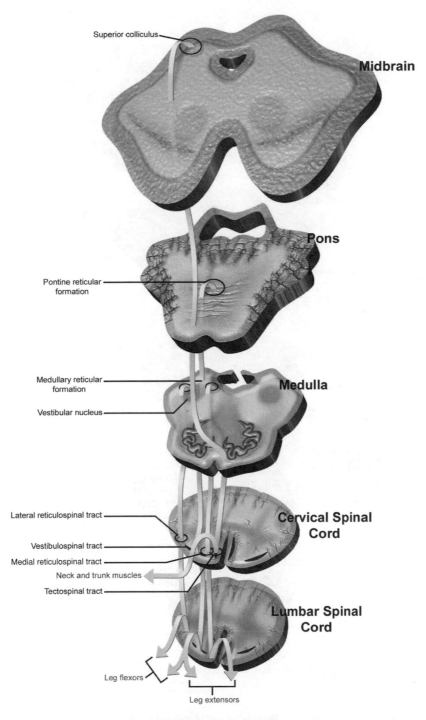

FIG. 4.2. Ventromedial pathway. Copyright Blausen Medical Communications. Reproduced by permission.

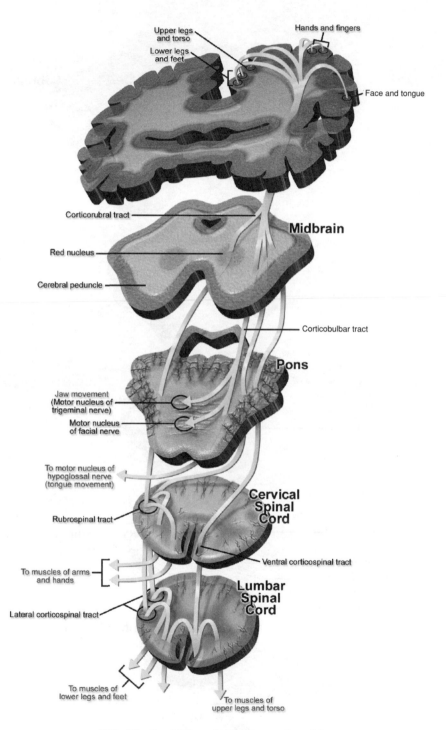

FIG. 4.3. Descending motor pathways. Copyright
Blausen Medical Communications. Reproduced by permission.

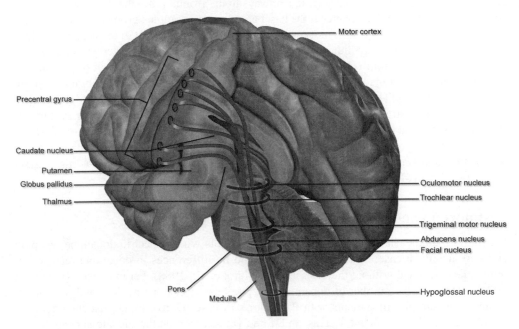

Corticobulbar Tract

Motor cortex

Precentral gyrus

Caudate nucleus

Putamen

Globus pallidus

Thalmus

Oculomotor nucleus

Trochlear nucleus

Trigeminal motor nucleus

Abducens nucleus

Facial nucleus

Pons

Medulla

Hypoglossal nucleus

FIG. 4.4.   Corticobulbar motor pathway. Copyright Blausen Medical Communications. Reproduced by permission.

Parkinson's Disease

Non-Parkinson's

red nucleus

reticular formation

cerebral aqueduct

Substantia nigra

Parkinson's

Superior colliculus

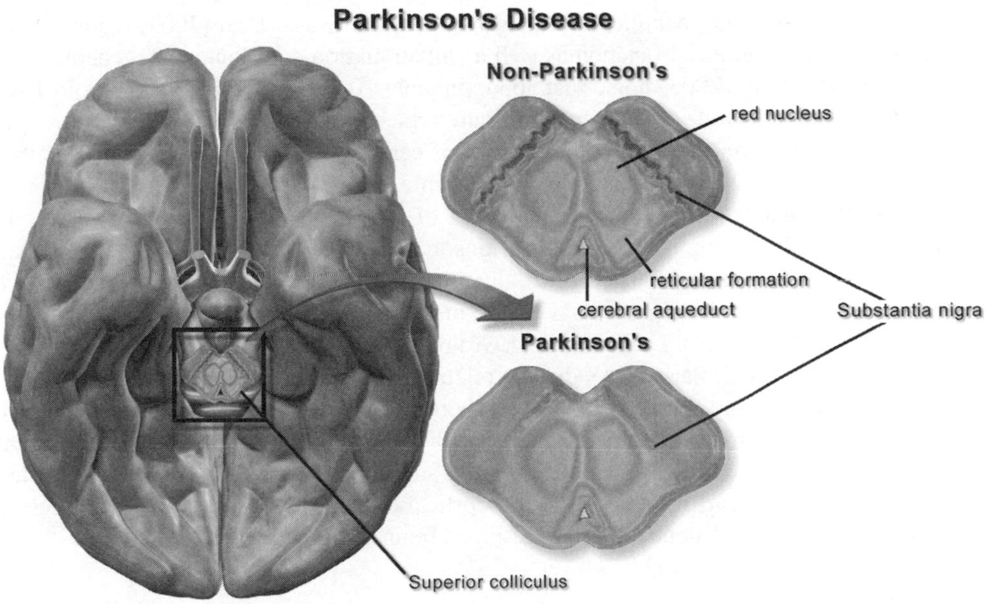

FIG. 4.5.   Location of substantia nigra and degeneration of cells characteristic of Parkinson's disease. Copyright Blausen Medical Communications. Reproduced by permission.

several interacting factors including genetic and environmental. The degeneration and death of dopaminergic neurons lead to dopamine reductions in the striatum (putamen, caudate nucleus, and nucleus accumbens) and projecting pathways to the frontal lobes that form parallel loops or circuits. As discussed in chapter 1, the basal ganglia are a complex group of subcortical cell bodies that play a critical role in movement. The basal ganglia consist of the caudate nucleus, putamen, and the globus pallidus. The caudate nucleus and putamen together are known as the striatum. The striatum receives input from the cortex and other structures (e.g., thalamus and amygdala) and projects information to widespread regions such as the brain stem and the prefrontal cortex. The nucleus accumbens is a group of cell bodies located adjacent to the striatum. The nigrostriatal system extends from the substantia nigra to the striatum. Parkinson's disease is associated with degeneration of dopaminergic cell bodies of the substantia nigra that affects functioning of the nigrostriatal system and results in slowness of movement and rigidity. Medication and surgical procedures for Parkinson's disease typically target the nigrostriatal region (see Kultas-Ilinsky & Ilinsky, 2000 for a review).

Postmortem and MRI Findings

Postmortem studies have produced contradictory results with respect to dopamine receptors and Parkinson's disease: increased, decreased, and no differences in dopamine receptors in individuals with and without the disease (e.g., Pierot et al., 1988). For example, Rinne et al. (1991) measured the number of dopamine receptors in the caudate nucleus and putamen in postmortem samples of patients with Parkinson's disease relative to age-matched controls. Results revealed a significant decrease in D1 and D2 receptors in the caudate nucleus but not the putamen, and age was not related to receptor densities. Studies have also reported decreased dopamine receptors in the cerebellum of patients with Parkinson's disease (Hurley, Mash, & Jenner, 2003). Based on postmortem studies, Fitzmaurice et al. (2003) have suggested that deficiencies in antioxidants such as glutathione in Parkinson's patients may contribute to the degeneration of dopamine neurons in the nigrostriatial pathways. Beal (2003) reported that impairment of mitochondrial function as well as inflammation contribute to degeneration of neurons. Mandel et al. (2003) noted that approximately 70–75% of dopamine neurons have died by the time Parkinson's disease symptoms are typically diagnosed.

MRI studies have revealed different patterns of cerebral atrophy depending on whether the disease is accompanied by dementia. For example, Burton and colleagues (2004) found reduced gray matter volume in the frontal lobes of patients with Parkinson's disease and no dementia relative to control subjects. Parkinson's patients with dementia, however, had significantly greater regions of atrophy including the occipital lobes. Other MRI studies have found hippocampal atrophy in patients with Parkinson's disease compared to control subjects (e.g., Camicioli et al., 2003). Laakso et al. (1996) reported significantly smaller hippocampal volumes in patients with Parkinson's disease relative to those with Alzheimer's disease and control subjects. Recently, Almeida et al. (2003) compared whole brain and caudate volume in subjects with Parkinson's disease and Alzheimer's disease and found that atrophy was present only in the latter group. Collectively, these findings suggest that structural changes associated with Parkinson's disease are more specific to subcortical structures, but as the disease progresses and is accompanied by dementia, more widespread brain atrophy is observed.

Neuroimaging Findings

A number of neuroimaging studies have substantiated a reduction in the density of dopamine transporters in individuals with Parkinson's disease, and this reduction is correlated with severity of symptoms (e.g., Davis et al., 2003; Seibyl et al., 1995). Reduction in dopamine transporters is not unique to Parkinson's disease, however, and some studies suggest that the reduction may be greater in other diseases of movement (e.g., Varrone et al., 2001). Studies consistently indicate that the reduction of dopamine transporters is greater in the putamen than the caudate in patients with Parkinson's disease, and greater reductions are found in the striatum contralateral to the side of the body with the most symptoms (Innis et al., 1993; Marek et al., 1996). Research also suggests that relatives of patients with Parkinson's disease who are greater risk of the disorder show decreased striatal uptake compared to control subjects, even when they are symptom-free (e.g., Maraganore et al., 1999). Although it is known that Parkinson's disease is characterized by a progessive loss of dopaminergic neurons in the striatum and that dopamine agonists can dramatically improve symptoms during the early stages of the disease, the mechanism by which this improvement occurs is uncertain. Tedroff et al. (1999) hypothesized that loss of dopamine-producing cells may be greater in the putamen and caudate and used PET to measure dopamine synthesis capacity in subjects with Parkinson's disease and control subjects. Results revealed a curious finding: Subjects with Parkinson's disease had a 198% rate of presynaptic dopamine activity in the dorsal putamen compared to control subjects. The researchers speculated that this increase reflects a compensatory response in reaction to the death of dopamine neurons in the substantia nigra.

Regional cerebral blood flow studies have found both reductions and increased activity in patients with Parkinson's disease in various regions relative to control subjects (Abe et al., 2003; Firbank, Colloby, Burn, McKeith, & O'Brien, 2003). For example, Turner and colleagues (2003) found increased blood flow and involvement of more cortical regions in patients with Parkinson's disease while performing eye tracking or limb movement tasks. The authors speculated that patients may recruit more cortical regions as a compensatory response to the degeneration of motor systems that accompany the disease. Playford et al. (1992) also found differential activation of brain regions in subjects with and without Parkinson's disease during motor tasks, and reported that those with the disease had impaired activation of subcortical as well as prefrontal and motor cortices. Lozza, Marie, and Baron (2002) used PET to measure glucose metabolism in patients with Parkinson's disease and found tremor was negatively correlated with activity in the putamen and cerebellum while rigidity was positively correlated with activity in the putamen. Kassubek and colleagues (2001) reported increased glucose metabolism in the ventrolateral region of the thalamus of patients with Parkinson's disease; this finding was positively correlated with degree of resting tremor. These findings were consistent with those reported by Hallett and Dubinsky (1993). Collectively, these findings support differential patterns of brain activity in patients with Parkinson's disease and indicate that more brain regions are recruited to perform cognitive and motor tasks compared to control subjects.

Neurotransmitter Findings

A number of studies have measured monoamine concentrations in the cerebral spinal fluid (CSF) of patients with Parkinson's disease and have found a significant relationship between severity of symptoms and monoamine metabolite reductions. For example, Tohgi et al. (1993) reported that reduced levels in the dopamine metabolites homovanillic acid were associated with rigidity, akinesia, and dementia, while reduced levels of norepinephrine were associated with freezing of gait. Tremor was not associated with metabolite levels, however. Cheng, Kuo, Chia, and Dryhurst (1996) also found lower levels of dopamine metabolites in patients with Parkinson's disease, which Engelborghs, Marescau, and De Deyn (2003) have suggested likely reflects dopaminergic cell loss.

In addition to disturbances in the dopaminergic system, other neurotransmitter systems are believed to play a role in the pathophysiology of Parkinson's disease. For example, Molina et al. (1997) found reduced levels of amino acids in patients with Parkinson's disease and suggested that these patients may have a dysfunction of amino acid transport from the blood to the brain. Studies have also compared patients with Parkinson's disease with and without depression and have found significantly lower serotonin levels in those with comorbid depression (Mayeux, Stern, Cote, & Williams, 1984). In a addition to degeneration of dopaminergic neurons, Kerenyi et al. (2003) found reduced density of serotonin transporters in the caudate, putamen, and striatum of patients with Parkinson's disease, using PET. Chia, Cheng, and Kuo (1993) reported that CSF epinephrine levels were higher in patients with Parkinson's disease than control subjects, while Eldrup and colleagues (1995) found epinephrine levels were reduced.

As mentioned previously, Parkinson's disease is often accompanied by dementia and psychosis, and the loss of cholinergic neurons in the nucleus basalis of Meynert is believed to play a critical role in the emergence of cognitive impairments (Bosboom, Stoffers, & Wolters, 2003). For example, many studies have found a relationship between greater severity of cognitive impairment and degree of reduction in acetylcholine-related activity in patients with Parkinson's disease as well as postmortem samples (e.g., Kuhl et al., 1996; Mattila et al., 2001; Whitehouse et al., 1988). Burghaus and colleagues (2003) recently found a significant decrease in acetylcholine binding sites and specific subunits of the nicotinic receptor at the level of the cortex in patients with Parkinson's disease, and similar results were reported by Pimlott and colleagues (2004). As reviewed by Zhou, Wilson, and Dani (2003), the striatum consists of a dense mingling of multiple types of neurotransmitter receptors including dopamine and cholinergic. Given these findings, studies have explored whether cholinesterase inhibitors are beneficial in the treatment of Parkinson's disease and, indeed, a number of studies have found improvements in cognitive impairments and psychotic symptoms in patients treated with these drugs (e.g., Leroi et al., 2004). Minett et al. (2003), however, recently discovered that withdrawal of cholinesterase inhibitors may result in acute cognitive and behavioral deterioration. Other neurotransmitters such as GABA and glutamate have also been implicated in Parkinson's disease, primarily due to their role in regulating dopamine release in the substantia nigra and surrounding structures (Cobb & Abercrombie, 2003; Plaitakis & Shashidharan, 2000; Pralong, Magistretti, & Stoop, 2002).

INTERVENTIONS FOR PARKINSON'S DISEASE

Pharmacological Interventions

Olson (2000) aptly noted that there are three main approaches to treating Parkinson's disease: replacing dopamine, replacing dopamine releasing neurons via transplantations, and halting neuronal loss. Today, the main form of treatment is pharmacological to increase dopamine production (levodopa) or to mimic the effects of dopamine at the level of the receptor (dopamine agonists). During the 1950s, Carlsson et al. (1957) demonstrated that treatment with levodopa (L-Dopa) improved Parkinsonlike symptoms induced in other animals. Today, levodopa is the most frequently used medication for Parkinson's disease and is converted by cells to dopamine. Approximately 95% of patients show a moderate to very good response to levodopa, but given that dopamine is increased throughout the brain and not only the striatum, it is associated with a number of unpleasant side effects (e.g., involuntary movements, psychosis, nausea; Webster, 2001). Dopamine agonists such as pramipexole (mirapex), pergolide (permax), and ropinirole (requip) that attach to postsynaptic receptors are also used to treat the disease, but are most effective in combination with drugs that promote the synthesis and release of dopamine (Webster, 2001). Although these medications have been found to reduce dyskinesia, their mode of action is not completely understood. Linazasoro and colleagues (1999) used PET to measure the density of postsynaptic dopmaine receptors (D2) after 6 months of treatment with a dopamine agonist (pergolide) in five patients with Parkinson's disease. Results revealed a reduction in the putamen and caudate following treatment, which the authors speculated may have been due to downregulation of receptors. Side effects associated with dopamine agonists include headache, gastrointestinal problems, hypotension, psychosis, and sleep disturbances.

Other drugs that prevent the breakdown of dopamine such as monoamine oxidase inhibitors (MAOIs, e.g., selegiline/eldepryl) and catechol-o-methyl transferase (COMT) inhibitors (e.g., entacapone/comtan) are also used to treat Parkinson's disease. A serious side effect associated with MAOIs is hypertension; users of COMT inhibitors may experience nausea, headaches, confusion, gastrointestinal problems, and involuntary muscle movements. For mild Parkinson's symptoms, amantadine (symmetrel) is sometimes used, which is thought to increase the release of dopamine from presynaptic neurons. Side effects associated with this drug include dizziness, insomnia, nausea, sleep disturbances, and gastrointestinal problems (Physicians Desk Reference, 2003).

Surgery, Deep Brain Stimulation, and ECT

According to Eskandar and colleagues (2003), there has been a shift from ablative procedures to deep brain stimulation in the surgical treatment of Parkinson's disease. For example, in 1996 0% of surgical procedures involved placement of brain stimulators, a figure that rose to 88% in 2000! In terms of ablative procedures, a pallidotomy involves destruction of part of the globus pallidus that is overactive in Parkinson's patients. A pallidotomy can be performed unilaterally or bilaterally and has been found to improve unwanted muscular contractions as well as rigidity. Skalabrin, Laws, and Bennett (1998) found that patients who received a pallidotomy responded more favorably to levodopa after the surgery, based on their performance on timed motor tasks and additional forms of evaluation. An uncommon side effect associated with levodopa treatment as well as pallidotomy surgery for Parkinson's disease is hypersexuality, presumably due to increased dopaminergic functioning (Mendez, O'Connor, & Lim, 2004). A thalamotomy involves destruction of part of the thalamus and has been found to improve tremor and, to a lesser extent, rigidity and unwanted excessive motor movements (Krack, Poepping, Weinert, Schrader, & Deuschl, 2000). The surgical approaches for pallidotomy and thalamotomy vary, and most patients respond well to the surgery (Niranjan, Jawahar, Kondziolka, & Lunsford, 1999). Recently, a gamma knife radiosurgery method has been developed that preliminary studies suggest is just as effective and safer than other thalamotomy methods (Ohye, Shibazaki, Zhang, & Andou, 2002; Young et al., 2000).

In contrast to ablative surgery, deep brain stimulation does not involve destruction of tissue. As discussed in chapter 3, a small lead with an electrode is inserted in specific target areas of the brain (i.e., globus pallidus, subthalamic nucleus) (Mazzone, 2003). The procedure can be performed under general or local anesthesia (Maltête et al., 2004), and the frequencies at which the stimulation is delivered can vary (Foffani et al., 2003). The lead and electrode remain in the brain and are connected to a programmed, battery-operated pulse generator implanted in the chest. The generator sends impulses directly to the target region of the brain. Many studies have substantiated that DBS improve tremors characteristic of movement disorders such as Parkinson's disease (Obeso et al., 2001; Vingerhoets et al., 2002). Interestingly, Ceballos-Baumann and colleagues (1999) found deep brain stimulation in the subthalamic nucleus resulted in decreased rCBF in the primary motor cortex of Parkinson's patients. A recent study by Pinto et al. (2004) supported these findings and also reported increased rCBF levels in the cerebellum, premotor cortex, and prefrontal cortex prior to subthalamic nucleus stimulation. Thobois and colleagues (2002), however, found that subthalamic stimulation increased rCBF in the putamen, thalamus, and prefrontal cortex of patients with Parkinson's disease. Long-term follow-up studies of deep brain stimulation have found sustained improvement in motor functions up to 2 years after the stimulation (Kleiner-Fisman et al., 2003). Anderson and Mullins (2003), however, reported patients with Parkinson's disease and dementia may experience further declines in cognitive functions following deep brain stimulation. In contrast, Gironell et al. (2003) found that neither bilateral or unilateral pallidotomy nor subthalamic brain stimulation had adverse effects on cognitive functioning.

Electroconvulsive therapy has also been found to improve motor symptoms of Parkinson's disease (Kennedy, Mittal, & O'Jile, 2003). According to a study of seven Parkinson's patients (Douyon, Serby, Klutchko, & Rotrosen, 1989), ECT resulted in significant motor improvements, especially in older patients. Recently, Shulman (2003) reported that ECT was associated improvement of psychotic symptoms as well as motor symptoms in patients with Parkinson's disease. Balldin and colleagues (1981) reported that ECT was particularly effective with patients who had responded inconsistently to medication. A number of studies have suggested that ECT should be continued in such cases (e.g., Aarsland, Larsen, Waage, & Langeveld, 1997; Fall & Granerus, 1999).

Neurotrophins and Transplantations

Numerous studies have discovered a reduction of brain-derived neurotrophic factor (BDNF) in several brain regions (e.g., substantia nigra, caudate, putamen, frontal cortex, cerebellum) of individuals with Parkinson's disease (e.g., Murer, Yan, & Raiman-Vozari, 2001; Parain et al., 1999). As discussed in chapter 1, BDNF is a neurotrophin that promotes the survival of neurons in the central nervous system. According to Howells et al. (2000), the reduction of BDNF is due in part to loss of dopamine neurons that produce the neurotrophin and because surviving dopaminergic neurons produce less BDNF than other types of neurons. Mogi and colleagues (1999) also found reductions in another type of neurotrophin—nerve growth factor (NGF)—in several brain regions of patients with Parkinson's disease compared to control subjects. They speculated that these neurotrophins are likely involved in the pathogenesis of the disease, although the direction of this relationship remains unclear. Momose and colleagues (2002), however, recently found that polymorphisms of the BDNF gene occur more frequently in patients with Parkinson's disease than controls, which supports a causal role for abnormalities of BDNF in the pathogenesis of the disease. Researchers have begun to explore whether delivery of neurotrophins to degenerating nigrostriatal neurons can influence cellular function. Kordower et al. (2000), for example, injected a neurotrophin (glial cell line derived neurotrophic factor) into the substantia nigra and striatum of other animals who had Parkinsonlike symptoms, and discovered regeneration of neurons in these regions. Georgievska and colleagues (2002) reported similar findings with rats. Although these findings appear promising, studies with human subjects are needed to explore the potential neurotrophic effects on patients with Parkinson's disease.

According to Clarkson and Freed (1999), since 1988 studies have been conducted on the efficacy of tranplantation of human fetal dompamine cells into the brains of individuals suffering from Parkinson's disease. Lindvall and colleagues (1990) at the University of Lund, Sweden, were among the first to transplant dopamine neurons from human fetuses (8 to 9 weeks gestational age) into the putamen of patients with severe Parkinson's disease and document behavioral improvement that correlated with increased dopamine synthesis in the transplanted area. Lindvall et al. (1994) followed up two patients with Parkinson's disease 3 years after the transplantation and reported that the dopaminergic neurons continued to survive and a continued reduction of clinical symptoms was observed. Sawle et al. (1992) also reported successful outcomes with two patients with Parkinson's disease who had received fetal tissue implants in the putamen. Mendez et al. (2002) recommended that fetal tissue be transplanted bilaterally into more than one area (i.e., putamen and substantia nigra) to improve the likelihood of greater clinical improvement, and preliminary findings by Mendez et al. with three patients support this hypothesis. In 1992, Freed and colleagues implanted fetal dopaminergic cells into the caudate and putamen of two patients with Parkinson's disease, and in the putamen of five patients. Results indicated that all seven patients reported improvement in symptoms 3 to 12 months following surgery. In 2001, Freed and colleagues randomly assigned 40 patients with severe Parkinson's disease to a transplant or sham-surgery group. Results revealed a significant difference in standardized tests of clinical improvement, with the transplant group performing significantly higher than the sham-surgery group. Results also indicated that younger, but not older, patients who had received the transplant demonstrated significant improvement relative to the sham-surgery group.

Despite these encouraging findings, other studies have not supported the efficacy of fetal transplants in the treatment of Parkinson's disease. Olanow et al. (2003), for example, recently conducted a 24-month double-blind, placebo-controlled trial of fetal bilateral transplantation. Findings revealed that 56% of the transplanted patients developed dyskinesia that persisted when dopamine-related medications were ceased. In addition, patients who received the transplant did not differ from patients who did not receive the transplant in scores on the Unified Parkinson's Disease Rating Scale. Freed et al. (2001) also reported that a significant percentage (15%) of transplant patients had developed persistent dyskinesias following the surgery. Ma et al. (2002) suggested that dyskinesias following transplantation surgery result from increased dopaminergic functioning in some, but not all, regions of the striatum. Research also indicates that cognitive performance does not appear to improve during the first year following bilateral fetal transplants (Trott et al., 2003) and that factors such as age of the fetal tissue and patient age may affect the clinical outcome (Freed et al., 2001). In general, fetal transplantation studies suggest that the procedure is generally safe with low morbidity but a significant percentage of patients may experience dyskinesias. Although the results vary, findings indicate that patients often experience short- and long-term clinical benefits of fetal transplant surgery (Hauser et al., 1999). Questions remain about the optimal procedures (i.e., unilateral or bilateral, locations) as well as the potential effects of variables such as fetal and patient age (Freed et al., 2003).

Environmental Factors

Although Parkinson's disease is due to a loss of dopaminergic neurons of the substantia nigra, the cause of the neuron loss remains speculative. As reviewed earlier, studies support a role for genetic factors in early-onset cases of Parkinson's disease, but most cases appear late in life and are not associated with a genetic basis. This finding has led researchers to identify possible environmental factors that might contribute to the disease. For example, Imaizumi (1995) reported the age-adjusted death rate for Parkinson's disease was higher in urban than rural areas in Japan during the years 1979–1985. In addition, the death rate was higher in the southwest than the northeast, and Imaizumi speculated that environmental factors might differ regionally and contribute to the development of Parkinson's disease. Gorell, Peterson, Rybicki, and Johnson (2004) conducted an epidemiological study of risk factors associated with Parkinson's disease and concluded that long-term exposure to lead, copper, and insecticide as well as a family history of the disease were significantly associated with development of Parkinson's disease. A plethora of studies have suggested that exposure to heavy metals and pesticides increases the risk of Parkinson's disease (e.g., Baldereschi et al., 2003; Menegon, Board, Blackburn, Mellick, & Le Couteur, 1998; Priyadarshi, Khuder, Schaub, & Shrivastava, 2000; Tan et al., 2003). Sherer, Betarbet, and Greenamyre (2002) have suggested that exposure to factors such as pesticides may result in oxidative stress and consequently increase the likelihood of neurotoxicity and cellular death, leading to further neurodegeneration.

In addition to genetic, metals, and pesticides, certain lifestyle factors have been associated with increased risk. For example, Abbott et al. (2002) reported a positive relationship between body fat and increased risk of Parkinson's disease, and Abbott et al. (2001) reported that infrequent bowel movements were also associated with an increased risk. Interestingly, a large number of studies have reported that moderate to high caffeine consumption is associated with a significantly lower incidence (e.g., Abbott et al., 2003; Ascherio et al., 2001; Ross et al., 2000). Alcohol and tea consumption are also associated with a lower risk (Checkoway et al., 2002; Ragonese et al., 2003; Tan et al., 2003), as is the presence of domestic animals in the home (Kuopio, Marttila, Helenius, & Rinne, 1999). A robust finding in the literature is that cigarette smoking is inversely associated with the risk of Parkinson's disease (Abbott et al., 2003; Hernan, Takkouche, Caamano-Isorna, & Gestal-Otero, 2002; Preux et al., 2000). Rybicki and colleagues (1999), however, found this finding held true only in subjects without a family history of the disease; it was *positively* associated with Parkinson's disease in those with a family history of Parkinson's disease. Perhaps one of the strongest pieces of evidence that environmental factors can induce Parkinsonism is the documented cases of drug users who rapidly developed the disease after using a substance contaminated with 1-methl-4-phenyl-1,2,3, 6-tetrahydropyridine (MPTP), which destroys the cells of the substantia nigra (Langston & Ballard, 1984; Weingarten, 1988). Overall, environmental factors have been linked to an increased as well as a decreased risk of developing Parkinson's disease. It is likely that genetic and environmental factors interact in a complex fashion that serves to increase or decrease an individual's susceptibility.

SUMMARY

In summary, Parkinson's disease is a progressive neurological disorder characterized by resting tremor, rigidity, postural instability, and slowed ability to start and continue movements (bradykinesia). Research indicates that men are at greater risk (1.5 times) for Parkinson's disease than women. It is estimated that 1 in 100 people over 65 years of age and 1 in 10 people over age 80 have Parkinson's disease although cross-cultural studies have reported differences in prevalence rates. Genetic factors have been implicated in early-onset cases of the disease although most cases have no known genetic basis. Environmental factors such as long-term exposure to heavy metals and pesticides are associated with increased risk of the disease while protective factors may include cigarette smoking and caffeine and alcohol consumption. Based on these findings, it appears as if an interaction between biological and environmental factors contributes to the development of Parkinson's disease. The manner, however, in which biological and environmental factors lead to increased vulnerability of the brain is poorly understood. Levodopa is the primary medication used to treat the symptoms of Parkinson's disease; other drugs such as dopamine agonists and MAO inhibitors are used as well. Ablative surgical procedures and, more recently, deep brain stimulation are often effective at decreasing severe symptoms. Other more controversial treatments include ECT and fetal tissue transplantations.

5

Schizophrenia

The DSM IV-TR (APA, 2000) identifies the following as psychotic disorders: schizophreniform disorder, schizoaffective disorder, delusional disorder, brief psychotic disorder, shared psychotic disorder, psychotic disorder due to a general medical condition, and substance-induced psychotic disorder. Given the large body of research that is available on schizophrenia, this chapter focuses on its pathophysiology and pharmacological treatment.

BACKGROUND, PREVALENCE, AND COURSE

According to the DSM IV-TR criteria (APA, 2000), the essential features of schizophrenia include the presence of both positive and negative symptoms for at least 6 months' duration (see Table 5.1). Positive symptoms reflect a distortion or excess of perceptions while negative symptoms reflect restrictions in the range and intensity of emotional expression, thought, and language and in the production of goal-directed behavior. Positive symptoms include hallucinations, delusions, disorganized thought and language, and grossly disorganized behavior. Hallucinations are distorted sensory perceptions that may involve any of the senses, although auditory hallucinations are by far the most common. Delusions include distorted, exaggerated thinking and erroneous beliefs. The most common are persecutory delusions. Disorganized thinking in schizophrenia is characterized by incoherence, tangentiality, or frequent changes in thought and expression of ideas. Grossly disorganized behavior may be manifested in lack of goal-directed behavior or unpredictable agitation. Negative symptoms include the absence of normal emotional expression—flat affect, lack of behavior, and social withdrawal. It is important to note that there is considerable heterogeneity of symptoms across individuals; symptoms may vary, however, by age and gender. Psychotic symptoms have also been found to be influenced by cultural factors such as ethnicity and religion (David, 1999). Positive and negative symptoms are not unique to schizophrenia and are sometimes present in disorders such as Parkinson's and Alzheimer diseases and temporal lobe epilepsy (Getz et al., 2002).

The current DSM IV-TR (APA, 2000) identifies five characteristic symptoms of schizophrenia and five subtypes. According to the DSM IV-TR, the subtypes have limited value in

TABLE 5.1

Diagnostic Criteria for Schizophrenia (DSM IV-TR, 2000)

1. *Characteristic symptoms:* Two (or more) of the following, each present for a significant portion of time during a 1-month period (or less if successfully treated):
   1) delusions
   2) hallucinations
   3) disorganized speech (e.g., frequent derailment or incoherence)
   4) grossly disorganized or catatonic behavior
   5) negative symptoms, i.e., affective flattening, alogia, or avolition
      Note: Only one Criterion A symptom is required if delusions are bizarre or hallucinations consist of a voice keeping up a running commentary on the person's behavior or thoughts, or two or more voices conversing with each other.
2. *Social/occupational dysfunction:* For a significant portion of the time since the onset of the disturbance, one or more major areas of functioning such as work, interpersonal relations, or self-care are markedly below the level achieved prior to the onset (or when the onset is in childhood or adolescence, failure to achieve expected level of interpersonal, academic, or occupational achievement).
3. *Duration:* Continuous signs of the disturbance persist for at least 6 months. This 6-month period must include at least 1 month of symptoms (or less if successfully treated) that meet Criterion A (i.e., active-phase symptoms) and may include periods of prodromal or residual symptoms. During these prodromal or residual periods, the signs of the disturbance may be manifested by only negative symptoms or two or more symptoms listed in Criterion A present in an attenuated form (e.g., odd beliefs, unusual perceptual experiences).
4. *Schizoaffective and Mood Disorder exclusion:* Schizoaffective Disorder and Mood Disorder With Psychotic Features have been ruled out because either (1) no Major Depressive, Manic, or Mixed Episodes have occurred concurrently with the active-phase symptoms; or (2) if mood episodes have occurred during active phase symptoms, their total duration has been brief relative to the duration of the active and residual periods.
5. *Substance/general medical condition exclusion:* The disturbance is not due to the direct physiological effects of a substance (e.g., a drug of abuse, a medication) or a general medication condition.
6. *Relationship to a Pervasive Developmental Disorder:* If there is a history of Autistic Disorder or another Pervasive Developmental Disorder, the additional diagnosis of Schizophrenia is made only if prominent delusions or hallucinations are also present for at least a month (or less if successfully treated).

Classification of longitudinal course (can be applied only after at least 1 year has elapsed since the initial onset of active-phase symptoms):

Episodic With Interepisode Residual Symptoms (episodes are defined by the reemergence of prominent psychotic symptoms); *also specify if:* **With Prominent Negative Symptoms**

Episodic With No Interepisode Residual Symptoms Continuous (prominent psychotic symptoms are present throughout the period of observation); *also specify if:* **With Prominent Negative Symptoms**

Single Episode In Partial Remission; *also specify if:* **With Prominent Negative Symptoms**

Single Episode In Full Remission

Other of Unspecified Pattern

predicting course and treatment response. Instead, research supports that three main dimensions of schizophrenia (psychotic, disorganized, and negative) may be present to different degrees among individuals with the disorder. Peralta and Cuesta (2001) have argued that schizophrenic symptoms can be further subdivided into eight dimensions: psychosis, disorganization, negative, mania, depression, excitement, catatonia, and lack of insight.

Schizophrenia is found worldwide, with a prevalence rate among adults between .5 and 1.5% (APA, 2000). The prevalence rates vary to some extent across countries (Jablensky, 1997). Research by van Os, Hanssen, Bijl, and Vollenbergh (2001) and Pedersen and Mortensen (2001) has found that the prevalence of psychotic symptoms and disorders is higher in urban relative to rural settings, a finding that is not accounted for by population differences. Equal numbers of males and females are diagnosed with the disorder in community-based samples, but a higher rate of schizophrenia is seen in males in hospital-based studies (APA, 2000). Contrary to popular belief, most individuals with schizophrenia do not commit violent crimes. Research indicates that those who do commit violent acts are more likely to abuse substances and suffer from acute psychotic symptoms (Walsh, Buchanan, & Fahy, 2001). Buckley and colleagues (2004) recently reported that individuals with schizophrenia who committed violent acts functioned at a lower level and had a prominent lack of insight concerning their illness, their behavior, and legal complications of their illness. Research also indicates that individuals with schizophrenia are at greater risk for cognitive impairment (e.g., memory, executive function deficits), comorbidity (e.g., anxiety, depression) suicide, illicit substance use and abuse, and sexual dysfunction compared to the general population. For example, Macdonald and colleagues (2003) recently reported that 96% of women and 82% of men with schizophrenia reported sexual problems such as less desire, erectile difficulties, and reduced pleasure. Duke, Pantelis, McPhillips, and Barnes (2001) reported that 16% of individuals with schizophrenia reported a lifetime history of nonalcohol substance abuse including cannabis, psychostimulants, LSD, and opiates.

The onset of schizophrenia typically occurs during late adolescence or young adulthood and may be either abrupt or gradual. According to the DSM IV-TR (APA, 2000), the median age of onset is early to mid-20s for men and late 20s for women, and most individuals display a slow and gradual progression of negative symptoms prior to the first psychotic episode. In rare cases, schizophrenia emerges in childhood and is characterized by delays and aberrations in cognitive, language motor, and social skills (Nicolson & Rapport, 2000). The course of schizophrenia is variable: Some individuals remain chronically ill while others experience periods of exacerbation or remission. Males are more likely to develop schizophrenia in late adolescence and females in young adulthood. Prior to menopause, women with schizophrenia tend to have less severe symptoms and respond better to pharmocological treatment than males (Gur, Petty, Turetsky, & Gur, 1996). In general, the earlier the onset, the greater the number of positive and negative symptoms and structural brain abnormalities, and hence the poorer the prognosis (APA, 2000).

The mere presence of psychotic symptoms is not necessarily indicative of schizophrenia, however. In addition to the presence of positive symptoms (i.e., hallucinations and delusions), most individuals with schizophrenia also experience negative symptoms (i.e., disruptions in affect) to a degree and frequency that causes distress and significant impairment in daily functioning. Recent research by Dhossche et al. (2002) suggests that hallucinations during adolescence are more common than previously believed and are not necessarily predictive of schizophrenia in later life. Indeed, Johns and van Os (2001) reviewed a number of studies of college students and other young adults that suggest that psychotic experiences are not unusual and, in fact, occur on a continuum in the general population. Many individuals reported having had hallucinations (e.g., hearing voices) or delusions (e.g., paranoia, parapsychological phenomena). Johns and van Os suggested that psychotic symptoms may be similar to hypertension in that once it reaches a certain threshold, problems increase exponentially.

Posey and Losch (1983) found that 71% of college students surveyed reported experiencing at least one auditory hallucination (e.g., hearing voices during periods of wakefulness). Tien (1991) reported that the lifetime prevalence of hallucinations (visual, auditory, tactile) in a community sample was 15% for women and 10% for men. Healthy individuals have also been found to hold delusional ideas (Johns & van Os, 2001). Fisman (1991) described musical hallucinations in two females aged 65 and 87 and reported that hallucinations of this type are often associated with age, deafness, and brain disease and occur more frequently in women. Recently, Yoshizumi and colleagues (2004) found that 21% of 380 Japanese children 11–12 years of age experienced a visual or auditory hallucination. Given these findings, research is needed to determine the factors that contribute to the progression from psychotic symptoms to a psychotic disorder. McGorry and colleagues (2002) found that medication and cognitive–behavioral therapy reduced the risk of transitioning from a nonpsychotic to psychotic state in young adults deemed at "ultra risk" for developing schizophrenia. The results of this study support Johns and van Os's (2001) hypothesis that psychotic symptoms may correspond to a continuum-threshold relationship and an exponential increase in risk factors may cause the threshold to be reached—that is, development of schizophrenia.

Several studies support that a longer duration of untreated psychosis is predictive of a poorer outcome in terms of rate of remission and level of positive and negative symptoms (e.g., Malla et al., 2002). In other words, early intervention is associated with a better prognosis and lower rates of remission. Interestingly, Beng-Choon et al. (2003) found that individuals who experienced a first episode of psychosis but did not receive treatment (untreated for 74.3 weeks) did *not* show evidence of brain tissue loss based on MRI scans. Conflicting results were reported by Kasai et al. (2003), however, who found significant decreases in the left superior temporal gyrus in individuals with a first episode of psychosis. They also noted a 9.6% further volume reduction of the left temporal gyrus within a one-and-a-half-year period. Inconsistencies across studies are likely due to a number of methodological differences such as sample characteristics and instrument selection.

PHYSIOLOGICAL EXPLANATIONS FOR PSYCHOSIS

The physiological mechanisms responsible for hallucinations and delusions are unknown although several theories have been proposed. Grossberg (2000), for example, suggested that visual hallucinations are the result of involuntary perceptual experiences in the absence of external stimuli, and that these involuntary perceptions arise from tonically hyperactive neuronal signals originating from the cortex. He noted that humans can voluntarily create conscious experiences that involve visual imagery, daydreams, and so on; with schizophrenia, these volitional signals no longer remain under control of the individual and occur at random, resulting in hallucinations. David (1999) reviewed neuropsychological and neuroimaging studies concerning auditory hallucinations and reported that distinct brain regions are activated with auditory hallucinations relative to inner speech. The complexities involved in these networks are poorly understood. Neuroimaging studies have found, for example, that during inner speech, localized regions in the left frontal lobe (i.e., Broca's area) increase in activity and that during auditory hallucinations, Broca's area and regions in the left temporal lobe (i.e., auditory association cortex and striatum) become more activated (McGuire et al., 1996; Musalek et al., 1989). Other imaging studies have found a significant correlation between the presence and intensity of auditory hallucinations and glucose metabolism in the striatum and anterior cingulate regions (Cleghorn et al., 1992). MRI studies have found a relationship between shrinkage of the left superior temporal gyrus and severity of auditory hallucinations (Barta, Pearlson, Powers, Richards, & Tune, 1990). Additional studies using single subjects have produced inconsistent results, however, with some subjects showing increased subcortical activity during auditory hallucinations while other subjects showed greater cortical activation (Silbersweig et al., 1995).

With respect to delusions, several neuroimaging studies have found a positive correlation between the degree of reality distortion and increased rCBF in the left prefrontal cortex, striatum, and several regions of the temporal lobe (Kaplan et al., 1993; Liddle et al., 1992). Blackwood, Howard, Bentall, and Murray (2001) conducted a comprehensive review of the literature and concluded that delusions fall on a belief continuum, similar to what Johns and van Os (2001) suggested of hallucinations. Blackwood and colleagues further asserted that formation of delusions, especially persecutory delusions, depend on (a) biased selection of threatening social data and (b) compromised inferential reasoning concerning the intention of others. As they pointed out, what remains unclear is how these cognitive processes interact with other psychological processes and neuroanatomical factors. The authors hypothesized that "excessive amygdala activation may contribute to the attentional bias toward threatening stimuli found in persecutory delusions and that excessive activation of the ventromedial prefrontal cortex may result in an aberrant emotional hunch in response to noisy social data, that is, a misrepresentation of body state resulting in the perception of threat where none actually exists" (p. 533).

It is important to note that studies investigating the physiological correlates of hallucinations and delusions have several methodological limitations. For example, several studies have used neuroimaging techniques while individuals with schizophrenia were actively psychotic. The content of the hallucinations likely varied across individuals and may have influenced areas of brain activation. Sample size is another problematic issue as many studies included small samples or even single cases. In addition, some studies included subjects who were not actively psychotic but had a history of psychosis. Comorbidity (e.g., anxiety disorders, depression, medical problems) is also a potential confound, as are medication use, age, and gender. Goodwin, Lyons, and McNally (2002), for example, reported that nearly half of those with schizophrenia also suffer from an anxiety disorder (panic attacks). Despite these limitations, research suggests that hallucinations involve cortical and subcortical regions. The specific dysfunctions within the auditory or visual regions that give rise to hallucinations are yet to be discovered.

ETIOLOGIC THEORIES

There is no known cause of schizophrenia. Research investigating the pathophysiology of schizophrenia has involved heritability, genetic, anatomical, neurotransmitter, neurodevelopmental, and neuroimaging studies.

Heritability Studies

Research on the heritability of schizophrenia has investigated the occurrence of schizophrenia in monozygotic and dizygotic twins, biological relatives, unrelated individuals, and adoption cases. The consensus across studies is that schizophrenia is more likely to occur in monozygotic twins than any other pairs. Specific results vary across studies, ranging from 41% to 87% in monozygotic twins (Cardno et al., 1999). Some investigations have reported monozygotic concordance rates of 45% and 10% for dizygotic twins (Holzman and Matthysse, 1990), while other studies have reported concordance rates of 48% and 17% for monozygotic and dizygotic twins, respectively (Gottesman, 1991). These rates drop substantially between siblings and unrelated individuals.

Further evidence from adoption studies supports a heritability factor in schizophrenia. Kety et al. (1994) studied the occurrence of schizophrenia in children who were adopted as well as their biological parents and siblings. Results indicated that 12.5% of the biological relatives developed schizophrenia while none of the adoptive relatives developed the disorder. Gottesman and Bertelsen (1989) examined the rates of schizophrenia in children whose parent was either a monozygotic or dizygotic twin and either had or did not have schizophrenia. These authors found that 16.8% of the children whose monozygotic parent had schizophrenia developed schizophrenia, while 17.4% of the children developed schizophrenia whose monozygotic parent did not have schizophrenia. In addition, 17.4% of the children developed schizophrenia whose dizygotic parent had schizophrenia, but only 2.1% of the children of the nonschizophrenic dizygotic parent. Davis, Phelps, and Bracha (1995) reported that the concordance rate for monochorionic monozygotic twins was 60% but only 11% for dichorionic monozygotic twins. Collectively, these results suggest that schizophrenia may be passed on genetically but that not everyone who has the inherited predisposition develops the disorder. These findings raise two important questions: What genes are involved in schizophrenia? What factors determine whether a person with this genetic vulnerability develops the disorder?

Studies suggest that genes play a substantial role in the transmission of schizophrenia (and other mental disorders) but that other factors also contribute to the disease. For example, if one identical twin has schizophrenia, the likelihood that the other twin will develop schizophrenia is about 45%. Thus, genes are important but not determinant. As Hyman (2003) stated, "Our brains, not our genes regulate our behavior, and our brains are the product of genes, environment and chance operating over a lifetime" (p. 99). Recently, Bassett, Chow, Waterworth, and Brzustowica (2001) reported that intrauterine factors, stochastic (random) factors, and mutations after conception may help to explain the discordant rate of schizophrenia in monozygotic twins.

Molecular Genetic Findings

To date, no single gene or collection of genes has been found to cause schizophrenia. Schizophrenia clearly has a genetic basis, however, based on the high heritability estimates discussed previously (45–87%). Rather than investigating the prevalence of schizophrenia in families, twins, and adoptees, molecular genetics examines the DNA of family members and individuals with schizophrenia. There are two main approaches to exploring the genetics of schizophrenia: *linkage studies* and *association studies*. *Linkage studies* attempt to locate chromosomal regions that are shared among individuals with schizophrenia but not among unaffected individuals. These regions of interest are defined by DNA markers located along the chromosome. Chromosomes contain DNA and DNA consists of four bases: adenine (A), guanine (G), cytosine (C), and thymine (T). These bases are connected systematically with A paired with T and G paired with C. Genes are segments of the DNA that have a specific function such as the creation of proteins that serve critical cellular functions. Only about 2% of human DNA contains genes, and each gene consists of thousands of base pairs (Tsuang, & Tsuang, 1999). DNA markers can be identified in individuals by establishing a pattern in the DNA sequence of base pairs. There are various methods available for establishing these DNA patterns, but they result in creating segments of varying length known as fragments. Individuals can be classified based on the pattern and length of fragments that result from these patterns of base pairs. Linkage studies seek to determine whether individuals with schizophrenia have specific DNA markers relative to those without the disorder.

It is important to understand that linkage studies reveal a region or regions of a chromosome that may be involved in schizophrenia but do not identify individual genes. After identifying specific chromosomal locations, nearby susceptibility genes within this region can be identified. These genes can then be screened for possible mutations in individuals with schizophrenia. The presence or lack of presence of the mutations in individuals without schizophrenia helps to determine whether the mutation is indeed associated with schizophrenia. Additional studies then explore how the gene and mutation may be involved in the etiology of schizophrenia (Basset et al., 2001).

Association studies involve the identification of "candidate genes," that is, genes suspected of being involved in schizophrenia based on theory. For example, the gene for a specific type of dopamine receptor has been studied based on the theory that schizophrenia involves dysfunction of the dopaminergic system. After candidate genes have been identified, they are examined to determine whether the gene is mutated in some way. Specifically, geneticists explore whether the base-pair sequence in the candidate gene differs significantly among those with and without schizophrenia. If individuals with schizophrenia were consistently found to show a base-pair sequence that differs from those without the disorder, a gene for schizophrenia would be discovered. The last step would be to determine precisely how the affected gene leads to schizophrenia. Genetic mutations are defined as any permanent change in the DNA sequence of a gene that can be caused during development or by environmental toxins (Faraone, Tsuang, & Tsuang, 1999). These mutations lead to changes in proteins that may result in disease. Examples of genetic mutations include deletions (a DNA segment is missing), translocation mutations (a DNA segment from one chromosome is tacked onto another), duplication mutations (a DNA segment is inserted twice into a chromosome), trinucleotide repeat mutations (a triplet sequence of base pairs is repeated within a gene), and others (see Tsuang & Tsuang, 1999 for a review). It is important to note that genetic mutations might alter proteins to some degree, but not enough to cause disease. For example, Egan, Weinberger, and Lu (2003) hypothesized that a variant on the gene for brain-derived neurotroic factor (BDNF) would be associated with increased risk for schizophrenia given that BDNF is important in hippocampal functioning. Three groups were included in their study: individuals with schizophrenia, siblings of these individuals, and healthy comparison subjects. Contrary to expectations, they found that although the presence of the gene variant had deleterious effects on cognitive performance and was associated with abnormal blood flow in the hippocampus during neuroimaging, it did *not* predict risk for schizophrenia. These findings demonstrate that it is critical for scientists to not only identify candidate genes but also to discover the process by which genes cause diseases such as schizophrenia.

Linkage and association studies have not yet yielded the chromosomal regions or genes responsible for schizophrenia, but they have produced encouraging findings. To assist in this process, new techniques such as "linkage disequilibrium" have been developed to help identify the location of susceptibility genes. Linkage disequilibrium can scan tens to hundreds of thousands of pairs of DNA, and its recommended use is with affected individuals and their parents (Kendler, 1999). Several regions of chromosomes have been linked to schizophrenia including chromosomes 5, 6, 8, 10, 12, 13, and 22 (Bassett, Chow, Waterworth, & Brzustowica, 2001; Mimmack et al., 2002; Pulvar, 2000). In general, these studies have provided inconsistent findings.

Recently, a genetic subtype of schizophrenia has been associated with a small deletion on chromosome 2211q. The genetic syndrome association with this deletion is known as 22qDS and is associated with multiple problems such as learning difficulties, mental retardation, and physical defects (Bassett et al., 2001). Research has found that 25% of individuals with this deletion develop schizophrenia (Murphy, Jones, & Owen, 1999). This deletion is associated with only a small percentage of individuals with schizophrenia, however. Most individuals with 22qDS syndrome do not develop schizophrenia. Bassett and colleagues (2003) recently compared adult with 22qDS syndrome with and without schizophrenia and concluded that the deletion in chromosome 22 likely leads to neurodevelopmental changes that result in the expression of schizophrenia, at least in a subgroup of individuals with the disorder.

Other regions of chromosome 22 have also been of interest. Specifically, chromosome 22q12 and six genes located in close proximity to each other in this region are associated with production of proteins that are of vital importance to normal cell functioning. Known as lipoproteins (apo L proteins), their function in the brain is poorly understood. Mimmack and colleagues (2002), however, discovered robust and reliable changes ("up-regulation") in the expression of three of the six genes located on chromosome 22q12 that control the production of lipoproteins. They hypothesized that alterations in these genes and production of lipoproteins may be related to abnormal cellular function in schizophrenia, particularly in the area of the prefrontal cortex.

A region on chromosome 2 (2p13-14) has also been associated with schizophrenia suscep- tibility. Novak, Kim, Seeman, and Tallerico (2002) examined postmortem brains of individuals with and without schizophrenia and discovered that a gene identified as Nogo on chromosome 2 was overexpressed in those with schizophrenia. This gene produces a protein found in myelin that is known to inhibit the outgrowth of developing neurons and nerve terminals. An elevated expression of Nogo, particularly in the frontal cortex, is hypothesized to contribute to abnor- mal cell migration and formation during development and neuronal function in adulthood. Additional genes have been linked to schizophrenia. For example, Kromkamp et al. (2003) found a decreased expression of a particular gene (homeobox gene DLX1) in postmortem brain tissue of adults with a history of schizophrenia that was not found in brain tissue samples of adults with a history of bipolar disorder. The decreased expression of the homeobox gene was hypothesized to be related to abnormal thalamic circuits sometimes found in individuals with schizophrenia. Recently, Kendler (2004) reported that at least five studies have found signifi- cant associations between markers on the DTNBP1 (i.e., dysbindin-1) gene and schizophrenia, suggesting that variations in the dysbindin gene influence the risk of schizophrenia.

As will be discussed later in this chapter, the dopamine system has been implicated in the pathophysiology of schizophrenia, with genes involved in the functioning of the dopamine sys- tem of particular interest. Researchers have focused on alterations in dopamine transmission as well as dopamine receptors. Dopamine receptors are regulated by genes, and several studies have reported associations between alterations in dopamine receptor genes and schizophrenia. For example, Williams et al. (1998) conducted a meta-analysis of 30 studies investigating the D3 receptor gene and concluded that a relationship exists between aberrations (e.g., polymor- phisms) of D3 receptor genes and schizophrenia (see Levant, 1997 for a review), although the complexities of this relationship are poorly understood. In addition, Glatt, Faraone, and Tsuang (2003) conducted a meta-analysis to summarize the findings concerning the gene for catechol O-methyltransferase (COMT) and its association with schizophrenia. Located on chromosome 22q, the gene is involved in the production of COMT, an enzyme that metabolizes dopamine. Based on the findings of 14 studies reviewed, Glatt and colleagues concluded that presence of a variant of the COMT gene may be considered a risk factor for schizophrenia but that additional, definitive studies are needed.

One of the difficulties in identifying a genetic basis for schizophrenia is that significant findings in one study frequently are not replicated in additional studies. For example, Brzus- towica, Hodgkison, Chow, Honer, and Bassett (2000) suggested that genes associated with susceptibility to schizophrenia can be found on chromosome 1. Recent findings by Levinson et al. (2002) failed to replicate these findings; they suggested that chromosomes 6, 8, and 13 be investigated. Other researchers have explored chromosomes 12, 15, and 16—to name only a few (e.g., Schwab et al., 1998; Straub et al., 1998). Recently, researchers studied the DNA from over 200 individuals from Canada and 183 individuals from Russia with schizophrenia and found two genetic markers from chromosome 13q34 that were associated with the disease in both the Canadian and Russian samples (Chumakov et al., 2002). In this study, researchers described a human gene, G72 located on chromosome 13q34, and found evidence that this gene interacts with second gene that regulates glutamate signaling in the NMDA receptor. The scientists speculated that G72 could trigger overproduction of proteins that could lower glutamate receptor activity substantially, thereby predisposing an individual to the development of schizophrenia. Chumakov et al. noted, however, that additional studies need to be conducted and that the susceptibility to schizophrenia could be "highly epistatic, with genes regulating each other in complex interconnected networks of interactions" (p. 13675).

Collectively, results across numerous molecular genetic studies indicate that genes are undoubtably implicated in the development of schizophrenia, although the specific genes involved remain inconclusive at this time. To complicate matters, research suggests that multiple genes may be involved in schizophrenia and that prenatal and environmental factors may modify gene expression. Additional chromosome locations and susceptibility genes are likely to be identified in the future.

Anatomical Studies

A large body of research exists concerning the neuroanatomy and neurochemistry of individuals with schizophrenia relative to individuals without the disorder. In general, the findings have been inconsistent among individuals with schizophrenia *and* across studies. In 1913, Emil Kraepelin was among the first to propose that individuals with schizophrenia follow a progressively deteriorating course. Current research suggests that the course can be highly variable, with some individuals showing chronic symptoms and others showing fewer symptoms that appear to remit. Whether these differences in symptomology are related to distinct brain differences is unclear.

Prior to the advancement of technology and neuroimaging techniques, researchers relied primarily on postmortem samples to investigate the brains of individuals with schizophrenia. For example, postmortem studies have reported that the brains of individuals with the disorder do not differ significantly by age (e.g., Selemon, Rajkowska, & Goldman-Rakic, 1995). A recent study by Hulshoff Pol et al. (2002) using MRI, however, found smaller gray matter volume in older patients with schizophrenia relative to younger patients. Thus, the issue of whether brain abnormalities become more prominent over time remains unresolved. It is plausible that the degree of progression is individually determined and is influenced by onset and severity of the disorder as well as treatment history. Research with postmortem samples has found additional anatomical differences between individuals with and without schizophrenia. For example, Haug (1962) examined postmortem samples of individuals with schizophrenia and was the first to describe the pattern of ventricular enlargement that is commonly associated with this disorder (Fig. 5.1).

Ventricular enlargement is thought to be the result of neuronal loss in various regions of the brain, but the cause of this loss is speculative. Weinberger (1995) found that ventricular size varied among individuals with schizophrenia, with some patients showing abnormally large ventricles while others showed ventricles of normal size. Interestingly, Seidman et al. (1997) found enlarged ventricles and other anatomical differences in nonpsychotic relatives of individuals with schizophrenia. These results were interpreted as supporting a genetic predisposition to schizophrenia that is triggered by either environmental events or other genes.

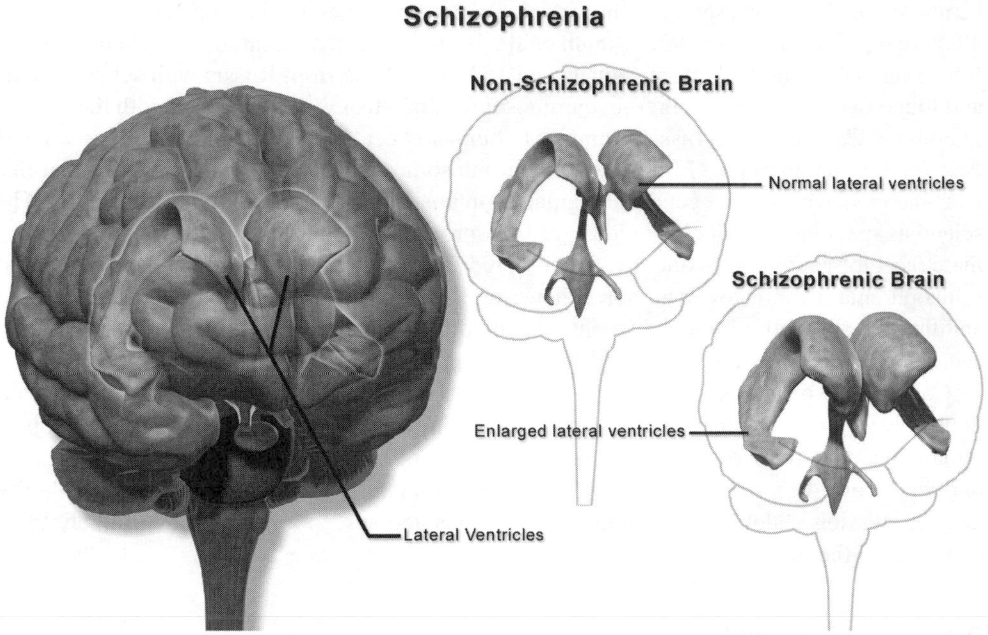

Schizophrenia

FIG. 5.1.   Enlarged ventricles sometimes found in individuals with schizophrenia. Copyright Blausen Medical Communications. Reproduced by permission.

Studies have also reported disorganized arrangements of neurons, neurons that are abnormally small in size, misplacement of neurons, and increased and decreased density of neurons in cortical and subcortical regions (e.g., Benes, Davidson, & Bird, 1986; Selemon, Rajkowska, & Goldman-Rakic, 1995). Other studies have found abnormally high levels of neurotrophic factors and enlarged ventricles and abnormalities of the hippocampus, amygdala, and additional areas of the temporal lobes as well as the frontal lobes (e.g., Honer et al., 1997).

In 1984 Kovelman and Scheibel discovered that neurons located within the hippocampus were not neatly arranged in columns as would be expected but were disorganized in appearance. The authors speculated that perhaps this anatomical abnormality resulted in faulty cortical–subcortical systems and consequent abnormalities in behavior. Recently, Rioux, Nissanov, Lauber, Bilker, and Arnold (2003) examined (postmortem) brain tissue from the anterior parahippocampal gyrus of individuals with and without schizophrenia. Results indicated that the individuals with schizophrenia showed a different pattern of neuronal placement (i.e., misplaced) in the anterior section of the parahippocampal gyrus. No group differences were found, however, with respect to morphological characteristics of neurons or density of neurons in this region. In addition, no relationship was found between brain tissue and age, duration of illness, age of onset, or medication usage. The authors interpreted the findings as supporting aberrant brain development in individuals with schizophrenia due to abnormalities in cell migration and/or pruning.

Other studies have reported differences in density of neuronal tissue in adults with schizophrenia. Selemon, Rajkowska, and Goldman-Rakic (1995), for example, reported abnormally high density of neurons in the prefrontal cortex and primary visual cortex of individuals with schizophrenia. Selemon and Goldman-Rakic (1999) argued that increased neuronal density in the cortex suggests that the actual number of neurons is not lower but that the neurons are atrophied (the reduced neuropil hypothesis). In other words, the neurons are packed closely together and have fewer dendritic branches and synaptic connections. Recently, Selemon (2004) suggested that the increase in neuronal density found in some studies may reflect either an increase in the number of neurons in the tissue sampled or a reduction in the overall volume of brain tissue and interneuronal spaces. Glantz and Lewis (2000) suggested that the synaptic connections are significantly altered in individuals with schizophrenia, particularly in the prefrontal cortex. Specifically, Glantz and Lewis found a decrease in dendritic spine density in patients with schizophrenia which compromises the number of excitatory inputs to neurons in this area. Interestingly, the prefrontal cortex does not fully mature until late adolescence or early adulthood, the period of onset for most individuals with schizophrenia. Therefore, it is plausible that problems that occur early in brain development (cell migration, proliferation, pruning) are cumulative and not observed until later in life.

To explore whether abnormal anatomical findings were unique to schizophrenia, Benes et al. (2001) investigated whether the density of neurons in the anterior cingulate cortex differed between the postmortem brains of individuals with schizophrenia and those with bipolar disorder and controls. Results revealed that glia cell density did not differ across groups. However, the clinical groups both showed decreased density of neurons but in different locations. Byne et al. (2002) and Danos et al. (2003) reported reduced number and reduced size of neurons in the region of the thalamus in postmortem samples of individuals with schizophrenia. Additional studies have found a reduction of neurons in the thalamus as well as reduced metabolic activity in this area for individuals with schizophrenia (e.g., Andreasen et al., 1994; Malaspina et al., 2004). Selemon, Kleinman, Herman, and Goldman-Rakic (2002) compared the postmortem brains of 14 individuals with schizophrenia to 19 normal brains. When total gray and white matter volumes of the cortex were measured, only the gray matter of the frontal lobes was found to differ between groups (12% smaller). The researchers interpreted their findings as supportive of previous studies implicating the frontal lobes and prefrontal cortex as a focal point for pathology in schizophrenia. In addition, the authors suggested that a smaller volume of gray matter in the frontal lobe is most likely reflective of reduced synapses, terminals, and pruning of dendritic arbors and spines—consistent with the neuropil hypothesis advanced by Selemon and colleagues (1995).

Protein Involvement in Schizophrenia

Researchers have also investigated various proteins involved in the establishment and maintenance of synapses in the area of the cingulate cortex (e.g., synaptophysin) and their possible role in schizophrenia. These studies suggest that synaptic pathology may exist in individuals with schizophrenia, but the findings are inconsistent and are characteristic of other disorders such as bipolar disorder (e.g., Eastwood & Harrison, 2001; Fatemi, Earle, Stary, Lee, & Sedgewick, 2001). Fatemi et al. (2001) recently reported that a protein (SNAP-25) that is important in presynaptic axonal growth and exocytosis, was significantly reduced in an area of the hippocampus in postmortem samples of individuals with schizophrenia but not those with clinical depression. Similar reductions were found as well in individuals with bipolar disorder, however, which suggests that SNAP-25 alterations are not unique to schizophrenia. In general, though, these findings imply that the connections among neurons and neural networks are aberrant in individuals with schizophrenia. Recently, Law and colleagues (2004) examined postmortem brain tissue of individuals with schizophrenia, bipolar and major depression, and control subjects and found that those with schizophrenia had decreased expression of a protein (spinophilin) known to be important in dendritic spine formation. The authors suggested that schizophrenia may be characterized by alterations in dendritic spine number that interfere with synaptic connections and neuronal communication.

Magnetic Resonance Imaging Studies (MRI)

Although many studies have found anatomical abnormalities in individuals with schizophrenia, the findings have been inconsistent and to date there are no specific structural abnormalities that are diagnostic or unique to schizophrenia. Nonetheless, postmortem and MRI studies do suggest that a number of structural abnormalities of the brain may be implicated in schizophrenia (see McCarley et al., 1999 for a review).

Recently, Cannon and colleagues (2002) used MRI to investigate patterns of gray matter loss in monozygotic twins discordant for schizophrenia. Results revealed gray matter deficits in those with schizophrenia in the areas of the prefrontal cortex, parietal lobe, and superior temporal gyrus. Gray matter loss was correlated with symptom severity and cognitive dysfunction but not with drug treatment or duration of the disorder. In 1995, Petty and colleagues examined a particular region of the temporal lobe—the planum temporale—that lies on the superior surface of the temporal lobe. The planum temporale is involved in the production and comprehension of langue, and in right-handed people the surface area of the left planum temporale is typically larger than the right. Petty et al. compared the right and left surface areas of the planum temporale in 14 right-handed individuals with schizophrenia relative to control participants. Results indicated that in all but one of the individuals with schizophrenia, a reversal of the expected asymmetry was found (i.e., the right was larger than the left). The authors suggested that these findings support a neurodevelopmental disturbance in schizophrenia that occurs prenatally, either as a result of genetic or environmental factors or the interaction of the two. Lim et al. (1996) proposed a similar neurodevelopmental explanation for their MRI findings that revealed a significant gray matter loss of the cortex and enlarged ventricles in individuals with first-episode schizophrenia. Recently, Onitsuka and colleagues (2004) used MRI to study the temporal gyrus (middle and inferior) in male patients with chronic schizophrenia relative to control male subjects. Results revealed that individuals with schizophrenia had significant gray matter volume reductions in the middle left temporal gyrus (13% reduction) as well as a 10% reduction in the bilateral inferior temporal gyrus. Interestingly, severity of hallucinations was significantly correlated with smaller volumes of the left temporal gyrus.

To explore whether schizophrenia is characterized by brain changes over time, Paul and colleagues (2001) used MRI to study a form of schizophrenia that begins in childhood. The researchers studied a small group of adolescents with schizophrenia relative to adolescents without the disorder (matched for age and gender) over a 5-year period. Three-dimensional maps of brain change were recorded by MRI and the amount and rate of cell loss determined with each scan. Results detected specific brain changes (loss of cells) and pattern of change from early to late adolescence. Specifically, individuals with schizophrenia were found to have a greater and faster rate of cell loss at the level of the cortex. In addition, the pattern of loss was specific—it began in the parietal lobe and progressed anteriorly into the temporal lobes, sensorimotor and dorsolateral prefrontal corices, and frontal eye fields. This pattern of loss correlated with severity of psychotic symptoms and cognitive impairments characteristic of schizophrenia. The pattern and rate of tissue loss were not associated with medical history, intelligence, or gender. These findings are remarkable because they substantiate that structural changes are progressive and are associated with cognitive and behavioral symptoms of schizophrenia, at least with the form that begins in childhood. Interestingly, this study also found evidence of cell loss throughout the superior frontal, motor, and parietal brain regions in normal adolescents. These findings are supportive of the theory that genes determine the framework for brain development, including periods of increased growth and pruning.

Keller et al. (2003) reported similar patterns of tissue loss in children, adolescents, and young adults (ages 8–24) with schizophrenia. Specifically, the volumes of the cortex and the cerebellum were significantly smaller in individuals with schizophrenia relative to those without the disorder. Recently, Kasai and colleagues (2003) used MRI to compare patients with first-episode schizophrenia to those without the disorder and a group of adults with psychotic symptoms but not schizophrenia. Findings indicated that the group with schizophrenia showed significant greater decreases in gray matter volume over time in the left superior temporal gyrus but not in other brain regions. Also using MRI, Gilbert et al. (2001) found that the left, right, and total volume of the thalamus were significantly smaller in individuals with newly diagnosed schizophrenia than those without the disorder. Other studies have found loss of gray matter volume in the temporal lobe of patients with schizophrenia—pattern of loss associated with the auditory hallucinations and thought and memory problems characteristic of the disorder (see Shenton, Dickey, Frumin, & McCarley, 2001 for a review).

Longitudinal studies can be used to help clarify whether brain changes associated with schizophrenia begin in childhood and continue throughout adolescence and adulthood. Only a handful of such studies have been conducted with adolescents and adults with schizophrenia and, in general, demonstrate a progressive loss of total brain tissue and cellular loss in specific regions such as the temporal lobes (e.g., DeLisi et al., 1995), frontal lobes (Gur et al., 1998), hippocampus and amygdala (Giedd et al., 1999), and basal ganglia (Rapoport et al., 1997). Loss of brain tissue has been found to correlate with symptom severity, with more severe symptoms associated with greater tissue loss. For example, Mathalon, Sullivan, Lim, and Pfefferbaum (2001) explored the level of brain tissue loss in adult males with and without schizophrenia over a 4-year period. Using MRI, the researchers found that brain tissue loss was faster in adults with schizophrenia, and a pattern of progression was found in the right frontal lobe and bilateral temporal lobe. Greater left lateral ventricle expansion was also found in the adults with schizophrenia. Similar to previous studies, cellular loss was associated with greater symptom severity. Hulshoff Pol et al. (2002) and Cahn et al. (2002) recently reported total brain, cerebral gray matter, prefrontal gray matter, and prefrontal white matter volumes were smaller in individuals with schizophrenia compared to control patients. The authors also reported that the lateral and third ventricles and peripheral cerebral spinal fluid volumes were larger in individuals with schizophrenia. Recently, Milev and colleagues (2003) found that temporal lobe tissue volume at the onset of schizophrenia was predictive of continued symptoms (hallucinations) 5 years later. They suggested that MRI scans may help to identify individuals who are at higher risk for poor outcome, especially if this information is gathered at the onset of the disease.

Structural abnormalities have also been found in other brain regions in individuals with schizophrenia. For example, Okugawa, Sedvall, and Agartz (2003) recently reported that part of the cerebellum was significantly smaller in both males and females with chronic schizophrenia compared to those without the disorder. These findings are consistent with the results from an earlier study (Okugawa et al., 2002) of males with chronic schizophrenia and lend additional support that cerebellar brain differences exist in those with the disease. Work by Keller et al. (2003) indicating that individuals with schizophrenia showed a progressive loss of cerebellar volume, particularly during adolescence, suggests that excessive loss of brain tissue in this region during adolescence may be a "trait marker" for schizophrenia (p. 132). Several studies have reported that the corpus callosum is smaller in individuals with schizophrenia (e.g., Woodruff et al., 1995), although recent findings by Panizzon et al. (2003) found that only male patients with schizophrenia differed from control subjects with respect to the size of the corpus callosum. Research also indicates that the olfactory system is highly influenced by genetic factors, and several studies have found odor detection, identification, and memory deficits in individuals with schizophrenia (e.g., Barinaga, 2001; Kopala, Good, Torrey, & Honer, 1998). Sallett et al. (2003) also found abnormalities in the cortical folds (i.e., reduced gyri) in individuals with schizophrenia, further supporting abnormalities in neurodevelopment process in individuals with schizophrenia.

To explore whether medication use was associated with brain tissue loss, Cahn et al. (2002) examined the relationship between antipsychotic medication and brain matter. Results revealed that decreases in cerebral gray matter volume correlated significantly with use of medication. Savas et al. (2002) found a relationship between hippocampal size and response to medication (risperidone). Specifically, individuals with schizophrenia who responded well to risperidone had significantly greater hippocampal volume than those who did not. Consistent with previous studies, the researchers also found hippocampal volume in individuals with schizophrenia was smaller than in normal adults.

MRI Findings in First-Degree Relatives

To explore whether genetic vulnerability for schizophrenia may be evidenced in the olfactory system, Turetsky, Moberg, Arnold, Doty, and Gur (2003) recently used MRI to investigate the structure of the olfactory bulbs in individuals with schizophrenia and their first-degree relatives. Distinct structural abnormalities of both the left and right olfactory bulbs were found in individuals with schizophrenia, related to olfactory deficits. First-degree relatives also showed structural abnormalities, but only of the right olfactory bulb and the findings were unrelated to olfactory deficits. The results were interpreted as supporting problems in neural system development in patients with schizophrenia that are influenced by genetic factors. Recently, Seidman et al. (2002) measured the hippocampal volumes in nonpsychotic first-degree relatives of individuals with schizophrenia. The study was based on their previous work that suggested that factual memory and hippocampal volume may be good predictors of increased vulnerability to schizophrenia. The results indicated that, compared to a control group, these first-degree relatives had significantly smaller hippicampi in the left hemisphere. Within families, however, the size of the hippocampus did not differ. In addition, hippocampal size and memory were correlated, with better memory performance associated with larger hippocampal volume. The results were interpreted as supporting the hypothesis that smaller left hippocampi and verbal memory deficits are indicative of neurodevelopmental compromise and may be a marker for vulnerability to schizophrenia.

In general, MRI findings suggest that schizophrenia is associated with a reduction in total brain volume, progressive gray matter loss that occurs in the early stages of the disorder particularly in the prefrontal and superior temporal lobes, enlargement of the lateral ventricles, and smaller thalamic and hippocampi volume. These results are not unique to schizophrenia, however, and although they reflect aberrant structural findings, they do not reveal etiologic information about schizophrenia.

Neuroimaging Studies

Results from several neuroimaging studies support the idea that schizophrenia is characterized by abnormalities in brain structure and function, but the specific nature of these abnormalities is poorly understood. As discussed in chapter three, fMRI and PET measure glucose metabolism or blood flow changes. Several studies using PET and fMIR have found evidence of reduced blood flow or glucose metabolism in adults with schizophrenia. Weinberger and Lipska (1995), for example, compared the performance of monozygotic twins, in which only one twin in each pair had schizophrenia, while performing a behavioral task (Wisconsin Card Sorting Test). The results indicated that the twins with schizophrenia displayed reduced blood flow in the prefrontal cortex while performing the task (i.e., hypofrontality). Bertolino et al. (2000) examined working memory performance in a group of adults with schizophrenia. Results were consistent with Weinberger and Lipska (1995). Less cortical activation was found in adults with schizophrenia during a behavioral task (Wisconsin Card Sorting Test) using PET. The authors interpreted the findings as supporting the theory that the prefrontal cortex and associated neural networks are dysfunctional in schizophrenia.

Using PET, Buchsbaum et al. (1990) also reported reduced rates of glucose metabolism in the frontal cortex and temporal–parietal regions in patients with schizophrenia relative to comparison participants during an attention task. Andreasen et al. (1992) reported decreased frontal activity only in individuals with schizophrenia who had significant negative symptoms. Using fMRI, Curtis et al. (1998) found hypofrontality in individuals with schizophrenia during a verbal fluency task. Pickar et al. (1990) found similar results and suggested that hypofrontality may be responsible for the negative symptoms observed in schizophrenia. Also, Taylor, Tandon, Shipley, Eiser, and Goodson (1991) suggested that negative symptoms are not necessarily related to hypfrontality but instead may be due to REM sleep disturbances frequently found in individuals with schizophrenia and the neurotransmitter systems (e.g., serotonin) involved in the control of REM sleep.

Many other studies, however, have not found evidence of reduced blood flow or glucose metabolism in individuals with schizophrenia—and in fact have reported normal or overactivity in this region. For example, when Callicott and colleagues (2003) explored fMRI response of siblings of individuals with schizophrenia during a memory task, results showed an exaggerated and inefficient response of the dorsolateral prefrontal cortex during the memory task, despite their normal performance on the task. The researchers suggested that this physiological inefficiency in memory processing may be related to a genetic risk factor for schizophrenia. Similarly, using PET, Kim et al. (2003) recently reported that adults with schizphrenia did not show hypofrontality but rather a distinct activation pattern in the prefrontal region compared to adults without schizophrenia. In a review of the literature, Berman and Weinberger (1991) found that only 60% of the 39 studies reviewed could be interpreted as showing hypofrontality in individuals with schizophrenia. Taylor (1996) conducted a similar review and also emphasized the lack of consensus in the literature. A number of factors may contribute to the inconsistent findings in the literature: methodological differences, testing and instrumentation differences, sample characteristic differences (e.g, substance abuse, severity of symptoms, onset of symptoms, treatment history), medication usage, and situational factors such as lack of motivation or effort and disengagement during behavioral tasks. It is also important to note that hypofrontality is not unique to schizophrenia and has been found in other disorders such as ADHD and dementia. In 2001, Curtis et al. explored whether hypofrontality findings were unique to schizophrenia or characteristic of bipolar disorders as well. Based on fMRI, the researchers concluded individuals with schizophrenia and bipolar disorders demonstrated clear differences in frontal activation, with individuals with schizophrenia showing greater hypofrontality. Thus, the question of whether hypofrontality is characteristic of schizophrenia remains equivocal.

Research has also found blood flow abnormalities in other brain regions of individuals with schizophrenia, including the cerebellum (Andreasen et al., 1996; Andreasen et al., 1997). Recently, Menon, Anagnoson, Glover, and Pfefferbaum (2001) using fMRI found significantly less activation of the basal ganglia in individuals with schizophrenia during a motor-sequencing task. These deficits of the basal ganglia were hypothesized to underlie the movement-related and goal-directed behavioral abnormalities commonly observed in individuals with the disorder. Jessen et al. (2003) reported that adults with schizophrenia showed significantly less activation of the hippocampus during a recognition task compared to adults without the disorder. These findings support MRI results and suggest that schizophrenia may be characterized by structural and functional abnormalities of the hippocampus.

In summary, neuroimaging studies suggest that individuals with schizophrenia show differences in brain activation relative to individuals without the disorder. These differences are characterized by increased and decreased levels of activation in various brain regions, particularly in the thalamus, hippocampus, cerebellum, and prefrontal cortex. These findings are not conclusive, however, nor are they unique to schizophrenia. In addition, patterns of blood flow or glucose metabolism only indirectly reflect cellular function and do not reveal information concerning the etiology of schizophrenia. In other words, neuroimaging findings are only correlational in nature and do not reflect directionality of the findings. For example, it is possible that changes in biochemistry result in behavioral changes, and it is also possible that environmental factors elicit behavioral changes that in turn result in changes in biochemistry.

Neurotransmitter Studies

To date, the most widely studied theory centers on the role of the neurotransmitter dopamine. The view that dopamine may be involved in schizophrenia arose from two main observations: (a) amphetamines, which increase the amount of dopamine that is available in the synaptic cleft, can induce positive psychotic symptoms and (b) antipsychotic medications that block dopamine receptors (D2) decrease psychotic symptoms. These observations led to the hypothesis that overactivity of the dopaminergic system may cause the symptoms characteristic of schizophrenia. For example, early theories of schizophrenia suggested that the symptoms of schizophrenia might be due to elevated levels of dopamine. Studies that have attempted to indirectly measure dopamine levels based on dopamine metabolites (i.e., homovanillic acid) found in the cerebral spinal fluid, however, have produced mixed results. This methodology has been criticized due to the unreliability of metabolite measures and the fact that metabolites reflect global dopaminergic activity rather than activity in specific brain regions or structures (Byne, Kemether, Jones, Haroutunian, & Davis, 1999). Current dopamine-related theories of schizophrenia focus on the role of dopamine receptors.

Dopamine Receptors

Based on the theory that the positive symptoms of schizophrenia may be due to hyperactivity of the dopaminergic system, researchers have explored whether individuals with schizophrenia may have increased density of dopamine receptors. To investigate this hypothesis, scientisits have relied primarily on postmortem samples and, more recently, neuroimaging techniques. In general, results indicate that individuals with schizophrenia tend to have a significant (but small) increase in dopamine receptor density (D2 receptors) and, compared to controls, show greater variability in these measures (see Laruelle, 1998 for a review).

Recently, Abi-Dargham and colleagues (2000) used SPECT to study the baseline levels (i.e., no medication) of D2 receptor occupancy in the striatum by dopamine in individuals with and without schizophrenia. The researchers also measured D2 receptor occupancy after acute dopamine depletion, which was reached by administering a drug that inhibited tyrosine hydroxylase over a 2-day period. Results indicated that individuals with schizophrenia showed a higher level of dopamine receptor occupancy relative to controls during the baseline condition and after acute depletion of dopamine. Specifically, dopamine depletion resulted in approximately a 19% increase in D2 receptor availability in individuals with schizophrenia but only 9% in control subjects. The results provided evidence that schizophrenia is associated with excessive stimulation of D2 receptors by dopamine. The study also found that greater occupancy of receptors at baseline was predictive of a better response to antipsychotic medication.

Further evidence of D2 involvement in schizophrenia was found by Gjedde and Wong (2001). Haloperidol was administered to three groups of adults: those with schizophrenia, those with bipolar disorder, and healthy controls. When the researchers measured the drug's affinity to dopamine receptors in the caudate nucleus, haloperidol binding was highest in individuals with schizophrenia. The authors speculated that higher rates of binding to D2 receptors in parts of the caudate nucleus are associated with psychosis. The D2 receptor has been implicated in schizophrenia as most antipsychotic medications have an affinity for the dopamine 2 receptor (D2). Results from several postmortem studies have found an elevated number of D2 receptors in individuals with schizophrenia both for those who have and have not taken antipsychotic medications. This finding suggests that the increase is not simply an artifact of up-regulation in receptor numbers due to the medication (e.g., Burt, Creese, & Snyder, 1977). With regard to living individuals with schizophrenia and D2 receptors, neuroimaging techniques using radioactive tracers that attach to dopamine receptors, have produced inconsistent findings. Some studies, for example, have reported increased numbers of D2 receptors while others have not (e.g., Farde et al., 1990; Wong et al., 1986). Other postmortem studies have found decreased numbers of D3 and D4 receptors in areas other than the prefrontal cortex and increased numbers in the prefrontal area (e.g., Schmauss et al., 1993; Seeman et al., 1995). Ilani et al. (2001) recently reported that individuals with schizophrenia show elevated levels of D3 receptors in their blood lymphocytes, an increase not affected by antipsychotic drugs (i.e., a similarly elevated level was found in nonmedicated individuals with schizophrenia). Iiani and colleagues proposed that D3 receptor levels on blood lymphocytes be used as a marker for the identification of schizophrenia.

Research has also investigated whether the abnormalities exist with presynaptic dopamine function as well. Using PET, Hietala et al. (1995) found increased uptake of dopamine in individuals with schizophrenia, and the negative symptoms of the disorder have been found to be negatively correlated with reuptake levels (Hietala et al., 1999). Lindstrom et al. (1999) also used PET and found increased rates of dopamine synthesis in the striatum and parts of the prefrontal cortex in individuals with schizophrenia relative to a group of adults without the disorder. Recently, Lavalaye et al. (2001) hypothesized that these findings may be due an elevated density of dopamine transporter proteins. Using SPECT, they examined the density of these reuptake proteins in the striatum in individuals with schizophrenia who had and had never taken antipsychotic medications compared to control subjects. Contrary to expectations, individuals with schizophrenia did not show an increased density of dopamine transporter proteins relative to control subjects, nor were significant differences found between medicated and nonmedicated individuals with schizophrenia. These null results are consistent with several postmortem studies that did not find alterations in dopamine transporter density in schizophrenia (e.g., Joyce et al., 1988). Lavalaye et al. speculated that increased decarboxylase activity (i.e., dopamine synthesis activity) might better explain the previous studies that found increased reuptake, rather than an increased number of dopamine transporters. Harper Mozley and colleagues (2001) recently found that dopamine reuptake differed between healthy males and females during several neuropsychological tasks. They suggested that these sex differences may be related to hormonal differences and that dopamine functioning might be enhanced by selectively manipulating hormonal systems.

Amphetamine Administration

Davis et al. (1991) found increased activity in the frontal regions of patients with schizophrenia following administration of dopamine agonists such as amphetamine. Laruelle et al. (1996) also administered amphetamines to individuals with schizophrenia and measured dopamine release in the striatum using PET. Results indicated that more dopamine receptors (D2) were occupied by dopamine following amphetamine administration in patients with schizophrenia compared to adults without the disorder. The increase in dopamine receptor occupancy was associated with the emergence and worsening of psychotic symptoms, supporting the theory of abnormal functioning of the dopaminergic system in individuals with schizophrenia. Laruelle noted, however, that the increase of dopamine in the extracellular fluid could be due to a number of factors and that their role in schizophrenia is poorly understood. For example, amphetamines may increase extracellular dopamine levels by facilitating the release of dopamine at the synapse, inhibiting reuptake of the neurotransmitter, increasing dopamine synthesis, or inhibiting enzymes that break down dopamine in the intracellular fluid (MAO). Laruelle and Abi-Dargham (1999) have also reported that the dopaminergic system in schizophrenia fluctuates over time and responds differently to amphetamine administration during psychotic and nonpsychotic episodes.

Weinberger (1987), Pliszka (2003), and others have suggested that the positive symptoms of schizophrenia may be due to hyperactivity of dopaminergic neurons in the nucleus accumbens and the negative symptoms to hypofrontality of the prefrontal cortex. Is it possible, for example, that neurodevelopmental aberrations lead to loss of neurons in the frontal regions and, consequently, dopaminergic systems are dysfunctional in this region? Consistent with this hypothesis, Daniel et al. (1991) found that blood flow increased in the prefrontal cortex of individuals with schizophrenia following the administration of amphetamines, and cognitive improvement was noted on an executive function task (Wisconsin Card Sorting Test). In addition, Okubo et al. (1997) found decreased numbers of D1 receptors in the prefrontal cortex of individuals with schizophrenia, and these were negatively correlated with positive symptoms.

Collectively, studies investigating the dopamine hypothesis indicate that the role of dopamine is far more complex than simply an overabundance of the neurotransmitter. Preliminary studies support the hypothesis that dopamine is likely involved in both the negative and positive symptoms associated with schizophrenia, with increased neural activation in subcortical areas and decreased activation in cortical areas. Evidence that supports a role of dopamine in schizophrenia includes: (a) cognitive and behavioral improvement with drugs that block dopamine receptors, (b) inducement of psychotic symptoms with dopamine agonists, (c) increased neural activity in the prefrontal regions following administration of amphetamines, and (d) neuroimaging studies showing a heightened rate of dopamine synthesis during periods of psychosis. Evidence that is inconsistent includes: (a) failure of all individuals with schizophrenia to show improvement with antipsychotic medications; (b) in addition to altering dopamine, amphetamines alter other neurotransmitters such as norepinephrine; (c) drugs that block other dopamine receptors or other neurotransmitter receptors can improve symptoms; and (d) inconsistency across studies concerning density of pre- and postsynaptic dopamine receptors.

Involvement of Other Neurotransmitters

Other neurotransmitter systems have been investigated due to their interactions with the dopaminergic system and because newer antipsychotic drugs have a greater affinity for receptors other than dopamine receptors. The serotonergic system, for example, is closely linked anatomically with both the dopaminergic and glutamate systems. Postmortem studies have produced inconsistent findings, with some studies reporting a significant elevation of serotonin receptors in the prefrontal cortex of individuals with schizophrenia (Sumiyoshi, Stockmeier, Overholser, Dilley, & Meltzer, 1996) that has not been replicated by other researchers (e.g., Cruz, Eggan, Azmitia, & Lewis, 2004; Tauscher et al., 2002). PET studies have also revealed elevated serotonin receptors in other regions in individuals with schizophrenia (e.g., Tauscher et al., 2002). The significance of these findings is difficult to interpret. As mentioned in chapter two, the cell bodies of serotonin neurons are located in several areas of the brain—two midbrain nuclei, the dorsal raphe nucleus, and the median raphe nucleus. These neurons project to the cortex and striatum as well as the limbic regions. At the level of the midbrain, striatum, and cortex, these serotonin neurons are believed to inhibit firing of dopamine neurons and perhaps inhibit glutamate release in the striatum. Thus, it is possible that the interaction of neurotransmitter systems is responsible for the therapeutic effects of antipsychotics. For example, the antipsychotic medication clozapine is known to block serotonin receptors as well as dopamine receptors, with a greater affinity for the serotonin receptors (Perrine, 1996). Drugs, however, that selectively target serotonin receptors (i.e., serotonin antagonists) do not improve psychotic symptoms. The result of decreasing serotonergic and dopaminergic activity in selective areas is behavioral improvement in positive as well as negative symptoms. This finding suggests that improvement of psychotic symptoms is likely the result of altering several neurotransmitter systems, not simply dopaminergic systems. Kapur and Seeman (2001) have argued that effectiveness of atypical antipsychotic medications such as clozapine is due to their modulation of the D2 receptor and not the blockade of serotonin receptors. More research is needed to better understand the role of serotonin and serotonin receptors in schizophrenia.

In addition to serotonin, glutamate, GABA, and other neurotransmitters have been investigated in the pathophysiology of schizophrenia as well. Glutamate became a focus of study after it was discovered that phencyclidine (PCP) could induce many of the same symptoms as schizophrenia (Javitt and Zukin, 1991). PCP occupies and blocks one subtype of the glutamate receptors—the NMDA receptor. It has also been found to worsen psychotic symptoms in individuals with schizophrenia (Javitt and Zukin, 1991). Research investigating the density of NMDA receptors, glutamate metabolite levels, and glutamate precursor levels has produced contradictory results. Recently, Law and Deakin (2001) found that in postmortem samples, individuals with schizophrenia, depression, and bipolar disorder, all had reductions in NMDA receptors. However, those, with schizophrenia had a reversed pattern of findings compared to the other two groups in the area of the hippocampus. Benes et al. (2001) also found glutamate receptor differences in the hippocampus between the postmortem brains of control subjects and individuals with schizophrenia and individuals with depression. Grace's (2001) model of dopaminergic function suggests that dopamine is released on a continual basis (*tonic release*) and that increased levels are released in response to stimulation (*phasic release*). Grace argued that these tonic and phasic releases of dopamine are modulated by several neurotransmitters, particularly glutamate, and therefore glutamate likely plays a critical in the pathogenesis of schizophrenia. Recently, Clinton, Haroutunian, Davis, and Meador-Woodruff (2003) suggested that abnormalities of the glutamate system may occur not only at the level of the glutamate receptor (NMDA receptor) but also within the intracellular pathways that interact with the NMDA receptors. In support of their theory, they found three proteins were abnormally expressed in the thalamus in patients with schizophrenia. As these proteins are involved in intracellular processes that impact the functioning of the NMDA receptor, any alteration therein can impede normal NMDA receptor functioning.

Several abnormalities of the GABA system have also been found in individuals with schizophrenia, including an increased density of GABA receptors and lower levels of enzymes that help to synthesize GABA (Akbarian et al., 1995). Dopamine release in the prefrontal cortex may facilitate the GABA inhibition that helps to mediate excitation in this region. If the dopamine systems are dysfunctional, the GABA systems are in turn affected and aberrant behavior may occur. As reviewed by Soares and Innis (1999), however, several studies found no evidence of GABA dysfunction when unmedicated individuals with schizophrenia were compared to control participants using neuroimaging techniques. Lewis (2000) noted that there are several classes of GABA neurons, which differ in a number of important respects (e.g., axonal targets, morphology). He found a decrease in density of a specific type of GABA transporter in individuals with schizophrenia that he suggested may alter GABA transmission in the prefrontal cortex.

Acetylcholine receptors (muscarinic) are also of interest in that a number of postmortem studies have reported fewer muscarinic receptors in the frontal cortex of individuals with schizophrenia (Bennett et al., 1979). Recently, Raedler and colleagues (2003) used SPECT to detect muscarinc receptor availability in the cortex, basal ganglia, thalamus, and pons in individuals with and without schizophrenia. Results revealed that the availability of multiple subtypes of muscarinic receptors was significantly less (20–30%) in the cortex, basal ganglia, and thalamus in individuals with schizophrenia. Reduced availability of muscarinic receptors in the striatum was also correlated with greater severity of positive symptoms. These results may help to explain why previous studies have found that anticholinergic drugs (e.g., Biperiden) worsen positive symptoms in patients with schizophrenia (Tandon, DeQuardo, Goodson, Mann, and Greden, 1992). Raedler et al. interpreted their findings as supporting a dysfunctional cholinergic system in schizophrenia but noted that this finding may be a secondary effect of other pathophysiological systems.

Carlsson et al. (2001) have proposed that several neurotransmitter systems affecting numerous neural networks underlie the positive and negative symptoms characteristic of schizophrenia. For example, glutamate deficiencies likely affect subcortical dopaminergic systems and elevated serotonin activity likely contributes to negative and positive symptoms. In addition, the researchers recommended that more attention be devoted to the role of neuropeptides, GABA, and acetylcholine in schizophrenia. Similarly, Cloninger (2003) recently emphasized that complex neural networks and interactions among these networks likely result in the positive symptoms of schizophrenia. Specifically, he reported that in certain brain circuits, glutamate actives receptors on GABA, serotonin, and noradrenergic neurons. These neurons in turn inhibit excitatory activity in pathways rich in glutamate and acetylcholine. The end result is that by reducing firing of glutamate and acetylcholine releasing neurons, neurons in the cortex and limbic brain regions are disinhibited, producing positive symptoms such as hallucinations. Because dopamine is thought to affect the activity of glutamate, NMDA receptors and medications that block dopamine receptors reduce glutamate activity and therefore reduce psychotic symptoms. Goff and colleagues (2004) recently reported that serum folate concentrations were significantly lower in patients with schizophrenia, a finding that correlated with the severity of negative symptoms. They suggested that low folate levels may interfere with synthesis of various neurotransmitters and advocated controlled trials of folate augmentation for individuals with schizophrenia.

In summary, it appears as though there is an intricate relationship among the neurotransmitters implicated in schizophrenia, and the nature and degree to which these neurotransmitters are involved remains unclear. Perhaps the most robust finding is that dopamine plays a critical role in positive symptoms but the complexities of its interaction with other neurotransmitter systems is poorly understood. In addition, the long-term effects of the cognitive and behavioral symptoms of schizophrenia on the plasticity of the brain is open to speculation and conceivably could result in neurochemistry alterations. Likewise, the long-term effects of medication on brain neurochemistry remain unclear as well the effects of medication that is taken sporadically or inconsistently.

Neurodevelopment Studies

The fact that only about half of monozygotic twins both develop schizophrenia clearly suggests that environmental factors play an important role in the development of the disorder. Although historically schizophrenia has been attributed to poor maternal parenting, there are absolutely no empirical findings in support of this hypothesis. Currently, environmental factors are once again a main focus of research—but primarily as they relate to fetal brain development. According to the neurodevelopmental hypothesis (Weinberger, 1987, 1996), during pre- or early postnatal development normal brain development is disrupted, leading to neural abnormalities that are later reflected in the behavioral symptoms associated with schizophrenia. A multitude of factors could contribute to abnormal brain development—viral infections, maternal stress, maternal health and diet, birth complications, a number of teratogens (i.e., prenatal exposure to toxic substances), among others. Possibly, prenatal factors interact with genetic information of the fetus that further affects cellular processes such as migration, differentiation, cell death, synaptic connections, and establishment of neural networks.

For example, in 1985 Bradbury and Miller reported that individuals born in the winter months have a greater risk of developing schizophrenia than individuals born at other times of the year. Additional studies have supported this finding (see Torrey, Miller, Rawlings, & Yoken, 1997 for a review). Davies and colleagues (2000) recently reported an excess of first admissions for schizophrenia during the summer months in the Northern Hemisphere and the winter in the Southern Hemisphere. Although the authors were unable to explain their findings, they suggested that research is needed to address the impact of latitude and season of peak admission to psychiatric inpatient facilities. One possible explanation for the seasonality of birth finding is that viral infections are most common during the fall. Although viruses cannot cross the placenta, women who conceive during this period and contract a viral infection may suffer from a fever, which can slow the division of fetal neurons and development (Laburn, 1996). A study by Mednick, Machon, and Huttunen (1990) supports the hypothesis that the flu virus increases the risk of schizophrenia as the researchers discovered that babies who were born 3 months after a major influenza epidemic developed schizophrenia at double the normal rate. It is important to note that these studies are only correlational. Many individuals whose mothers were exposed to the flu virus during pregnancy do not develop the disorder and, similarly, individuals also develop the disorder whose mothers did not contract the flu virus. In addition, studies have found that prenatal risk factors and influenza are associated with other disorders such as bipolar disorder and depression (Torrey, Miller, Rawlings, & Yoken, 1997).

Karlsson et al. (2001) recently examined the cerebral spinal fluid of individuals with recent-onset schizophrenia and regions of the frontal lobe in postmortem brains to explore whether evidence of retroviruses could be detected. Cerebral spinal fluid findings revealed that 28% of individuals had retroviral sequences that were not found in comparison participants. Furthermore, evidence of viral infection (retroviral RNA) was found in 100% of the postmortem brain tissue of those with schizophrenia and only 6.7% of the comparison brains. The authors speculated that retroviruses could be one of the agents involved in the etiology of schizophrenia. Dickerson and colleagues (2003) recently found that individuals with schizophrenia who were also infected with human herpes virus 1 had more pronounced short-term memory deficits than noninfected adults with schizophrenia.

Recently, additional environmental factors have become the focus of research. For example, Cannon et al. (1999) and Dalman (2001) found that infants deprived of oxygen during birth (i.e., *anoxia*) were at greater risk for developing schizophrenia later in life than infants who did not experience anoxia (see Boksa & El-Khodor, 2003 for a review). Dalman et al. (2001) also discovered that premature and low birth weight babies were twice as likely to develop the disorder as term and normal weight babies. Wahlbeck, Forsen, Osmond, Barker, and Eriksson (2001) found an association between low maternal body mass index, small size at birth, and thinness during childhood and schizophrenia. Studies have also found a number of minor physical abnormalities in individuals with schizophrenia, lending further support for a neurodevelopmental model of schizophrenia. For example, Trixler et al. (2001) reported that individuals with schizophrenia have higher rates of furrowed tongue, a greater distance between toes one and two, and misshapen ears compared to controls. Schiffman et al. (2002) reported that children with three or more physical anomalies (e.g., wideset eyes, lowset ears, webbed toes) were significantly more likely to develop the disorder than children without the anomalies. Kopala and colleagues (2001) found olfactory deficits in adults with schizophrenia and their family members compared to families without schizophrenia. Levine and colleagues (2002) found elevated homocysteine levels in the blood of individuals with schizophrenia that may be related to prenatal factors. Malaspina et al. (2001) investigated the relationship between paternal age and the development of schizophrenia and reported that the risk increased fourfold when the father was 50 years or older at the time of conception. It is crucial to note that, similar to the viral studies, these findings are only correlational. However, they do suggest that environmental factors in conjunction with genetic factors lead to the development of schizophrenia.

Keshavan, Anderson, and Pettegrew (1994) asserted that schizophrenia could be due to excessive pruning of synapses, particularly in the prefrontal cortex, as well as failure of pruning to occur in other brain regions. According to the researchers, schizophrenia may result when the level of synaptic pruning reaches a certain threshold that disrupts the prefrontal–limbic circuits. Hemmingsen, Madsen, Glenthoj, and Rubin (1999) also hypothesized that schizophrenia is the result of a genetic predisposition that is manifested through aberrant proliferation and pruning of synapses during brain development. They emphasized, however, that this process differs among individuals depending on their genetic profile and may be influenced by external factors such as the intrauterine environment. Hypothetically, the abnormal synaptic connections affects behavior and social interactions, which in turn lead to storage of abnormal experiences of the world that exacerbate the psychotic states that later emerge. In other words, Hemmingsen and colleagues suggested that schizophrenia is the result not of abnormal neurons but rather abnormal neuronal networks. McGlashan and Hoffman (2000) concurred with the abnormal network view and suggested that early interventions could possibly delay or even prevent the onset of schizophrenia. For example, during the prodromal phase of schizophrenia—when individuals show early signs of developing the disorder—antipsychotic medication may be effective at preventing the onset of the first psychotic episode. McGlashan and Hoffman emphasized that more information is needed on the neurobiology of synaptic connectivity and pruning as well as interventions that may foster or alter this process.

SUMMARY

Despite decades of research, the cause of schizophrenia remains unknown. Findings from various lines of research implicate several brain structures and regions as well as a complex relationship between neurotransmitter systems. Increased activity of dopaminergic neurons of the mesolimbic system has been implicated in the positive symptoms of schizophrenia and reduced activity of dopaminergic neurons of the prefrontal cortex in the negative symptoms. In addition, a substantial body of research suggests that schizophrenia is a disorder of reduced synaptic connectivity, particularly in the prefrontal–limbic pathways. It is important to note that most studies concerning the pathophysiology of schizophrenia are based on group results, which do not reveal information about individuals. In addition, it is critical to emphasize that much of the research concerning schizophrenia is based on correlational studies that cannot— and do not—address causation. Advances in technology and molecular genetics will likely help to elucidate the physiological underpinnings of schizophrenia. Eventually, researchers may be able to combine genetic information with neuroimaging techniques to detect schizophrenia at an earlier stage or identify those at risk of developing the disorder. Answers concerning causation may be found in future molecular genetic studies, although, as addressed previously in this chapter, the relationship between genetic and environmental factors is likely highly complex.

PHARMACOLOGICAL INTERVENTIONS FOR SCHIZOPHRENIA

In addition to medication, a variety of therapies have been found to improve the cognitive and behavioral functioning of individuals with schizophrenia (e.g., Hogarty et al., 2004; Penn et al., 2004). Coverage of this material is beyond the scope of this chapter, however. Instead, the following focuses on medication and its physiological effects on individuals with schizophrenia.

Insulin was one of the first medications discovered to improve psychotic symptoms (LeDoux, 2002). In 1933, Manfred Sake, a Viennese physician, administered a small dose of insulin to patients with schizophrenia to stimulate their appetite. An unexpected benefit was improvement in the psychotic symptoms. It was not until 1952 that Delay and Deniker found that chlorpromazine (Thorazine) reduced psychotic symptoms in patients with schizophrenia. Today, the two main types of medications used to treat schizophrenia are *typical* (first-generation antipsychotics) and *atypical* neuroleptics (second-generation antipsychotics) (see Table 5.2; Lohr & Braff, 2003). Typical refers to neuroleptics that (a) are dopamine antagonists, (b) produce extrapyramidal side effects, and (c) improve positive symptoms. Atypical neuroleptics (a) have an affinity for several types of neurotransmitter receptors, (b) produce fewer extrapyramidal side effects, and (c) improve both positive and negative symptoms.

Typical and atypical neuroleptics are similar in that both are effective at improving psychotic symptoms due to their affinity for D2 receptors. The affinity for other dopamine subtypes (e.g., D1, D3, D4, D5) varies widely among neuroleptics. An affinity for D2 receptors is positively correlated with the potency of neuroleptics, while an affinity for D4 receptors is associated with fewer extrapyramidal side effects and improvement in negative symptoms (Carvey, 1998). Typical and atypical neuroleptics differ in a number of ways. Typical neuroleptics tend to produce greater extrapyramidal side effects due to their widespread blockage of dopamine in the subcortical structures that are important in movement (e.g., basal ganglia). These effects include slowed movements, decreased facial expression, resting tremor, muscle spasms of the

TABLE 5.2

Antipsychotic Medications

Typical Neuroleptics	thioridazine (Mellaril)
acetophenazine (Tindal)	thiothixene (Navane)
chlorpromazine (Thorazine)	trifluoperazine (Stelazine)
chlorprothixene (Taractan)	ziprasidone (Geodon)
fluphenazine (Prolixin)	
Haldol (haloperidol)	
loxapine (Loxitane)	**Atypical Neuroleptics**
mesoridazine (Serentil)	aripiprazole (Abilify)
molindone (Moban)	clozapine (Clozaril)
perphenazine (Trilafon)	quetiapine (Seroquel)
pimozide (Orap)	risperidone (Risperdal)
	Zyprexa (olanzapine)

Please refer to the Physician's Desk Reference for physicians and mental health professionals for additional information concerning these and other drugs.

neck and shoulder, and restlessness. Over time, tardive dyskenisia may develop and more severe tardive dyskenisia effects are associated with typical neuroleptics.

Neuroleptics also differ in their affinity for other types of neurotransmitter receptors such as serotonergic, muscarinic, noradrenergic, and histraminergic. An affinity for these receptors is associated with various side effects such as sedation, dry mouth, blurred vision, intestinal slowing, sexual dysfunction, and weight gain. As mentioned previously, the precise mode of action for decreasing psychotic symptoms is not well understood. Kapur (2003) recently suggested that antipsychotic medications do not cure psychotic symptoms but instead decrease the salience of the distressing ideas and perceptions. In other words, during treatment with neuroleptics, a patient's hallucinations and delusions do not disappear but instead are in remission. During relapse, these delusions and hallucinations become more salient and return to their previously distressing state. Kapur also suggested that dopamine dysregulation underlies psychosis but "a subject's own cognitive, psychodynamic, and cuntural context gives form to the experience" (p. 17). Recently, Davis, Chen, and Glick (2003) conducted a meta-analysis of the efficacy of typical and atypical antipsychotic medications and concluded that some, but not all, atypical antipsychotic medications are more efficacious than typical antipsychotics, alleviating a greater variety of symptoms. Despite the clinical reputation of atypical antipsychotics as the first line of choice for the treatment of schizophrenia—particularly clozapine—research by Woerner et al. (2003) found that clozapine had no benefit over typical antipsychotics.

Typical Neuroleptics

Although the mode of action of typical neuroleptics differs to some degree with the type of medication, they are all dopmaine-receptor antagonists. Grace, Bunney, Moore, and Todd (1997) suggested that dopamine receptor antagonism in the mesolimbic system results in a decrease of positive symptoms but that the receptor antagonism in the nigrostriatal system produces the unwanted extrapyramidal side effects. Typical neuroleptics are often effective at decreasing positive symptoms of schizophrenia but not particularly efficacious at improving negative ones. In fact, when Salokangas, Honkonen, Stengard, Koivisto, and Hietala (2002) investigated the association between neuroleptic treatment and negative symptoms in 1,528 patients with schizophrenia, they found that patients with catatonic symptoms experienced significantly more negative symptoms when taking these medications. Negative symptoms were assessed with the Positive and Negative Syndrome Scale (PANSS) on dimensions such as lack of spontaneity and flow in conversation, blunted affect, passive or apathetic social withdrawal, and stereotypical thinking. This worsening of negative symptoms was found despite the fact that the daily dose of neuroleptic medications was lower in these individuals relative to the other subtypes of schizophrenia. The authors speculated that patients with catatonic schizophrenia may have significantly lower levels of presynaptic dopaminergic activity in certain brain regions (e.g., basal ganglia) compared to other types of schizophrenia. Neuroleptics further reduce this activity and lead to increased levels of negative symptoms.

It has been estimated that 80% of the brain's D2 receptors are occupied within an hour of neuroleptic administration (Farde et al., 1989). This occupancy rate varies to some degree with the type of medication and among individuals. Notable improvement in positive symptoms, however, typically occurs after several weeks of taking the drug. This delayed effect is poorly understood and although several theories have been advanced, no single explanation accounts for this anatomical and behavioral discrepancy. Research also indicates that the antipsychotic effects of these medications occur when approximately 60% of the dopamine receptors are occupied and that extrapyramidal side effects such as tremors begin when approximately 80% of the receptors are occupied (i.e., therapeutic window; Haan et al., 2003; Strange, 2001). Kapur et al. (2000), however, found significant variability among individuals with schizophrenia with respect to range of D2 occupancy (38–87%) after a 2-week period of taking haloperidol. The degree of symptom improvement was positively correlated with receptor occupancy level but also with extrapyramidal side effects: As occupancy increased, psychotic symptoms improved but extrapyramidal behaviors worsened. As mentioned previously, extrapyramidal side effects are due to dopamine receptor occupancy in subcortical regions (basal ganglia, striatum) that are important for movement. When these receptors are blocked, tremor, stiffness, and slowness of movement result.

Atypical Neuroleptics

Lieberman et al. (2003) reported that atypical antipsychotic medications have become the most commonly used class of drugs in clinical practice. The mode of action of atypical neuroleptics is not well understood, but they are believed to have an affinity for dopamine and other neurotransmitter receptors. In addition, atypical neuroleptics have a greater affinity for dopamine receptors in the prefrontal cortex and other areas and less so in the striatum. Therefore, atypical neuroleptics are generally associated with fewer extrapyramidal side effects. Halliday and colleagues (2002) examined the prevalence of movement disorders among 136 individuals with schizophrenia and found that 43% of the patients had probably tardive dyskinesia, 35% Parkinsonism, and 15% akathisia. Contrary to expectations, there was no difference in the prevalence of the movement disorders based on type of medication used (typical vs. atypical neuroleptics). Jest et al. (1999) found that the risk of tardive dyskinesia was higher in older patients with schizophrenia even with low doses and short-term treatment. In addition, they reported that risperidone was less likely to result in tardive dyskinesia than haloperidol. Mamo et al. (2002) also reported a correlation between increasing age and risk of tardive dyskinesia in patients treated with antipsychotic medications.

With regard to receptor affinity, clozapine has been shown to have a substantially higher affinity for serotonin receptors (5-HT2) than D2 or D4 receptors. A study by Arango and colleagues (2003) found that patients with schizophrenia who had larger brain volumes (prefrontal, hippocampus and caudate regions) showed greater improvement in positive and negative symptoms when treated with clozapine than those with schizophrenia who had smaller brain volumes. Arango and colleagues suggested that there is an abundance of serotonin receptors in the prefrontal cortex and by blocking these receptors, dopamine release may be increased in this region, hence improvement in the negative symptoms of schizophrenia. In addition to reducing psychotic symptoms, a study by Meltzer et al. (2003) suggests that clozapine may also reduce the rate of suicide and hospitalization.

Risperidone also has a greater affinity for serotonin (5-HT2 and 5-HT7) than dopamine receptors, although risperidone has also been found to block D4 receptors to some degree. Clozapine, risperidone, and other atypical neuroleptics have been found to improve both negative and positive symptoms. Recent research by Conley and Mahmoud (2001) compared the efficacy of two atypical neuroleptics—olanzapine (Zyprexa) and risperidone (Risperidol)—in 377 subjects with schizophrenia. Results indicated that olanzapine and risperidone did not differ with respect to extrapyramidal symptoms, but olanzapine was more efficacious at reducing positive and negative symptoms. Olanzapine was also associated with greater weight gain than risperidone. Csernansky et al. (2002) compared a typical neuroleptic, haloperidol, and an atypical neuroleptic, risperidone, and found that the occurrence of relapse was significantly lower in individuals with schizophrenia who were treated with the latter. Lieberman et al. (2003) compared the efficacy and safety of a typical antipsychotic, haloperidol, and a typical antipsychotic, olanzapine, in patients with first-episode psychosis. Results indicated that although both drugs were effective at decreasing psychotic symptoms, those who received olanzapine were more likely to continue with treatment. In addition, those treated with olanzapine experienced fewer extrapyramidal side effects but had significantly more weight gain than those treated with haloperidol. As mentioned previously, the atypical neuroleptics have fewer extrapyramidal side effects, but because of their affinity to several types of neurotransmitter receptors (e.g., acetylcholine, histamine, norepinephrine), they do have other side effects such as sedation, weight gain, increases in prolactin, restlessness, fatigue, and cognitive impairment.

In November 2002, the FDA approved the use of Aripiprazole (Abilify) for the treatment of schizophrenia. Aripiprazole is an atypical antipsychotic medication that is a partial dopamine (D2) and serotonin (5-HT1A) *agonist* and has been demonstrated to improve negative and positive symptoms of schizophrenia (Marder et al., 2003). Relative to typical antipsychotic medications, Aripiprazole has fewer side effects and minimal extrapyramidal symptoms. Although the precise mechanism of Aripiprazole is unknown, it is thought to have the ability to block or stimulate receptors as needed if they are either over- or understimulated (Marder et al., 2003). In addition, Silver (2003) has suggested that antipsychotic medications can be augmented with antidepressant medications (i.e., selective serotonin reuptake inhibitors) to treat the negative symptoms of schizophrenia.

Mode of Action

Kapur and Seeman (2001) have argued that effectiveness of atypical antipsychotic medications is due to their modulation of the D2 receptor and not the blockade of other dopamine or serotonin receptors, as has been suggested in the literature. Specifically, they asserted that all antipsychotics—whether typical or atypical—block a some but not all D2 receptors. These medications differ, however, with respect to the rapidity at which they occupy and leave the D2 receptor (Pilowsky, Costa, & Eli, 1992). Furthermore, many atypical antipsychotic medications (e.g., risperidone, olanzapine, clozapine, quetiapine, ziprasidone) show a greater serotonin (5-HT2A) occupancy than D2 occupancy, but they do not reduce psychotic symptoms until D2 occupancy exceeds 65% (similar to haloperidol). Thus, Kapur and Seeman argued that blockade of serotonin receptors is "neither necessary nor sufficient for antipsychotic response" (p. 362); however, "low affinity at the D2 receptor in and of itself is sufficient for producing atypical antipsychotic activity" (p. 363). As noted by Kapur and Seeman, drugs that selectively target serotonin or other dopamine receptors are not effective at reducing psychotic symptoms. They did not suggest, however, that other neurotransmitter systems are irrelevant in psychosis and drug action but argued that the relevance of these systems cannot be determined until the effect of D2 occupancy is considered and controlled for. Finally, Kapur and Seeman proposed that atypical antipsychotic medications that have appropriate levels of receptor blockade and fast dissociation from the D2 receptor improves functioning of neurotransmitter systems. The result is improvement in psychotic symptoms and fewer extrapyramidal side effects, relative to typical antipsychotic medications. Although clozapine is associated with fewer extrapyramidal side effects presumably due to its rapid release from D2 receptors, Seeman and Tallerico (1999) have suggested that this rapid release may help explain the higher rate of relapse (five times higher) individuals with schizophrenia experience upon withdrawal of the medication. Recently, Tauscher and colleagues (2004) used PET to investigate D1 and D2 receptor occupancy in 25 patients with schizophrenia who were receiving one of four atypical antipsychotic medications: clozapine, risperidone, olanzapine, or quetiapine. Results revealed that clozapine had the highest rate of D1 occupancy in the striatum (55%) and quetiapine the lowest (12%). Risperidone had the highest D2 occupancy (81%) and quetiapine the lowest (30%); clozapine, however, had the highest ratio of striatal D1/D2 occupancy of the four medications. These findings may help to explain why many patients who are treatment-resistant to other antipsychotic medications respond favorably to clozapine.

Optimal Dosing

Recently, researchers have questioned the practice of administering dosages of medication to achieve a continuously high occupancy of D2 receptors to improve psychotic symptoms (e.g., Kapur & Seeman, 2001). This practice is based on the concept of a therapeutic window, that is, continual occupancy of 60–70% of D2 receptors is needed to substantially improve psychotic symptoms. Tauscher-Wisniewski and colleagues (2002), however, found that patients with a first episode of schizophrenia responded well to treatment with a single daily dose of antipsychotic medication (quetiapine) that resulted in only transiently high dopamine receptor occupancy. Merlo and colleagues (2002) reported similar findings when comparing smaller and larger doses of risperidone in the treatment of first-episode psychosis. Using SPECT, Bressan et al. (2003) also found that modest D2 receptor occupancy, without serotonin receptor antagonism, was sufficient to explain the effectiveness of an atypical antipsychotic drug, Amisulpride (not yet approved for use in the United States). These results are consistent with Kapur and Seeman's (2001) work suggesting that transient occupancy allows the dopaminergic system to function more optimally.

No "ideal" medication for the treatment of schizophrenia is currently available. Webster (2001) suggested that the ideal neuroleptic would (a) reduce dopamine activity in the mesolimbic system to reduce positive symptoms, (b) increase dopamine activity in the prefrontal cortex to improve negative symptoms, and (c) have no effect on the striatum to avoid inducing extrapyramidal symptoms. Perhaps, in addition to Webster's criteria, drugs should: (d) have minimal affinity for other neurotransmitter receptors so as to minimize non-extrapyramidal side effects and (e) achieve a balance between neurotransmitter systems that produces optimal behavioral effects. Undoubtedly, newer drugs will be developed for the treatment of schizophrenia. A greater understanding of the mode of action of all antipsychotic medications *may* help to elucidate the pathophysiology of schizophrenia. Although medications can certainly improve behavioral and cognitive symptoms characteristic of schizophrenia, they are not without side effects nor are they curative in nature.

SUMMARY

The essential features of schizophrenia reflect a distortion or excess of perceptions and a restriction in the change and intensity of emotion, thought and behavior. The onset typically occurs during late adolescence or young adulthood. There is no definitive cause of schizophrenia. Research investigating the pathophysiology of the disorder has focused on genetic, heritability, anatomical, neurotransmitter, neurodevelopmental, and neuroimaging studies. Treatment of schizophrenia typically involves antipsychotic medication although the mode of action of these drugs is not completely understood. What is clear is that medication can certainly improve the cognitive and behavioral symptoms of schizophrenia but medications are not curative and are accompanied by side effects.

6

Mood Disorders

The DSM IV-TR (2000) classifies mood disorders into depressive disorders and bipolar disorders, and two disorders based on etiology—mood disorder due to a general medical condition and substance-induced mood disorder. The depressive disorders include major depressive disorder, dysthymic disorder, and depressive disorder not otherwise specified, while the bipolar disorders include bipolar I, bipolar II, cyclothymic disorder, and bipolar disorder not otherwise specified. The distinguishing feature between major depression and bipolar disorder is the lack of a manic episode (see DSM IV-TR criteria Tables 6.1 & 6.2). Given that the majority of studies have investigated major depressive disorder and bipolar disorder, these disorders are the focus of this chapter. Specifically, this chapter reviews information on diagnositic criteria, prevalence, gender, and other relevant findings pertaining to major depression and bipolar disorder and discusses the genetic, anatomical, neurochemical, and neuroimaging findings associated with these disorders. Information is also presented concerning medication and other physiologically based treatment approaches for major depression and bipolar disorder.

MAJOR DEPRESSIVE DISORDER

Background Information

According to the DSM IV-TR, 10–25% of women and 5–12% of men will experience an episode of major depression, and 1–2% will experience bipolar disorder at some point in their lives. Kessler and colleagues (2003) recently conducted an epidemiology study of depression in 9,090 adults from 48 states and reported the lifetime prevalence of major depression was 16.2% (women) and 6.6% (men) within the last 12 months. The majority of subjects described their level of impairment during depression as severe, and over 70% of cases involved at least one additional psychiatric disorder. Symptoms of depression typically develop over time and, untreated, can last 4 months or longer (APA, 2000). Kessler et al. reported the average duration of depression is 16 weeks. In the majority of cases, depression remits within a few months although some (5–10%) continue for 2 or more years. According to Greenberg et al. (2003), the economic burden of depression is also increasing as reflected in costs associated with depression in the

TABLE 6.1

DSM IV-TR Criteria for Major Depressive Episode (DSM IV-TR, 2000)

A. Five (or more) of the following symptoms have been present during the same 2-week period and represent a change from previous functioning; at least one of the symptoms is either (1) depressed mood or (2) loss of interest or pleasure.
   Note: Do not include symptoms that are clearly due to a general medical condition, or mood-incongruent delusions or hallucinations.
   (1) depressed mood most of the day, nearly every day, as indicated by either subjective report (e.g., feels sad or empty) or observation made by others (e.g., appears tearful).
       Note: in children and adolescents, can be irritable mood.
   (2) Markedly diminished interest or pleasure in all, or almost all, activities most of the day, nearly every day (as indicated by either subjective account or observation made by others)
   (3) Significant weight loss when not dieting or weight gain (e.g., a change of more than 5% of body weight in a month), or decrease or increase in appetite nearly every day.
       Note: in children, consider failure to make expected weight gains.
   (4) Insomnia or hypersomnia nearly every day
   (5) Psychomotor agitation or retardation nearly every day (observable by others, not merely subjective feelings of restlessness or being slowed down)
   (6) Fatigue or loss of energy nearly every day
   (7) Feelings of worthlessness or excessive or inappropriate guilt (which may be delusional) nearly every day (not merely self-reproach or guilt about being sick)
   (8) Diminished ability to think or concentrate, or indecisiveness, nearly every day (either by subjective account or as observed by others)
   (9) Recurrent thoughts of death (not just fear of dying), recurrent suicidal ideation without specific plan, or a suicide attempt or a specific plan for committing suicide
B. The symptoms do not meet criteria for a Mixed Episode.
C. The symptoms cause clinically significant distress or impairment in social, occupational, or other important areas of functioning.
D. The symptoms are not due to the direct physiological effects of a substance (e.g., a drug of abuse, a medication) or a general medical condition (e.g., hypothyroidism)
E. The symptoms are not better accounted for by Bereavement, i.e., after the loss of a loved one, the symptoms persist for longer than 2 months or are characterized by marked functional impairment, morbid preoccupation with worthlessness, suicidal ideation, psychotic symptoms, or psychomotor retardation.

workplace, mortality costs from depression-related suicides, and direct costs. They reported that as the treatment rate of depression increased by nearly 50% between 1990–2000, the associated costs rose from $77.4 billion in 1990 to $83.1 billion in 2000. Papakostas and colleagues (2004) recently reported that adults suffering from major depression are more likely to report a poorer quality of life. Studies exploring the effectiveness of treatment in improving quality of life are lacking. According to the DSM IV-TR, cultural differences exist in the experience and communication of symptoms of depression. In some cultures, depression may be experienced largely in physical complaints rather than emotions. Fava (2003), for example, reported that approximately 76% of patients with depression report various somatic symptoms such as stomachaches, headaches, and back pain. Oquendo et al. (2001) recently reported that the 1-year prevalence rates for major depression were 3.6% for whites, 3.5% for blacks, 2.8% for Mexican Americans, 2.5% for Cuban Americans, and 6.9% for Puerto Ricans. Suicide rates were highest in white males. Depression often co-occurs with other disorders such as anxiety, attention, and behavior disorders in childhood and adolescence (DSM IV-TR, APA, 2000) and anxiety and substance use disorders in adulthood (Zimmerman, Chelminski, & McDermut, 2002).

Depression is more common in adult females than males, according to Steiner, Dunn, and Born (2003), perhaps up to 50% greater. Gold (2003) noted that the majority of patients treated for mood disorders are women of childbearing age. Recently, Hegarty, Gunn, Chondros, and Small (2004) reported that physical, emotional, and sexual abuse are strongly associated with depression in women, and approximately 24% of women have experienced abuse in an intimate adult relationship. Grupp-Phelan, Whitaker, and Naish (2003) found 18% of mothers who brought their children (age 6 months to 18 years) to an emergency room or pediatric primary care clinic had major depression and 5% reported suicidal ideation. Maternal depression is associated with intellectual and behavior problems in their children's early childhood and adolescence. Hay (2001), for example, found that children of mothers who were depressed at 3 months postpartum had markedly lower IQ scores, significant attentional problems, and difficulties with mathematical reasoning. More recently, Hay and colleagues (2003) reported that maternal depression was strongly associated with violence and anger management difficulties in their children during adolescence.

Although gender differences in the rate of depression exist in adulthood, prior to puberty, the incidence of depression is similar among boys and girls (Kazdin & Marciano, 1998). Goodyer, Park, and Herbert (2001) suggested that endocrine processes such as higher cortisol levels are associated with depression in adolescents but not younger children. They also found that personal disappointments were associated with persistent depression in adolescents and argued that adverse life events may result in a hypersecretion of cortisol, which may lead to memory distortions and cognitive rumination. These cognitive processes may in turn amplify the negative feelings and contribute to the progression of depression during adolescence. Additional developmental differences have been reported between adult and childhood depression; for example, studies indicate that antidepressants are less effective at treating depression in children than adults (Ryan, 2003). Birmaher and colleagues (1996) reported that childhood depression is associated with poor psychosocial and academic outcome and increased risk for bipolar disorder, suicide, and substance abuse in adolescence. Collectively, these findings suggest that the nature and treatment of depression differ in children and adults and that more research is needed to better understand these differences.

Researchers have also recently begun to study late-onset depression. According to Fountoulakis and colleagues (2003), 2% of the general population over age 65 suffers from depression. Similar to the childhood literature, research suggests that depression differs in many aspects in older individuals than young and middle-aged adults. For example, physiological and neuropsychological studies have found an increased severity of subcortical vascular disease and greater cognitive impairment in those over 65 who suffer from depression (Baldwin et al., 2004; Salloway et al., 1996). Ballmaier et al. (2004) suggested that depression in elderly patients may be characterized by specific brain changes such as reductions in gray matter, white matter, and cerebral spinal fluid. Late-onset depression is also associated with a number of neurologic conditions such as stroke (Narushima, Kosier, & Robinson, 2003), Alzheimer's disease and Parkinson's disease (Reynolds, 1992), HIV infection (Elliott & Roy-Byrne, 1998), diabetes (Lustman, Clouse, & Freedland, 1998), and multiple sclerosis (Feinstein et al., 2004).

Etiologic Theories

Genetic Studies

Family and twin studies of major depression clearly implicate genetic factors in childhood and adult depression (Kendler, Prescott, Myers, & Neale, 2003). For example, Glowinski, Madden, Bucholz, Lynskey, and Heath (2003) studied a sample of 3,416 female adolescent twins and reported a genetic risk of 40.4% for major depression. A meta-analysis of twin studies by Sullivan, Neale, and Kendler (2000) reported an overall heritability of 37% for major depression. Other studies have reported much higher heritability estimates (i.e., 78% for females, 57% for males; Kendler, Pedersen, Johnson, Neale, & Mathe, 1995). Maher et al. (2002) reported that first-degree relatives are two times more likely to suffer from major depression, which led them to argue that major depression is likely due to a major locus rather than multiple genes. Lieb and colleagues (2002) followed up 2,427 adolescents and young adults for whom diagnostic information was available for both parents and calculated the risk of depression in their offspring. Results indicated that major depression in parents increases the risk for depression as well as other psychiatric disorders. Specifically, offspring of depressed parents reported higher persistence of depression, more depressive episodes, higher social impairment, and increased rates of seeking treatment. Surprisingly, having either or both parents with depression influenced equally the offspring's risk for depression. Individuals with major depression are at greater risk for attempting suicide, with the rate of suicide twice as high in families of suicide victims compared to families without this history (Runeson and Åsberg, 2003). Brent et al. (2003) also reported that suicidal behavior is mediated by familial transmission but noted that impulsive, aggressive tendencies is the most powerful predictor of suicide attempts, particularly at an early age.

In terms of specific candidate genes, Llerena and colleagues (2003) analyzed the frequency of three genetic polymorphisms of the CYP2C9 gene in patients suffering from major depression relative to those with schizophrenia and healthy control subjects. Results indicated that one polymorphism (CYP2C9(*)3) was higher in patients with major depression. A number of studies have linked the COMT gene (catechol-O-methyltransferasae) to major depression (e.g., Ohara, Nagai, Suzuki, & Ohara, 1998). COMT is an extracellular enzyme that breaks down dopamine and norepinephrine into inactive metabolites, and polymorphisms of this gene have been associated with major depression and bipolar disorder (e.g., Li et al., 1997). Some studies, however, have not supported an association between COMT gene variants and major depression or bipolar disorder (e.g., Frisch et al., 1999). Studies exploring the role of various serotonin receptor genes in depression have reached inconsistent results. Huang and colleagues (2003), for example, reported that major depression and substance abuse disorder were associated with a polymorphism of a specific serotonin receptor gene (5-HT1B, G861C polymorphism) but this gene variant was not associated with bipolar disorder, schizophrenia, or suicide attempts. Bondy and colleagues (2002) found that the presence of two gene variants (angiotensin I converting enzyme and the G-protein B3 T-allele) typically associated with increased risk of cardiovascular disease were associated with a fivefold increased risk for major depression.

Some studies have suggested that polymorphisms of the serotonin transporter gene are associated with susceptibility to major depression and that a polymorphism of the transporter gene may predict medication effectiveness (Perlis et al., 2003). Ito et al. (2002), however, failed to find an association between antidepressant response (SSRI) and polymorphism of the serotonin transporter gene. Anguelova, Benkelfat, and Turecki (2003) recently conducted a meta-analysis of 86 studies investigating the role of serotonin receptor and transporter genes in major depression and bipolar disorder. Results supported a relationship between two polymorphisms of the serotonin transporter gene and bipolar disorder but an association was not found for major depression. Caspi and colleagues (2003) recently reported that a polymorphism of the serotonin transporter gene modulated the influence of stress on major depression. Specifically, individuals with the polymorphism displayed more symptoms of depression and suicidality in relation to stressful life events than individuals who did not have the polymorphism. Glatt, Tampilic, Christie, DeYoung, and Freimer (2004) recently reported that certain gene variants for serotonin receptors may be unique to specific populations such as depression and schizophrenia. Glatt and colleagues noted, however, the genes for serotonin receptors are highly complex and this complexity may contribute to the inconsistencies found among clinical studies.

In addition to serotonin genes, other genes associated with the GABA, acetylcholine, and glutamate neurotransmitter systems have recently been implicated in depression as well (Oswald, Souery, & Mendlewicz, 2003). When Merali et al. (2004) compared postmortem brains of depressed suicide victims to nondepressed, nonsuicide individuals, they discovered lower density and structural abnormalites of the GABA receptor in the brains of suicide victims. They speculated that these differences may have been due to gene regulation that contributed to depression and/or suicidality. Kosel and colleagues (2004) also reported reduced GABA receptor binding and altered GABA receptor functioning in a case study of a severely treatment-resistant, 42-year-old male with major depression and generalized anxiety disorder. This patient received electroconvulsive therapy (ECT) and relative to a control subject who also received ECT, the patient evinced an insensitivity to anesthesia. Genetic analyses revealed the presence of a gene variant that contributed to the altered GABA receptor functioning and was associated with the patient's insensitivity to anesthesia. The authors speculated that the gene variant and altered GABA receptor functioning may help to explain depression cases who do not respond to traditional pharmacological treatments. Similarly, Yamada, Wtanabe, Iwayama-Shigeno, and Yoshikawa (2003) reported polymorphisms of two GABA receptor genes were associated with depression in females and suggested that GABA receptor genes play an important role in the susceptibility to develop mood disorders. Given findings that indicate that individuals with depression are more likely to smoke cigarettes than the general population, Lai, Hong, and Tsai (2001) explored whether a specific gene variant for the nicotinic acetylcholine receptors (alpha7 nAChR) was associated with major depression. Results revealed a modest difference between subjects with major depression and controls, suggesting that the variation in the acetylcholine receptor gene may influence the risk of major depression. Finally, Schiffer (2002) proposed that mutations in glutamate receptor genes may increase the risk of developing major depression.

In summary, a number of genes and gene variants have been associated with major depression but the results have often been conflicting. It is also important to note that association studies merely establish a relationship between genes, chromosomal regions, and disorders; they do not reveal causal or etiologic information about the disorders. Anguelova, Benkelfat, and Turecki (2003) recently reviewed 86 association studies that focused on genetic variation and major depression as well as bipolar disorder, and reported that most of the studies did *not* find a significant association between serotonin receptor variants and depression. Oswald, Souery, and Mendlewicz (2003) reached a similar conclusion but argued that better-designed studies and the use of new molecular genetic methods will lead to better understanding of the role of genetic variants in depression. As technology advances and additional studies that are theory-driven and incorporate larger sample sizes are conducted, a role for specific genes in the development of major depression will likely be revealed. At best, the current literature suggests that a number of genes and gene variants are associated with major depression, but the findings are inconclusive. In addition, genetic factors can be modified by environmental factors. For example, as Kaufman and Charney (2001) noted, stress early in life can promote functional and structural changes in the brain that are associated with an increased risk of depression in later life. Relatively little in known, however, about the interaction between genetic and environmental factors and the ways in which these factors might be modified to promote adaptive changes at the cellular level.

Monoamine Hypothesis

Since the early 1960s, researchers have proposed that major depression results from dys-function of neurotransmitter systems, in particular the serotonergic system. As mentioned in chapter 1, the serotonergic system extends from nuclei located in the brain stem and projects widely throughout the brain. Serotonergic neurons are involved in many physiological func-tions such as appetite, sleep, libido, immune and endocrine system functioning, and mood, most of which are compromised in major depression (Nemeroff, 1998). Physiological evi-dence implicating serotonin in depression has come from a number of sources. Schildkaut (1965), for example, noted that pharmacological agents that reduce availability of serotonin and norepinephrine could *induce* depression in some individuals. In addition, studies have found decreased levels of serotonin metabolites in the cerebral spinal fluid of individuals with major depression, particularly those with a history of suicide attempts (Coccaro et al., 1989; Rao, Hawellek, Papassotiropoulos, Deister, & Frahnert, 1998). A reduction of serotonin trans-porter binding sites has also been found in depressed individuals, and a myriad of studies have demonstrated that increasing levels of monoamines is associated with improvement of symptoms. Collectively, these findings lead to the monoamine hypothesis of depression, which, in essence, predicts that depression is due to reduced levels of neurotransmitters, particularly serotonin and norepinephrine (Delgado, 2000).

If serotonin levels are directly related to depression, then altering levels should reliably af-fect mood. Pharmacological agents, however, that deplete serotonin and norepinephrine levels do not induce depression in healthy individuals (Duman, Heninger, & Nestler, 1997; Stimpson, Agrawal, & Lewis, 2002). Futhermore, when Delgado et al. (1991) investigated the effects of depletion of the serotonin precursor tryptophan in 43 depressed patients, they found that tryp-tophan depletion did not rapidly worsen patients' symptoms. However, as Delgado et al. (1991) and Bell, Abrams, and Nutt (2001) reported, in most patients who have responded favorably to antidepressants, tryptophan depletion causes a rapid relapse of depression. Interestingly, Miller et al. (1996) found a relapse of depression in subjects who responded to norepinephrine reup-take inhibitors (but not SSRIs) following treatment with agents that blocked norepinephrine and dopamine synthesis. Given that depression occurs more often in females, it is telling that tryptophan depletion studies have found that women are more likely to experience "mood low-ering" (but not depression) than men (Nishizawa et al., 1997). Some, but not all, studies have reported an increased vulnerability to mood lowering in subjects who have a family history of mood disorders (e.g., Klaassen et al., 1998). Morris et al. (1999) used PET to investigate tryptophan depletion in depressed patients and found decreased brain metabolism in several regions—dorsolateral prefrontal cortex, orbitofrontal cortex, thalamus, and amygdala. Tryp-tophan depletion has also been investigated in OCD, panic disorder, bulimia, bipolar disorder, schizophrenia, and dementia. As reviewed by Bell, Abrams, and Nutt (2001), tryptophan de-pletion is associated with worsening of symptoms in bulimia, increased levels of anxiety in panic disorder when combined with pharmacological agents that induce panic attacks, impaired cognitive functioning in dementia, and worsening of negative symptoms in schizophrenia, but has no obvious effect on bipolar disorder or OCD symptoms.

What can be concluded from the tryptophan depletion studies? Given that depression does not worsen following depletion, serotonin may play a modulatory role in depression rather than a primary causal role. Based on studies that indicate some depressed individuals respond to different types of antidepressants that target different neurotransmitter systems (e.g., serotonin versus norepinephrine), depression may have multiple origins or at least multiple mechanism for attenuating symptoms. Serotonin has been implicated in a number of other disorders and, in some cases, tryptophan depletion is associated with a worsening of symptoms but not in others. For example, Huwig-Poppe and colleagues (1999) found that tryptophan depletion led to sleep disturbances in individuals with OCD relative to healthy subjects, and Smith, Fairburn, and Cowen (1999) reported that tryptophan depletion caused a worsening of symptoms in individuals with bulimia. Johnson and colleagues (2001), however, reported that mood was unaffected by tryptophan depletion in patients with major depression or bipolar disorder, all of whom had been taking lithium for at least a year. A number of explanations are possible for these findings. For example, as severity of symptoms is associated with the effects of tryptophan depletion, perhaps a threshold of neurotransmitter depletion is need to induce symptoms and such threshold may be individually dependent. It is also possible that the effects of reductions in serotonin may be offset by other neurotransmitter or intracellular systems.

Serotonin Receptors

Serotonin receptor abnormalities have also been the focus of studies exploring the physiological basis of depression. For example, Drevets et al. (2000) used PET to study serotonin autoreceptor (5-HT1A) binding in individuals suffering from depression (major depression and bipolar) relative to controls and reported a 42% binding reduction in the midbrain raphe and 25–33% reduction in limbic and cortical regions in patients with depression. These findings suggest that both types of depression might be characterized by a reduction of autoreceptors that play a critical role in detecting the presence of serotonin in the extracellular fluid and triggering the presynaptic neuron to alter release of the neurotransmitter. Sargent and colleagues (2000) used PET and a serotonin autoreceptor antagonist to measure 5-HT1A receptor binding in patients with major depression before and during treatment with SSRIs. Results revealed widespread reductions in 5-HT1A receptor binding, but, contrary to expectations, receptor binding was not changed during treatment with antidepressants. Bhagwagar, Montgomery, Grasby, and Cowen (2003) tested the hypothesis that elevated cortisol levels may cause a reduction in serotonin (5-HT1A) receptors in patients recovered from depression. Hydrocortisone and placebo were administered to 14 individuals who had recovered from depression and the 5-HT1A binding was measured using PET. Results revealed that females had a higher receptor binding than males but that hydrocortisone treatment did not reduce serotonin receptor binding in regions observed, including the hippocampus. The authors argued that the findings do not support the theory that decreased serotonin autoreceptor binding is the result of elevated stress hormones such as cortisol.

With regard to postsynaptic receptor binding, Yatham and colleagues (2000) reported substantially reduced binding potential (22–27%) in frontal, temporal, parietal, and cortical regions in patients with depression relative to healthy volunteers. Similar results were reported by Larisch et al. (2001). A number of studies have investigated the effects of antidepressants on serotonin receptors. Massou et al. (1997), for example, used PET to study the adaptive changes of serotonin postsynatpic receptors (5-HT2A) in patients with depression who were and were not treated with antidepressants. Results indicated that serotonin receptor binding was higher in treated than untreated individuals, suggesting that antidepressants may promote up-regulation of serotonin receptors. Interestingly, Yatham et al. (1999) reported that after 3–4 weeks of antidepressant treatment (desipramine), patients with depression showed a significant *reduction* in serotonin postsynaptic receptor binding (5-HT2) in frontal, temporal, parietal, and occipital regions based on PET scans before and after antidepressant treatment. These results suggest that serotonin postsynaptic receptors down-regulate with chronic antidepressant treatment and that this down-regulation corresponds with symptom improvement. Meyer and colleagues (1999), however, did not find a difference in serotonin binding potential

(5-HT2) in individuals with and without depression after the effect of age was removed. These findings are consistent with recent results reported by Sheline, Mintun, Moerlein, and Snyder (2002), who found that 5-HT2 receptor binding in healthy volunteers decreased dramatically in a variety of brain regions with increasing age, notably during midlife. It is important to note that decreased serotonin receptor binding is not unique to depression but is characteristic of other clinical disorders such as schizophrenia as well (Ngan, Yatham, Ruth, & Liddle, 2000).

Postmortem studies concerning the role of serotonin receptors in major depression have been inconclusive. Meador-Woodruff, Hogg, and Smith (2001), for example, recently examined postmortem brain tissue from persons with major depression (and other disorders) to determine whether abnormalities of the glutamate receptor existed. Surprisingly, no significant differences were found in brain tissue from individuals with major depression or with other disorders such as schizophrenia and bipolar disorder relative to controls. As Stockmeier (2003) noted, however, methodological differences may contribute to the conflicting findings in postmortem studies such as cause of death, long-term medication usage, substance use and abuse, smoking history, and differences in postmortem sample locations.

In summary, the monoamine hypothesis of depression does not adequately explain the pathophysiology of depression for several reasons. For example, many disorders (e.g., bulimia nervosa, obsessive compulsive disorder, panic disorder) respond favorably to antidepressants and neurotransmitter systems other than serotonin have been implicated in these disorders (Hirschfeld, 2000). In addition, approximately a third of patients with depression do not improve with antidepressants, even though neurotrotransmitter levels increase immediately. Finally, structural studies receptors and monoamine metabolites have been inconsistent, with some studies reporting metabolite differences between individuals with and without major depression and others no differences (van Heeringen, 2003).

Neuroimaging Studies

Neuroimaging studies of depression are plentiful. Many studies have found blood flow and glucose metabolism abnormalities in various brain regions, especially prefrontal and limbic regions, in subjects with depression relative to healthy controls (Drevets, 2000; Kennedy, Javanmard, & Vaccarino, 1997). Results have been conflicting, however, with some studies finding increased metabolism in various brain regions while most studies have found decreased metabolism rates (Bonne et al., 2003; Drevets, Ongur, & Price, 1998; Kimbrell et al., 2002; Soares & Mann, 1997). For example, numerous studies have reported reduced blood flow and glucose metabolism in the prefrontal cortex of individuals with depression relative to control subjects, and many studies have found increased activity in subcortical structures such as the thalamus and amygdala (Drevets, 1998). Murata, Suzuki, Higuchi, and Oshima (2000) reported regional cerebral blood flow was significantly lower in patients with major depression relative to control subjects in the right anterior frontal cortex, temporal cortex, thalamus, and putamen. Silfverskiold and Risberg (1989), however, found a positive relationship between global cerebral blood flow and symptoms of depression. In addition, Drevets et al. (1992) reported *increased* blood flow in the left prefrontal cortex and left amygdala using PET and suggested that a circuit involving the prefrontal cortex, amygdala, and regions of the striatum is involved in the neuroanatomy of major depression. Biver et al. (1994) also reported increased rates of glucose metabolism in the orbital frontal lobe but decreased metabolism in the dorsolateral region of the frontal lobe and parietal cortex of patients with major depression relative to control subjects. Kimbrell et al. (2002) recently studied glucose metabolism in patients with a range of severity of symptoms of major depression using PET. Results revealed that significantly reduced widespread regions of glucose metabolism in subjects with depression relative to control subjects. In addition, Kimbrell et al. found that severity of symptoms was negatively correlated with glucose metabolism in cortical and subcortical regions.

Meyer et al. (2003) compared PET scans and dysfunctional attitude levels before and after administration of a serotonin agonist (d-fenfluramine) in individuals with major depression and control subjects. Results revealed that individuals with depression had significantly higher dysfunctional attitudes, a finding that was correlated with serotonin binding potential. Interestingly, dysfunctional attitudes decreased in both depressed and healthy control subjects following administration of the serotonin agonist, suggesting a role for serotonin in negative attitude formation. Harmer and colleagues (2003) administered a single dose of an antidepressant (reboxetine) or placebo to 24 healthy volunteers and measured their mood and responses to a facial expression task and an emotional categorization task. Results revealed that following administration of the antidepressant, subjects were better able to process emotional information. The authors speculated that antidepressants may reduce negative biases in information processing in nondepressed volunteers, which may help to explain cognitive attitude changes found in previous studies.

In addition to comparing PET scans of depressed individuals with nondepressed individuals, studies have examined PET scans of individuals with various clinical disorders relative to depression. For example, Kegeles et al. (2003) used PET to compare glucose metabolism in various brain regions in subjects with major depression or bipolar disorder relative to controls. All of the subjects with depression and bipolar disorder had at least one first-degree relative with a history of major depression. The researchers measured glucose metabolism during placebo and following adminstration of a serotonin agonist (dl-fenfluramine). Results indicated that subjects with depression and bipolar disorder had lower glucose metabolism in ventromedial prefrontal regions relative to control subjects during baseline and following administration of the serotonin agonist. No differences were found between the clinical groups with respect to glucose metabolism at baseline or with the serotonin agonist. The results indicated that subjects with depression had lower than normal regional glucose metabolism at baseline and that this metabolism rate was suppressed *even further* with the serotonin agonist. As the researchers noted, this finding appears paradoxical and why metabolic inhibition contributes to mood improvement remains to be elucidated. Nobler et al. (2001) suggested that further suppressing neuronal activity produces an anticonvulsant and antidepressant effect, although the particulars of this effect are poorly understood.

Sackeim et al. (1993) compared global and regional areas of cerebral blood flow in 30 adults with major depression, 30 patients with Alzheimer's disease, and 30 normal controls. Results indicated that the two clinical groups both showed reduced global blood flow but distinct regions were associated with depression (prefrontal) versus Alzheimer's (parieto–temporal). Liotti, Mayberg, McGinnis, Brannan, and Jerabek (2002) studied provocation of sadness in individuals with major depression who were in remission, individuals with major depression, and healthy volunteers using cerebral blood flow and PET. Results revealed decreases in blood flow in the orbitofrontal cortex in those with depression or in remission relative to control subjects. In addition, healthy subjects showed increased blood flow in areas not observed in the clinical groups (subgenual anterior cingulate and right prefrontal cortex). The authors suggested that provocation of sadness unmasks a marker for depression, and that disease-specific modification of neural pathways appears to be consistently present in individuals with depression as well as those with a history of the disease.

Davidson, Irwin, Anderle, and Kalin (2003) used fMRI to measure areas of brain activation while affective and neutral visual stimuli were presented to individuals with major depression before and after 2 and 8 weeks of treatment with an antidepressant (venlafaxine). Results indicated that individuals with depression as well as control subjects showed bilateral activation in the visual cortex, prefrontal cortex, and amygdala. Relative to healthy control subjects, the group with major depression showed greater activation in the visual cortex and less activation in the left prefrontal cortex in response to negative versus neutral stimuli. In addition, depressed subjects treated with antidepressants showed significant increases in various brain regions after 2 weeks, similar to the level observed in control subjects, and increased activity was correlated with symptom improvement. According to Davidson and colleagues, these findings implicate a neural circuit that underlies emotional responses to visual stimuli, and alterations of this circuitry may be characteristic of major depression. Antidepressants may normalize abnormalities of this faulty circuitry. In a related study, Siegle et al. (2002) used fMRI to measure activity in the amygdala during negative, positive, and neutral visually presented words in seven depressed and ten healthy control subjects. They hypothesized that individuals with depression would demonstrate more sustained activation in brain areas previously associated with processing of emotions. Results indicated that compared to healthy controls, individuals with depression showed greater bilateral sustained amygdala activation for negative words than positive words. This finding was also correlated with self-reported rumination, suggesting that individuals with depression tend to process negative information for a significantly longer period of time than nondepressed individuals. This study also found a negative correlation between activity of the prefrontal cortex and the amygdala, which supports previous studies that found reduced activity in the frontal regions (e.g., Sackeim et al., 1993). Siegle et al. speculated that therapies that invoke cortical control, such as attention control training, could decrease sustained activity of the amygdala and thereby reduce the cognitive rumination characteristic of depression.

Saxena et al. (2003) used PET to measure glucose metabolism in individuals with major depression or OCD and a group of individuals who had both disorders. All subjects were treated with an serotonin reuptake inhibitor (paroxetine) and pre and post antidepressant scans were compared. Results indicated that individuals with OCD who showed increased activity in the right caudate responded better to antidepressants, while those with major depression who showed reduced activity in the right amygdala and increased activity in the prefrontal region responded better to antidepressants. Overall, these findings suggest that although OCD and major depression tend to respond well to the same antidepressant, the neurophysiological substrates that predict drug response appear to be quite different. Recently, Ravnkilde et al. (2003) compared neuropsychological test performance and PET scans in a group of individuals with depression relative to control subjects. Based on a principal components analysis (PCA) of the neuropsychological tests in comparison with PET scans, the authors concluded that those with depression process information in a qualitatively, rather than quantitatively, different manner than healthy control subjects.

Given the lack of consistency among neuroimaging studies, it is difficult to draw conclusions concerning brain regions involved in the pathophysiology of major depression. Drevets (1998) suggested that two interconnected circuits appear to be particularly involved in depression: a limbic–thalamo–cortical circuit, which includes the amygdala, medial thalamus, and ventral prefrontal cortex; and the limbic–striatal–pallidal–thalamic circuit, which includes the thalamus, striatum, and pallidum. According to Drevets, neurotransmission within these circuits likely differs among individuals with different manifestations of depression. Pizzagalli et al. (2003) agreed with this proposition or hypothesis and suggested that given the heterogeneity of symptoms associated with depression, more refined subtyping of depression may help to uncover neural correlates associated with the disorder. As discussed in chapter 3, results of neuroimaging studies may be influenced by technical issues such as neuroimaging methods used (e.g., PET, fMRI, SPECT) and statistical analysis procedures. Sample characteristics such as gender, age, and comorbidity can also influence findings. In addition, structural abnormalities can affect PET and SPECT images as well as blood flow indices (Drevets, 1998). All these factors may help to explain the inconsistencies across neuroimaging studies of depression.

Anatomical Findings (MRI)

Similar to the neuroimaging studies, structural MRI findings have been inconsistent in major depression. Many researchers have proposed that depression may result from death of hippocampal cells and indeed several studies have found the hippocampus is smaller in patients with major depression relative to control subjects (e.g., Bremner et al., 2000; Frodl et al., 2002a). Hippocampal cells are thought to be particularly vulnerable to stress and associated increases in glucocorticoid levels and may contribute to the hippocampal volume reduction found in these studies. Other studies, however, have not found size differences in the hippocampus between individuals with and without depression (e.g., Vakili et al., 2000). Campbell, Marriott, Nahmias, and MacQueen (2004) recently conducted a meta-analysis of MRI hippocampal volume studies in patients with depression and concluded that the hippocampus does tend to be smaller in those suffering from depression compared to control subjects. Similarly, Videbech and Ravnkilde (2004) conducted a meta-analysis of studies that investigated hippocampal volume in patients with major depression and patients with bipolar disorder and concluded that hippocampal volume was reduced only in the former group. Posener et al. (2003) noted that the shape of the hippocampus was significantly different in patients with major depression compared to control subjects, although no difference was found in hippocampus volume. This study did find, however, a negative correlation between total brain volume and lifetime number of depressive episodes, perhaps due to degenerative changes. These findings are consistent with Stahl's (2000) suggestion that recurrent depression may contribute to structural brain changes. Posener et al. also suggested that structural defects contribute to the shape abnormalities, which in turn may have widespread effects on neural projections and circuits that stem from the hippocampus. Ehnvall and colleagues (2003) proposed that recurrent episodes of depression over time may alter the brain's catecholamine systems, resulting in chronically increased levels of neurotransmitters such as norepinephrine. Engström and colleagues (1999), for example, reported that individuals with depression who attempted suicide had significantly lower levels of CSF dopamine metabolites (homovanillic acid) than healthy controls, but no differences were found in CSF serotonin or norephinephrine metabolites. Recently, Levine and colleagues (2000) found elevated glutamate metabolites in the CSF of unmedicated patients with major depression relative to control subjects, which led them to speculate that the glutaminergic system may be involved in the pathophysiology of depression.

To explore whether hippocampal size varied among individuals with different clinical disorders, Damadzic et al. (2001) compared postmortem hippocampal samples from individuals with major depression, bipolar disorder, and schizophrenia as well as normal control subjects. Contrary to expectations, cell density differences were not found between these groups. Muller and colleagues (2001) also examined postmortem hippocampal tissue of individuals with major depression and bipolar disorder and did not find evidence of cell loss or structural abnormalities. Recently, Frodl et al. (2004) used MRI to measure hippocampal volume in 40 patients with depression relative to healthy controls. Results indicated that patients with depression who had a specific polymorphism of the serotonin transporter gene (5-HTTLPR) had significantly smaller hippocampal volumes than control subjects. The researchers speculated that an impairment in the serotonin system may interact with excitatory neurotransmitters as well as neurotrophic factors and thereby affect the structure of the hippocampus. Alternatively, dysfunction of the glutamate system may lead to exotoxicity and hippocampal malformation (Belsham, 2001).

Additional anatomical structures have been implicated in major depression. For example, subjects with major depression have demonstrated impairment in facial expression recognition and production of emotional expression (Gur et al., 1992). This impairment has been linked to the amygdala, which plays a critical role in the expression and interpretation of emotion. PET studies, for example, have found increased blood flow in the amygdala in individuals with major depression (Drevets et al., 1992) and decreased hippocampal volumes in those with depression relative to control subjects (Sheline et al., 1996). Sheline, Mokhtar, and Price (1998) used MRI to compare amygdala volumes in 40 adults with and without depression between the ages of 23–86 years. No differences were found between the groups with respect to whole-brain volume or total amygdala volume, but those with depression did show a bilaterally reduced core volume of the amygdala. The core volume of the amygdala consists of nuclei that are highly connected with subcortical and cortical structures. The authors speculated that a reduced core volume of the amygdala may have widespread implications for emotional aspects of memory, attention, and perception, which may in turn be related to the pathogenesis of depression. Contrary to expectations, however, Frodl et al. (2002b) and Frodl et al. (2003) found enlarged amygdala volumes in patients with major depression relative to controls. The authors speculated that increased blood flow in this region, as found by neuroimaging studies of patients suffering from depression, may contribute to the enlarged size of the amygdala.

Global brain size has also been measured in depressed individuals, resulting in inconsistent findings. For example, Vythilingam et al. (2003) did not find global brain size differences in adults with major depression, but did report reduced neuronal viability in the putamen and caudate using proton magnetic resonance spectroscopy. Some studies have reported smaller frontal lobes in patients with depression relative to control subjects (Coffey et al., 1993). Elkis, Friedman, Wise, and Meltzer (1995) conducted a meta-analysis of structural findings in mood disorders and reported that 97% of the studies found evidence of ventricular enlargement in subjects with depression relative to control subjects. In addition, the meta-analysis supported that subjects with depression have greater sulci enlargement relative to control subjects. Ventricular and sulci enlargement are not unique to depression, however, and have also been reported in schizophrenia (Elkis, Friedman, Wise, & Meltzer, 1995), Alzheimer's disease (Fazekas et al., 1989), anorexia nervosa (Krieg, Pirke, Lauer, & Backmund, 1988), and alcoholism (Lishman, 1990).

Baumann et al. (2002) recently examined 12 postmortem brains of 6 individuals with major depression and 6 with bipolar disorder and reported that all showed a reduced number of neurons in the ventrolateral subnucleus of the dorsal raphe. As the main neurotransmitter produced by cells in this area is serotonin, the authors speculated that impairment of the dorsal raphe may affect serotonergic and other neurotransmitter systems implicated in depression. This hypothesis is supported by neurodegenerative disorders such as Alzheimer's disease and Parkinson's disease that are characterized by cell loss in this region and are frequently accompanied by depression (e.g., Paulus & Jellinger, 1991). Miguel-Hidalgo and Rajkowska (2003) compared postmortem studies of pathology of the prefrontal cortex in those who suffered from depression versus chronic alcohol abuse. Findings suggested that neuronal and glial cell pathology is present in both groups, but cellular changes tended to be more prominent and widespread in cortical areas of those who abused alcohol. Depression was characterized by a significant reduction in glial cell distribution in the prefrontal cortex, and Miguel-Hidalgo and Rajkowska suggested that this reduction compromised support to the surrounding neurons and presumably affected neuronal function.

Because major depression can often be successfully treated with antidepressants that block the serotonin transporters, studies have explored the density of the transporters in postmortem tissue and living subjects. Results of postmortem studies that have measured serotonin transporter binding sites in individuals with depression have been mixed, with some studies reporting reductions in the transporter (e.g., Malison et al., 1998) and other studies no differences between serotonin binding sites in those with and without depression (e.g., Klimek, Roberson, Stockmeier, & Ordway, 2003; Little et al., 1997). Dahlstrom et al. (2000) measured serotonin transporter availability in children and adolescents with depression who were not treated with antidepressants using SPECT. Results revealed that children and adolescents with depression had significantly *higher* serotonin transporter availability in the midbrain region than children without the disorder. No differences were found with respect to dopamine transporter availability in the striatum. Bligh-Glover et al. (2000) measured density of the serotonin transporter in the midbrain region of suicide victims with major depression and age-matched controls and found no differences between the groups. Arango et al. (2001) also examined postmortem tissue of suicide victims and reported that, in general, the concentration of serotonin transporter binding sites did not differ between control subjects and suicide victims. In the dorsal raphe nucleus of the brain stem, however, the volume of the tissue was 40% smaller than controls.

Factors other than depression have been associated with reduced availability of serotonin transporter binding sites, however. For example, Neumeister and colleagues (2000) used SPECT to study possible variations in availability of serotonin transporters in 11 females. Results indicated that the concentration of the binding sites in the hypothalamus and thalamus varied over time, with significant reductions during the winter months. The authors speculated that this variation may help to explain seasonal mood-related depression but additional, larger studies including males are needed to further explore this hypothesis. Age-related declines in the availability of serotonin transporters have also been reported. For example, van Dyck et al. (2000) used SPECT with 126 healthy subjects (18–88 years) and found that the binding potential of serotonin transporter declined 4.2% per decade. Jacobsen and colleagues (2000) suggested that age-related declines in serotonin transporter binding might explain the poor response to SSRIs observed in some adult and elderly patients with depression.

In addition to age-related changes in serotonin transporters, Tafet et al. (2001) suggested that the chronic stress that often accompanies depression may further reduce the density of serotonin transporters. In addition to serotonin, dopamine transporters have also been investigated in depression. For instance, Brunswick, Amsterdam, Mozley, and Newberg (2003) recently reported that independent of age and gender, individuals with depresssion had greater dopamine uptake in the basal ganglia (i.e., 23% increase in right anterior putamen, 35% in right posterior putamen, 18% left posterior putamen, and 12% left caudate nucleus) relative to control subjects. Thus, the question of whether serotonin transporters play a role in major depression remains equivocal and additional, well-designed studies are warranted.

Depression and Cerebrovascular Functioning

Research with depression in elderly subjects has produced evidence of structural brain changes in this population. Ballmaier et al. (2004) were the first to measure the entire brain surface using MRI in elderly patients with and without major depression. Results revealed a significantly smaller frontal cortex in depressed patients as well as increased gray matter in the temporal and parietal cortices. The authors speculated that complex cortical brain changes may contribute to the observed gray matter increases in depressed elderly subjects. Levy et al. (2003) followed 259 elderly patients for 5 years and found that those with geriatric depression (mean onset was 45 years) who had severe deep white matter lesions on MRI scans were at substantially higher risk for death compared to elderly patients without these lesions. The authors speculated that deep white matter brain changes may be due to cerebrovascular events that increase the likelihood of depression and mortality. The specifics of the relationship between cerebrovascular disease and depression, however, have not been fully elucidated. Recently, some researchers have speculated that reduced blood flow findings in depression may be associated with faulty responses of cerebral blood vessels to neuronal and chemical stimuli (Matsuo, Kato, & Kato, 2002). For example, Neu, Schlattmann, Schilling, and Hartmann (2004) measured cerebrovasular reactivity (CVR) in patients suffering from depression—that is, the capacity of cerebral arterioles to dilate in response to a dilatory stimulus. Their assessment of 33 patients with major depression and 26 healthy controls found a significant reduction in cerebrovascular reactivity in the depressed patients. The authors noted that impaired CVR is associated with increased risk of stroke and suggested that future studies investigate CVR in depression.

Tiemeier, Bakker, Hofman, Koudstaal, and Breteler (2002) investigated cerebral blood flow velocity in 2,093 elderly subjects and found that blood flow velocity was significantly reduced in subjects who suffered from depression. Rechlin, Weis, and Claus (1994) investigated heart rate variability in patients with depression relative to control subjects and did not find differences between these two groups. Matsuo, Kato, and Kato (2002), however, reported differences in oxygen consumption in patients with major depression and patients with bipolar disorder relative to healthy comparison subjects in the frontal regions during a neuropsychological task. Epidemiological studies have reported that 21 to 41% of stroke victims suffer from depression following the stroke (Andersen, Vestergaard, Riis, & Lauritzen, 1994; Burvill et al., 1995), further supporting a relationship between cerebrovascular disease and depression. Jorge and colleagues (2004) recently reported that in a sample of 91 patients with traumatic brain injury (TBI), 33% developed major depression within a year after the injury. The authors speculated that TBI may induce reduced metabolic activity in the prefrontal region and increased activity in subcortical structures such as the amygdala and limbic region. Collectively, results from these studies suggest that a difference in cerebral blood vessel functioning may contribute to the reduced blood flow results frequently found in patients suffering from depression and are consistent with the assertion by Thomas et al. (2001) that depression, particularly late-life onset, is associated with vascular disease processes. Tiemeier (2003) recently noted, however, the relationship between depression and vascular pathology is bi-directional as depressive symptoms earlier in life increase the risk of vascular disease later in life, and vascular disease such as stroke is associated with the onset of depression.

Depression also occurs in elderly subjects with Alzheimer's disease and subjects with dementia with notable structural pathology such as Lewy bodies (Samuels et al., 2004). Wilson and colleagues (2003) examined a group of 130 Catholic priests, nuns, and brothers who underwent annual clinical evaluations and brain autopsy after death. Results indicated that depressive symptoms were unrelated to structural pathology observed in Alzheimer's disease such as plaques and tangles. The authors concluded that major depression co-occuring with Alzheimer's disease is independent of plaques and tangles. According to Rajkowska (2003), postmortem studies generally find alterations in neuronal and glial cell density in the frontal and limbic regions of patients with major depression.

In summary, studies have found a number of structural brain differences in individuals with depression relative to those without the disorder. These findings have not been replicated in all studies, however, and there is no structural difference that is consistently found in patients with depression relative to healthy comparison subjects. Furthermore, structural differences that have been reported are not unique to depression, nor do they reflect the cause of the observed differences. In other words, structural findings are based on correlational findings and do not provide information about the causes of the differences or the etiology of depressive symptoms. Although it is possible that anatomical differences contribute to the expression of depression, it is also possible that long-term depressive symptoms contribute to anatomical changes in the brain.

Additional Theories of Depression

In addition to genetic and neurotransmitter studies, researchers have also explored the role of the immune system in depression. Specifically, some studies have reported that major depression is accompanied by activation of the immune system which leads to autoimmune abnormalities in neurotransmitter receptors and impaired functioning of the hypothalamic–pituitary–adrenal (HPA) axis (Tanaka et al., 2003; Tiemeier, 2003). For example, Tanaka and colleagues (2003) measured serum antibodies to human neurotransmitter receptors (e.g., muscarinic, mu-opiod, serotonin, and dopamine) in patients with mood disorders and other psychiatric disorders and reported an association between autoantibodies and psychiatric symptoms. With regard to the HPA axis, Raison and Miller (2003) found reduced production of cortisol and responsiveness to glucocorticoids in patients suffering from major depression. Jozuka, Jozuka, Takeuchi, and Nishikaze (2003), Maes et al. (1992), and Trzonkowski et al. (2004) also reported reduced levels of cortisol and other immunological and hormonal markers in individuals with depression relative to control subjects. Leonard (2000) suggested that depression is caused by an interaction of immune, endocrine, and neurotransmitter systems that results in inflammatory response in the brain. Research by Heiske, Jesberg, Krieg, and Vedder (2003), Lima et al. (2003), and Szuster-Ciesielska and colleagues (2003) indicates that antidepressants influence the neuroendocrine system and may normalize the altered function of the HPA axis, thereby improving symptoms characteristic of depression. Khanzode, Dakhale, Khanzode, Saoji, and Palasodkar (2003) suggested that depression is characterized by altered antioxidant defense systems and that antidepressants such as fluoxetine and citalopram (SSRIs) may help to normalize this system. When they measured blood serum levels in 62 patients with major depression and 40 healthy volunteers, patients with depression had higher levels of superoxide dismutase (SOD) activity and lower ascorbic acid concentrations, levels that improved significantly following treatment with antidepressants.

Steiner, Dunn, and Born (2003) noted that the lifetime prevalence of depression in women is twice that of men and argued that fluctuating levels of estrogen and other sex steroids may underlie the development of mood disorders in some women. Bhagwagar, Whale, and Cowen (2002) investigated endocrine response (i.e., changes in prolactin and cortisol) to citalopram in individuals with major depression, individuals recovered from major depression, and control subjects. Citalopram is a serotonin reuptake inhibitor that produces dose-related increases in prolactin and cortisol due to acute increases of serotonin in the hypothalamus. Bhagwagar and colleagues sought to determine whether impairments in serotonin functioning were evident and whether these impairments persisted following recovery. All subjects received citalopram intravenously and blood prolactin and cortisol levels recorded during baseline, placebo, and medication conditions. Results indicated no significant differences between baseline prolactin and cortisol levels across the three groups. Following administration of citalopram, however, subjects with depression showed a significantly blunted response with respect to cortisol levels relative to the recovered and control groups. In addition, both the depressed group and recovered group showed significant decreases in prolactin following citalopram compared to the control group. These findings suggest that prolactin and cortisol responses are impaired in patients with major depression and that following recovery, prolactin responses remain abnormal while cortisol levels return to normal functioning. Given that citalopram produces predictable, dose-related changes in prolactin and cortisol due to acute changes in the serotonergic system, these findings support an aberration of the serotonin system. The nature of this impairment and whether it is related to serotonin transporters, postsynaptic receptors, or inhibited release of serotonin are unknown.

Bottiglieri et al. (2000) and others have suggested that a folate deficiency may occur in nearly a third of patients with severe depression, impairing biosynthesis of neurotransmitters such as serotonin, dopamine, and norepinephrine. To further explore whether individuals with depression suffer from folate deficiency, Bottiglieri and colleagues measured a number of blood serum measures including homocysteine levels (previous studies have found that homocysteine levels are a sensitive marker of folate deficiency) in patients with major depression, neurological disorders, and a control group. Results indicated that total plasma homocysteine levels were significantly higher in those with depression relative to the other two groups. In addition, those with depression and high homocysteine levels had significantly lower CSF metabolites for serotonin, dopamine, and norepinephrine, and the authors speculated that these findings suggest an impairment in the biosynthesis of these neurotransmitters. As they explained, antidepressants may be less effective when homocysteine levels are low and therefore homocysteine measures should be implemented more routinely with patients with depression.

Smith (1991) hypothesized that abnormal fatty acid composition, largely due to a diet lacking omega-3 fatty acids, may trigger an inflammatory response by the immune system and underlie the pathophysiology of major depression. Maes and Smith (1998) suggested that changes in fatty acids, immune system activation, and an inflammatory response may interact with neurotransmitter systems such as serotonin and result in depression. Several studies have reported that treatment with omega-3 fatty acids improved symptoms of major depression and bipolar disorders (e.g., Murck, Song, Horrobin, & Uhr, 2004; Stoll et al., 1999). Logan (2003) recently suggested that omega-3 fatty acids may increase cAMP, CREB, and BDNF in humans suffering from major depression. Larger, methodologically well-designed studies, however, have failed to find an association between omega-3 fatty acids and depression as well as other psychiatric disorders (e.g., Fux, Benjamin, & Nemets, 2004; Hakkarainen et al., 2004). Marangell and colleagues (2003) recently randomly assigned 36 patients with depression to receive omega-3 fatty acid supplements or placebo for 6 weeks. Results indicated that symptoms of depression did not improve in either condition, suggesting that omega-3 fatty acids are not an effective method for treating depression. Hakkarainen et al. (2004) conducted a population-based study in Finland of dietary intake of omega-3 fatty acids and self-reported low mood, episodes of major depression, and suicide rates in 29,133 men aged 50–69 years. Based on dietary history and self-report data, the researchers concluded that there were no associations between dietary intake of omega-3 fatty acids or fish consumption and level of mood, suicide rates, or episodes of major depression.

Physiologically Based Treatment Methods for Depression
Antidepressants and Neuroimaging Studies

The vast amount of information available on the effectiveness of therapy in the treatment of depression is beyond the scope of this text. The following section focuses on physiologically based interventions for depression.

As covered in chapter 2, three broad classes of antidepressants are used to treat depression: monoamine oxidase inhibitors, tricyclic, and atypical antidepressants. Stahl (1998) described four additional classes of antidepressants, three of which increase serotonin but also have other effects. For example, venlafaxine inhibits reuptake of both serotonin and norepiephrine. Nefazodone, a serotonin receptor antagonist, prevents reuptake, and mirtazapine, is a serotonin autoreceptor and postsynaptic (5-HT2 and 5-HT3) antagonist. Bupropion has no direct effect on the serotonin system and instead blocks reuptake of dopamine and norepinephrine

(Learned-Coughlin et al., 2003). The mode of action differs with each class of antidepressant. Monoamine oxidase inhibitors are drugs that prevent monoamine oxidase from breaking down neurotransmitters within the terminal button and consequently more neurotransmitter is available for release and for activating postsynaptic receptors. Use of MAOIs is associated with improvement of depression symptoms although the precise cellular mechanisms that result in behavioral improvement are not well understood. Monoamine oxidase inhibitors are prescribed less frequently than other depressants due to their interaction with the amino acid tyramine, commonly found in foods such as cheese, coffee, and chocolate. Specifically, when MAO is inhibited, tyramine is not broken down and accumulates in the intracellular and extracellular fluid. The accumulation of tyramine increases blood pressure and can cause hypertension and stroke (PDR, 2003).

Tricyclic antidepressants (e.g., imipramine, desipramine) block the reuptake of norepinephrine and, to a lesser degree, serotonin by binding to the presynaptic transporter proteins. The major limitation of tricyclic antidepressants is their adverse side effects (e.g., sedation, dry mouth, blurred vision, dizziness; PDR, 2003). The atypical antidepressants—selective serotonin reuptake inhibitors (SSRIs) such as fluoxetine and Paxil—are the most commonly prescribed antidepressant medications, accounting for 50% or more of such prescriptions (Stahl, 1998). Relative to tricyclic antidepressants, SSRIs produce fewer side effects, have a greater compliance rate, and can be used to treat a large number of disorders. According to a meta-analysis completed by Edwards and Anderson (1999) involving five SSRIs (citalopram, fluoxetine, fluvoxamine, paroxetine, and sertraline), fluoxetine has a slower onset but otherwise there is no difference in the clinical efficacy of the drugs. Quitkin and colleagues (2003) studied 840 patients in a 12-week trial of fluoxetine and reported that symptom improvement may not be observed for 6 to 8 weeks. Although many studies suggest that older tricyclic antidepressants and newer SSRIs have equivalent efficacy in treating depression (Song et al., 1993), Parker (2002) recently suggested that older tricyclic antidepressants may be more effective than new SSRIs in older patients with major depression. In addition, Bruijn, Moleman, Mulder, and van den Broek (1999) reported that the tricyclic imipramine was more efficacious and had fewer side effects than mirtazapine. These studies suggest that efficacy of antidepressants is likely influenced by a number of factors and thus their selection and use should be individually determined.

As mentioned in chapter 2, the mode of action of SSRIs is not completely understood but appears to initially involve a four-step process that implicates the serotonergic system in the pathophysiology of depression: (a) SSRIs immediately attach to the serotonin transporter (SERT) and prevent the reuptake of serotonin, (b) this blockage causes a rapid increase of serotonin in the soma, (c) autoreceptors become desensitized to the increased levels of serotonin and more serotonin is released from the terminal button, and (d) after several weeks the postsynaptic receptors also desensitize which is associated with alleviation of symptoms. Chronic antidepressant treatment appears to promote intracellular changes that lead to an increased expression of nerve growth factors, dendritic expansion, and neurogenesis in restricted brain regions such as the hippocampus (Manji, 2003).

Approximately two thirds of individuals with depression respond to a single antidepressant, and nearly 95% respond to a combination of antidepressants (Stahl, 2000). Antidepressant use has increased in the United States as well as many other parts of the world. Poluzzi et al. (2003) studied prescriptions of antidepressants in Italy, a country that prior to 2000 had a low consumption of antidepressants. Results indicated that after antidepressants were admitted for reimbursement without restrictions, prescriptions increased significantly, albeit at lower than recommended daily doses; women were prescribed antidepressants more often than men; 63% of prescriptions were SSRIs; and SSRIs were prescribed less frequently with increasing age. During the past decade, use of antidepressants with children and adolescents has also increased. El-Mallakh, Peters, and Waltrip (2000) have raised concerns over the use of antide-pressants with this population given the unknown long-term structural and cellular side effects of antidepressants. As these authors noted, the child and adolescent brain is still developing and it is unknown whether antidepressants can alter normal developmental processes such as dendritic expansion and synaptic pruning. Furthermore, the specific effects of antidepressants on neurotransmitter and cellular processes are not well understood. For example, Nobler, Ol-vet, and Sackeim (2002) reported that antidepressants reduce rCBF in prefrontal brain regions, and Davies, Lloyd, Jones, Barnes, and Pilowsky (2003) reported decreased rCBF in the left occipital lobe, right cerebellum, and bilateral temporal cortex. Davies and colleagues also found, however, increased rCBF bilaterally in the thalamus in depressed patients treated with an antidepressant (venlafaxine). These changes in rCBF were associated with improvement of depressive symptoms.

Little et al. (1996) also found decreased glucose metabolism in frontal regions was associated with a favorable response to antidepressants (venlafaxine or bupropion) and that nonresponders showed a different pattern of glucose metabolism. Mayberg et al. (2000) used PET to measure glucose metabolism changes with fluoxetine treatment in patients with major depression over a 6-week period. Results indicated that improvement of symptoms was associated with a decrease in glucose metabolism in the striatum and limbic regions and increases in glucose metabolism in the prefrontal, parietal, anterior, and posterior cingulate regions. Individuals who did not improve with fluoxetine showed an inverse pattern of glucose response, leading the researchers to speculate that failure to increase and decrease glucose metabolism in specific brain regions may underlie nontreatment response. Bonne et al. (1999) investigated the effects of fluoxetine on cerebral blood flow in 15 healthy volunteers using SPECT. Compared to baseline and placebo conditions, results revealed no significant changes in cerebral blood flow following 6 weeks of treatment. Gelfin, Gorfine, and Lerer (1998) also investigated the effects of fluoxetine in normal volunteers over a 7-week, placebo controlled trial and found no significant changes in mood or other psychological variables. Leuchter et al. (2002) and Cook et al. (2002) recently investigated quantitative electroencephalography (QEEG) changes in individuals with major depression who were taking either antidepressant medication or placebo. Results indicated that 52% of the subjects responded to antidepressant medication and 38% responded to placebo. Both groups had similar rates of decline in depression symptoms, but QEEG findings revealed different physiological patterns in those receiving antidepressants. Depressed subjects responding to antidepressants showed decreased frontal activity (consistent with blood flow studies) while those who responded to placebo showed an increase in prefrontal activity. The researchers suggested that subjects with depression who have increased metabolic activity in the frontal regions as found by some PET studies, may show improvement in symptoms based on a placebo response, while medication responders have a different pattern of activity.

Follow-up studies indicate that depression has a recurring course but use of antidepressants may reduce relapse rates. According to Hirschfeld and Schatzberg (1994), approximately 30% of adults with depression will relapse within a year; for adults who have experienced at least two episodes of depression, the relapse rate is 70–80%. According to Stahl (2000, p. 8), five factors increase the risk of relapse: (a) multiple prior episodes, (b) severe episodes, (c) long-lasting episodes, (d) episodes with bipolar disorder or psychotic features, and (e) incomplete recovery between two consecutive episodes. Studies indicate that antidepressants significantly reduce relapse rates by as much as 50%, particularly if the medication is taken for 1 year (Reimherr et al., 1998). Frank et al. (1990) found that relapse rates were also reduced over a 3-year period, as only 15% of adults taking an antidepressant (imipramine) had a reoccurrence of depression compared to 90% who took a placebo. Nelson and colleagues (2004) recently reported that combining SSRIs (e.g., fluoxetine) and norepinephrine reuptake inhibitors (e.g., desipramine) significantly increases remission rates than either antidepressant used alone during a 6-week study. Hall and colleagues (2003) analyzed trends in suicide rates and trends in antidepressant prescribing in Australia between 1991–2000 and concluded rates of suicide in that country decreased significantly with the introduction of antidepressants. However, research also suggests that although depressive symptoms may improve, nearly half of patients who respond to antidepressants fail to reach remission (nonsymptomatic) and even fewer attain recovery—that is, remission lasting for 6–12 months (Stahl, 2000). Stahl (2000) has suggested that patients who do not reach remission are at an increased risk for relapse, suicide, and impairment. He also noted that left untreated, depression may "have a long-lasting or even irreversible neuropathological effect on the brain, rendering treatment less effective if symptoms are allowed to progress than if they are removed by appropriate treatment early in the course of the illness" (p. 18).

Antidepressants and Suicidal Behavior

Teicher, Glod, and Cole (1993) suggested that treatment with some antidepressants may actually increase suicidality in patients with depression, and numerous studies and theoretical articles have attempted to address this controversial question. For example, Healy (2003) reviewed clinical studies and meta-analyses concerning antidepressants and suicide and concluded that SSRIs may double the risk of suicide attempts and completed suicides compared to older antidepressants or no treatment. Cheeta and colleagues (2004) reviewed antidepressant-related deaths in England and Wales between 1998–2000 and reported that 80% of deaths from antidepressants were suicides and that suicide deaths were even higher when SSRIs were used in combination with tricyclic antidepressants. Rossi, Barraco, and Donda (2004), however, reviewed studies involving 9,087 patients who were treated with an SSRI (fluoxetine) and found that fluoxetine was not associated with an increased risk of suicide. Khan, Khan, Kolts, and Brown (2003) examined suicide rates in 48,277 depressed patients who took SSRIs, placebo, or other antidepressants. Results indicated that there was no difference in suicide risk among those taking placebo or any of the antidepressants. Balon (2003) argued that articles which claim that antidepressants increase the risk or cause suicide in depressed patients can be viewed as propaganda, and stated that "the evidence seems to be in the eye of the beholder" (p. 298). As mentioned in chaper 2, Khan and colleagues (2003) reported that of 48,277 depressed individuals treated with antidepressants, 77 committed suicide. Similar rates were found among those who received an SSRI or a placebo. Kahn et al. concluded that the findings did not support an increased risk between antidepressants and suicide. These findings may not apply to children, however. As discussed in chapter 2, in 2004 the FDA reviewed 24 trials involving over 4,400 children and adolescents treated with 9 different antidepressant drugs (or placebo) for OCD, major depression, or other psychiatric disorders and reported an average suicide risk of 4% compared to 2% for placebo (no suicides actually occurred during the trials). As a result of these findings, the FDA directed manufacturers of all antidepressant drugs to include a boxed warning statement about the increased risk of suicidal thinking or behavior among children and adolescents treated with these medications. Empirically, the relationship between treatment with antidepressants and suicide is difficult to assess, but overall, studies do not support a causal relationship.

Pregnancy and Antidepressants

According to Gold (2003), the majority of patients treated for mood disorders are women of childbearing age. Nonacs and Cohen (2003) reported that depression is common during pregnancy and that women with a history of depression are at even greater risk. Wisner, Perel, Peindl, and Hanusa (2004) reported that 41% of women who have suffered one episode of postpartum depression experience a recurrence within a year of giving birth. Bonari, Bennett, Einarson, and Koren (2004) reported that untreated depression during pregnancy is associated with a higher risk of maternal morbidity, suicide ideation, postpartum depression, and adverse fetal outcome. Given these findings, treatment for depression during pregnancy is crucial. Preliminary studies suggested that antidepressants are relatively safe during late pregnancy. For example, Hendrick and colleagues (2003a, b) measured 38 maternal blood cord samples for presence of maternal antidepressant concentrations. Results indicated that 86% of the cord samples had detectable antidepressant metabolites, at levels generally lower than corresponding maternal concentrations. These findings suggest the fetus is able to metabolize and eliminate antidepressants, but not completely. All of the infants were full-term and of average weight. Nonacs and Cohen (2003) reported that none of the antidepressants are thought to increase the risk of congenital malformations in infants. Recently, however, Sanz, De-las-Cue vas, Kiuku, Bate, and Edwards (2005) used the World Health Organization's database to investigate whether the use of SSRIs were associated with withdrawal symptoms in newborns. Results revealed that a number (i.e., 93) of cases of neonatal convulsions and withdrawal were associated with the drugs, most often involving paxil (paroxeline), Oberlander et al. (2005) observe the pain reactivity of 2 month old infants who had been exposed to SSRIs prenatally and postnatally (breast milk) in response to a painful event (heel-lance). Results revealed those infants who had been exposed to SSRIs had significantly few facial reactions to the heel-lance and their heart rate was significantly lower immediately following the painful events. The authors suggested that SSRIs may alter pain modulation in infants exposed to SSRIs prenatally and postnatally; however, additional studies are needed to understand the potential long-term effects.

With regard to breast milk and medications, Gardiner and colleagues (2003) studied maternal drug doses (olanzapine) used to treat postpartum psychosis and breast milk concentrations in seven mother–infant nursing pairs. Results indicated that the amount of drug in breast milk was 1% of the maternal dose and was not detectable in the plasma samples of the infants. All of the infants in the study were healthy and no side effects of the medication were observed. Suri and colleagues (2002) estimated the percentage of maternal fluoxetine (Prozac) that nursing infants receive in breast milk, and reported that over the course of a year, the maximum dose that an infant receives is 47% of the maternal daily dose of fluoxetine. Hendrick and colleagues (2003a) found that breast-fed infants of mothers taking antidepressants were of average weight 6 months after birth, and Misri and Kostaras (2002) concluded that, with a few exceptions, no serious side effects have been reported in infants exposed to antidepressants via breast milk.

Intracellular Changes and Antidepressants

In addition to neurotransmitter, immune system, and endocrine systems, second messenger systems have been implicated in major depression as well. Duman, Heninger, and Nestler (1997), for example, proposed that depression is due to complex molecular and intracellular changes. For example, intracellular processes include intricate second messenger pathways that are involved in a neuron's ability to receive, process, and respond to information (Bhalla & Iyengar, 1999). Abnormalities in signaling pathways have been implicated in a number of human diseases (Spiegel, 1998) and, more recently, psychiatric disorders including addiction, anxiety, and mood disorders (Pandey, 2003; Warsh, Young, & Li, 2000). One intracellular pathway—the cAMP pathway—has received considerable attention in major depression as well as bipolar disorder. The cAMP pathway is part of a complex second messenger system that is activated when neurotransmitters including serotonin and norepinephrine occupy receptors. Activation of cAMP induces a series of intracellular changes, including changes in the cAMP response element binding protein (CREB), which in turn triggers changes in gene expression. Fujioka, Fujioka, and Duman (2004) recently reported that activation of cAMP and cascading events increased the proliferation, survival, and maturation of newborn neurons in the hippocampus of adult rats. Postmortem studies with humans have found increased levels of several proteins associated with blunted cAMP functioning (Garcia-Sevilla et al., 1999), and Stewart et al. (2001) suggested that dysregulation of second messenger systems are implicated in major depression in humans. Stewart et al. examined postmortem brain tissue samples of individuals with major depression, bipolar disorder, schizophrenia, and control subjects and reported both major depression and bipolar disorder are characterized by faulty cAMP functioning.

Treatment with antidepressants may improve functioning of the cAMP pathway (i.e., increase CREB levels), and mood-stabilizing drugs such as lithium may decrease CREB levels and decrease intracellular signaling (Duman, Heninger, & Nestler, 1997). For example, Nibuya, Nestler, and Duman (1996) found that chronic administration of antidepressants increased cAMP and CREB activation in the hippocampus of rats. Other studies have found that antidepressants lead to a down-regulation of cAMP in other brain regions such as the locus coeruleus (Nestler, Alreja, & Aghajanian, 1999). Other animal studies have also found that antidepressants increase the expression of brain-derived neurotrophic factors (BDNF) that enhance the growth and survival of neurons (Morcuende et al., 2003). Altar, Whitehead, Chen, Wortwein, and Madsen (2003) recently reported that antidepressants significantly increased BDNF levels in rats, with some areas of the brain showing greater increases than others (i.e., 29% in neostriatum and 18% in the frontal cortex). Duman (2002) suggested that down-regulation of cAMP and CREB may contribute to the pathophysiology of depression in humans and methods (e.g., antidepressants) that increase these transcription factors likely contribute to a therapeutic response. Exercise has also been reported to improve symptoms of depression (e.g., Blumenthal et al., 1999; Dimeo, Bauer, Varahram, Proest, & Halter, 2001) in many but not all studies (e.g., Martinsen, Hoffart, & Solberg, 1989). Although the mechanisms responsible for improvement of depressive symptoms with regular exercise are not fully understood, intracellular changes in cAMP and CREB activation may be involved. Alternatively, as Blumenthal et al. (1999) noted, reduced activity of the HPA axis and increased secretion of endorphins and opioid peptides may also contribute to the improvement of depression during exercise. Given the research findings that support a link between vascular disease and depression, increased oxygen during aerobic training may also be related to improvement of symptoms (Martinsen, Hoffart, & Solberg, 1989).

Recently researchers have begun to focus on the molecular theory that stress can down-regulate the expression of proteins and other substances that are crucial for the viability and plasticity of neurons (Duman, Malberg, & Thome, 1999). This research is particularly exciting in that it suggests that antidepressants may correct or even prevent adverse cellular changes. D'Sa and Duman (2002), Miguel-Hidalgo and Rajkowska (2002), and others have suggested that antidepressants may be capable of reversing some of the morphological brain changes associated with depression in other animals. According to Miguel-Hidalgo and Rajkowska, research with other animals has found that antidepressants can increase neurgenesis and lead to increased growth of dendrites and axons. D'Sa and Duman noted that antidepressants increase production of neurotrophins, and as discussed in chapter 2, these substances are intimately involved in cell plasticity and survival. Duman, Nakagawa, and Malberg (2001) reported that antidpressants can also promote neurogenesis in the hippocampus of adult rodents and may be able to reverse the effects of stress on hippocampal neurons. Studies with humans are sparse, however. Eriksson and colleagues (1998) was among the first to demonstrate that contrary to popular belief, hippocampal neurons do regenerate in adult humans, although his sample consisted of cancer patients who did not receive treatment with antidepressants. Reid and Stewart (2001) have proposed that stress may induce a series of effects ranging from mild structural changes to neuronal death. Depending on an individual's genetic factors, early childhood experience, previous episodes and duration of stress, and unique experiences such as head injury and so on, the physiological effects of stress at any given point in life will differ among individuals. They suggested that neurotransmitter systems may play a secondary rather than primary role in the etiology of depression, but nonetheless serve as a mechanism for attenuating the symptoms of depression.

Antidepressants and Neurotrophic Factors

Preliminary studies with other animals suggest that antidepressants can induce structural changes such as dendritic expansion as well as intracellular changes that lead to an increase in neurotrophic factors such as BDNF. Laifenfeld, Klein, and Ben-Shachar (2002) recently reported that norepinephrine alters the expression of genes and promotes cellular changes such as neuronal sprouting and increased connectivity in human cells. Manji (2003) noted that drugs that increase neurotrophic growth factors are currently under development for the treatment of mood disorders. The effects of antidepressants in humans have recently been investigated using neuroimaging techniques. For example, Sheline, Gado, and Kraemer (2003) used MRI to measure the effects of antidepressant treatment on hippocampal volumes of 38 adult females and found that longer durations of untreated depression were associated with reductions in volume. The authors suggested that antidepressants serve a neuroprotective effect during depression that may be due to CREB activation and increased levels of neurotrophic factors generated by antidepressants. Indeed, Duman (1998) suggested that stress decreases the production of neurotrophic factors (i.e., BDNF), which may contribute to atrophy and altered function of neurons in the hippocampus. Vaidya and Duman (2001) hypothesized that antidepressants may increase the expression of BDNF and consequently reverse or attenuate the toxic effects of stress-induced neuronal changes. Shimizu and colleagues (2003) recently measured BDNF serum levels of patients with major depression who had not been treated with antidepressants, those with major depression who were currently treated with antidepressants, and healthy controls. Results indicated that BDNF levels were significantly lower in the antidepressant-naïve group relative to the antidepressant-treated group and control subjects. In addition, BDNF levels increased substantially after treatment with antidepressants. These findings support a role for low BDNF levels in depression and suggest that antidepressants may help to normalize levels.

Recently, Lai, Hong, and Tsai (2003) compared CREB expression in 21 individuals with major depression before and after antidepressant treatment relative to control subjects. Results revealed that initial CREB levels were similar in untreated individuals with major depression and control subjects. After 8 weeks of antidepressant treatment, however, CREB expression was significantly *decreased* in individuals with depression, unrelated to therapeutic response. Manji and colleagues (2003) have suggested that drugs which target intracellular processes, promote the activity of neurotrophic growth factors, and enhance functioning of the second messenger pathways (e.g., cAMP phosphodiesterase inhibitors) hold promise for the treatment of severe, treatment-resistant depression. It is important to note that there are many intracellular pathways and it is possible that several contribute to symptoms of depression. Preliminary results suggest that when antidepressants are administered, the cAMP pathway plays a critical role in the alleviation of depressive symptoms. It is possible, however, that other pathways are also involved in antidepressant effects and may be affected by other nonpharmacological treatments for depression. Additional studies are needed to better understand the role of the cAMP pathway and other intracellular pathways in the pathophysiology of depression.

It is also important to note that intracellular changes are not unique to antidepressants. Schmitt, Weber, Jatzko, Braus, and Henn (2004) recently reported that chronic use of the antipsychotic haloperidol increased glial cell expansion, leading to a significant increase in the size of the hippocampus in rats. Coyle and Duman (2003) noted that lithium, used to treat bipolar disorder, and ECT, used to treat major depression as well as other disorders, activate intracellular signaling and promote neurogenesis and synaptic plasticity in other animals. Chen et al. (1999) reported that both antidepressants and mood stabilizers regulate intracellular changes and gene expression but do so by different intracellular pathways (cyclic adenosine monophosphate pathway and protein kinase C signaling pathway, respectively). Given that antidepressants and mood stabilizers are often effective at ameliorating symptoms of depression and bipolar disorder, Chen and colleagues (2001) suggested that mood disorders are likely characterized by impaired cell resiliency and impaired neuroplasticity. Zarate et al. (2003) reported that mood disorders are associated with structural changes such as reduction in density and size of glia and neurons in specific brain areas and that glutamate may play a major role in these changes. Therefore, they suggested, drugs that block the NMDA receptor or inhibit glutamate release may prove useful in the future treatment of depression.

Brain Stimulation and Nonpharmacological Treatments

As noted previously, a substantial number of individuals with depression do not respond to antidepressants. Michalak and Lam (2002) reviewed approaches used to treat chronic, resistant depression and concluded that antidepressants used in conjunction with psychotherapy are superior to either treatment approach used in isolation. They noted that psychotherapy alone does not appear to be efficacious for treating severe, chronic depression. Stimpson, Agrawal, and Lewis (2002) conducted a systematic review of all randomized controlled trials that measured the efficacy of medication or psychological intervention for treatment-resistant depression and located 16 studies. None of the studies included psychotherapy, however, and according to the authors, all of the studies were limited by serious methodological problems. Stimpson et al. concluded that empirical information is currently lacking concerning the management of treatment-resistant depression. Electroconvulsive therapy (ECT) is frequently used with patients who do not respond to traditional approaches, and although ECT can often improve depressive symptoms, the mechanism by which this occurs is unclear.

Patients with major depression who have undergone ECT can be evaluated with PET to measure glucose metabolism and regional cerebral blood flow (rCBF) before and after treatment. In 1994, Nobler and colleagues used PET to measure global and regional cerebral blood flow and glucose metabolism in patients with major depression and patients with bipolar disorder 30 minutes before, 50 minutes after, and a week after ECT. Results indicated larger blood flow reductions were associated with better outcome for both groups of patients. More recently, Nobler et al. (2001) studied glucose patterns in patients with major depression before and 5 days after bilateral treatment with ECT. Results indicated that following ECT, widespread decreases in cerebral glucose metabolism were found. The researchers suggested that ECT reduces neuronal activity in subcortical and cortical regions, which potentially explains its antidepressant effects. A study by Milo et al. (2001) reported that prior to ECT, patients with depression had reduced blood flow of the frontal regions relative to controls. Following ECT, those who showed improvement in depressive symptoms had significant increases (toward normal) in blood flow and those who showed minimal response no significant change in rCBF. Blumenfeld, McNally, Ostroff, and Zubal (2003) measured rCBF *during* bilateral ECT (bifrontal or bitemporal) in patients with major depression. Results indicated blood flow increases in the prefrontal and anterior cingulate regions with bifrontal ECT, with the greatest increase in the prefrontal regions.

Bitemporal ECT was associated with blood flow increases in the lateral frontal cortex and anterior temporal lobes. Research with other animals suggests that ECT increases sensitivity of serotonin postsynaptic receptors in the hippocampus and increases release of neutransmitters such as GABA and glutamate (Ishihara, Amano, Hayakawa, Yamawaki, & Sasa, 1999; Ishihara & Sasa, 2001). ECT may decrease the sensitivity of serotonin autoreceptors, however, resulting in an increased release of neurotransmitters (Gur, Lerer, & Newman, 1997; Gur et al., 2002). Although the underlying mechanisms of ECT that lead to symptom improvement are not fully understood, research suggests that ECT may be superior to antidepressants in reducing relapse rates over time. For example, Gagné and colleagues (2000) examined survival rates of chronically depressed adults who received either long-term ECT or antidepressant treatment. Results indicated that the probability of surviving without relapse was 93% for those who received ECT and only 52% for those who received antidepressants. At 5 years, survival rates were 73% for those who continued to receive ECT and 18% for those who received antidepressants only.

Additional nonpharmacological—but largely experimental—treatments for depression include vagus nerve stimulation (VNS), transcranial magnetic stimulation (TMS), and magnetic seizure therapy (Trivedi, 2003). As reviewed in chapter 3, VNS was approved by the FDA for treatment of epilepsy given its effectiveness at attenuating seizures. VNS is also approved for treatment of resistant depression (major and bipolar) in Europe and Canada, where several studies have shown improvement in 30% or more of patients who received such treatment (Goodnick, Rush, George, Marangell, & Sackeim, 2001). Sackeim and colleagues (2001) recently studied 60 individuals with treatment-resistant major depression for 12 weeks (2 weeks baseline, 10 weeks post-VNS implantation) and concluded that VNS is most effective with patients with low to moderate antidepressant resistance. In addition, patients who had never received ECT were nearly four times more likely to respond favorably to VNS. Marangell et al. (2002) followed 30 patients with major depression for a year to explore the long-term effectiveness of VNS. Results indicated that VNS was associated with a sustained response and increased rates of remission in patients with major depression. Carpenter, Friehs, and Price (2003) recommended that additional, longer-term studies be conducted with VNS, as well as short-term studies to explore its effectiveness in conjunction with antidepresssants. Although the mechanisms responsible for therapeutic improvement following VNS are poorly understood, they suggested that VNS increases afferent inputs to limbic and higher cortical brain regions and that this increased activity may contribute to symptom improvement.

Relative to VNS, more studies have been conducted with repetitive transcranial magnetic stimulation (rTMS). For example, Padberg et al. (1999) compared the effectiveness of fast rTMS to slow rTMS in 18 patients with treatment-resistant major depression. Results revealed a 19% reduction of depression scores after slow rTMS but only a 6% reduction after fast rTMS. These results suggest that slow rTMS may be more effective than fast rTMS and, as noted by the researchers slow rTMS can be safely applied at higher intensities. According to Nahas et al. (1998), slower yet higher rTMS intensities are associated with a more marked antidepressant effect. However, when Garcia-Toro and colleagues (2001) examined the effectiveness of rTMS compared to antidepressants and when used in conjunction with antidepressants, they found that rTMS was no more efficacious than standard antidepressant medication and appeared to have no additive effects. Janicak et al. (2002) compared rTMS to ECT in 25 patients with depression (major depression and bipolar). Patients were randomly assigned to receive rTMS (10–20 sessions) or ECT (4–12 sessions); after 2–4 weeks, results indicated that rTMS and ECT produced similar therapeutic effects. Loo et al. (2001) explored whether side effects emerged after a 2–4-week course of rTMS in depressed individuals with respect to cognitive functioning and hearing. No mean changes were observed in auditory threshold, and improvement was found on neuropsychological tasks. Thus, these results suggest that rTMS is safe, at least over a 4-week period. Similarly, a 3-week study by Martis et al. (2003) reported no deleterious effects associated with rTMS and like improvements on neuropsychological tasks. Not all studies have supported the use of rTMS in the treatment of depression, however. For example, Martin et al. (2003) recently conducted a meta-analysis of the effectiveness of rTMS for the treatment of depression. Based on their review of 14 studies, which they criticized for the quality of the research, they concluded that "there is currently insufficient evidence to suggest that rTMS is effective in the treatment of depression" (p. 483). In addition to VNS and rTMS, researchers have begun to explore the effectiveness of other brain stimulation techniques in the treatment of depression such as deep brain stimulation (DBS) and magnetic seizure therapy (MST; e.g., Lisanby, Luber, Schlaepfer, & Sackeim, 2003).

Recently, Rohan et al. (2004) reported that mood improvement occurred in 23 of 30 subjects with bipolar disorder and 4 of 14 healthy controls who had participated in a study using echo-planar magnetic resonance spectroscopic imaging (EP-MRSI). According to the researchers, in a previous study of conventional and nonconventional interventions on mood and brain chemistry in patients with bipolar disorder, subjects had reported anecdotally that they had experienced mood improvement after the EP-MRSI scans. EP-MRSI is similar to fMRI in that oscillating magnetic fields are used to obtain a brain scan, but it differs in field direction, waveform frequency, and intensity. The researchers tested a hypotheses that EP-MRSI scans have mood-enhancing effects in subjects with bipolar disorder relative to control subjects and relative to sham EP-MRSI scans. Based on subject responses on a depression questionnaire (the Brief Affect Scale) administered immediately before and after the scans, the authors concluded that EP-MRSI does appear to improve mood in patients with bipolar disorder. Athough most of these brain stimulation methods appear promising in the treatment of bipolar disorder and depression, little empirical information is currently available concerning their efficacy and safety.

Although more empirical studies are available concerning the effectiveness of pharmacological treatments for depression, a number of alternative approaches have also been studied. For example, many studies have reported benefits of the medicinal plant St.-John's-wort in the treatment of mild to moderate depression (e.g., Kirsch, 2003). Similar to antidepressants, however, the mode of action of St.-John's-wort is poorly understood, but neuroendocrine studies suggest it may affect the genes that control the functioning of the HPA axis (Butterweck, 2003). Smith, Leenerts, and Gajewski (2003) reported that a therapeutic writing intervention was effective at reducing reactive depression, and Jones and Field (1999) suggested that massage and music therapies may be helpful at reducing symptoms of depression in adolescents. Numerous studies have attested to the effectiveness of bright-light exposure and aerobic exercise in improving depressed mood (e.g., Leppamaki, Partonen, & Lonnqvist, 2002). Nutritional therapies are more controversial, but some studies have found increased mood stabilization with mineral and other supplements (e.g., Kaplan et al., 2001). Additional, well-designed studies are needed, however, to further explore the effectiveness and physiological basis of alternative interventions for the treatment of depression, including mild, moderate, and severe forms.

SUMMARY

As discussed in chapter 1, the prefrontal and limbic regions are involved in cognitive processes such as higher-order thinking and motivational and emotional processing, and are highly interconnected by neural networks and circuits. Dysfunction in these connections is thought to result in the emotional, cognitive, motivational, and behavioral symptoms characteristic of major depression. Functional studies have supported this hypothesis as patients with depression typically show reduced blood flow and glucose metabolism in frontal and limbic regions. Antidepressants have been found to further reduce this activity, which is correlated with symptom relief. Structural findings have been inconsistent, with some studies reporting reduced volume of the hippocampus and amygdala while other studies have not replicated these findings. It is plausible that dysfunction, whether it be increased or decreased activity or structure, causes abnormalities of complex neural circuits extending from subcortical to cortical regions. These disturbances affect cognitive, emotional, and behavioral systems and in the case of depression are characterized by lack of motivation, profound sadness, and reduced social and behavioral functioning. Familial and genetic studies suggest that genes likely play a major role in the risk of major depression, although given the recent findings concerning intracellular processes and depression, many genes may be involved. Environmental factors and exposure to stress may also play a role such as altering functioning of the HPA axis which causes release of hormones that are toxic to hippocampal cells and consequently may predispose an individual to depression. Additional life-event stressors or cerebrovascular events such as stroke may further disrupt neuroendocrine and neurotransmitter systems and result in symptoms of major depression. It is also possible that nonpharmacological interventions affect brain functioning and improve symptoms expression. For example, Paquette et al. (2003) recently reported that cognitive-behavioral therapy can induce metabolic changes in the brains of individuals with major depression or obsessive compulsive disorder. Relative to physiologically based intereventions, less is known about the brain-based effects of therapy, and future studies are likely to continue to explore this area. Clearly, the pathophysiology of major depression is complex and likely involves interactions among genetic, cellular, neurochemical, psychological, and environmental factors.

BIPOLAR DISORDER

The distinguishing feature between major depression and bipolar disorder is the presence of mania. A manic episode is characterized by an abnormally and persistently elevated, expansive, or irritable mood. The diagnostic criteria for a manic episode appear in Table 6.2. The DSM IV-TR identifies several types of bipolar disorder that are distinguished according to the frequency of manic episodes and degree of functional impairment. According to the DSM IV-TR, 1–2% of men and women will experience bipolar disorder at some point in their lives. Approximately 10–15% of individuals with bipolar disorder will commit suicide, and the disorder is often accompanied by associated problems such as occupational failure, marital difficulties, school failure, and substance use and abuse. According to the DSM IV-TR, bipolar disorder is also associated with anxiety disorders (e.g., panic disorder, social phobia), ADHD, and eating disorders (e.g., anorexia and bulimia nervosa). For example, MacKinnon et al. (2002) reported that more than a third of individuals with bipolar disorder or major depression had experienced at least one panic attack, and panic disorder was diagnosed more frequently in families of individuals with bipolar disorder relative to a control group. Freeman, Freeman, and McElroy (2002) reported that bipolar disorder is comorbid with anxiety disorders (panic disorder, obsessive compulsive disorder, social phobia, posttraumatic stress disorder) at rates significantly higher than the general population.

In addition to social and occupational impairments, individuals with bipolar disorder often demonstrate deficits on neuropsychological tasks such as those that measure problem solving, verbal memory, and executive functions. Studies are inconsistent, however, as to whether the level of impairment is worse during episodes of depression or mania (Basso, Lowery, Neel, Purdie, & Bornstein, 2002). Lagace, Kutcher, and Robertson (2003) recently reported that

TABLE 6.2

DSM IV-TR Criteria for Bipolar Disorder (DSM IV-TR, 2000)

DSM IV-TR Criteria for Manic Episode

A. A distinct period of abnormally and persistently elevated, expansive, or irritable mood, lasting at least 1 week (or any duration if hospitalization is necessary)

B. During the period of mood disturbance, three (or more) of the following symptoms have persisted (four if the mood is only irritable) and have been present to a significant degree:
   (1) inflated self-esteem or grandiosity
   (2) decreased need for sleep (e.g., feels rested after only 3 hours of sleep)
   (3) more talkative than usual or pressure to keep talking
   (4) flight of ideas or subjective experience that thoughts are racing
   (5) distractability (i.e., attention too easily drawn to unimportant or irrelevant external stimuli)
   (6) increase in goal-directed activity (either socially, at work or school, or sexually) or psychomotor agitation
   (7) excessive involvement in pleasurable activities that have a high potential for painful consequences (e.g., engaging in unrestrained buying sprees, sexual indiscretions, or foolish business investments)

C. The symptoms do not meet criteria for a Mixed Episode

D. The mood disturbance is sufficiently severe to cause marked impairment in occupational functioning or in usual social activities or relationships with others, or to necessitate hospitalization to prevent harm to self or others, or there are psychotic features.

E. The symptoms are not due to the direct physiological effects of a substance (e.g., a drug of abuse, a medication, or other treatment) or a general medical condition (e.g., hyperthyroidism).
   Note: Manic-like episodes that are clearly caused by somatic antidepressant treatment (e.g., medication, electroconvulsive therapy, light therapy) should not count toward a diagnosis of Bipolar I Disorder.

DSM IV-TR Diagnostic Criteria for 296.0x Bipolar I Disorder, Single Manic Episode

A. Presence of only one Manic Episode and no past Major Depressive Episodes.
   Note: Recurrence is defined as either a change in polarity from depression or an interval of at least 2 months without manic symptoms.

B. The Manic Episode is not better accounted for by Schizoaffective Disorder and is not superimposed on Schizophrenia, Schizophreniform Disorder, Delusional Disorder, or Psychotic Disorder Not Otherwise Specified.

Specify if:
   Mixed: If symptoms meet criteria for a Mixed Episode

If the full criteria are currently met for a Manic, Mixed, or Major Depressive Episode, *specify* its current clinical status and/or features:
   Mild, Moderate, Severe Without Psychotic Features/Severe With Psychotic Features
   With Catatonic Features
   With Postpartum Onset

If the full criteria are not currently met for a Manic, Mixed, or Major Depressive Episode, *specify* the current clinical status of the Bipolar I Disorder or features of the most recent episode:
   In Partial Remission, In Full Remission
   With Catatonic Features
   With Postpartum Onset

DSM IV-TR Diagnostic Criteria for 296.89 Bipolar II Disorder

A. Presence (or history) of one or more Major Depressive Episodes
B. Presence (or history) of at least one Hypomanic Episode
C. There has never been a Manic Episode or a Mixed Episode.
D. The mood symptoms in Criteria A and B are not better accounted for by Schizoaffective Disorder and are not superimposed on Schizophrenia, Schizophreniform Disorder, or Psychotic Disorder Not Otherwise Specified.
E. The symptoms cause clinically significant distress or impairment in social, occupational, or other important areas of functioning

Specify current or most recent episode:

Hypomanic: if currently (or most recently) in a Hypomanic Episode
Depressed: if currently (or most recently) in a Major Depressive Episode

If the full criteria are currently met for a Major Depressive Episode, *specify* its current clinical status and/or features:

Mild, Moderate, Severe Without Psychotic Features/Severe With Psychotic Features.
Note: Fifth-digit codes specified on p. 413 cannot be used here because the code for Bipolar II Disorder already uses the fifth digit.

Chronic
With Catatonic Features
With Melancholic Features
With Atypical Features
With Postpartum Onset

If the full criteria are not currently met for a Hypomanic or Major Depressive Episode, *specify* the clinical status of the Bipolar II Disorder and/or features of the most recent Major Depressive Episode (only if it is the most recent type of mood episode):

In Partial Remission, In Full Remission.
Note: Fifth-digit codes specified on p. 413 cannot be used here because the code for Bipolar II Disorder already uses the fifth digit.

Chronic
With Catatonic Features
With Melancholic Features
With Atypical Features
With Postpartum Onset

Specify

Longitudinal Course Specifiers (With and Without Interepisode Recovery)
With Seasonal Pattern
With Rapid Cycling

---

adolescents with bipolar disorder have specific mathematics deficits relative to a control group and relative to adolescents with major depression. They speculated that these deficits might be related to neuroanatomical abnormalities (e.g., underactivation of the dorsolateral prefrontal cortex). However, this study did not use brain imaging techniques to explore this hypothesis.

According to the DSM IV-TR, the incidence of bipolar disorder is steady across ethnic groups. The average age of onset for bipolar disorder is 20 for both sexes and is equally common in males and females (DSM IV-TR, 2000). Children and adolescents with recurrent major depression are at increased risk for bipolar disorder. Bipolar disorder is a lifelong disorder as greater than 90% of individuals who experience a manic episode continue to experience them in the future (DSM IV-TR, 2000). Fagiolini, Kupfer, Houck, Novick, and Frank (2003) reported that obesity is associated with a poorer outcome in individuals with bipolar disorder as obese patients with bipolar disorder experienced a greater number of depressive and manic episodes and their symptoms tended to be more severe. According to Yildiz and Sachs (2003), psychotic symptoms are also common in bipolar disorder. In a sample of 328 patients with bipolar disorder, they found that 42% had experienced psychotic symptoms. Males experienced psychotic symptoms at a significantly younger age than females, a finding the authors suggested may indicate that the underlying phyisiological basis of bipolar disorder differs in males and females. Jones and Craddock (2001) recently reported that approximately 20 to 30% of women with a history of bipolar disorder experience an episode of mania or psychosis following childbirth. Potash et al. (2001) compared bipolar patients with and without psychotic symptoms and found that 64% of those with psychotic symptoms had at least one relative with an affective disorder with psychotic symptoms. Only 28% of the nonpsychotic bipolar patients had a relative with such symptoms, leading the researchers to conclude that bipolar disorder with psychotic symptoms is likely a subtype that may have an overlapping genetic basis with schizophrenia.

Kupfer and colleagues (2002) recently studied 2,839 patients with bipolar disorder and found that 85% were hospitalized at least once (43% for mania episodes and 69% for depressive episodes). Greater than 50% had attempted suicide, typically during a depressed episode. One third of the sample were married; one third were never married; and the remaining subjects were divorced, widowed, or separated. Approximately 45% of the subjects had children under the age of 18. More than 90% of the group had completed high school, and 11% had earned a graduate or professional degree. Nearly 65%, however, were unemployed at the time of the study and 40% were receiving public assistance or disability support. Over 17% of the sample had received ECT and 75% were taking one to three medications (40% were taking anticonvulsants, one third lithium, and 25% benzodiazepine). According to Kupfer et al., over 50% of the subjects reported having at least one family member with bipolar disorder and/or depression. The mean age of onset of bipolar disorder was 19.8 years, with the majority reporting depression as the first episode experienced. Over 50% of the sample reported that they did not receive any treatment during their first episode of depression or mania. Of those who did receive treatment, 28.2% were hospitalized, one third received medication, and one third received psychotherapy. Collectively, these findings suggest that bipolar disorder has a relatively early onset and tends to run in families. This study also suggests that most individuals with the disorder attain a high school education or above but do not maintain employment in adulthood. Finally, the results suggest that most individuals with bipolar disorder take multiple medications such as mood stabilizers and anticonvulsants, and that for most individuals, bipolar disorder is a chronic condition characterized by social, interpersonal, and occupational struggles.

Genetic Studies

Genetic studies have consistently reported a high heritability estimate for bipolar disorder, and according to Smoller and Fin (2003), first-degree relatives have a tenfold increase of developing bipolar disorder. McGuffin et al. (2003) recently studied 30 monozygotic and 37 dizygotic twin pairs and concluded that the heritability estimate for bipolar disorder was 85%. The specific concordance rates were .67 for monozygotic and .19 for dizygotic twin pairs. These findings are consistent with Bertelsen, Harvald, and Hauge (1977), who reported bipolar concordance rates of .79 and .19 for monozygotic and dizygotic twins. Kendler, Pedersen, Neale, and Mathe (1995) studied a sample of 486 twin pairs and provided a heritability estimate of 79% for bipolar disorder. Smoller and Finn (2003) recently completed a thorough review of family, twin, and adoption studies and concluded that the recurrence risk for bipolar disorder in first-degree relatives is 8.7%. Kieseppa and colleagues (2004) reported a concordance rate of .43 for monozygotic twins and .06 for dizygotic twins in a population-based study in Finland. Childhood or adolescent onset of bipolar disorder appears to represent a unique subtype and, according to Schurhoff et. al. (2000) and Faraone, Glatt, and Tsuang (2003), may have a stronger genetic basis. Adoption studies also support a heritability component for bipolar disorder as frequency of the disorder is significantly greater in biological parents than adoptive parents of children who later develop bipolar disorder (Smoller & Fin, 2003).

Similar to major depression, a number of chromosomal regions and candidate genes have been investigated for bipolar disorder. Badner and Gershon (2002) recently conducted a meta-analysis of linkage studies for bipolar disorder and schizophrenia and reported that chromosome regions 13q32 and 22q12 were most often linked to bipolar disorder and to schizophrenia. Potash and colleagues (2003) recently reported similar findings and suggested that these regions may be particularly relevant to both disorders given the overlapping symptom of psychosis. Because similar genes and neurotransmitters have been implicated in bipolar disorder and schizophrenia and both disorders are often characterized by psychotic symptoms that are alleviated by antipsychotic medications, Moller (2003) proposed that bipolar disorder and schizophrenia are not distinct disorders but instead fall on a continuum of psychiatric disturbance. Additional chromosomes have been linked to bipolar disorder, including regions on chromosomes 10 and 18 (Berrettini et al., 1994; Foroud et al., 2000; McMahon et al., 2001). Blackwood and colleagues (1996) studied 12 families with bipolar disorder and suggested that there was a linkage with chromosome 4 (4p), while other studies have reported markers on chromosomes 11 and 16 (e.g., Egeland et al., 1987; Ewald et al., 1995). Detera-Wadleigh and colleagues (1999) conducted a genome-wide scan on 396 individuals to identify chromosomal regions associated with increased vulnerability to bipolar disorder. Results of this study supported previous linkages reported in the literature and also identified new linkage regions (1q32 and 18p11.2). Ophoff and colleagues (2002) also conducted a genome-wide association study but focused on 109 subjects with severe bipolar disorder. Their findings suggested that the chromosome 8p was linked to bipolar disorder but multiple regions (D8s503 to D8S520) could contain a bipolar susceptibility gene.

With respect to candidate genes, genes that are involved in the formation of neurotransmitters have been of primary focus. For example, the gene that encodes the enzyme catechol-O-methyltransferase (COMT) which deactivates dopamine and norepinephrine has received considerable attention. Initially, researchers hypothesized that a polymorphism of this gene may be linked to bipolar disorder, but studies failed to support this association (e.g., Lachman et al., 1996a; Tunbridge, Burnet, Sodhi, & Harrison, 2004). Lachman et al. (1996b), however, suggested that although a polymorphism of the COMT gene may not be responsible for bipolar disorder, it may increase the frequency of manic to depressive episodes ("rapid cycling"). Kirov and colleagues (1998) tested this hypothesis and explored whether a gene variant that causes low COMT activity would be more frequent among individuals with rapid-cycling bipolar disorder than those with nonrapid cycling. Results supported the hypothesis and suggested that the COMT gene is in fact linked to the frequency of rapid cycling in bipolar disorder. However, recently Rotondo et al. (2002) reported that subjects with bipolar disorder, relative to control subjects and those with panic disorder, showed significantly higher frequencies of a polymorphism of the COMT gene (COMT Met158) as well as the serotonin transporter gene (5-HTTLPR). Given the inconsistencies, it is difficult to draw any firm conclusions about the role of the COMT gene in bipolar disorder. It is possible that COMT gene variants are linked to more refined subtypes of bipolar disorder (e.g., rapid-cycling) or that two or more gene variants (e.g., serotonin transporters and COMT) result in physiological conditions that increase vulnerability to bipolar disorder. Recently, Geller and colleagues (2004) reported that a polymorphism (Val66MET) of the brain-derived neurotrophic factor gene is associated with increased susceptibility to bipolar disorder in children and adolescents, but also noted that this particular polymorphism may be associated with other childhood disorders such as obsessive compulsive disorder.

Several studies have reported that antidepressants can induce mania in perhaps 20% or more of individuals with bipolar disorder (e.g. Angst, 1985; Solomon, Rich, & Darko, 1990). Given that most antidepressants affect the serotonin system, related studies have explored the role of serotonin-related genes in bipolar disorder. For example, Collier et al. (1996) suggested that a polymorphism of the serotonin transporter gene (SLC6A4) was linked to bipolar disorder, although subsequent studies failed to find this association (e.g., Furlong et al., 1998; Mundo et al., 2000). Mundo et al. (2001) investigated the prevalence of a polymorphism of the serotonin transporter gene (SLC6A4) in 27 patients with bipolar disorder who experienced antidepressant-induced mania relative to 29 bipolar patients who had been treated with antidepressants but did not experience mania. Results indicated that 63% of patients with induced mania showed a particular polymorphism (5HTTLPR) compared to 29% of the bipolar patients who did not experience antidepressant-induced mania. The authors suggested that the presence of this polymorphism may be a predictor for antidepressant-induced mania in patients with bipolar disorder, but additional replication studies are necessary. Quintin et al. (2001) studied the effects of acute tryptophan depletion in nonsymptomatic relatives of patients with bipolar disorder. Results revealed that prior to tryptophan depletion, relatives of patients with bipolar disorder had lower serotonin concentrations, lower affinity, and fewer serotonin transporter binding sites than control subjects. Following tryptophan depletion, nonsymptomatic relatives experienced greater mood lowering and increased impulsivity. The authors speculated that abnormal serotonergic functioning may be heritable and increase vulnerability to affective disorders such as bipolar disorder.

Other types of genes have also been studied in relation to bipolar disorder. For example, Nygaard et al. (2002) recently considered whether polymorphisms of the gene that regulates the somatostatin receptor were associated with bipolar disorder. Somatostatin functions as a neuropeptide in the brain and helps to modulate the release of neurotransmitters and other neuropeptides. According to Nygaard et al., somatostatin receptors interact with dopamine receptors and enhance binding of neurotransmitters to the receptors. Given that dopamine antagonists are sometimes used to treat bipolar disorder, the reserarchers explored whether polymorphisms of the somatostatin gene were linked to bipolar disorder, and based on their analyses, concluded that a linkage did exist between the gene variants studied and bipolar disorder. Mood stabilizers such as lithium and valproate are thought to affect glutamate transmission, and therefore the gene that regulates a glutamate receptor (N-methyl-D-aspartate receptor, NDMAR) has been investigated. Mundo et al. (2003), for example, explored whether there was an association between three polymorphisms of the glutamate gene found on chromosome 9q34.3. Results revealed that two of the gene variants were significantly linked to the presence of bipolar disorder. Recently, Chen et al. (2004) and others have reported that variants of genes G72 and G30 on chromosome 13q33 are associated with an increased risk of bipolar disorder.

Ranade et al. (2003) reported a linkage between polymorphisms of the serotonin 2A receptor gene and bipolar disorder, whereas Murphy et al. (2000) reported a linkage between the gene for the serotonin transporter (region 17q11.1-q12) and bipolar disorder. Given that calcium plays a critical role in a variety of cellular functions including neurotransmitter release and second messenger systems, Yoon et al. (2001) suggested that the gene (TRPC7 gene) that is involved in intracellular calcium functioning may be implicated in bipolar disorder. Estrogen has also been linked to depression and bipolar disorder as some women with low levels of estrogen have reported improvement in depressive symptoms following hormone replacement therapy (Sichel et al., 1995). According to Kealey and colleagues (2001), the gene that regulates one of the two identified estrogen receptors (ER B) is located within a particular region of chromosome 14 (14q22-24). They explored whether a genetic variation within this region was linked to bipolar disorder based on a sample (102) of individuals with the disorder and their parents. Results did not support a linkage between variations of the estrogen gene and susceptibility to bipolar disorder. Craddock and Jones (2001) conducted a review of molecular genetic findings and bipolar disorder and concluded that although several chromosomal regions and candidate genes have generated intense interest, no robust positive findings have yet emerged from the literature.

In summary, although several chromosomal regions and candidate genes have been linked to bipolar disorder, no single or group of genes is definitively responsible for an increased susceptibility to bipolar disorder. Familial studies clearly support a strong heritability component for bipolar disorder, but the etiology is likely complex and may involve multiple genes working singly or in combination (Mathews & Reus, 2003). As Becker (2004) suggested, common gene variants may play a different role in psychiatric disorders depending on environmental conditions as well as the genetic backgrounds of individuals.

Anatomical Findings

Similarly, to major depression, structural imaging studies with bipolar disorder have produced mixed results. Some studies, for example, have found bipolar subjects to have increased ventricular size relative to control subects (e.g., Lim, Rosenbloom, Faustman, Sullivan, & Pfefferbaum, 1999; Zipursky et al., 1997), but other studies have not found this difference (Brambilla et al., 2001). Andreasen, Swayze, Flaum, Alliger, and Cohen (1990) found increased ventricular size in male patients with bipolar disorder relative to those with depression and healthy controls. In this study, ventricular enlargement was not related to previous ECT or medication history. Ali et al. (2001) explored the severity of bipolar disorder with the size of the hippocampus, temporal lobes, third ventricles, and lateral ventricles using MRI. Contrary to expectations, results revealed that greater length of time and severity of symptoms were associated with a significantly larger—rather than smaller—left temporal lobe, and differences were not found on the remaining anatomical measures. The authors speculated that abnormalities in brain development or exposure to mood-stabilizing medications may have contributed to enlargement of the temporal lobe. Recently, Strakowski and colleagues (2002) compared MRI scans of patients with first-onset bipolar disorder, those with multiple episodes, and control subjects. Results revealed that the lateral ventricles were significantly larger in bipolar subjects with multiple episodes relative to the other two groups. In addition, bipolar subjects with multiple episodes had smaller cerebral volumes relative to control subjects and first-onset bipolar subjects. The putamen of the first-onset bipolar subjects, however, was significantly larger than the putamen of control subjects. Although the study was cross-sectional in design and longitudinal studies are needed, the results suggest that anatomical changes may occur during the course of the disorder.

Subcortical abnormalities have also been reported in individuals with bipolar disorder. For example, Aylward et al. (1994), Figiel et al. (1991), and Dupont et al. (1995) reported abnormalities of subcortical white matter (e.g., signal hyperintensity and lesions) in patients with bipolar disorder relative to control subjects. Bearden, Hoffman, and Cannon (2001) noted that white matter hyperintensities (also known as lesions) are not usually present in the brains of healthy adults until middle age and when present reflect a change of water content in the brain and tissue abnormality. White matter hyperintensities are associated with a number of brain-based medical conditions and cognitive impairment (Mangone, Gorelick, Hier, & Ganellen, 1990). Dupont et al. (1995) found that individuals with bipolar disorder had greater white matter abnormalities in the frontal regions compared to control subjects and subjects with major depression. In addition, individuals with bipolar disorder had a significantly larger thalamus than those with major depression, and degree of white matter abnormality was positively correlated with increased ventricular size. Dupont et al. proposed that the increased white matter volume, hyperintensities, and enlarged thalamus found in the bipolar group suggest abnormalities of neurodevelopment. Caetano et al. (2001), however, compared the thalamus of 25 patients with bipolar disorder, 17 with major depression, and 39 healthy controls using MRI and did not find thalamic size differences among the three groups. Several studies have found evidence of increased size of brain structures in individuals with bipolar disorder relative to control subjects, such as the amygdala (Altshuler, Bartzokis, Grieder, Curran, & Mintz, 1998; Brambilla et al., 2003), caudate (Aylward et al., 1994), pituitary volume (Sassi et al., 2001), and thalamus (Altshuler et al., 1998).

Overall brain volume has also been explored in bipolar disorder, and most studies have reported no significant differences between individuals with bipolar disorder relative to control subjects (e.g., Harvey, Persaud, Ron, Baker, & Murray, 1994). Studies have found differences, however, with respect to specific regions and structures. For example, Lim, Rosenbloom, Faustman, Sullivan, and Pfefferbaum (1999) examined MRI scans of individuals with bipolar disorder, schizophrenia, and controls and reported that both clinical groups had widespread reductions in cortical gray matter but not white matter. The reductions were more pronounced in the subjects with schizophrenia. Zipursky et al. (1997) and Harvey, Persaud, Ron, Baker, and Murray (1994), however, found cortical gray matter loss in patients with schizophrenia but not bipolar disorder. Bearden, Hoffman, and Cannon (2001) reported that approximately 8–25% of individuals with bipolar disorder have some degree of cortical or cerebellar brain tissue loss. Gilmore and Bouldin (2002) examined postmortem tissue from the lining of a section of the temporal lobes (temporal horn) in individuals with bipolar disorder, schizophrenia, and control subjects to determine whether evidence existed of early brain insults (i.e., ependymal abnormalities). Results revealed that subjects did not differ in number of ependymal abnormalities. The authors cautioned that control subjects had an unexpectedly high rate of these cellular abnormalities and that consequently ependymal abnormalities may not be a useful marker of psychiatric disorders in postmortem brain tissue.

Bearden, Hoffman, and Cannon (2001) recently conducted an exhaustive review of structural findings in bipolar disorder and concluded that abnormalities are common. The etiology of structural abnormalities found in bipolar disorder is unknown but could reflect either neurodevelopmental abnormalities or cellular degeneration over the course of the disorder. Using fMRI, Blumberg and colleagues (2003) studied ten adolescents with bipolar disorder and found significantly greater activity in the left putamen and thalamus during a color-naming task (Stroop) compared to control subjects. In addition, control subjects were found to have increased activity in the prefrontal cortex with increasing age, a finding not evident in the group with bipolar disorder. According to the researchers, the findings support that adolescents with bipolar disorder have prefrontal and subcortical abnormalities consistent with a developmental disturbance in brain function.

Other developmental studies have focused on neurological soft signs and prenatal factors. Trixler, Tényi, Csábi, and Szabó (2001), for example, reported that a furrowed tongue was significantly more common in individuals with bipolar disorder than control subjects and suggested that this finding was consistent with a neurodevelopmental involvement in bipolar disorder. Gutiérrez and colleagues (1998) reported that individuals with bipolar disorder showed significantly more abnormal hand features (e.g., ridge dissociation) than control subjects and argued that disruptions in normal prenatal development increase the risk for the disorder. Sigurdsson, Fombonne, Sayal, and Chekley (1999) and others have suggested that bipolar disorder may due to prenatal and postnatal neurodevelopmental abnormalities. For example, Sigurdsson and colleagues (1999) found delays in language and motor development were more common in individuals with bipolar disorder relative to control subjects, and Friedman et al. (1999) found that adolescents with bipolar disorder had larger ventricles and sulci and smaller thalamic volume than control subjects. Unlike studies that support a neurodevelopmental hypothesis of schizophrenia, however, studies with bipolar disorder do not generally find prenatal or birth complications, neurological soft signs, or evidence of prenatal exposure to influenza virus (Bearden, Hoffman, & Cannon, 2001). Moore and colleagues (2001), however, recently explored the presence of deep subcortical and ventricular white matter lesions in 79 patients with bipolar disorder and found that of those who exhibited subcortical lesions, 69.2% were born in the winter months. The researchers concluded that bipolar disorder, birth season, and white matter lesions are all related and may reflect a problem during prenatal development.

Postmortem Findings

Numerous postmortem studies have been conducted on biploar disorder and, like the MRI findings, results have been inconclusive. Ongur, Drevets, and Price (1998) examined the number and size of neurons and glial cells in brain tissue of individuals with bipolar disorder, major depression, or controls. Results indicated that the number of glial cells was significantly reduced in mood disorders, particularly in subgroups of subjects with bipolar disorder (24% reduction) or major depression (41% reduction) relative to control subjects. Knable and colleagues (2004) recently analyzed multiple measures from postmortem hippocampi of individuals with bipolar disorder and schizophrenia and concluded that molecular abnormalities were found in synaptic density, glutamate, and other neurotransmitter receptors in both disorders. Selemon and Rajkowska (2003), however, noted that although cellular pathology is characteristic of both bipolar disorder and schizophrenia, differences in prefrontal pathology exist with respect to magnitude and involvement of glial and neurons. For example, Rajkowska, Halaris, and Selemon (2001) examined postmortem samples of individuals with bipolar disorder and individuals with schizophrenia and reported that bipolar disorder was characterized by reduced neuronal density in layer III of the dorsolateral prefrontal cortex as well as reduced pyramidal cell density in layers III and V. In addition, glial cells in multiple layers were enlarged and misshapen in bipolar disorder samples. Schizophrenia was characterized by increased, rather than reduced, neuronal density in this study. Altshuler (1993) and Stahl (2000) proposed recurrent episodes of depression or mania may cause cellular death and toxicity that result in brain tissue loss and cognitive impairment. Longitudinal studies are needed to explore this hypothesis.

Cotter, Mackay, Landau, Kerwin, and Everall (2001) examined postmortem tissue and reported no differences in glial cell and neuronal density in postmortem tissue from the anterior cingulate cortex in patients with bipolar disorder relative to control subjects. Benes, Vincent, and Todtenkopf (2001) also reported that glial cell density was similar across bipolar, schizophrenia, and control tissue samples, but the tissue from bipolar subjects revealed a substantial (27%) reduction in the density of nonpyramidal neurons in the anterior cingulate cortex. Chana and colleagues (2003) found reduced neuronal density in layers V and VI of the anterior cingulate cortex in postmortem tissue, but this reduction was found in bipolar disorder, major depression, and schizophrenia. Recently, Thomas and colleagues (2004) compared postmortem samples from the anterior cingulate of individuals with bipolar disorder, major depression, schizophrenia, and control subjects and reported that the bipolar sample had evidence of elevated immunoreactivity in the gray and white matter. The authors speculated that an inflammatory response may be present in patients with bipolar disorder. Iwamoto, Kakiuchi, Bundo, Ikeda, and Kato (2004) also compared postmortem brain tissue (prefrontal cortices) in bipolar disorder, major depression, schizophrenia, and control subjects and examined evidence of altered gene expression. Results were consistent with distinct and shared changes in each disorder, and bipolar disorder was characterized by down-regulation of genes that encoded receptors and transporter proteins and up-regulation of genes that encoded stress response proteins.

In summary, a number of structural differences have been found in living and postmortem brains of individuals with bipolar disorder. These findings have been inconsistent, however, and are likely influenced by methodological factors. It is also important to note that none of the structural abnormalities found in individuals with bipolar disorder are unique to the disorder and are sometimes found in other psychiatric disorders and medical conditions. In addition, the cause of the structural differences remains unknown and may be unrelated to the expression of bipolar disorder. In other words, the disorder itself may lead to structural changes or the structural differences may be due to disturbances elsewhere in the brain.

Neurotransmitter and Neuroimaging Studies

Neurotransmitter Studies

As mentioned previously, the role of serotonin in bipolar disorder is inconclusive. Genetic studies, for example, have been inconsistent with respect to the relationship between serotonin gene variants and bipolar disorder. Postmortem studies have found reductions in serotonin metabolites in the frontal and parietal regions (e.g., Young et al., 1994), and cerebral spinal fluid studies of living subjects with bipolar disorder have also reported significantly lower levels of serotonin metabolites during depressive episodes (e.g., Asberg et al., 1984). Metabolite studies performed during manic periods have been inconsistent (Yildiz, Sachs, Dorer, & Renshaw, 2001). With respect to serotonin transporters, Leake and colleagues (1991) reported fewer serotonin reuptake sites in postmortem samples of bipolar patients. O'Connell et al. (1995), however, used SPECT with 11 individuals with bipolar disorder and found significantly higher levels of serotonin reuptake in these individuals relative to control subjects. Mahmood and Silverstone (2001) recently reviewed the physiological evidence concerning serotonin and bipolar disorder and concluded that serotonin activity appears to be reduced during the depression state of bipolar disorder but during mania, the results are inconsistent. They suggested that chronic treatment with lithium and anticonvulsants increases serotonin levels in patients with depression and mania and may help to explain their mood-stabilizing effects.

Other neurotransmitters have also been implicated in bipolar disorder. Ali and Milev (2003) and others, for example, have reported that abrupt antidepressant withdrawal and drugs that result in excessive levels of norepinephrine are associated with the induction of manic symptoms. Bhanji, Margolese, Saint-Laurent, and Chouinard (2002) recently reported that the antidepressant mirtazapine, which blocks serotonin and norepinephrine autoreceptors, can also induce mania in a minority of individuals. Montgomery (1995), however, reported that mirtazapine induced mania in only 25% of clinical trials worldwide. Similarly, Bunney and Garland (1982) proposed that dopamine abnormalities may be implicated in bipolar disorder, especially given that dopamine antagonists can effectively reduce mania and perhaps improve symptoms of depression. Goldberg, Burdick, and Endick (2004) recently treated 22 depressed patients with bipolar disorder with a dopamine agonist (pramipexole) typically used in the treatment of Parkinson's disease. Results indicated that 67% of patients treated with pramipexole improved at least 50% on a depression rating scale (those taking placebo improved 21%). It is unclear, however, whether dopamine pre- or postsynaptic neurons play a role in bipolar disorder as relatively few receptor studies have been conducted. Pearlson et al. (1995) investigated dopamine receptor binding in individuals with and without psychotic symptoms and bipolar disorder and reported that receptor binding was increased in those with bipolar disorder and psychotic symptoms but not in those with nonpsychotic bipolar disorder. These findings suggest that dopamine may play a greater role in psychosis than depression and mania. Anand et al. (2000) investigated 13 patients with bipolar disorder using PET, and measured dopamine release before and after administration of amphetamine. Results indicated that individuals with bipolar disorder and control subjects did not differ with respect to dopamine release and binding in the striatum. The authors suggested that the results indicate that mania symptoms are not likely related to increases in dopamine release but may instead be related to postsynaptic functioning.

In addition to serotonin, norepinephrine, and dopamine, gamma-amino butyric acid (GABA) has also been implicated in bipolar disorder. For example, Petty et al. (1993) reported that GABA plasma levels were significantly reduced in patients with bipolar disorder (mania and depression) and in patients with major depression. However, similar research by Roy et al. (1991) did not find differences in cerebral spinal fluid GABA metabolites. Research that most implicates GABA in the pathophysiology of bipolar disorder is the effectiveness of anticonvulsants in reducing manic symptoms. As White (2003) noted, because bipolar disorder is episodic like epilepsy, it is not surprising that anticonvulsants can be effective mood stabilizers in its treatment. Although the precise mode of action has not been identified, many anticonvulsants enhance the activity of the (GABA) neurotransmitter system by preventing the enzymatic degradation of GABA or facilitating postsynaptic transmission. Given the specific effects of anticonvulsants on the GABA system, researchers have recently begun to explore whether polymorphisms of GABA receptor genes are associated with bipolar disorder. For example, Horiuchi et al. (2004) investigated presence of 13 polymorphisms of the GAGRA1 gene (that encodes one of the subunits of the GABA-A receptor) in 24 Japanese patients with bipolar disorder, 147 with major depression, and 191 control subjects. Results supported an association between variations of the GABRA 1 gene and bipolar disorder. Additional replication studies are needed to further explore the GABRA 1 gene as well as other GABA-related genes in bipolar disorder before conclusions can be deduced. GABA is also thought to play a critical role in anxiety disorders, and the high rate of comorbidity between bipolar and anxiety disorders further implicates GABA in the pathophysiology of bipolar disorder.

In summary, a number of neurotransmitters have been implicated in bipolar disorder—serotonin, norepinephrine, dopamine, and GABA. It is unlikely that any one of these neurotransmitters is responsible for the symptoms of bipolar disorder. Instead, it is more probable that these (and other) neurotransmitters interact in a complex fashion that influences intracellular functioning including gene expression and complex intracellular signaling.

Intracellular Processes

As discussed in the previous section on major depression, intracellular processes include complex signaling pathways that are involved in a neuron's ability to receive, process, and respond to information (Bhalla & Iyengar, 1999). Abnormalities in signaling pathways have been implicated in psychiatric disorders and have received considerable attention in both major depression and bipolar disorder. Bezchlibnyk and Young (2002) recently reviewed studies that used either blood samples or postmortem brain tissue of individuals with bipolar disorder and concluded that the disorder is likely due, at least in part, to abnormalities in signal transduction pathways. Specifically, altered levels of functioning of intracellular G-proteins, protein kinase A, and protein kinase C have consistently been associated with bipolar disorder (e.g., Chang, Li, & Warsh, 2003). In additional, second messenger pathways such as the ERK pathway are presumably activated by lithium and anticonvulsants and, according to Einat and colleagues (2003), the ERK pathway may play a critical role in modulating manic behavior. Young (2001) suggested that norepinephrine plays a critical role in manic behavior, as norepinephrine activates complex second messenger systems including G-protein and levels of G-proteins have been found to be elevated in patients with bipolar disorder (Young et al., 1993). G-protein activates a series of events along the second messenger pathway including cAMP response element binding protein (CREB), which in turn triggers changes in gene expression. Young et al. (1993) reported greater cAMP activity in subjects with bipolar disorder and suggested that increased activity in G-proteins, cAMP, and other transcription factors along the norepinephrine pathway are likely associated with manic symptoms in bipolar disorder. Stewart and colleagues (2001) examined postmortem tissue of individuals with bipolar disorder and suggested that mood stabilizers blunt overactive signaling pathways. Although these work is promising and may eventually lead to the physiological basis of the disorder, additional work is needed to better understand the role of intracellular signaling pathways in the development and expression of bipolar disorder.

Neuroimaging Studies

Numerous glucose metabolism and blood flow studies are available concerning the performance of individuals with bipolar disorder relative to those with other disorders and control groups. Again, like the neuroimaging findings with major depression, glucose metabolism and blood flow differences have been found between those with and without bipolar disorder—but the findings have been inconsistent. For example, Silfverskiiold and Risberg (1989) measured rCBF in patients with major depression or bipolar disorder and found that both groups showed normal rCBF when compared to control subjects. A negative correlation was found, however, between medication dosage and rCBF in subjects with bipolar disorder. Nobler et al. (1994), however, reported significant cortical and rCBF reductions in patients with bipolar disorder and in patients with major depression. Furthermore, these reductions were further reduced in both groups following treatment with ECT, and were especially prominent in those who responded favorably to ECT. Rubin et al. (1995) measured rCBF in patients with acute mania or major depression and found similar cortical blood flow reductions in both groups relative to control subjects. Tutus and colleagues (1998) also measured rCBF in patients with bipolar disorder relative to healthy control subjects and patients with major depression. Unlike previous studies, Tutus et al. reported no differences between bipolar and control subjects but did report increased left frontal rCBF in patients with major depression relative to the other groups.

Kruger and colleagues (2003) recently suggested that individuals with bipolar disorder are more sensitive to environmental stressors such as emotional stimuli than control subjects. To explore this hypothesis, they used PET and included subjects with bipolar disorder who were experiencing a depression episode or were in remission. When regional cerebral blood flow (rCBF) changes were measured during a task designed to induce sadness, results revealed changes unique to each group. Specifically, bipolar patients who were in remission displayed increased blood flow in the dorsal anterior cingulate and premotor cortex while those who were depressed displayed lateral prefrontal decreases in blood flow. Both groups demonstrated decreased blood flow in the bilateral frontal cortex (dorsal–ventral–medial) during the task. The authors speculated that unique changes in blood flow during active depression states (or remission) may reflect important underlying pathological substrates of bipolar disorder. One potential confound in many bipolar studies is that patients are often taking medication at the time of the study. Ketter et al. (2001) investigated 43 individuals with bipolar disorder who were medication-free, and compared glucose metabolism in these patients relative to control subjects. Results indicated that, relative to control subjects, bipolar subjects had decreased glucose metabolism globally as well as in the limbic cortex and prefrontal cortex. Glucose metabolism was increased, however, in several subcortical structures (thalamus, right amygdala, ventral striatum) in bipolar subjects compared to control subjects. The researchers suggested that the frontal hypometabolism findings represent a common neural substrate characteristic of depression and that the hypermetabolism observed in the subcortical structures may represent a congenital abnormality characteristic of rapid-cycling bipolar disorder. In an earlier study, Baxter and colleagues (1989) also found that glucose metabolism rates in the bilateral prefrontal cortex were significantly reduced in patients with bipolar disorder and in patients with major depression relative to control subjects and subjects with obsessive compulsive disorder.

Several studies have also reported blood flow and glucose abnormalities in the basal ganglia of individuals with bipolar disorder. For example, Caligiuri et al. (2003) recently used fMRI to measure cortical and subcortical brain activity in individuals with bipolar disorder relative to healthy control subjects. Results indicated that both depressed and manic bipolar subjects had significantly elevated blood oxygen levels in cortical and subcortical regions compared to controls. In addition, medication-free subjects with bipolar disorder (manic state) had significantly higher activity in the left globus pallidus and significantly lower activity in the right globus pallidus compared to depressed bipolar subjects. A positive correlation was found between mania symptoms and level of activity in the globus pallidus and caudate. Subjects who were not taking mood-stabilizing medications had significantly higher levels of activity in the basal ganglia, thalamus, and motor cortex than those who were taking medication. The authors suggested that mania is related to a disinhibition within the basal ganglia and that antimania medications (e.g., mood stabilizers, antipsychotics) may normalize functioning within these regions and subsequent pathways to and from the cortex. Dunn et al. (2002) studied the relationship between subcortical and cortical activity and self-reported symptoms of depression using PET and the Beck Depression Inventory. Results revealed a negative correlation between depression symptoms and glucose metabolism in several brain regions in individuals with major depression as well as those with bipolar disorder. Dunn and colleagues and others (e.g., al-Mousawi et al., 1996) have suggested that unipolar and bipolar depression may have common physiologically substrates that appear to involve cortical and subcortical regions (e.g., frontal and temporal cortices, caudate, putamen, anterior cingulate).

DelBello and colleagues (2004) studied whether anatomical abnormalities could be identified in the globus pallidus, caudate, putamen, thalamus, and amygdala in adolescents with bipolar disorder using MRI. Findings indicated that overall cerebral volume and the amygdala were smaller in adolescents with bipolar disorder than control subjects. The putamen, however, was larger in subjects with bipolar disorder. As discussed previously, Aylward and colleagues (1994) also used MRI and reported larger caudate volumes in males with bipolar disorder relative to control subjects, but no size differences were found in total brain volume, putamen, or globus pallidus. Cecil, Delbello, Sellars, and Strakowski (2003) used proton magnetic resonance spectroscopy to measure concentrations of various metabolites thought to reflect impairments in cellular metabolism and function in the frontal region and cerebellum in children between the ages of 8–12 with bipolar disorder. Compared to healthy control children, children with bipolar disorder were found to have elevated levels (16% higher) in the frontal regions and lower levels of metabolites (8% lower) in the vermis of the cerebellum. The researchers argued that these neurochemical abnormalities are similar to those found with adults and are evidence of abnormal brain functioning early in life. Davanzo et al. (2003) recently reported that adolescents with bipolar disorder have elevated levels of of the enzyme myo-inositol in the anterior cingulate cortex, levels that are significantly higher than control subjects and adolescents with intermittent explosive disorder. The researchers suggested that although intermittent explosive disorder and bipolar disorder in children and adolescents overlap in clinical symptoms, myo-inositol levels may physiologically differentiate the two groups. Elevated levels of myo-inositol are thought to reflect abnormalities of cellular functioning, and acute lithium treatment has been found to significantly reduce myo-inositol levels (Davanzo et al., 2001). Harwood (2003) recently reported that the most commonly used mood-stabilizing drugs—lithium, valporate, and carbamazepine—all suppress inositol signaling. Sjøholt and colleagues (2000) from the University of Bergen, Norway, recently reported that several variants of the gene that regulates the enzyme myo-inositol (IMPA2) are associated with bipolar disorder, at least in a small sample of bipolar Norwegian subjects. Future studies are needed to further explore the role of cellular enzymes such as myo-inositol in bipolar disorder.

In summary, studies suggest greater subcortical involvement in bipolar disorder relative to major depression. Discrepancies exist across neuroanatomical, neurotransmitter, and neuroimaging studies, however, and no single finding is unique to bipolar disorder. As Videbech (2000) noted, inconsistencies among structural and neuroimaging studies are likely influenced by methodological differences such as sample size, subject selection, imaging protocol, and imaging analyses. Additional potential confounds include age and sex of subjects, severity of illness, medication usage and history, and comorbid disorders. Future, well-designed studies with larger samples and more stringent inclusionary will likely help to elucidate the structural and neurochemical underpinnings of bipolar disorder.

Mood Stabilizers and Anticonvulsant Medications

The three main types of medication used in the treatment of bipolar disorder are mood stabilizers (e.g., lithium), anticonvulsants (e.g., carbamazepine), and antipsychotic medications (e.g., thioridazine). Although these classifications are based on the chemical structure and pharmokinetics of the drugs, some anticonvulsants (e.g., carbamazepine, divalproex) also have mood-stabilizing properties. According to Bauer and Mitchner (2004), the term "mood stabilizer" is not officially recognized by the FDA. They proposed that drugs that effectively treat acute mania and depressive symptoms and prevent these symptoms from emerging over time be recognized as mood stabilizers. Based on a review of 551 studies that used lithium, valproate, or olanzapine, Bauer and Mitchner concluded that lithium should be used as a first-line agent in the treatment of bipolar disorder. As discussed in chapter 2, the precise mode of action of mood stabilizers is poorly understood. Many of these drugs are thought to attenuate glutamate excitatory transmission (Ketter & Wang, 2003) and perhaps inhibit toxicity of excessive glutamate release (Bown, Wang, & Young, 2003). Lithium is thought to affect second messenger systems and perhaps serve neuroprotective functions by increasing neurotrophic factors. For example, Moore and colleagues (2000) found that after 4 weeks of lithium treatment gray matter volume increased in patients with bipolar disorder. Pardo, Andreolotti, Ramos, Picatoste, and Claro (2003) reported that lithium inhibited certain intracellular pathways in glial cells but activated these same pathways in neurons. The authors suggested that lithium may therefore facilitate neuronal repair and reduce the buildup of glial cells in response to traumatic injury. Bown, Wang, and Young (2003) reported that decreased neuronal and glial cell densities sometimes occur in the brains of patients with bipolar disorder and that chronic treatment with mood stabilizers such as lithium may inhibit the death of the cells. The mode of action of anticonvulsants (e.g., carbamazepine, divalproex) is also unclear, but research suggests they inhibit norepinephrine reuptake and block sodium channels. Research also indicates that effectiveness varies among types of medication depending on factors such as severity of symptoms and comorbidity.

Ketter and Wang (2002) reviewed clinical symptoms of bipolar disorder and responsiveness of these symptoms to three mood stabilizers: lithium, divalproex, and carbamazepine. They concluded that individuals are more likely to have a better response to lithium if they have a pattern of mania followed by depression, euphoric mania, fewer episodes, and recovery between episodes. Those who have a pattern of depression followed by mania, frequent episodes, rapid cycling, and severe mania tend to respond better to divalproex or carbamazepine. Ketter and Wang also reviewed brain imaging and medication findings and concluded that increases and decreases in glucose metabolism in various brain regions are associated with medication responsiveness, but that due to limited sensitivity and specificity, brain imaging techniques should not be used as clinical tests for medication responsivity. Some research suggests that patients with bipolar disorder and comorbid anxiety are less likely to respond to lithium and more likely to respond to anticonvulsants such as valporate. According to Freeman, Freeman, and McElroy (2002), antipsychotics are frequently used to treat manic symptoms, and although their principal mode of action is blockage of dopamine receptors, Ketter and Wang (2003) suggested that they also affect GABA and glutamate neurotransmission to a lesser extent. Newer anticonvulsant medications (e.g., gabapentin) may also be effective at decreasing mania and stabilizing mood over time. However, empirical studies are needed to better understand the role of these medications in the treatment of bipolar disorder.

Given the effectiveness of anticonvulsant medications at decreasing bipolar symptoms, researchers have explored the possibility that the glutamate system is hyperactive in bipolar disorder. Postmortem studies, for example, have examined the density of glutamate receptors in the hippocampus, but contrary to expectations, results have not yielded differences between individuals with bipolar disorder and control subjects (Scarr, Pavey, Sundram, MacKinnon, & Dean, 2003). Michael and colleagues (2003), however, used proton magnetic resonance spectroscopy to measure glutamate levels in living patients with bipolar disorder relative to control subjects. Results indicated that individuals with bipolar disorder had significantly higher glutamate levels in the dorsolateral prefrontal cortex, which may be related to symptoms of mania. GABA (y-aminobutyric acid), is the principal inhibitory neurotransmitter in the brain, has also been implicated in bipolar disorder. Research with other animals, for example, has found that chronic treatment with mood stabilizers results in an increase of GABA receptors in the limbic region, and some mood stabilizers (e.g., valproate) increase the release of GABA (Ketter & Wang, 2003).

Bowden (2000) reported that lithium and other mood stabilizers help to prevent relapse and therefore may reduce suicidal risk in patients with bipolar disorder. Maj (2003) reviewed studies concerning the effectiveness and antisuicidality effects of lithium and concluded that lithium can drastically reduce affective morbidity and appears to exert an antisuicidal effect in individuals with bipolar disorder. Yerevanian, Koek, and Mintz (2003) reported that anti-convulsant mood stabilizers were equally efficacious as lithium at reducing the risk of suicidal behavior in patients with bipolar disorder. Goodwin and colleagues (2003) recently compared suicide death rates in patients with bipolar disorder treated with lithium or the anticonvulsant divalproex (depakote). After correcting for age, sex, comorbid psychiatric conditions, and other factors, they found that risk of suicide death was 2.7 times higher with divalproex treatment than with lithium. Finally, Baldessarini, Tondo, and Hennen (2001) reviewed 33 lithium studies conducted between 1970–2000 and reported that long-term lithium treatment was associated with a thirteenfold lower rate of suicide compared to no lithium treatment or a discontinuation of lithium treatment. Collectively, these studies suggest that mood stabilizers may help to reduce suicidal behavior in patients with bipolar disorder.

Adjunctive Medications

Kupfer et al. (2002) reported that most individuals with bipolar disorder take more than one type of medication due to the heterogeneity of symptoms and comorbidity associated with the disorder. For example, approximately 20% of individuals with bipolar disorder have panic disorder (MacKinnon et al., 2002), and many are prescribed benzodiazepines in addition to mood stabilizers. Long-term use of benzodiazepines is dangerous, however, as they can lead to tolerance, addiction, withdrawal, and possibly even neurotoxicity (Michelini et al., 1996). Antidepressants are also used as adjuncts to mood stabilizers in the treatment of bipolar disorder and, according to Ketter and Wang (2003), may enhance GABAergic neurotransmission and reduce glutamatergic neurotransmission. As mentioned previously, antidepressants can exacerbate mania symptoms and precipitate rapid cycling in individuals with bipolar disorder. Ghaemi and colleagues (2004) recently compared outcomes of a wide range of antidepressant trials with 41 patients with bipolar disorder and 37 patients with major depression. Results indicated that mania was induced in 48.8% of patients with bipolar disorder and rapid cycling was accelerated in 25.6% of the bipolar patients (neither of these symptoms occurred in any of the patients with major depression). In addition, tolerance (i.e., loss of favorable response) was 3.4 times as frequent in patients with bipolar disorder compared to those with major depression. The researchers concluded that antidepressants have greater psychiatric risks and fewer benefits with individuals with bipolar disorder.

With regard to the treatment of bipolar disorder in children, Swann et al. (1997) suggested that anticonvulsants may be more effective than lithium given that children and adolescents are more likely to experience rapid cycling than adults (Geller et al., 2000). DelBello, Schwiers, Rosenberg, and Strakowski (2002) recently reported that a combination of an antipsychotic (quetiapine) and anticonvulsant (divalproex) was more effective at treating adolescents with bipolar disorder than an anticonvulsant used alone. Zito and colleagues (2003) examined the use of psychotropic medication patterns with children and adolescents in the United States and reported that use of these drugs nearly reached adult utilization rates during the 1990s. Compared to the number of studies that have been conducted with adults, however, relatively little information is available concerning the appropriate use, safety, and long-term effects of psychotropic medications with children and adolescents.

SUMMARY

Bipolar disorder is reported to have a strong genetic basis with a heritability estimate of approximately 85%. A number of susceptibility genes have been identified for bipolar disorder, but results have been inconclusive. Structural and neuroimaging studies have reported differences between individuals with and without bipolar disorder, but these findings have also been inconsistent. Preliminary studies suggest that bipolar disorder may be characterized by abnormalities such as heightened activity and structural enlargement of subcortical structures as well as reduced cellular activity of frontal regions. Several neurotransmitter systems have been implicated in bipolar disorder, and given the effectiveness of mood stabilizers and anticonvulsant medications at reducing manic symptoms, glutamate and GABA likely play a role in the pathophysiology of bipolar disorder. It is critical to note that anatomical and neurochemistry findings are based on correlational studies and therefore do not reveal causation. Additional genetic, neuroanatomical, neurochemical, and neuroimaging studies are needed to better understand the pathphysiological substrates of bipolar disorder as well as the effect of environmental factors on the expression of the disrder. As Manji and Lenox (2000) recently reported, the underlying pathophysiology of bipolar disorder consists of independent yet complex interacting systems that are continually evolving.

7

Anxiety Disorders

Anxiety disorders identified by the DSM IV-TR (2000) include panic disorder with agoraphobia, agoraphobia without history of panic disorder, specific phobia, social phobia, OCD, posttraumatic stress disorder, acute stress disorder, generalized anxiety disorder, anxiety disorder due to a general medical condition, substance-induced anxiety disorder, and anxiety disorder not otherwise specified. Given the voluminous amount of information available on anxiety disorders, this chapter focuses on two disorders: panic disorder and obsessive compulsive disorder (OCD).

Like previous chapters, this chapter presents background information and genetic, anatomical, neurochemical, and neuroimaging findings associated with each disorder. Research on treatment approaches is also discussed for panic disorder and obsessive compulsive disorder. Although a plethora of information is available concerning therapy approaches for these disorders, this information is beyond the scope of this text and will not be presented here. In keeping with the nature of the text, the primary focus will be on physiologically based treatment approaches for panic disorder and OCD.

PANIC DISORDER

Background Information

According to the DSM IV-TR, the lifetime prevalence rate of panic disorder (PD) in the general population is between 1 and 2%, but considerably higher in clinical samples (e.g., 10%). The distinguishing feature of panic disorder is the presence of recurrent, unexpected panic attacks. A panic attack is characterized by a discrete period of intense fear in the absence of danger, accompanied by a number of cognitive or somatic symptoms (Table 7.1). DSM IV-TR criteria also specify that following the panic attack, a pervasive fear about having another often colors thoughts and behavior. The frequency and severity of panic attacks vary widely among individuals, with the age of onset typically between adolescence and young adulthood (mid-30s)—although panic disorder does occur in children (e.g., Goodwin, Pine, & Hoven, 2003; Muris, Schmidt, Engelbrecht, & Perold, 2002). Flint (1994) reported that anxiety disorders, including panic disorder, are significantly less common in the elderly. The course of

TABLE 7.1

DSM IV-TR Diagnostic Criteria for Panic Disorder (DSM IV-TR, 2000)

DSM IV-TR Criteria for Panic Attack

A discrete period of intense fear or discomfort, in which four (or more) of the following symptoms developed abruptly and reached a peak within 10 minutes:

   (1) palpitations, pounding heart, or accelerated heart rate
   (2) sweating
   (3) trembling or shaking
   (4) sensations of shortness of breath or smothering
   (5) feeling of choking
   (6) chest pain or discomfort
   (7) nausea or abdominal distress
   (8) feeling dizzy, unsteady, lightheaded, or faint
   (9) derealization (feelings of unreality) or depersonalization (being detached from oneself)
  (10) fear of losing control or going crazy
  (11) fear of dying
  (12) paresthesias (numbness or tingling sensations)
  (13) chills or hot flashes

DSM IV-TR Diagnostic Criteria for 300.1 Panic Disorder Without Agoraphobia

A. Both (1) and (2):
   (1) recurrent and unexpected Panic Attacks
   (2) at least one of the attacks has been followed by a 1 month (or more) of one (or more) of the following:
     (a) persistent concern about having additional attacks
     (b) worry about the implications of the attack or its consequence (e.g., losing control, having a heart attack, "going crazy")
     (c) a significant change in behavior related to attacks
B. Absence of Agoraphobia
C. The Panic Attacks are not due to the direct physiological effects of a substance (e.g., a drug of abuse, a medication) or a general medical condition (e.g., hyperthyroidism).
D. The Panic Attacks are not better accounted for by another mental disorder, such as Social Phobia (e.g., occurring on exposure to feared social situations), Specific Phobia (e.g., on exposure to a specific phobic situation), Obsessive-Compulsive Disorder (e.g., exposure to dirt in someone with an obsession about contamination), Post-traumatic Stress Disorder (e.g., in response to stimuli associated with a severe stressor), or Separation Anxiety Disorder (e.g., in response to being away from home or close relatives).

---

panic disorder is usually chronic but is sometimes characterized by periods of remission and recurrent episodes. Approximately one third to 50% of individuals with panic disorder are also diagnosed with agoraphobia—anxiety about (or avoidance of) places or situations where a person fears it may be difficult to escape or help may be unavailable. Starcevic and colleagues (1993) reported that frequent and severe panic attacks along with fears about future panic attacks likely contribute to the development of agoraphobia in many patients with panic disorder.

Panic disorder is diagnosed at least two times more often in women than men. According to Smoller et al. (2003), panic attacks are relatively common among postmenopausal women, regardless of use of hormone replacement therapy. The researchers also found that panic attacks were often associated with medical problems (e.g., migraines, emphysema, cardiovascular disease) and stressful life events. Karajgi et al. (1990) found that 8% of outpatients with chronic obstructive pulmonary disease had a diagnosis of panic disorder. Several studies have reported provocation of panic disorder following exposure to solvents, cocaine, and Ecstasy

TABLE 7.2

DSM IV-TR Diagnostic Criteria for 300.3 Obsessive-Compulsive Disorder (DSM IV-TR, 2000)

A. Either obsessions or compulsions:
 Obsessions as defined by (1), (2), (3), and (4)
  (1) recurrent and persistent thoughts, impulses, or images that are experienced, at some time during the disturbance, as intrusive and inappropriate and that cause marked anxiety or distress
  (2) the thoughts, impulses, or images are not simply excessive worries about real-life problems
  (3) the person attempts to ignore or suppress such thoughts, impulses, or images, or to neutralize them with some other thought or action
  (4) the person recognizes that the obsessional thoughts, impulses, or images are a product of his or her own mind (not imposed from without as in thought insertion.)
 Compulsions as defined by (1) and (2):
  (1) repetitive behaviors (e.g., hand washing, ordering, checking) or mental acts (e.g., praying, counting, repeating words silently) that the person feels driven to perform in response to an obsession, or according to rules that must be applied rigidly
  (2) the behaviors or mental acts are aimed at preventing or reducing distress or preventing some dreaded event or situation; however, these behaviors or mental acts either are not connected in a realistic way with what they are designed to neutralize or prevent or are clearly excessive.
B. At some point during the course of the disorder, the person has recognized that the obsessions or compulsions are excessive or unreasonable. **Note:** This does not apply to children.
C. The obsessions or compulsions cause marked distress, are time consuming (take more than 1 hour a day), or significantly interfere with the person's normal routine, occupational (or academic) functioning, or usual social activities or relationships.
D. In another, Axis I disorder is present; the content of the obsessions or compulsions is not restricted to it (e.g., preoccuption with food in the presence of an Eating Disorder; hair pulling in the presence of Trichotillomania; concern with appearance in the presence of Body Dysmorphic Disorder; preoccupation with drugs in the presence of a Substance Use Disorder; preoccupation with having a serious illness in the presence of Hypochondriasis; preoccupation with sexual urges or fantasies in the presence of Paraphilia; or guilty ruminations in the presence of Major Depressive Disorder).
E. The disturbance is not due to the direct physiological effects of a substance (e.g., a drug of abuse, a medication) or a general medical condition.
 Specify if
  With Poor Insight: if, for most of the time during the current episode, the person does not recognize that the obsessions and compulsions are excessive or unreasonable.

(Dager et al., 1997; Louie et al., 1996; Pallanti & Mazzi, 1992). Panic disorder occurs throughout the world (Gater et al., 1998). For example, when Carlbring, Gustafsson, Ekselius, and Andersson (2002) studied the prevalence of panic disorder in 1,000 randomly selected adults from Sweden, they found a 12-month prevalence of 2.2%. Consistent with other gender-related studies, panic disorder was more common in Swedish women (5.6%) than men (1%). According to a study by the World Health Organization conducted in 14 countries, patients who have both panic disorder and depression are at increased risk for disability and suicide. Some research suggests that the experience of panic attacks differs across cultures. For example, Hollifield, Finley, and Skipper (2003) reported modest differences between a sample of Caucasians and Hispanics with respect to prevalence, frequency, and severity of panic attack symptoms, and Neerakal and Srinivasan (2003) found that certain DSM-IV criteria were rarely identified as problematic by patients from India.

Panic disorder is often comorbid with other anxiety disorders (e.g., generalized anxiety disorder, simple phobias, social phobia) as well as other clinical disorders such as depression and bipolar disorder (Freeman, Freeman, & McElroy, 2002; Pary, Matuschka, Lewis, Caso, & Lippmann, 2003). The DSM IV-TR reports that 10 to 65% of individuals with panic disorder also have major depression. Goodwin and Hoven (2002) reported that the co-occurrence of panic disorder and bipolar disorder was associated with childhood onset of panic attacks and greater severity of panic disorder, and Goodwin, Fergusson, and Horwood (2004) recently found that panic attacks during adolescence were associated with psychoticism in young adulthood. Panic disorder also commonly occurs with chronic medical conditions such as hypertension, pulmonary disease, lipid disorders, and asthma (McLaughlin, Geissler, & Wan, 2003).

Early Childhood Issues

A number of studies have reported that panic disorder is associated with childhood separation anxiety disorder (SAD) (e.g., Hayward, Killen, & Taylor, 2003), although a recent 7-year longitudinal study did not find a relationship between the two (Aschenbrand, Kendall, Webb, Safford, & Flannery-Schroeder, 2003). Interestingly, Aschenbrand and colleagues (2003) did find that children with a history of SAD were more likely to develop other anxiety disorders such as OCD, PTSD, or specific phobias. Panic disorder is also associated with traumatic experiences. Safren, Gershuny, Marzol, Otto, and Pollack (2002), for example, found that adults with panic disorder had significantly higher rates of childhood sexual or physical abuse than adults with other anxiety disorders. Bandelow and colleagues (2002) also found a relationship with traumatic life events (e.g., death of parent, family violence, parental substance abuse) in 115 adult patients with panic disorder. Hagengimana and colleagues (2003) studied the presence of anxiety disorders in a group of widows who were traumatized by the 1994 genocide in Rwanda. Results indicated that 35% of the women suffered from panic disorder and that an even greater percentage experienced panic attacks.

Research also suggests that dysfunctional parenting is associated with panic disorder. For example, Pacchierotti et al. (2002) reported that patients with panic disorder rated their parents as significantly less caring on the Parental Bonding Instrument relative to a control group. Using the same instrument, however, Turgeon and colleagues (2002) did not find this difference but reported that parental overprotective behaviors were associated with OCD and panic disorder in adulthood. Someya et al. (2000) also found a significant relationship between overprotective parenting and panic disorder later in life in a sample of Japanese patients with panic disorder. They reported a relationship as well between "rejecting" parenting and adult panic disorder. Of course, these studies are correlational in design and suggest only that parental style may be one contributing factor in the complex etiology of panic disorder.

Genetic Studies

In general, family and twin studies suggest a genetic influence in the development of panic disorder. Kendler, Neale, Kessler, Heath, and Eaves (1993), for example, reported a heritability estimate of 30 to 40% for panic disorder in a population-based twin registry of 2,163 women. Skre and colleagues (1993) examined the prevalence of anxiety disorders in a sample of 20 monozygotic and 29 dizygotic twins and found the concordance ratio for panic disorder in monozygotic twins relative to dizygotic twins was greater than 2:1. Weissman (1993) reported population-based lifetime rates of panic disorder range from 1.2/100 to 2.4/100, while the lifetime rates for first-degree relatives of those with panic disorder was substantially higher (7.7/100 to 20.5/100). Scherrer et al. (2000) noted that other anxiety disorders such as generalized anxiety disorder often coexist with panic disorder, suggesting a common genetic influence. Chantarujikapong et al. (2001) studied the presence of panic disorder, generalized anxiety disorder, and posttraumatic stress disorder in 3,327 male monozygotic and dizygotic twin pairs. Based on genetic model fitting, they concluded that these anxiety disorders display significant genetic and environmental overlap but also have distinct etiologic components. Kendler, Gardner, and Prescott (2001) also concluded that panic disorder has a moderate level of heritability but that familial and environmental factors likely contribute to its development. Finally, a meta-analysis of family and twin studies conducted by Hettema, Neale, and Kendler (2001) concluded that panic disorder as well as generalized anxiety disorder, phobias, and OCD all have a significant heritability component.

A number of chromosomal regions and specific genes have been investigated as potential candidates for panic disorder. As reviewed by Crowe (2004), other animal studies have targeted genes regulating serotonin, dopamine, and corticotropin releasing hormone receptors and have found evidence implicating all of these systems in the expression of anxiety symptoms. With regards to humans, Gratacòs et al. (2001) proposed that a region of chromosome 15 is associated with several anxiety disorders including panic disorder. Specifically, they discovered that a genetic mutation (DUP25) in this region that resulted in duplication of the gene was present in 90% of individuals in the study with anxiety disorders. Interestingly, this same duplication was found in 87% of a sample of double-jointed individuals but only 7% of control subjects. The researchers suggested that DUP25 is a susceptibility factor for anxiety disorders and joint laxity. Several follow-up studies, however, have failed to find DUP25 involvement in panic disorder (e.g., Schumucher et al., 2003; Tabiner et al., 2003; Zhu et al., 2004). Other chromosomal regions that have been implicated in panic disorder include chromosome 10 (10p11) (Hamilton et al., 2004).

Genes that are involved in regulating the catecholaminergic system have also been investigated in the pathogenesis of panic disorder. For example, Domschke et al. (2004) and others have explored whether polymorphisms of the catechol-O-methyl-transferase (COMT) gene are associated with panic disorder. As discussed in the previous chapter, catechol-O-methyl-transferase is an enzyme that breaks down catecholamines and—if over- or underactive—can lead to dysfuction of neurotransmitter systems such as dopamine, norepinephrine, and serotonin. Domschke et al. studied 115 men and women with panic disorder and measured the presence of a single polymorphism of the COMT gene (472GA = V158M). Results revealed an association with panic disorder in women but not men. Hamilton et al. (2002) also studied polymorphisms of the COMT gene and suggested that a susceptibility locus for panic disorder involved the COMT gene or a nearby region of chromosome 22. Woo, Yoon, and Yu (2002) concurred with Domschke et al. and Hamilton et al. Based on a study of 51 patients with panic disorder and 45 controls, they reported that 19.6% of those with panic disorder versus 2.2% of controls had a specific COMT polymorphism. Rotondo and colleagues (2002), however, found that subjects with bipolar disorder had a greater frequency of a polymorphism of the COMT gene as well as the serotonin transporter gene, but these results were not characteristic of subjects with panic disorder and comorbid bipolar disorder. Ohara and colleagues (1998) and Henderson et al. (2000) reported that polymorphisms of the COMT gene were not associated with anxiety disorders. Variants of the COMT gene have also been associated with a number of disorders such as schizophrenia (Park et al., 2002), violent behavior (Kotler et al., 1999) and personality characteristics (Benjamin et al., 2000). Given the inconsistencies among studies, the role of the COMT gene in panic disorder remains uncertain.

Other candidate genes that have been studied in panic disorder include those that regulate the adenosine 2A receptor (ADORA2A), dopamine transporter, dopamine receptors, or cholecystokinin receptors—to name only a few. Adenosine is released by neurons and glial cells and serves as a neuromodulator in the brain by activating second messenger systems and increasing neuronal inhibition. Hamilton et al. (2004) explored whether polymorphisms in and around the ADORA2A gene were associated with panic disorder in 70 patients. Following linkage and association analyses, they concluded that a susceptibility locus for panic disorder was likely contained within the ADORA2A gene or nearby region of chromosome 22. Hamilton et al. (2000) also investigated the association between gene variants of the dopamine receptor and dopamine transporter in patients with panic disorder but concluded that these polymorphisms did not appear to play a role in the disorder. Recently, Sand et al. (2002) investigated whether patients with panic disorder had a higher frequency of gene variants of the norepinephrine transporter gene (NET) and found no significant difference between 87 patients with panic disorder and 89 healthy control subjects. In summary, despite the apparently strong familial component of panic disorder, genetic studies have not identified a gene or group of genes that are clearly implicated.

Provocation of Panic

Given their random nature, it is difficult to study panic attacks as they occur. It has been well documented, however, that several substances can induce panic symptoms in humans and other animals. For example, cholecystokinin (CCK)—a neuropeptide secreted in the brain—appears to play a critical role in anxiety-related behaviors as injections of pharmacological CCK (CCK-4) and CCK receptor agonists (e.g., pentagastrin) can provoke anxiety symptoms in humans (Bradwejn & Koszycki, 1994). The mechanism by which CCK increases cerebral blood flow and anxiety is poorly understood, however. Bradwejn and Koszycki (2001) recently reported that CCK metabolism is different in patients with panic disorder relative to control subjects and that CCK receptors (CCK-2) are hypersensitive to stimulation in individuals with panic disorder. Sánchez-Fernández et al. (2003) suggested that CCK may induce cerebral blood flow via presynaptic receptors and found that the effects of CCK-4 were blocked by an antagonist that targeted a specific type of presynaptic CCK receptors (CCK2R). Interestingly, according to Flint et al. (2002), age-related changes in the brain's CCK system lead to a diminished cardiovascular response to CCK-4, which may help to explain the comorbidity of panic disorder with chronic medical conditions such as hypertension and pulmonary disease.

Javanmard et al. (1999) were among the first to study changes in rCBF following injections of pharmacologcially induced panic with CCK-4 (panicogen cholecystokinin-4) in healthy volunteers. Using PET, results indicated that CCK-4 quickly induced increases in rCBF in the hypothalamic region while later scans revealed increased rCBF in another area of the limbic region (claustrum-insular region). Also found were reductions in blood flow in the frontal regions following CCK-4. The authors suggested that these changes in rCBF as a function of time may reflect a neurocircuitry specific to panic attacks. Zwanzger et al. (2003) recently reported that an antiepileptic drug, tiagabine, reduced symptoms of panic in healthy volunteers following administration of CCK-4. Accoriding to Zwanzger et al., tiagabine is a GABA reuptake inhibitor and therefore dysregulation of the GABA system likely plays a role in panic disorder.

Given the relationship between CCK and panic disorder, researchers have investigated whether there is an association between CCK receptor genes and panic disorder. For example, Ise and colleagues (2003) explored whether a polymorphism of the CCK-A receptor gene (CCKAR) was more frequent in patients with panic disorder relative to healthy control subjects. Contrary to expectations, no significant difference between patients with panic disorder and control subjects was found. Hattori et al. (2001) explored whether a relationship existed between polymorphisms of another CCK receptor gene, CCK-B receptor, and panic disorder, and also failed to find a relationship between this gene and panic disorder. Hamilton et al. (2001) reported similar null findings. Ebihara and colleagues (2003), however, recently reported that a specific gene variant was present significantly *less* frequently in patients with panic disorder relative to healthy control subjects and argued that this gene variant may act as a protective factor against panic by reducing the expression of anxiety-producing CCK.

Yohimbine has also been found to increase anxiety and induce panic attacks in humans, especially those with panic disorder relative to healthy adults or adults with other anxiety disorders (Charney, Woods, Goodman, & Heninger, 1987). Yohimbine, derived from an African tree herb (Corynanthe yohimbe), is an alpha 2-adrenergic receptor antagonist and results in increased norepinephrine release. Sallee, Sethuraman, Sine, and Liu (2000) found that yohimbine significantly increased anxiety symptoms in children with anxiety disorders relative to control subjects. Yeragani, Tancer, and Uhde (2003) recently measured heart rate variability and the effects of yohimbine as well as clonidine (an alpha-2 andrenoreceptor *agonist*) in patients with and without panic disorder. Results revealed significant heart rate increases and decreases following administration of yohimbine and clonidine, respectively, changes not observed in the control group. Individuals with panic disorder also became more anxious than the control group following yohimbine administration. Other studies (e.g., Charney & Heninger, 1986; Puzantian & Hart, 1993) have also found decreased anxiety in patients with panic disorder treated with clonidine. Cameron and colleagues (2000) found significant increases in blood pressure, increases in norepinephrine release, and decreases in the thalamus, cerebellum, and whole-brain blood flow in healthy volunteers. Subjects who experienced a panic attack following yohimbine administration, however, showed an increase in whole-brain blood flow. Collectively, yohimbine studies with healthy and clinical subjects support a hypersensitivity of the noradrenergic neurotransmitter system in children and adults with panic disorder.

Inhalation of carbon dioxide (CO_2) is also commonly used to induce panic symptoms in individuals with panic disorder and in healthy volunteers. When carbon dioxide is inhaled, the level of carbon dioxide in the blood goes up and the individual breathes faster to get more out and to bring in more oxygen. Individuals with panic disorder are generally more sensitive to the effects of CO_2 and experience more severe symptoms than control subjects and subjects with other anxiety disorders such as OCD and generalized anxiety disorder. The mechanism for this heightened sensitivity in panic disorder is not well understood (Griez, de Loof, Pols, Zandbergen, & Lousberg, 1990; Verburg, Griez, Meijer, & Pols, 1995). Bailey, Argyropoulos, Lightman, and Nutt (2003) recently proposed that the noradrenergic system, particularly the locus coeruleus (an area rich in norepinephrine cell bodies), is involved in activation of the hypothalamic pituitary axis and in mediating increases in blood pressure, increases in cortisol, and increases in subjective fear responses following CO_2 inhalation in individuals with and without panic disorder. Sanderson, Rapee, and Barlow (1989) found that individuals with panic disorder reported lower levels of panic symptoms if they falsely believed they could decrease the amount of CO_2 inhaled by turning a dial. The researchers concluded that psychological factors such as perceived level of control affect the severity of panic attacks. Antidepressants such as fluvoxamine (luvox) have been found to decrease the sensitivity of individuals with panic disorder to CO_2 inhalation and effectively reduce the frequency and severity of attacks (Perna et al., 2002; Pols, Hauzer, Meijer, Verburg, & Griez, 1996).

Neurotransmitter Studies
Serotonin, GABA, Dopamine

Serotonin has also been implicated in panic disorder largely due to the efficacy of antidepressants in reducing anxiety symptoms (e.g., Asnis et al., 2001). Pollack and colleagues (2003) recently noted that SSRIs are the most desirable treatment for panic disorder given their effectiveness at decreasing anxiety symptoms, limited side effects, and lack of physical dependency. A study by Den Boer and Westenberg (1990) further implicates serotonin in panic disorder as patients treated with an SSRI (fluvoxamine) showed a dramatic reduction in frequency of panic attacks, but treatment with a serotonin antagonist was ineffective at improving symptoms. The role that serotonin plays in panic disorder is unclear, but Martini et al. (2004) suggested that intracellular pathways of serotonin receptors (1A and 2A) may be dysregulated in individuals with panic disorder. Along these same lines, Coplan and Lydiard (1998) indicated that anxiety may result from diminished or heightened serotonergic neurotransmission and that, depending on the specific pathways involved, serotonin can have an inhibitory or excitatory effect on neuronal activity. They also noted that serotonin and norepinephrine systems function interactively and thus an abnormality in this interactive system may manifest as pathological anxiety. For example, serotonergic neurons project from median raphe nuclei to the locus coeruleus and have an inhibitory effect on neurons in this area. The locus coeruleus is rich in norepinephrine-releasing neurons that project to midbrain and forebrain regions that play an important role in modulating fear and anxiety responses. Norepinephrine-releasing neurons, however, project from the locus coeruleus to neurons in the median raphe and have an excitatory effect, resulting in changes such as increased heart rate and blood pressure (Gorman et al., 2000). Therefore, factors that disrupt the homeostasis of the serotonin system can have deleterious effects for other neurotransmitter systems and ultimately behavior.

Treatment with SSRIs has been found to alter both serotonin and norepinephrine cerebral spinal fluid metabolite levels and lead to symptom improvement (De Bellis, Geracioti, Altemus, & Kling, 1993; Lucki & O'Leary, 2004; Sheline, Bardgett, & Csernansky, 1997). Gorman et al. (2000) suggested that SSRIs may reduce release of stress-related hormones from the hypothalamus and adrenal gland, thereby decreasing firing rate in the locus coeruleus (which leads to increased heart rate, blood pressure, and so on). They also speculated that SSRIs may inhibit excitatory projections from the amygdala to the hypothalamus and brain stem and consequently mitigate the anxiety response. In addition to being rich in norepinephrine-releasing neurons, the locus coeruleus contains cells that release neuropeptides and other neurotransmitters such as GABA. Benzodiazepines, which act on GABA receptors, also improve anxiety symptoms and are often used in the treatment of panic disorder. Cox, Norton, Dorward, and Fergusson (1989) found that over 83% of individuals who experienced panic attacks and were being treated for alcohol or drug abuse, used alcohol—a GABA agonist—to self-medicate their attacks, and 72% described this method as effective at reducing or preventing panic attacks. Benzodiazepines are also effective at reducing panic symptoms by enhancing GABA transmission. As Ströhle et al. (2002) demonstrated, however, GABA receptors and the effects of GABA are modulated by other factors such as peptides and neurosteroids, and thus the way in which neurotransmitters interact and contribute to panic symptoms is complex and poorly understood. Given the apparent interactive effects of neurotransmitters and the fact that pharmacological agents which target vastly different neurotransmitter systems can improve symptoms of anxiety, these studies suggest that parallel and interactive changes in neurotransmitter systems may underlie pathological states such as panic disorder.

Dopamine also appears to play a role in panic disorder. For example, Higuchi and colleagues (1999) reported that panic disorder was present in 20% of a sample of patients suffering from chronic schizophrenia, and Chen, Liu, and Yang (2001) recently reported a similar 25% finding. As discussed in chapter 5, dysregulation of the dopaminergic system is strongly implicated in schizophrenia. In addition, dopamine agonists such as cocaine have been found to produce paniclike symptoms (Hebert, Blanchard, & Blanchard, 1999) in other animals, and Louie et al. (1996) found in a sample of adults who had used cocaine and developed panic disorder, 60% believed the drug had caused the panic symptoms. Pallanti and Mazzi (1992) reported an association between recreational use of Ecstasy (3,4-methylenedioxymethamphetamine), a dopamine agonist, and precipitation of panic disorder. Pitchot et al. (1992) measured the growth hormone response to a dopamine agonist (apomorphine) in individuals with panic disorder or depression and discovered that following administration of the drug, those with panic disorder had a significantly higher growth hormone response than those with depression. The researchers interpreted these findings as implicating overactivity of the dopaminergic system in panic disorder. Antipsychotic medications that block dopamine receptors, however, are not effective at reducing panic symptoms and may, in fact induce or worsen panic symptoms, which suggests that the relationship between panic disorder and dopamine is likely complex (Anfinson, 2002; Higuchi et al., 1999).

Anxiety Systems

A single, universally accepted anatomical theory explaining panic disorder does not yet exist. Gorman, Liebowitz, Fyer, and Stein (1989) were among the first to propose such a unifying theory, but recently Gorman et al. (2000) revised their model and proposed a new hypothesis for the neuroanatomical basis of panic disorder. Specifically, Gorman, Kent, Sullivan, and Coplan (2000) emphasized that sensory input from multiple regions such as the cortex, brain stem, and subcortical structures projects through the amygdala, which in turn projects to many areas of the brain and results in autonomic and behavioral responses. With regards to panic, Gorman and colleagues suggested that a deficit may exist in "relay and coordination of upstream (cortical) and downstream (brainstem) sensory information, which results in heightened amygdalar activity with resultant behavioral, autonomic, and neuroendocrine activiation" (p. 495). In other words, individuals with panic disorder may process sensory information in a faulty manner that triggers physiological changes resulting in an extreme anxiety response—panic. The researchers also noted, however, that the pattern of autonomic and neuroendocrine responses varies among patients with panic disorder and that not all panic attacks are characterized by activation of neuroendocrine and autonomic systems. Consistent with this hypothesis, Brambilla et al. (2003) recently measured plasma concentrations of neurosteroids (e.g., progesterone, dehydroepiandrosterone) in individuals with panic disorder relative to controls and found that several neurosteroids were elevated in individuals with panic disorder. They speculated that the brain may hypersecrete neurosteriods in an attempt to counteract a hyperactive hypothalamic–pituitary–adrenal system. In their recently revised hypothesis, Gorman et al. acknowledged that in addition to abnormal autonomic and neuroendocrine factors, panic disorder is also highly familial and that environmental factors such as early childhood trauma and disruptions in infant–parent attachment increase the risk of developing it. Specifically, they proposed that individuals with panic disorder inherit a central nervous system that is overly sensitive to fear, and structures such as the amygdala, hypothalamus, thalamus, and locus coeruleus as well as environmental factors play a critical role in the development of panic attacks and panic disorder.

Shekhar et al. (2003) proposed that a complex, reciprocal network extending from the cortex, particularly the temporal and frontal cortices, to structures of the limbic system may regulate the panic response in patients with the disorder. According to Shekhar and colleagues, a regulatory dysfunction within this network could lead to abnormal responsivity to external (e.g., crowded places, highways) or internal (e.g, CO_2 inhalation) stimuli. They stressed the role of various regions of the amygdala in panic, but emphasized the basolateral nucleus of the amygdala (BLA). According to the authors, repeated activation of the BLA by stress hormones (e.g., corticotropin-releasing factor) induces a chronic state of anxiety that increases susceptibility to panic attacks following stimulation by external or internal factors. Quirk and

Gehlert (2003) also emphasized the role of the amygdala in panic and suggested that lack of appropriate inhibitory tone in the amygdala may lead to pathological responses. Similarly, Coplan and Lydiard (1998) proposed that dysregulation of the serotonin system and projections to the amygdala could result in overexcitation of neurons in the region of the amygdala. Malizia (1999) pointed out, however, that pathways extending from the orbitofrontal cortex to subcortical structures are likely involved in most forms of anxiety and therefore are not uniquely implicated in panic disorder. In a recent review of the neurobiological basis of anxiety, Charney (2003) also focused on the amygdala but expanded his discussion to include the prefrontal cortex, temporal cortex, and HPA axis. As discussed in chapter 7, the HPA axis is involved in the stress response and the release of stress-related hormones such as corticotropin releasing factor (CRF). CRF, in turn, increases the release of norepinephrine as well as other peptides and steroids (Arborelius, Owens, Plotsky, & Nemeroff, 1999). Antidepressants are hypothesized to normalize functioning of a hyperactive hypothalamic–pituitary–adrenal system in both depression and panic disorder (Ströhle & Holsboer, 2003). Recently, Massana et al. (2002a) found lower concentrations of brain metabolites (creatine and phosphocreatine) in the lower right medial temporal lobe region (amygdala–hippcampus region) but not in the prefrontal cortex region of patients with panic disorder. Massana et al. (2003b) also reported that the gray matter density of the left region of the hippocampus (parahippocampal gyrus) was significantly lower in subjects with panic disorder compared to control subjects. Collectively, these findings further support involvement of temporal lobe structures in the pathogenesis of panic disorder.

Not all studies have found physiologic abnormalities in patients with panic disorder, however. For example, Stein and Uhde (1989) did not find EEG abnormalities in 35 medication-free patients with panic disorder relative to control subjects, in contrast to Dantendorfer et al. (1996), who reported that patients with panic disorder displayed a higher than expected rate of EEG abnormalities. According to Charney (2003), inconsistencies abound across biologic investigations of anxiety, and he recommended that future genetic, neuroimaging, and neurochemical studies address the heterogeneity of anxiety disorders in their experimental designs. As with other clinical disorders, factors such as age, gender, medication history, length and severity of symptoms, comorbidity, and methodological and statistical procedures likely contribute to the inconsistencies across studies investigating panic disorder.

Additional Theories

Several studies have suggested that low levels of total cholesterol levels are associated with increased risk of death from injury and suicide (e.g., Papassotiropoulos, Hawellek, Frahnert, Rao, & Rao, 1999). Agargün et al. (1998) reported an association between low cholesterol and the presence of major depression in patients with panic disorder and suggested that cholesterol level may serve as an important psychiatric marker. Recently, Ozer and colleagues (2004) studied the relationship between suicide and cholesterol levels in individuals with panic disorder. Relative to control subjects, patients with panic disorder had lower serum cholesterol levels and greater risk for suicide. Other studies, however, have not substantiated this relationship (e.g., Deisenhammer et al., 2004) and, in fact, have found increased cholesterol levels in patients with panic disorder (e.g., Bajwa, 1992; Peter et al., 2002). Higher levels of cholesterol in panic disorder are hypothesized to be a result of increased noradrenergic activity that may underlie the physiological basis of panic disorder. In a recent review, Katerndahl (2004) suggested that regardless of cholesterol levels, recurrent panic attacks may increase the risk of coronary artery disease. Elevated plasma cholesterol levels have also been linked to Alzheimer's disease but, again studies have yielded conflicting results (Zaldy et al., 2003). In summary, the role of cholesterol in panic disorder remains unclear.

BRAIN IMAGING STUDIES AND PANIC DISORDER

Magnetic Resonance Imaging (MRI)

In a recent review of the MRI literature from 1966–2002, Brambilla, Barale, Caverzasi, and Soares (2002) concluded that different patterns of anatomical brain abnormalities appear to be involved with anxiety and mood disorders. The most consistent finding with respect to panic disorder was temporal lobe reduction, although the researchers cautioned that longitudinal studies with unmedicated individuals are necessary to better understand the disorder's underlying pathophysiology. Fontaine, Breton, Déry, Fontaine, and Elie (1990) were among the first to extensively study the anatomy of the temporal lobes in patients with panic disorder relative to control subjects: over 100 MRI images per individual with particular emphasis on temporal lobe scans. Results indicated a significantly higher number of abnormalities in patients with panic disorder compared to healthy volunteers (40% and 10%, respectively). These results are consistent with a previous study by Ontiveros et al. (1989), who also found a positive correlation between number of abnormalities and severity of panic symptoms. Uchida and colleagues (2003) and Vythilingam et al. (2000) reported smaller temporal lobe volume (9% reduction) in patients with panic disorder relative to control subjects. Massana et al. (2003a) found smaller left and right hemisphere amydalar volumes differences in medication-free patients with panic disorder compared to controls. No size differences were found in temporal lobe or hippocampi volumes.

It is important to note that factors unrelated to panic disorder are also associated with anatomical changes in the brain. Using MRI, Convit et al. (1995) found age-related reductions in medial and lateral temporal lobe volumes as well as age-related reductions in the hippocampus region. In addition, reduced hippocampal and amygdala volumes have been found in other disorders (Anand & Shekhar, 2003; Rauch, Shin, & Wright, 2003) and may reflect the diverse functions of these structures. For example, Schmahl, Vermetten, Elzinga, and Bremmer (2003) recently found that patients with bipolar disorder had a 21% and 13% smaller amygdala and hippocampal volume compared to control subjects. Nutt and Malizia (2004) reported that significant neurobiologic differences have been found in the hippocampus, amygdala, and medial frontal cortex in patients with PTSD. Ghadirian, Gauthier, and Bertrand (1986) described a case of a woman who suddenly began to experience panic attacks as well as hallucinations and depersonalization. A tumor was discovered in the right temporal lobe; upon its removal, all panic and visual hallucination symptoms disappeared. Matthews, Bell, and Fowlie (1996) treated a woman with abnormal EEG activity, visual hallucination, and panic attacks with an anticonvulsant medication (carbamazepine) and, according to the authors, the symptoms remitted.

Functional MRI (fMRI) Studies

Although the many fMRI and PET studies conducted with patients with panic disorder generally implicate subcortical structures (e.g., amygdala, hypothalamus), several problems characterize such studies (Gorman et al., 2000). For example, deep cortical structures are more difficult to image than cortical regions, unprovoked panic attacks often occur at random and are therefore difficult to capture, provocation of panic attacks often leads to hyperventilation and vasoconstriction which may obfuscate blood flow changes in the brain, and patients with panic disorder may be more sensitive to substances that induce panic (e.g., CO_2). Also, it is possible that the experience of being inside an MRI scanner could influence glucose metabolism and blood flow in the brain. In fact, Nazemi and Dager (2003) reported that patients with panic disorder are able to effectively cope with being confined in an MRI scanner but tend to maintain higher suffocation fears compared to control subjects. Thus, neuroimaging studies of panic disorder should be interpreted with these methodological issues in mind.

Several fMRI studies have found increased activation in the right frontal lobe when subjects with panic disorder were shown anxiety-relevant stimuli compared to neutral stimuli (e.g., Wiedemann et al., 1999). Furthermore, compared to control subjects, asymmetries in frontal activation characterize patients with panic disorder while at rest and during anxiety-provoking situations (Akiyoshi, Hieda, Aoki, & Nagayama, 2003). Wiedemann et al. and others have suggested that patients with panic disorder demonstrate avoidance–withdrawal behavior and that the pattern of greater right frontal activation may reflect an underlying dysfunctional system unique to patients with the disorder. Bystritsky et al. (2001) compared fMRI scans of six patients with panic disorder and six control subjects while they viewed imagery of neutral, moderate, and high-anxiety situations. Subjects with panic disorder displayed significantly higher bilateral activity in the hippocampus, cingulate, and orbitofrontal cortex during the moderate and high-anxiety conditions than the neutral condition. Bystritsky and colleagues proposed that this pattern of activity may be associated with retrieval of strong emotional memories and traumatic experiences and therefore leads to panic disorder in vulnerable individuals. Using fMRI, Maddock, Buonocore, Kile, and Garrett (2003) recently found patients with panic disorder showed significantly greater activation of the right mid-hipppocampal and prefrontal regions in response to threat-related stimuli. Consistent with previous hypotheses, the authors suggested patients with panic disorder process threat-related stimuli more extensively than those without the disorder.

Whalen et al. (2001) found increased activity occurred in the amygdala when healthy volunteers were shown pictures of fearful facial expressions compared to neutral or angry facial expressions. Based on fMRI scans, Thomas et al. (2001) found that children with panic disorder showed an exaggerated amygdala response (i.e., increased activity) to fearful faces compared to healthy controls and children with depression. The researchers speculated that this finding may reflect increased activity in withdrawal or avoidance neural networks in children with anxiety disorders, which is consistent with Wiedemann et al.'s proposal that panic disorder in adults is characterized by a physiologically based avoidance–withdrawal system that strongly influences behavior. Indeed, Lundh, Thulin, Czyzykow, and Ost (1998) found that individuals with panic disorder showed a recognition bias for safe versus neutral faces, a preference that correlated with their avoidance of feared situations. In general, results from fMRI studies suggest that patients with panic disorder have a heightened sensitivity to anxiety-provoking stimuli which is characterized by increased activity in the amygdala and decreased activity in frontal regions.

Positron Emission Tomography (PET) Studies

Findings from PET and single photon emission computed tomography (SPECT) studies have generally been consistent with fMRI studies, implicating subcortical and cortical structures in the pathophysiology of panic disorder. De Cristofaro, Sessarego, Pupi, Biondi, and Faravelli (1993), for example, compared SPECT scans of seven nonmedicated individuals with panic disorder and five age-matched controls following an injection of a panic-inducing substance (sodium lactate). Results indicated that those with panic disorder showed significant reductions in blood flow in the right and left hippocampus and increased blood flow in the left occipital cortex following the lactate infusion. The authors speculated that the increased blood flow in the occipital cortex was related to hypervigilance, whereas the reduction in blood flow to the hippocampus could reflect abnormal neuronal function in such patients. Fischer, Andersson,

Furmark, and Fredrikson (1998) reported on a case study of a healthy female volunteer who unexpectedly experienced a panic attack during a rCBF study. Results revealed decreased blood flow in several regions including the right orbitofrontal, anterior cingulate, and anterior temporal cortex.

Nordahl et al. (1990) used PET to measure glucose metabolism rates in patients with panic disorder while they performed an auditory task. Results indicated that subjects with panic disorder showed glucose metabolism decreases in the left parietal lobe and an increase in the orbital frontal cortex. In a later study, Nordahl et al. (1998) compared glucose metabolism rates in patients with and without panic disorder and found that activity in the left hippocampus and prefrontal regions was significantly lower than the right. Bisaga et al. (1998) also examined glucose metabolism but only included women with panic disorder in the study. Scans taken while subjects were at rest indicated a significant increase in glucose metabolism in the left hippocampus of patients with panic disorder relative to controls and a significant decrease in the right temporal and parietal regions. In a recent study, Eren and colleagues (2003) found a significant relationship between the severity of panic disorder and right hemisphere activation based on rCBF changes.

Studies have also compared PET scans of subjects with several other types of clinical disorders. For example, Lucey et al. (1997) compared rCBF changes in patients with panic disorder, OCD, and PTSD and found a positive correlation between whole-brain blood flow and anxiety symptoms. Results were similar among patients with panic disorder and control subjects with respect to blood flow measures in the caudate and frontal cortex. Boshuisen and colleagues (2002) compared areas of activation of patients with panic disorder and control subjects during an anticipatory anxiety condition. Findings indicated multiple areas of higher activity and reduced activity in patients with panic disorder relative to control subjects, supporting the hypothesis of brain processing differences in subjects with panic disorder. Meyer, Swinson, Kennedy, Houle, and Brown (2000) compared rCBF measurements of nine women with panic disorder and control subjects before and after administration of a serotonin agonist. Those with panic disorder showed a lower level of rCBF in the temporal cortex relative to controls as well as significantly higher blood flow in this region following administration of the serotonin agonist. The authors suggested that serotonin increases may modulate an underlying functional pathology of the left temporal cortex in patients with panic disorder. In a recent review of neuroimaging studies and the efficacy of SSRIs (paroxetine/Paxil), Kilts (2003) suggested that chronic administration of SSRIs may help to address the underlying pathophysiology of anxiety disorders. Neumeister et al. (2004) examined degree of binding of a serotonin tracer to presynaptic serotonin autoreceptors (5-HT1A) in 16 unmedicated patients with panic disorder and 15 healthy control subjects. Findings supported a role for serotonin in panic disorder as patients with the disorder showed significantly lower binding volumes in several regions (anterior and posterior cingulate, raphe) compared to control subjects.

As mentioned previously, neuroimaging studies are useful in helping to identify brain regions of increased or decreased glucose metabolism or blood flow in panic disorder, but the findings are not necessarily unique to panic disorder (e.g., Bonne et al., 2003). In addition, these findings *do not reveal the cause* of the functional differences between those with and without panic disorder. Wiesel (1992) stated that comparisons among neuroimaging (glucose metabolism) studies are severely limited due to large differences in clinical and experimental methodology. He advocated standardization of experimental factors (e.g., design issues) as well as clinical factors (e.g., gender, course of the disorder, comorbidity). Nevertheless, a general theme emerges from the MRI, fMRI, and PET studies to date: Panic disorder is often characterized by abnormal regional increases and decreases in activity, and pathways that extend from the amygdala and hippocampal regions to the frontal cortex appear to be particularly involved in its pathophysiology. It is important to emphasize that many of the studies reviewed are correlational in nature and thus do not reflect causation. In other words, the anatomical, neuroimaging, and neurochemistry findings associated with panic disorder may not be directly linked to the expression of the disorder. Additional studies are needed to tease apart the complex relationship between genetic, biological, and environmental factors that may contribute to the development and maintainence of panic disorder.

Pharmacological and Nonpharmacological Treatment Approaches

According to Pary, Matuschka, Lewis, Caso, and Lippmann (2003), the primary treatment approach for anxiety disorders is pharmacological. The four main classes of medications used in the treatment of panic disorder are benzodiazepines (e.g., Valium, Xanax, klonopin), SSRIs (e.g., Prozac, Paxil, Zoloft), tricyclic antidepressants (e.g., anafranil, tofranil), and MAOIs (e.g., marplan, nardil). According to the American Psychiatric Association, the current first-line of treatment for panic disorder is SSRIs due to their efficacy in reducing symptoms as well as their relative safety. A number of SSRIs are used to treat panic disorder, and most are equally effective in reducing panic symptoms. Bandelow et al. (2004) recently compared the efficacy of two SSRIs (sertraline/Zoloft and paroxetine/Paxil) in the acute treatment of panic disorder in over 200 subjects. Over a 12-week period, results indicated that the SSRIs were equally efficacious at reducing symptoms but sertraline was associated with fewer side effects. Paxil (paroxetine) is considered relatively safe and effective, although in rare cases overdoses have resulted in death (Vermeulen, 1998).

Historically, panic disorder has been treated with tricyclic antidepressants, monoamine oxidase inhibitors (MAOIs), and benzodiazepines. However, given the side effects associated with tricyclic antidepressants and MAOIs, as well as the risk of dependency and withdrawal that can occur with benzodiazepines, many experts now recommend the use of SSRIs. Research suggests these recommendations are often not followed in clinical practice. For example, Bruce et al. (2003) examined the prescribing practice of benzodiazepines over the last 10 years by studying 443 patients who were followed as part of a longitudinal study. Despite practice guidelines for treating panic disorder, the researchers found that benzodiazepines were most commonly used to treat panic disorder, SSRI treatment alone had increased only modestly, and approximately two thirds of the patients studied were taking benzodiazepines in combination with SSRIs. In addition, Valenstein et al. (2004) recently reported that benzodiazepines are frequently—but inappropriately—prescribed in the treatment of depression, particularly among elderly patients. They found that 36% of 46,244 depressed veterans and 41% of 12,819 elderly depressed veterans had received a prescription for benzodiazepines during the past year. Furthermore, 94% were taking antidepressants in conjunction with the benzodiazepines and the majority received long-term benzodiazepine prescriptions. These findings suggest that many patients with anxiety and depressive disorders are not currently being treated in accordance with practice guidelines and thus are at increased risk of experiencing the negative side effects associated with long-term use of benzodiazepines.

The mode of action of the two most frequently prescribed medications for panic disorder—benzodiazepines and SSRIs—is substantially different. As discussed in chapter 2, SSRIs are serotonin agonists while benzodiazepines are GABA agonists. Although both SSRIs and benzodiazepines are effective at treating panic disorder, benzodiazepines carry a high risk for tolerance and withdrawal. Benzodiazcpincs bind to part of the GABA receptor, and several studies have found lower GABA receptor binding levels in patients with panic disorder compared to control subjects. Specific areas of reduction have included the hippocampus (Bremner et al., 2000), left temporal lobes (Kaschka, Feistel, and Ebert, 1995), prefrontal cortex

(Bremmer et al., 2000), and global reduction in benzodiazepine binding throughout the brain (Malizia et al., 1998). Other studies, however, have reported increased receptor density in the prefrontal cortex in patients with panic disorder (Brandt et al., 1998) and greater right versus left hemisphere receptor binding in the prefrontal cortex (Kuikka et al., 1995). Decreased levels of benzodiazepine receptor binding have also been found in other disorders such as PTSD (Bremmer et al., 2000) and in subjects with alcoholism (Abi-Dargham et al., 1998). Roy-Byrne et al. (2003) reported that personality variables (e.g., harm avoidance) are associated with greater benzodiazepine withdrawal symptoms. Given the effectiveness of SSRIs at improving panic symptoms and their selectivity for the serotonin and not GABA receptor, as well as the inconsistencies among studies concerning density of benzodiazepine binding receptors, the role of GABA transmission in panic disorder remains unclear.

Long-term treatment of panic disorder typically involves medication in conjunction with cognitive-behavioral therapy to improve treatment response (Doyle & Pollack, 2004). Many studies have found that a combination of pharmacological intervention and cognitive-behavioral therapy is effective at improving panic symptoms, but given methodological limitations of studies, it is often difficult to determine whether the effects are additive (Gelder, 1998; Spiegel & Bruce, 1997). In addition, some researchers have argued that cognitive-behavioral therapy is preferable to pharmacological interventions (e.g., Rayburn & Otto, 2003), while others advocate for the management of panic disorder with short-term use of benzodiazepines and long-term use of SSRIs (Sheehan, 2002).

Alternative Interventions

Although pharmacological interventions are the most well studied intervention approach for panic disorder, a number of other techniques have been studied as well. For example, neurosurgery has been used in rare cases of treatment-resistant anxiety disorders. Rück et al. (2003) followed up 26 individuals who had not responded to pharmacological or behavioral interventions and had undergone neurosurgery for anxiety disorders (5 with social phobia, 13 with generalized anxiety disorder, and 8 with panic disorder). All of the patients had undergone capsulotomy, which involves bilateral lesioning of an area deep in the brain (internal capsule). Results indicated that 67% of the patients responded favorably to the procedure and displayed a significant reduction in anxiety symptoms. Seven of the 26 subjects, however, demonstrated adverse symptoms following the procedure such as neuropsychological impairment on executive function tasks and emotional apathy. The authors suggested that capsulotomy is an effective treatment for severe cases of anxiety disorder including panic disorder but noted the significant risk of adverse symptoms associated with the procedure.

A less invasive intervention that has recently received empirical attention is exercise. Broocks et al. (1998), for example, found that a 10-week exercise program was associated with significant improvement in symptoms of panic disorder but less effective than treatment with an antidepressant (clomipramine). In addition, Broman-Fulks, Berman, Rabian, and Webster (2004) compared the effects of high-intensity and low-intensity 20-minute treadmill exercise and found that high-intensity was associated with more rapid decreases in measures of global anxiety and fear of physiological sensations associated with anxiety and panic. Dratcu (2001) suggested that regular physical exercise should serve as an adjunctive treatment for panic disorder. Alternative interventions such as acupuncture have also been explored. Spence et al. (2004) found that acupuncture was associated with significant reductions in anxiety in individuals with subsyndromal anxiety symptoms and speculated that acupuncture increases melatonin secretion—which may modulate endogenous opioid production, facilitate GABA transmission, and consequently reduce anxiety symptoms. Inositol, an essential nutrient that is part of the B complex family of vitamins, has been found in a few studies to have therapeutic effects on depression, OCD, and panic disorder (Levine, 1997). Recently, Palatnik, Frolov, Fux, and Benjamin (2001) performed a double-blind study to compare the efficacy of an SSRI (fluvoxamine) and inositol in the treatment of panic disorder. Results revealed that the two were equally efficacious at reducing anxiety symptoms but that fewer side effects were associated with inositol. These findings are consistent with those reported in an earlier study comparing inositol versus placebo at reducing panic disorder symptoms (Benjamin et al., 1995). Meuret, Wilhelm, and Roth (2004) recently reported that a biofeedback program was effective at facilitating voluntary control of breathing and reducing symptoms of hyperventilation in patients with panic disorder. Although additional empirical studies are necessary, these findings suggest that alternative interventions may hold promise for the treatment of panic disorder.

SUMMARY

Panic disorder affects approximately 1 to 2% of the population and is more common in females. Familial and twin studies support a heritability component of the disorder. Molecular genetic studies have identified a number of candidate genes although no single or group of genes has been conclusively linked to panic disorder. Anatomical and neuroimaging studies suggest that subcortical limbic structures and pathways extending to and from the frontal cortex are strongly associated in the pathophysiology of panic disorder. A number of neurotransmitter and neuroendocrine systems have been implicated in the disorder, particularly GABA and serotonin. Unfortunately, much of the research concerning panic disorder is based on correlational studies and hence does not reveal causal factors involved in its pathophysiology. Acute treatment of panic disorder typically involves use of benzodiazepines, and a combination of SSRIs and cognitive behavioral therapy is often recommended for long-term management.

OBSESSIVE COMPULSIVE DISORDER (OCD)

Recurrent obsessions or compulsions that are time-consuming or cause significant distress and impairment in daily living characterize OCD (Table 7.2). According to the DSM IV-TR, *obsessions* are persistent ideas, impulses, thoughts, or images that an adult, but not necessarily a child, experiences as intrusive and inappropriate. *Compulsions* are repetitive overt or mental behaviors committed for the purpose of preventing or reducing anxiety or distress related to the obsessions. The most common adult obsessions with OCD are thoughts about contamination, doubts, order and symmetry, and aggressive and sexual images, while contamination and symmetry are common in children (Shafran, Ralph, & Tallis, 1995). The most common compulsions in both adults and children include cleaning and washing, counting, checking, requesting assurances, repeating actions, and ordering (DSM IV-TR, 2000). Leckman et al. (1997) described OCD as a multidimensional, etiologically heterogenous disorder, and based on a principal components analysis of the Yale-Brown Obsessive Compulsive Scale, suggested that four dimensions are especially characteristic: (a) obsessions and checking, (b) symmetry and ordering, (c) cleanliness and washing, and (d) hoarding. Saxena et al. (2002) recently found patients with OCD who had a problem with compulsive hoarding had greater functional impairment than those who did not hoard. The researchers also reported that patients who hoarded tended to be older than those with OCD who did not hoard. Tolin, Abramowitz, Brigidi, and Foa (2003) found that patients with OCD who had checking compulsions scored higher on a intolerance of uncertainty instrument than patients with OCD who did not have a checking compulsion. According to Okasha et al. (1994), most patients with OCD have both obsessions and compulsions.

OCD is equally common in adults of both sexes but more common in boys in childhood. Bogetto and colleagues (1999) found that males tend to have an earlier onset of OCD and that females are more likely to have an acute onset of OCD symptoms. The researchers also found that OCD is more likely to occur in males with tic or other anxiety disorders such as phobias. OCD typically begins in adolescence or adulthood with a gradual onset. Heyman et al. (2001) reported an average age of childhood onset from 7.5 to 12.5 years. In the majority of cases, OCD is chronic with periods of waxing and waning (DSM IV-TR, 2000). Lyoo et al. (2001) found patients with OCD had significantly higher harm-avoidance scores and significantly lower scores on novelty seeking and self-directedness than control subjects. They also found that severity of OCD symptoms correlated with harm avoidance, which the authors speculated was related to excessive concern for objects that could potentially cause harm.

According to the DSM IV-TR, stress often exacerbates OCD symptoms. Tarumi and Tashiiro (2004) reported that the majority of adults (70%) with chronic OCD reported problems with stress-related safety needs. The prevalence of the disorder varies among studies, with estimates ranging from .5 to 2.1% in adults and 1 to 2.3% in children and adolescents, across many cultures throughout the world (DSM IV-TR, 2000). Guerrero et al. (2003), however, reported that Native Hawaiians have a twofold higher risk for OCD than other ethnicities. Maggini et al. (2001) reported that 3% of nearly 3,000 Italian adolescents reported significant OCD symptoms, whereas Heyman et al. (2001) found only .25% of British children aged 5–15 reported significant OCD symptoms. Lemelson (2003) argued that cultural factors can influence the nature of obsessions and compulsions. For example, the most common obsessions in a sample of OCD patients from Bali, Indonesia, included the need to know information about passersby, somatic obsessions, and obsessions concerning witchcraft and spirits. Several studies have reported a relationship between religiosity and OCD. For example, Okasha et al. (1994) found that the most common obsessions in 90 patients with OCD attending an outpatient clinic in Cairo, Egypt, were religious and contamination obsessions and the most common compulsion repeating rituals. Tek and Ulug (2001) reported that 42% of a sample of 45 patients with OCD had religious obsessions. Abramowitz and colleagues (2002) used a self-report scale designed to measure religious obsessive compulsive symptoms—the PIOS (Penn Inventory of Scrupulosity)—with a group of college students and found that highly devout participants (i.e., Catholics, Protestants) evidenced higher scores on the PIOS than less religious participants. Greenberg and Witztum (1994) reported that religious symptoms were found in 13 of 19 ultraorthodox Jewish patients with OCD but only 1 of 15 non-ultraorthodox Jewish patients with OCD. Collectively, these studies suggest that OCD may be expressed in religious practices but is not a determinant of the disorder.

OCD is associated with a number of psychiatric disorders including other anxiety disorders, depression, eating disorders, and Tourette's disorder. Several studies have found differences in OCD symptoms between clinical groups. For example, George and colleagues (1993) compared obsessions and compulsions in a group of individuals with OCD only and a group with OCD and comorbid Tourette's disorder. Results indicated that subjects with comorbid OCD and Tourette's reported significantly more sexual, violent, and symmetrical obsessions and counting, blinking, and touching compulsions. Those with OCD reported significantly more contamination obsessions and cleaning compulsions. Similarly, Holzer et al. (1994) reported that patients with OCD and comorbid tic disorder compared to those with OCD only, had significantly more rubbing, touching, tapping, blinking, and staring compulsions—but the two groups did not differ with respect to obsessions. Perugi et al. (2002) found that OCD patients with comorbid bipolar disorder had a significantly higher rate of sexual obsessions and significantly fewer ordering compulsions than those with OCD alone. McDougle and colleagues (1995) compared the obsessions and compulsions of adults with autistic disorder and adults with OCD and found that the latter group was more likely to experience contamination, sexual, aggressive, and religious obsessions. Results also revealed that touching, tapping, rubbing, hoarding, ordering, and self-mutilating behaviors were more common in the autism group. Finally, Matsunaga et al. (1999) compared the obsessions and compulsions of patients with OCD and patients with anorexia nervosa and comorbid OCD and found patients with anorexia and OCD had a higher need for symmetry and ordering than those with OCD alone. Subjects with OCD, however, reported more aggressive obsessions and checking compulsions than the other two groups of patients. Masi et al. (2004) recently investigated the comorbidity of OCD and bipolar disorder in 102 children and adolescents and found that age of onset of OCD was significantly younger in adolescents with both OCD and bipolar disorder. Subjects with OCD alone had significantly more compulsions but a similar number of obsessions as those with OCD and bipolar disorder. Subjects with both disorders, however, had significantly more existential, philosophical, or superstitious obsessions than children and adolescents with only OCD. Collectively, these studies suggest that the obsessions and compulsions of patients with comorbid OCD differ from those with OCD alone. These behavioral differences may reflect differential neurophysiological underpinnings of the disorders.

Genetic Studies

In general, familial studies support a genetic component to OCD (Hettema, Neale, & Kendler, 2001). For example, Okasha et al. (1994) reported that 20% of patients with OCD in their cross-cultural study had a family history of OCD. Nestadt et al. (2001) examined the relationship between OCD, other anxiety disorders, affective disorders, and substance use disorders in 80 adults with OCD and their 343 first-degree relatives compared to a control group. Results indicated that other anxiety disorders (e.g., generalized anxiety disorder, panic disorder, specific phobias) and depression are frequently present in individuals with OCD. In addition, these disorders occurred significantly more frequently in relatives of patients with OCD than control subjects. The researchers suggested that other anxiety disorders, particularly GAD and agoraphobia, may share a common familial etiology with OCD.

Twin studies also support a role for genetics in OCD. Eley et al. (2003) recently factor analyzed mother-reported anxiety behaviors in 4,564 4-year-old twin pairs and found five factors: general distress, separation anxiety, fears, shyness, and obsessive compulsive behaviors. The obsessive compulsive factor was the least correlated with the other factors. The authors suggested that genetic and environmental influences contribute to the development of anxiety disorders, including OCD, in young children. Jonnal, Gardner, Prescott, and Kendler (2000) investigated a sample of 1,054 female twins and reported a heritability estimate of 33% for obsessions and 26% for compulsions. Additional twin studies with substantially smaller samples have also reported a high degree of concordance for OCD (e.g., McGuffin & Mawson, 1980). Hoaken and Schnurr (1980) noted, however, that for every ten monozygotic twin pairs that are concordant for OCD, four or so are discordant, and thus nongenetic factors clearly also play a role in the development of the disorder.

With respect to specific candidate genes, a number of genes are currently being investigated but no specific gene or group of genes is conclusively inculpated in OCD. Millet et al. (2003) compared polymorphisms of a dopamine postsynaptic receptor gene (DRD4) in patients with OCD relative to ethnically matched control subjects and found a significantly lower frequency of a gene variant (allele 2) in patients with OCD. Camarena et al. (2001a) and Lochner et al. (2004) found that polymorphisms of the MAO gene occurred significantly more frequently in females than males with OCD and suggested that gender differences may exist in genetic susceptibility to the disorder. Alsobrook et al. (2002) and Schindler et al. (2000) found an association between polymorphisms of the COMT gene and OCD, and Karayiorgou et al. (1997, 1999) suggested that variants of the COMT gene may lead to a three- to fourfold reduction in activity of COMT at the cellular level. Bengel et al. (1999) found that patients with OCD were more likely to have a specific serotonin transporter gene variant (two copies of the long allele) than control subjects and suggested that this polymorphism may increase OCD susceptibility. Mundo et al. (2000) suggested a relationship between OCD and a variant of the serotonin autoreceptor gene (5-HT1DB). Myoclonus-dystonia is an autosomal dominant genetic disorder characterized by involuntary slow, twisting, and jerking movements and is linked to chromosome region 7q21 and specifically gene DYT11 (Nygaard et al., 1999; Saunders-Pullman et al., 2002). Studies have found that myoclonus-dystonia is often associated with alcohol abuse, depression, and anxiety disorders including OCD. Saunders-Pullman et al. (2002) investigated whether OCD was present in manifesting as well as nonmanifesting carriers of myoclonus dystonia and found that 25% of manifesting carriers, 9% of nonmanifesting carriers, and 0% of noncarriers had OCD. Based on these findings, the researchers postulated that OCD is associated with the DYT11 gene.

Not all studies have found relationships between genetic polymorphisms and OCD, however. For example, Hemmings et al. (2003) investigated the frequency of several gene variants affecting dopamine and serotonin receptors as well as MAO gene variants in 71 patients with OCD and 129 control subjects. Contrary to expectations, results did not reveal any association between these gene variants and OCD. Similarly, Erdal et al. (2003) and Kinnear et al. (2001) failed to find a relationship between polymorphisms of the COMT gene and susceptibility to OCD. It is also important to note that polymorphisms of the COMT gene have been associated with other disorders such as anorexia nervosa (Frisch et al., 2001). Camarena et al. (2001b) explored whether variants of the serotonin transporter gene were associated with OCD given the effectiveness of SSRIs in treating OCD symptoms, but results did not reveal a significant difference between OCD patients and control subjects. Similar null results were reported by Billett and colleagues (1997), who compared the frequency of polymorphisms of the serotonin transporter gene in 72 patients with OCD and matched control subjects. In summary, OCD is occurs more often in first-degree relatives than the general population and, based on familial and twin studies, appears to have a genetic component. Despite efforts to identify genes that increase susceptibility to OCD, results have been inconsistent across genetic studies.

Neurotransmitter Studies

Serotonin

Because antidepressants such as SSRIs (e.g., Prozac) and tricyclics (e.g., clomipramine) are often highly effective at reducing OCD symptoms, serotonin has been a focus of study in the pathophysiology of OCD. For example, Pogarell et al. (2003) used SPECT to assess serotonin transporter availability in unmedicated individuals with OCD and healthy volunteers. Results indicated that individuals with OCD had a 25% higher SERT binding in the midbrain–pons region relative to control subjects, and binding was highest in individuals with early-onset OCD. There was no significant binding difference between groups with respect to striatal regions. The researchers speculated that elevated binding could reflect a higher density of serotonin transporters in subjects with OCD resulting in an increased capacity of serotonin reuptake or that the higher density of serotonin transporters may be a compensatory response to low serotonin levels. Whatever the case, the elevated binding in the midbrain–pons region supports serotonergic dysfunction in patients with OCD. Interestingly, Ozaki et al. (2003) reported that a specific mutation of the SERT gene (Ile-425Val) was strongly associated with OCD in a small study of family members with OCD. Tauscher et al. (2001) recently found a negative correlation between postsynaptic serotonin receptor binding potential and anxiety symptoms in a group of healthy volunteers, which helps to explain the antianxiety properties of serotonin agonists. Simpson et al. (2003), however, recently reported that reductions in SERT availability are associated with OCD with comorbid depression but may not be associated with OCD alone.

Other indices of serotonin functioning such as cerebral spinal fluid metabolite studies have produced mixed results. For example, a number of studies have reported decreased serotonin metabolite levels in subjects with OCD relative to control subjects (Altemus et al., 1994; Thorén et al., 1980), while other studies (e.g., Insel et al., 1985) have reported increased levels. Similarly, studies that have attempted to induce OCD symptoms have produced inconsistent findings. For example, several studies have found that serotonin autoreceptor agonists worsen OCD symptoms (e.g., Koran, Pallanti, & Quercioli, 2001; Stein et al., 1999) while other studies have not reported worsening of symptoms with serotonin agonists or antagonists (e.g., Goodman et al., 1995; Pian et al., 1998; Zohar et al., 1988). Stein and colleagues (1999) used SPECT to measure blood flow changes in patients with OCD following administration of sumatriptan, a serotonin autoreceptor agonist (5-HT 1D), compared to placebo. Results indicated a significant association between OCD symptom exacerbation and decreased neuronal activity in the frontal regions. Approximately half of the subjects with OCD, however, demonstrated a reduction in OCD symptoms following sumatriptan. The authors speculated that responses to sumatriptan are heterogenous and that this heterogeneity helps to explain the inconsistencies in the literature concerning the effects of serotonin autoreceptor agonists. Graf and colleagues (2003) have also demonstrated that compulsive self-grooming behavior can be induced in rats with the administration of serotonin autoreceptor agonists.

Interestingly, other nonpharmacological factors have been found to elicit OCD symptomology as well, including visual stimulation in the form of pictures. Shapira et al. (2003), for example, showed subjects with OCD and healthy volunteers pictures from the International Affective Picture System while they underwent fMRI scans. Results indicated that subjects with OCD showed a different pattern of brain activation during disgust-inducing pictures but a similar pattern to control subjects during threat-inducing pictures. Specific areas of increased activation in OCD subjects during the disgust condition included the right insula, parahippocampal region, and inferior frontal regions. Phillips et al. (2000) compared fMRI scans of subjects with OCD washing compulsions or subjects with OCD checking compulsions while they observed disgusting, washing-relevant, and neutral pictures. Results indicated that subjects with checking and washing compulsions showed different areas of activation depending on the type of picture observed and that these patterns differed significantly from the pattern displayed by control subjects. Berthier, Kulisevsky, Gironell, and Heras (1996) reported that acquired brain lesions in the basal ganglia or areas of the cerebral cortex (frontal, temporal, cingulate) were associated with inducement of OCD and argued, therefore, that damage specifically to the frontal–limbic–subcortical circuitry is involved in the pathogenesis of acquired OCD. Several studies have reported onset or worsening of OCD symptoms in women following childbirth (e.g., Abramowitz, Schwartz, Moore, & Luenzmann, 2003; Brandes, Soares, & Cohen, 2004). Most of these studies have found postpartum women with OCD experience intrusive obsessional thoughts to harm their infants and many suffer from depression (Sichel, Cohen, Dimmock, & Rosenbaum, 1993). Leckman et al. (1999) suggested that intrusive thoughts associated with harm-avoidant behaviors following the birth of a child serve an adaptive purpose (care and relationship building), and therefore OCD may be partially explained from an evolutionary perspective. Arnold (1999) reported that OCD that develops during the postpartum period may become chronic and interfere with the parent–child relationship, but antidepressants can be highly effective at reducing the symptoms of postpartum OCD. In summary, given the effectiveness of antidepressants, particularly SSRIs, at improving OCD symptoms, it appears that serotonin plays a role in the pathogenesis of the disorder. Whether serotonin's role in OCD is primary or secondary, however, has yet to be determined.

Dopamine

Several lines of research strongly implicate dopamine in the mediation of OCD symptoms. Other animal studies have demonstrated that dopamine agonists can induce behavior that resembles OCD behavior in humans. Rats treated with the dopamine receptor agonist quinpirole have been found to develop checking behavior (Tizabi et al., 2002) as well as excessive lever pressing (Joel, Avisar, & Doljansky, 2001). In addition, OCD observed in cats and dogs as well as other animals has been successfully treated with antidepressants such as clomipramine (Overall & Dunham, 2002) and, in some cases, dopamine antagonists. Dopamine antagonists have recently received attention for treatment of OCD in patients who do not respond to SSRIs. For example, Metin, Yazici, Tot, and Yazici (2003) recently reported that the antipsychotic drug amisulpiride was associated with significant reductions in OCD behavior in patients when used in conjunction with SSRIs. Dopamine agonists are also associated with provocation of OCD symptoms, however. For example, the antipsychotic agent risperidone has been recommended for patients with OCD who do not respond to SSRIs (Fountoulakis, Nimatoudis, Iacovides, & Kaprinis, 2004). Risperidone has an antagonistic effect on both dopamine and serotonin receptors, although the mechanisms by which it diminishes OCD symptoms are unclear. Alevizos and colleagues (2002), however, described six cases in which risperidone actually induced or worsened OCD symptoms and cautioned that patients receiving the drug should be closely monitored.

Perhaps the most convincing evidence of a relationship between dopamine and OCD stems from neurologic disorders affecting the basal ganglia such as Parkinson's disease and Tourette's disorder. For example, Müller et al. (1997) found that patients with Parkinson's disease scored higher than control subjects on the ordering subscale of the Hamburg Obsessive-Compulsive Inventory. Patients with Tourette's had higher scores on numerous subscales including checking, ordering, and counting/touching. Alegret et al. (2001) found that patients with mild Parkinson's disease did not differ from controls on an OCD inventory. However, those with severe Parkinson's did report significantly more symptoms than control subjects with respect to checking, doubting, and cleaning. The researchers proposed that OCD symptoms could be a result of a subset of neurochemical changes that occur at the level of the basal ganglia as Parkinson's disease progresses in patients with this disease. Recently, Maia, Pinto, Barbosa, Menezes, and Miguel (2003) studied the frequency of OCD in 100 patients with Parkinson's disease and reported that OCD symptoms were not higher in patients with the disease relative to control subjects. But, the researchers did find an association between left-side motor problems and OCD symptoms consistent with previous studies that have emphasized right hemisphere involvement in OCD. Kim and colleagues (2003) investigated the density of the dopamine transporter in the basal ganglia in patients with OCD and control subjects. Results indicated that patients with OCD had increased levels of DAT binding in the right basal ganglia relative to controls, supporting basal ganglia and dopamine involvement in OCD.

Yaryura-Tobias, Mancebo, and Bubrick (2001) have suggested that OCD, Tourette's disorder, and ADHD all involve pathology of the basal ganglia that may stem from two infectious etiologic factors: streptococcal virus and encephalitis. Tourette's disorder is a neurologic condition characterized by motor and vocal tics, and between 35% to 50% of individuals with

Tourette's disorder also have OCD (DSM IV-TR, 2000). The underlying pathophysiology of Tourette's disorder is not completely understood but appears to involve dysfunction of the pathways extending to and from the basal ganglia–thalamocortical regions (Segawa, 2003). Dysfunction of the basal ganglia has also been implicated in ADHD, and some studies suggest that individuals with ADHD have a higher incidence of comorbid OCD than individuals without ADHD (Geller, 2004). Interestingly, psychostimulants often used to treat ADHD, and primarily affecting the dopaminergic system, have been found to induce OCD symptoms in children as well as adults (Borcherding, Keysor, Rapoport, Elia, & Amass, 1990; Serby, 2003). Research has also found that a relationship between use of cocaine, a dopamine agonist, and increased risk of OCD in adults (Crum & Anthony, 1993). Collectively, these studies suggest that dopamine plays a role in OCD symptomology but that the intricacies of this relationship are poorly understood. As Micallef and Blin (2001) noted, the serotonergic and dopaminergic neurotransmitter systems function interactively and it is possible that decreased inhibitory influences of serotonin on dopaminergic neurons could result in hyperactivity dopapminergic neurons within the basal ganglia. Thus, OCD may be the consequence of dysfunctional interactive neurotransmitter systems within the basal ganglia and associated circuitry, and highly comorbid syndromes such as Tourette's disorder and ADHD may represent derivations of this faulty system.

Additional neurotransmitters implicated in OCD include GABA and opioids. GABA appears to play a role in OCD given the adjuctive effectiveness of benzodiazepines in reducing OCD symptoms in treatment-resistant adults and children (Francobandiera, 2001; Leonard et al., 1994). As reported by Hollander, Kaplan, and Stahl (2003) and D'Amico et al. (2003), however, benzodiazepines (clonazepam, olanzapine) used in isolation do not appear effective at reducing OCD symptoms but are associated with substantial improvement when used in conjunction with SSRIs. Rocca et al. (2000) suggested that a gene variant of the benzodiazepine receptor may be related to OCD and even subtypes of OCD (chronic versus episodic symptoms). With respect to the role of endogenous opioids in OCD, Friedman, Dar, and Shilony (2000) and Fals-Stewart and Angarano (1994) found that the rate of OCD was four times higher in individuals addicted to opioids. A few studies have found that the opioid antagonist naltrexone is effective at reducing some types of OCD symptoms (Grant & Kim, 2001).

Magnetic Resonance Imaging (MRI)

Many studies have found structural abnormalities in patients with OCD, most often in the subcortial and cortical regions. For example, Rosenberg et al. (1997) compared MRI scans of 19 children and adolescents with OCD to control subjects and found significantly smaller volumes of the prefrontal cortex, caudate nucleus, putamen, and lateral and third ventricles in patients with OCD. Robinson et al. (1995) also found that adult patients with OCD had significantly smaller caudate nucleus volumes than control subjects, but no volume differences were found with respect to the size of the prefrontal cortex or lateral or third ventricles. Bartha et al. (1998) did not find differences in left or right caudate volumes between patients with OCD and healthy control subjects. They did report metabolite reductions in the striatum of patients with OCD and speculated that neuronal density may be lower in this region. Consistent with this hypothesis are findings by Jenike and colleagues (1996), who reported significantly less white matter in patients with OCD than control subjects. Contradicting this perspective are findings by Mac Master, Keshavan, Dick, and Rosenberg (1999) and Rosenberg et al. (1997), who reported increased volumes of the corpus callosum as well as increased myelination in patients with OCD relative to control subjects.

Kwon et al. (2003b) recently used MRI to compare volumes of the hippocampus, amygdala, and thalamus in patients with OCD to patients with schizophrenia and healthy controls. Results revealed that the left amygdala was significantly larger in patients with OCD compared to the other two groups, and the hippocampus volume was significantly reduced in those with OCD and schizophrenia. No group differences were found with regard to the size of the thalamus. The researchers suggested that hippocampal reduction may be characteristic of both OCD and schizophrenia and enlargement of the amygdala may be unique to OCD. Szeszko and colleagues (1999), however, reported that the amygdala volume was significantly smaller in patients with OCD than healthy control subjects. Berthier and colleagues (2001) reported that patients who developed OCD following traumatic brain injury had contusions in subcortical structures (caudate nucleus) as well as frontal regions. It is important to note that significant size reductions of the subcortical structures (e.g. caudate nucleus) have also been found in children and adults with Tourette's disorder (Peterson et al., 2003) as well as other disorders. As Saxena, Brody, Schwartz, and Baxter (1998) noted, however, the heterogeneity of MRI findings in OCD may reflect differences among OCD patients such as age of onset, comorbid disorders, family history of OCD, or medication confounds. In summary, structural findings suggest that differences often exist in subcortical and cortical regions in patients with OCD relative to control subjects. These findings are not consistent among studies, however, and are not unique to OCD.

Neuroimaging Studies

A number of PET, fMRI, and SPECT studies have found functional differences between individuals with OCD and healthy volunteers. For example, Kwon et al. (2003a) recently reported that subjects with OCD showed increased metabolic activity in the right orbitofrontal cortex and decreased activity in the left parietal–occipital regions, and the level of activity was positively correlated with severity of OCD symptoms. The researchers also reported a significant correlation between activity in the prefrontal cortex and putamen and neuropsychological test performance in subjects with OCD. Additionally, studies suggest that the underlying pathphysiology of OCD may differ depending on the age at which OCD symptoms begin. For example, Busatto et al. (2001) compared rCBF in two groups of adults with OCD—those who developed the disorder prior to age 10 (early-onset) and those who developed OCD after age 12 (late-onset). Based on SPECT scans, both groups showed decreased rCBF in the right orbitofrontal regions. Subjects with early-onset OCD, however, had reduced rCBF in the left anterior cingulate and increased rCBF in the right cerebellum compared to control subjects. In addition, compared to late-onset OCD subjects, subjects with early-onset OCD showed reduced rCBF in the right thalamus. Other studies have also reported structural and functional abnormalities of the thalamus in patients with OCD. Gilbert et al. (2000), for example, investigated the volume of the hypothalamus of 21 children and adolescents (8 to 17 years) with OCD who had never taken medication for the disorder. Compared to control children, those with OCD had significantly larger thalamic volumes. Following 12 weeks of treatment with SSRI, the size of the hypothalamus decreased substantially in patients with OCD. Fitzgerald and colleagues (2000) also examined pediatric patients (8 to 15 years) with OCD and found functional abnormalities (i.e., reduced activity) in the left and right thalamus in children and adolescents with OCD relative to control subjects. Lacerda et al. (2003a) recently found a positive correlation between rCBF in the right thalamus and errors on neuropsychological tests in adults with OCD. Collectively, these studies implicate dysfunction of the thalamus in both childhood-onset and adult OCD.

A number of neuroimaging studies have substantiated involvement of prefrontal–subcortical pathways in the pathophysiology of OCD (Busatto et al., 2000; Castillo et al., 2005; Saxena, Brody, Schwartz, & Baxter, 1998). Kwon et al. (2003a), for example, reported increased glucose metabolism in the right orbitofrontal cortex in patients with OCD relative to control subjects, and increased activity in the right hippocampus and left putamen was positively correlated with severity of OCD symptoms. Lacerda et al. (2003b) also found a positive correlation between severity of OCD symptoms and rCBF in the right basal ganglia and right and left inferior frontal lobes in adult, medication-free Brazilian patients with OCD. A negative correlation was found, however, between severity of OCD symptoms and rCBF in the right thalamus. Diler, Kibar, and Avci (2004) recently measured rCBF in 18 medication-free children and adolescents with OCD prior to and after 12 weeks of treatment with an SSRI (paroxetine). Compared to control subjects, subjects with OCD had significantly higher rCBF in the right and left caudate, right and left dorsolateral prefrontal region, and cingulate. Following treatment with paroxetine, these regions showed significant reductions in rCBF, providing futher support of a dysfunction of the prefrontal–subcortical pathways in patients with OCD. Kang et al. (2003) reported similar findings and also observed that following 4 months of treatment, glucose metabolism changes of the putamen, cerebellum, and hippocampus were significantly associated with improved performance on neuropsychological tasks.

Diler, Kibar, and Avci's (2004) study has also been replicated in adults. For example, Hansen, Hasselbalch, Law, and Bolwig (2002) measured glucose metabolism using PET in 20 patients with OCD before and after 3 months of treatment with an SSRI (paroxetine). Results revealed a significant reduction in activity in the right caudate nucleus but no difference in global glucose metabolism before and after SSRI treatment. Saxena et al. (2001, 2002) performed similar studies and used PET to measure glucose metabolism patterns in subjects with OCD, subjects with major depression, and subjects with OCD and comorbid depression, prior to and after 8 to 12 weeks of SSRI treatment (paroxetine). Results indicated that subjects with OCD and subjects with depression showed differential patterns of response to the SSRI. Specifically, subjects with OCD alone showed glucose metabolsim decreases in the right caudate nucleus, right ventrolateral prefrontal cortex, and thalamus. SSRI treatment was associated with a decrease in glucose metabolism in the striatum in subjects with OCD alone. Subjects with depression and subjects with both disorders showed decreases in the left ventrolateral prefrontal cortex and increases in the right striatum. SSRI treatment was not associated with glucose metabolism decreases in the striatum but rather increased activity in both subjects with depression and OCD and comorbid depression. Hoehn-Saric et al. (2001) found that higher rCBF in the prefrontal and subcortical regions was associated with a better response to medication treatment in adult patients with OCD and comorbid major depression. Hoehn-Saric et al. also found that after 12 weeks of antidepressant treatment, subjects who showed substantial reductions in symptoms of OCD and depression also showed a diffuse reduction of rCBF in the prefrontal regions. These results were similar to those reported by Rauch et al. (2002), who used PET and rCBF measurements to predict antidepressant treatment response in adult patients with OCD.

Glutamate has also been implicated in OCD. For example, Rosenberg and colleagues (2000) measured glutamate concentrations in the caudate nucleus in children and adolescents with OCD before and after paroxetine treatment. Results revealed glutamate concentrations were significantly higher in patients with OCD than control subjects and that after 12 weeks of treat-ment, glutamate concentrations were reduced to a level similar to control subjects as were OCD symptoms. Hansen and colleagues (2002) reported similar findings with 20 patients with OCD treated with paroxetine, as did Bolton et al. (2001) in the case of an 8-year-old girl with OCD who was treated with paroxetine. The medication was discontinued after 14 months of treatment but follow-up results revealed that the decrease in OCD symptoms and glutamate lev-els persisted postmedication. Bolton et al. suggested that dysfunction of the glutamate system within the caudate nucleus may be reversible with antidepressant treatment.

Overall, studies suggest that OCD symptoms are mediated by overactivity in pathways extending from the subcortical structures (e.g., basal ganglia, thalamus) to and from the frontal cortex and that treatment with SSRIs decreases activity within these regions. Provocation studies such as those by Breiter et al. (1996) and more recently Adler et al. (2000) support the involvement of faulty frontal–subcortical circuitry in OCD. Adler et al. studied medication-free patients with OCD and exposed to them to stimuli designed to provoke OCD symptoms. Results indicated that patients with OCD, relative to control subjects, had increased neuronal activity in several regions of the frontal cortex (e.g., orbitofrontal, dorsolateral frontal) as well as the right cingulate cortex. Inconsistencies do exist across studies, however, and may reflect subject differences as well as measurement differences. As Reba (1993) noted, significant differences exist between imaging techniques that can affect the type of data obtained from neuroimaging scans of subjects with OCD. Trivedi (1996) pointed out that OCD studies have generally assessed subjects under three conditions: (1) while at rest, (2) during a challenge condition, or (3) during treatment. Clearly, results can vary substantially depending on the type of condition subjects were evaluated under during the study. Overall, however, the general theme that emerges from structural and functional studies is that OCD is characterized by abnormalities of subcortical and cortical structures and circuitry and that these abnormalities in function can often be remediated by pharmacological treatment. Nevertheless, these findings are correlational in nature and do not reveal the underlying source of the differences. In other words, structural differences are not necessarily related to or responsible for OCD symptoms, and disturbances in neural circuitry may be influenced by symptoms and behaviors associated with the disorder rather than causative.

Additional Theories

Pandas

Several lines of evidence have linked the development of OCD in some children and adults to an autoimmune response to streptococcal infections (Bodner, Morshed, & Peterson, 2001; Orvidas & Slattery, 2001; Swedo et al., 1998). Specifically, PANDAS (pediatric autoimmune neuropsychiatric disorders associated with streptococcal infections) has been used to describe children (and possibly adults) who have abrupt onset of tics or OCD (or both) following documented streptococcal infections. According to Arnold and Richter (2001) and Peterson et al. (2000), children who have had streptococcal infections and subsequently developed OCD often have increased basal ganglia volumes, presumably due to increased antibodies within the basal ganglia. Murphy and Pichichero (2002) found a relationship between PANDAS-related OCD and acute GABHS tonsillopharyngitis in 12 school-aged children. According to the researchers, treatment with antibiotics eradicated the GABHS infection as well as the OCD symptoms. Other studies, however, have not found antibiotics helpful in either preventing or decreasing PANDAS-related OCD symptoms (Arnold & Richter, 2001). It is important to note that most cases of OCD are not linked to streptococcal infenctions and, as Snider and Swedo (2003) recently pointed out, it is likely that individuals who develop OCD in reaction to streptococcal infections are genetically susceptible to the illness. Additional studies are needed to better understand the role of PANDAS in OCD and to identify genetic markers that may be associated with increased risk of PANDAS.

Interventions for OCD

Pharmacological

Numerous reviews are available concerning the pharmacological treatment of OCD in children, adolescents, and adults (e.g., Geller et al., 2003; Hollander et al., 2002). Antidepressants are the most commonly used medications for OCD, including clomipramine and SSRIs.

In general, research suggests that both medications are effective at reducing OCD symptoms but clomipramine is often superior to SSRIs (Geller et al., 2003). Clomipramine is associated with more side effects than SSRIs, however, and consequently SSRIs tend to have a higher compliance rate (Pigott & Seay, 1999). Several studies suggest that the SSRIs (e.g., paroxetine, fluoxetine, fluvoxamine, sertraline) are equally efficacious at treating OCD symptoms (Geller et al., 2003). Hollander et al. (2002) noted that it is not uncommon for patients with OCD to not respond to treatment with SSRIs and recommended that other medications be tried such as another SSRI or a serotonin–norepinephrine reuptake inhibitor. Hollander et al. and others have also recommended augmentation with neuroleptics or cognitive-behavioral therapy in treatment-resistant OCD. McDougle et al. (2000) recently examined the effectiveness of the antipsychotic medication risperidone in treating OCD and found that 50% of patients with OCD showed a favorable response to the medication. Figueroa and colleagues (1998) reported that a combination of SSRI and clomipramine was more effective at decreasing OCD symptoms than either drug used alone in children and adolescents with OCD. As mentioned previously, however, a greater risk of side effects is associated with clomipramine and antipsychotic medications compared to SSRIs.

Nonpharmacological Interventions

Cognitive-Behavioral Therapy

Cognitive-behavioral therapy has been widely investigated as a form of treatment for children, adolescents, and adults with OCD and will therefore be briefly mentioned. March, Mulle, and Herbel (1994) were among the first to develop a cognitive-behavioral treatment protocol for children and adolescents with OCD and demonstrated that the program can result in at least a 50% reduction in OCD symptoms. Adherence to the program helped to prevent reoccurrence of symptoms over time (18 months), they reported. Franklin et al. (1998) examined the efficacy of cognitive-behavioral therapy that involved the techniques of exposure and ritual prevention for children and adolescents with OCD. Results indicated that 67% of the subjects showed substantial improvement in symptoms and 62% maintained this reduction for at least 9 months. Similar positive findings have been reported by Benazon, Ager, and Rosenberg (2002) with children and adolescents, and Waters, Barrett, and March (2001) found that a structured family component enhanced the effectiveness of a 14-week cognitive-behavioral treatment protocol for children with OCD. In a recent review of the literature, Arnold et al. (2003) concluded that cognitive-behavioral interventions are often effective at treating OCD in children and adolescents and recommended cognitive-behavioral therapy alone or in conjunction with medication (e.g., SSRIs). De Haan and colleagues (1998) compared the effectiveness of medication (clomipramine) and behavior therapy for the treatment of OCD in children and adolescents and noted that both approaches reduced OCD symptomology but behavior therapy produced more significant changes.

Studies have also supported the use of cognitive-behavioral therapy with adults with OCD (Volpato et al., 2003). Cottraux et al. (2001) compared cognitive therapy with behavior therapy in adults with OCD and found that both approaches were equally effective at reducing OCD symptoms but cognitive therapy was superior at decreasing comorbid depression symptoms. Some studies have reported that the use of SSRIs in conjunction with cognitive-behavioral therapy results in even further reduction of OCD symptoms, while other studies have not found that SSRIs enhance treatment response to cognitive-behavioral therapy (e.g., Kampman, Keijsers, Hoogduin, & Verbraak, 2002; Simpson, Gorfinkle, & Liebowitz, 1999; Volpato et al., 2003). Marks (1997) reported that cognitive-behavioral therapy results in slightly more improvement of OCD symptoms than antidepressant medication and is associated with lower relapse rates. Van Balkom et al. (1998), however, compared cognitive-behavioral interventions and antidepressants in the treatment of OCD in adults and concluded the approaches were equally effective and a combination of medication and cognitive-behavioral therapy was not superior to either approach used in isolation. Conversely, Neziroglu, Yaryura-Tobias, Walz, and McKay (2000) reported that a combination of antidepressants and behavior therapy was more effective than medication alone at reducing OCD symptoms in children and adolescents. Abramowitz and colleagues (2003) recently reported that cognitive-behavioral therapy was less effective at treating patients with OCD who had hoarding compulsions compared to other types of OCD symptoms. Foster and Eisler (2001) recommended an integrative approach to the treatment of OCD by using both cognitive-behavioral therapy and medication, but tailoring the use of these approaches to meet the individual needs of patients with OCD. Because for some individuals the development of OCD is precipitated by environmental factors and for others it may be more neurobiologically based, the emphasis on behavioral or pharmacological interventions may differ, they said.

In 1996, Schwartz and Beyette published a book, "Brain Lock," which detailed a four-step self treatment method based on cognitive-behavioral principles. According to Schwartz and Beyette, their four-step program can effectively treat OCD by altering brain chemistry and modifying one's genetic disposition. Recent research has begun to investigate structural and functional brain changes in patients with OCD before and after cognitive-behavioral therapy. For example, Rosenberg, Benazon, Gilbert, Sullivan, and Moore (2000) used MRI to measure thalamic volume in medication-free children and adolescents with OCD prior to and after 12 weeks of cognitive-behavioral therapy. Unlike previous studies that reported functional and structural changes in the thalamus following paroxetine treatment, results did not reveal a change in thalamic volume. Similarly, Benazon, Moore, and Rosenberg (2003) failed to find metabolic changes in the caudate following 12 weeks of cognitive-behavioral therapy despite improvement of OCD symptoms. Nakatani et al. (2003), however, measured rCBF in 31 patients with treatment-resistant OCD, 22 patients with OCD who responded favorably to cognitive-behavioral therapy, and 22 control subjects. Results indicated that both groups of patients with OCD demonstrated increased rCBF in the right and left basal ganglia compared to controls, but only OCD subjects who responded to cognitive-behavioral therapy showed a significant decrease in rCBF in the right head of the caudate. Collectively, these findings suggest that greater functional and structural brain changes are associated with pharmacological interventions but some functional changes are associated with cognitive-behavioral treatment for OCD. Despite these physiological differences, both approaches are often effective at treating OCD.

Psychosurgery

According to Greenberg et al. (2003), there is considerable interest in the use and further development of neuroanatomically based treatments for OCD due to the fact that some patients do not respond to pharmacological or behavioral interventions. In the early 1930s, Egas Moniz coined the phrase "psychosurgery" to describe brain operations he performed to treat institutionalized patients with severe mental illness (Moniz, 1937). Today, psychosurgery is most often used with patients with chronically severe and treatment-refractory mental illness including mood and anxiety disorders, especially OCD (Cosgrove & Rauch, 1995). Given the physiological evidence suggesting that OCD symptoms originate from disturbances in the pathways projecting to and from subcortical to cortical regions (orbitofrontal cortex, thalamus, anterior cingulate, and striatum), surgical procedures typically target regions within this circuity. Four surgical procedures are used in patients with severe treatment-resistant OCD: (a) subcaudate tractotomy, (b) anterior capsulotomy, (c) anterior cingulotomy, and (d) limbic leucotomy. *Subcaudate tractotomy* involves lesioning an area under the head of the caudate nucleus to interrupt connections between subcortical and orbitofrontal regions, while an *anterior capsulotomy* targets pathways connecting the thalamus and the frontal lobes. An *anterior cingulotomy* involves lesioning an area of the cortex of the anterior cingulate, and a *limbic leucotomy* involves lesioning the anterior cingulate as well as an area of the caudate nucleus. According to Greenberg et al. (2003), lesioning procedures are effective at reducing intractable OCD symptoms in 35 to 75% of cases.

A substantial number of studies have examined the effectivenss of psychosurgery in improving OCD symptoms. For example, Baer et al. (1995) followed up 18 patients who had undergone cingulotomy for OCD approximately 27 months after the procedure. Results indicated that 28% responded well to the procedure while 17% were classified as partial responders. Similar results were reported by Jenike et al. (1991), who followed up 33 patients with OCD who had received cingulotomy at Massachusetts General Hospital. Sachdev and colleagues (2001) used PET to measure glucose metabolism in a 37-year-old female 18 days and 3 years after a bilateral orbitomedial leucotomy for her severe OCD. Results indicated a significant reduction in the head of the caudate, anterior cingulate, thalamus, and several frontal regions 18 days following the procedure and a sustained reduction in glucose metabolism in many of these regions after 3 years. These reductions in activity were strongly associated with improvement of symptoms and, according to the researchers, the case supports a dysfunction of subcortical–cortical circuitry in OCD. Kim et al. (2001) measured rCBF in patients who had undergone a limbic leukotomy for intractable OCD and found significant decreases in the medial frontal cortex, cingulate, and striatum.

Recently, Dougherty et al. (2002) followed a large sample (44) of patients who underwent one or more bilateral anterior cingulotomies and found that 32 to 45% of the patients responded favorably to the cingulotomy after approximately 32 months follow-up. Nearly 20% reported at least one negative side effect after the procedure (e.g., memory deficits, apathy, seizures). In a similar study but with fewer subjects, Montoya et al. (2002) followed up 21 patients with OCD or major depression who had undergone limbic leukotomy after 26 months. Findings revealed that 36 to 50% of the patients responded favorably to the procedure and showed a substantial reduction of OCD and depression symptoms. According to the researchers, a minority of patients experienced side effects that included urinary incontinence, memory problems, and apathy. Collectively, these studies suggest that a significant percentage of individuals who do not respond to traditional treatment methods for OCD may respond to neurosurgery. Given the risks associated with brain surgery and the potential side effects, psychosurgery is obviously reserved for severe, intractable cases of OCD.

Deep Brain Stimulation (DBS) and Electroconvulsive Therapy (ECT)

As an alternative to psychosurgery, DBS and ECT have been used to treat severe, treatment-resistant OCD. However, studies in this area are limited and those that have been conducted tend to involve small sample sizes. Nuttin and colleagues (1999), for example, studied the effectiveness of DBS in four patients with chronic, treatment-resistant OCD and reported that three of the four showed significant improvement of symptoms. More recently, Gabriëls et al. (2003) reported that two of three patients treated for OCD with DBS showed sustained improvement of symptoms over time (33 months) with no harmful side effects. Location of DBS depends on a number of factors and, as McIntyre and colleagues (2004) recently noted, small deviations in the placement of the DBS electrode can substantially alter the degree of activation and structures involved. Sturm et al. (2003) studied the effects of DBS in the right nucleus accumbens and also reported that three of the four patients treated benefited from DBS. Chronic DBS has also been studied in patients with OCD. For example, Anderson and Ahmed (2003) described the case of a woman who was treated with bilateral electrical stimulators that were placed in the interior limbs of the internal capsules (between the thalamus and caudate nucleus). Placement of the stimulators resulted in chronic electrical stimulation, and findings revealed short- and long-term improvement in the woman's OCD symptoms and general functioning. Nuttin et al. (1999) reported similar findings with placement of bilateral stimulators in four patients with OCD, and recently Nuttin et al. (2003) reported that during stimulation (compared to stimulation-off periods) bilateral stimulators led to decreased metabolism in the frontal regions of six patients with treatment-refractory OCD.

A number of studies have found that adult patients treated with ECT have shown short- and long-term reduction in OCD symptoms. According to Russell, Tharyan, Kumar, and Cherian (2002), there is reluctance among psychiatrists to use ECT with children and adolescents with any psychiatric illness including OCD, and its use with this population is controversial. With respect to adults, Mellman and Gorman (1984) described a case of a man with treatment-resistant OCD who showed significant reduction in OCD symptoms following ECT. Maletzky, McFarland, and Burt (1994) reported that nearly all of the 32 patients with intractable OCD benefited from ECT and that improvement in their symptoms was sustained over a 1-year period. Recently, Thomas and Kellner (2003) reported that a single, unilateral treatment with OCD resulted in remission of symptoms in an adult with severe OCD. As Datto (2000) reported, a number of side effects are associated with ECT—headaches, memory impairment, nausea, and muscle aches—although most of these symptoms are thought to be transitory.

SUMMARY

OCD affects approximately .5 to 2% of the population and is equally common in adult females and males. OCD is characterized by obsessions and/or compulsions that cause impairment in daily living. Based on familial and twin studies, OCD appears to have a genetic component although molecular genetic studies have not identified a gene or group of genes that cause OCD. Anatomical and neuroimaging studies suggest that circuitry involving subcortical structures such as the striatum, anterior cingulate, and thalamus and projections to and from the orbitofrontal cortex are strongly implicated in the pathophysiology of OCD. Several neurotransmitter systems have also been implicated in the disorder, particularly serotonin and dopamine. It is important to note that although these findings are associated with OCD, they do not reveal the underlying cause of the disorder. Treatment of OCD typically involves antidepressants (SSRIs and clomipramine) and cognitive-behavioral therapy. For severe, refractory OCD, psychosurgery and ECT have been found to reduce symptoms in 25 to 75% of cases.

8

Drug Addiction and Eating Disorders

This chapter reviews theories of addiction and research findings on neurotransmitter systems involved in drug addiction and eating disorders. Particular attention is given to structural changes associated with drug addiction as well as genetic, anatomical, and neuroimaging findings. Background information on eating disorders is included along with genetic, anatomical, neurochemical, and neuroimaging findings. Pharmacological treatment approachs to addiction and eating disorders are also discussed.

DRUG ADDICTION

According to Wise and Gardner (2004) there is no single, generally accepted definition of addiction. Nestler (2004) defined drug addiction as "the compulsive seeking (drug craving) and administration of a drug despite grave adverse consequences or as a loss of control over drug intake" (p. 698). The American Psychiatric Association (DSM IV-TR, APA, 2000) has divided substance-related disorders into two groups: substance use disorders and substance induced disorders. Substance induced disorders include substance intoxication, substance withdrawal, substance induced delirium, substance induced persisting dementia, substance induced persisting amnestic disorder, substance induced psychotic disorder, substance induced mood disorder, substance induced anxiety disorder, substance induced sexual dysfunction disorder, and substance induced sleep disorder (refer to DSM IV-TR for additional information). Substance use disorders include substance abuse and substance dependence. As defined by the DSM IV-TR, substance dependence involves a cluster of cognitive, behavioral, and physiological symptoms as well as continued use of the substance despite significant substance-related problems (Table 8.1).

Substance dependence is accompanied by tolerance and withdrawal symptoms. *Tolerance* refers to the need for increased amounts of the substance to achieve the desired effect and varies across substances and among individuals. *Withdrawal* refers to the aversive physiological effects that ensue when the addictive substance is removed or reduced and may include insomnia, anxiety, agitation, and digestive problems. Withdrawal symptoms vary by substance

TABLE 8.1

DSM IV-TR Criteria for Substance Dependence (DSM IV-TR, 2000)

A maladaptive pattern of substance use, leading to clinically significant impairment or distress, as manifested by three (or more) of the following, occurring at any time in the same 12-month period:

1) tolerance, as identified by either of the following:
    a) a need for markedly increased amounts of the substance to achieve intoxication or desired effect
    b) markedly diminished effect with continued use of the same amount of the substance
2) withdrawal, as manifested by either of the following:
    a) the characteristic withdrawal syndrome for the substance (refer to Criteria A and B of the criteria sets for Withdrawal from the specific substances)
    b) the same (or closely related) substance is taken to relieve or avoid withdrawal symptoms.
3) the substance is often taken in large amounts or over a longer period that was intended
4) there is a persistent desire or unsuccessful efforts to cut down or control substance use
5) a great deal of time is spent in activities necessary to obtain the substance (e.g., visiting multiple doctors or driving long distances), use the substance (e.g., chain-smoking), or recover from its effects
6) important social, occupational, or recreational activities are given up or reduced because of substance use
7) the substance use is continued despite knowledge of having a persistent or recurrent physical or psychological problem that is likely to have been caused or exacerbated by the substance (e.g., current cocaine use despite recognition of cocaine-induced depression, or continued drinking despite recognition that an ulcer was made worse by alcohol consumption)

Specify if:
   With Physiological Dependence: evidence of tolerance or withdrawal (i.e., either item 1 or 2 is present)
   Without Physiological Dependence: no evidence of tolerance or withdrawal (i.e., neither item 1 nor 2 is present)

Course specifiers (see text for definitions):
   Early Full Remission
   Early Partial Remission
   Sustained Full Remission
   Sustained Partial Remission
   On Agonist Therapy
   In a Controlled Environment

but generally, according to the DSM IV-TR, are opposite those observed with intoxication. In this chapter, the terms addiction and dependence are used interchangeably.

Background, Prevalence, and Course

According to the National Institute for Drug Abuse (NIDA), commonly abused drugs include cannabinoids, depressants, hallucinogens, opioids, stimulants, and alcohol. Addictive drugs include alcohol, barbituates, benzodiazepines, cannabinoids, nicotine, PCP, and stimulants. Although hallucinogens such as LSD, mescaline, and psilocybin are also frequently abused, they are nonaddictive (Hyman & Malenka, 2001). Preston, O'Neal, and Talaga (2002) reported that at least 5% of Americans are addicted to alcohol. Gonzalez-Castro, Barrington, Walton, and Rawson (2000) compared addiction patterns of cocaine and methamphetamine and reported that methamphetamine induces a faster rate of progression toward regular use and need for treatment. Research also indicates that substance use disorders often co-occur with psychiatric disorders and increase the complexity of providing effective treatment interventions. For example, Havassy, Alvidrez, and Owen (2004) studied over 400 patients from the public mental health system and a substance abuse treatment system and found that 54% had comorbid psychiatric and substance use disorders. A significantly larger percentage of public health patients met the criteria for comorbidity than those from the substance abuse settings (65% and 49%, respectively). According to the DSM IV-TR, the presence of co-occurring psychiatric disorders (e.g., bipolar disorder, major depressive disorder) increases the risk of a poor prognosis.

Although males are more likely than females to suffer from substance-related disorders, recent research indicates that substance abuse is increasing among females, the initiation of the substance use is occurring at younger ages, and females appear to have an accelerated progression to dependence (Zilberman, Tavares, & el-Guebaly, 2003). Greenfield and colleagues (2003) noted that among boys and girls aged 12–17 years, there is a comparable rate of use and initiation for alcohol, cocaine, heroin, and tobacco. The researchers also reported that women are particularly vulnerable to the medical, physical, mental, and social consequences of substance use and dependence and have the added potential risk of drug induced complications during pregnancy. Howell, Heiser, and Harrington (1999) reported that approximately 5% of pregnant women abuse illicit drugs during their pregnancy, but very little information is available concerning successful treatment approaches with this population.

Andrews and colleagues (2003) investigated the prevalence of substance use and future intentions among elementary school children and found that with most substances, prevalence and intention to use substances increased with grade level. For cigarettes and alcohol, intention to use at younger grades was related to subsequent use of the substance, suggesting that intention may be an early warning sign of substance use among children and adolescents. Mohler-Kuo, Lee, and Wechsler (2003) examined patterns of illicit drug use among college students from 1993–2001 and reported significant increases in the percentage of students using marijuana during this time period. Significant increases were also found in use of other illicit drugs, with greater than 98% of drug users using more than one substance.

According to the DSM IV-TR, there are wide cultural variations in attitudes toward substance use as shown by patterns of use both within and between countries. Individuals between the ages of 18–24 have relatively high prevalence rates for alcohol and illicit drugs, whereas the onset for most drugs of abuse and dependence occurs during the 20s—40s. The course of substance dependence (i.e., addiction) is variable, but usually chronic with periods of exacerbation and remission. Age and psychosocial factors have been associated with the clinical course and outcome of substance dependence (Chung et al., 2003), with depression serving as a major trigger for relapse in both men and women (Coelho et al., 2000; Snow & Anderson, 2000). A multisite longitudinal study conducted by Miller and colleagues (1997) of individuals undergoing outpatient alcohol and dependence treatment found that the most powerful predictors of relapse were posttreatment factors (support group attendance and a continuing care program). Wu and colleagues (2003) recently reported that in the United States uninsured persons aged 12–64 years have increased rates of alcohol and drug dependence for which only a minority receive treatment. Although psychosocial factors are crucial in the onset, development, and prognosis of substance use and dependence, this chapter's focus is the pathophysiology of addiction.

Reinforcement Theories

There is no single cause of addiction. Like many other psychiatric disorders, substance dependence is thought to be a product of environmental and physiological factors (Crabbe, 2002). Research into the physiological basis of substance dependence is conducted via genetic and heritability studies as well as neurotransmitter and neuroimaging studies. Much of the knowledge of the neurobiology of addiction is based on animal models but, as Wise and Gardner (2004) noted, there is no universally accepted animal model of addiction. Furthermore, animal models are severely limited by the fact that animals become addicted to a substance only when a human creates the addiction condition. As Wise and Gardner stated, "addiction is a uniquely human phenomenon . . . each animal model is an approximation that captures some but not all of the characteristics of the human condition" (p. 683).

The two main models of addiction are the positive reinforcement model and the negative reinforcement model (Maldonado, 2003). According to the positive reinforcement model, addiction involves the desire for pleasure or euphoria, whereas the negative reinforcement model emphasizes the desire to alleviate pain or discomfort. According to the negative reinforcement model of addiction, over time, compulsive drug-taking behavior results from a need to achieve a state of homeostasis. In other words, drugs are taken in order for the individual to feel normal. Both positive and negative reinforcement models can be applied to help explain addiction—drugs initially create a state of pleasure and are therefore reinforcing, but over time physiological changes occur and the drug is needed to alleviate withdrawal symptoms (negative reinforcement). Thus, addiction can be partially explained as a result of positive reinforcement and maintained as a result of negative reinforcement. Di Chiara (1999) noted that the rewarding properties of drugs do not justify the negative consequences that accompany their repeated use, and therefore secondary, conditioned stimuli must act as incentives of drug-taking behavior. Robinson and Berridge (2000) also argued that traditional positive and negative reinforcement principles of addiction are neither necessary nor sufficient to explain drug-seeking and drug-taking behavior, and instead proposed a more complex, incentive-sensitization model of addiction. In essence, they proposed that repeated drug use induces cellular changes that sensitize various brain systems to the drug. The systems most affected are those involved in incentive motivation and reward, and gradually these systems become hypersensitive to addictive drugs and to environmental stimuli associated with drug use—which leads to drug craving. According to Robinson and Berridge, addiction is the result of neuroadaptive, physiological changes that lead to alterations in motivational, attentional, and cognitive processes that interact to produce drug-seeking and drug abuse behavior. The authors suggested that medical and psychotherapeutic treatments that can reverse the neuroadaptive changes or prevent neuronal sensitization will be the most effective at successfully treating addiction. In summary, addiction can best be explained from the integration of several perspectives that encompass psychological and learning theories as well as neurobiological adaptations.

Neurotransmitter Systems

As mentioned in chapter 2, drugs exert their effects by enhancing (agonist) or interfering with (antagonist) the brain's neurotransmitter systems. These effects occur at the level of the synapse and, depending on the drug, the mode of action varies. For example, opiates attach to opioid receptors and mimic the effects of naturally occurring opioids. Nicotine is an agonist at the level of the nicotonic receptor (acetylcholine). Alcohol is a GABA agonist and attaches to a portion of the benzodiazepine receptor and enhances the effects of GABA. Alcohol also has antagonisitic effects as it inhibits functioning of the NMDA glutamate receptor, which is associated with the intoxicating effects of alcohol (Nestler, 2004). Stimulants such as cocaine prevent reuptake of dopamine and, to a lesser extent, serotonin and norepinephrine (Cami & Farre, 2003), whereas barbituates and benzodiazepines are GABA agonists. Cannabinoids attach to cannabionoid CB1 receptors that activate second messenger systems and enhance the release of dopamine in the midbrain and forebrain (Gardner, 2002). The receptors for various neurotransmitters are differentially distributed throughout the brain, and thus the behavioral effects of drugs differ depending on the targeted brain regions. For example, opioid receptors are located in various regions throughout the brain and include different subtypes: mu, delta, and kappa receptors. These receptors are located throughout the central nervous system but are heavily concentrated in the locus coeruleus, brain stem, and spinal cord, which explains why opiates such as morphine and oxycotin can have profound effects on respiration (Leino, Mildh, Lertola, Seppala, & Kirvela, 1999).

Sora and colleagues (2001) emphasized that substantial individual differences exist in human and other animals in terms of mu receptor levels and that this difference could be related to distinct opiate drug effects. The mu receptor appears to be particularly involved in addiction as mice without mu-opioid receptors lack opiate-induced tolerance and dependence (Sora et al., 2001). However, depending on factors that are not well understood, opioid agonists may have opposite behavioral actions depending on the type of opioid receptor that is activated. For example, Margolis, Hjelmstad, Bonci, and Fields (2003) recently reported that activation of the mu-opioid receptor in the ventral tegmental area of the brain stimulates dopaminergic neurons while activation of the kappa opioid receptor inhibits dopaminergic neurons in this same region. Additional research is needed to understand the role of these different types of opioid receptors in addiction. Differences also exist among humans with regard to the quantity and distribution pattern of other types of receptors such as dopamine and serotonin (Cravchik & Goldman, 2000), which may help to explain interindividual drug effects.

It is important to note that the modulating effects of other neurotransmitters on dopamine and opioid neurotransmission are not well understood and may play an important role in drug addiction. For example, Vollenweider, Vontobel, Hell, and Leenders (1999) studied the effects of a serotonin receptor agonist (psilocybin) on dopamine receptor (D2) binding and found that serotonin receptor activation helped to modulate (increase) dopamine release in the striatum. A few studies have found that in addition to affecting the dopaminergic system, cocaine is associated with alterations in serotonergic function. Buydens-Branchey and colleagues (1999), for example, reported that male cocaine addicts treated with a serotonin reuptake inhibitor showed a greater change in hormonal systems (i.e., elevated prolactin response) than controls. Interestingly, similar findings were reported by Wolfe and colleagues (2000) when they compared serotonin-mediated prolactin responses in individuals with active bulimia and in recovery. These findings suggest that different forms of addiction may alter the normal functioning of several regulatory systems including the serotonergic system.

The opioid system interacts with other neurotransmitter systems such as the glutamate system and the NMDA receptor. For example, according to Mao (1999), there is an overlap between distribution patterns of opioid receptors and NMDA receptors, and some neurons contain both types of receptors. Although poorly understood, opioid receptors have been found to interact with the NMDA receptor and this interaction may play a critical role in aspects of addiction (Mao, 1999). For example, NMDA receptor antagonists have been found to prevent morphine dependence in other animals (Fundytus & Coderre, 1994). A few studies suggest that opioid tolerance can also be prevented by an NMDA antagonist, although these findings are inconclusive. Mao (1999) suggested that pain involves the activation of NMDA receptors and that this activation may modulate opioid receptors and could contribute to structural changes at the cellular level believed to underlie tolerance, dependence, and withdrawal. Shalev, Grimm, and Shaham (2002) recently reviewed the neurobiology of relapse and suggested that most neurotransmitter systems—including dopamine, serotonin, GABA, glutamate, noradrenaline, acetylcholine, and endogenous opioids and cannabioids as well as the corticotropin-releasing endocrine system—may all play a critical role in stimulant and opioid relapse in humans.

Mesolimbic and Frontal Pathways

Despite the different neurotransmitter systems targeted by drugs, the fact that all drugs of abuse are positively reinforcing often leads to repeated use. Although the neurobiological underpinnings of addiction are not fully understood, most research on the reinforcing properties of drugs implicates the mesolimbic pathway and the dopaminergic system. As discussed in chapter 2, the mesolimbic pathway arises from dopaminergic neurons in the midbrain (ventral tegmental area) and projects to the nucleus accumbens and structures in the forebrain including the prefrontal cortex (Self, 2004). These regions contain highly complex neural networks and circuits that are rich in a variety of neurotransmitters such as dopamine, glutamate, serotonin, and GABA as well as different types of peptides. Nestler (2002) suggested that complex circuits involving the hippocampus, cerebral cortex, ventral and dorsal striatum, and amygdala are implicated in addiction, and Goldstein and Volkow (2002) recently emphasized the role of frontal regions in drug addiction. As discussed in chapter 1, the frontal regions of the brain are important in higher-order cognitive functions as well as the ability to monitor one's own behavior and inhibit impulsive responding (i.e., executive functions). Individuals suffering from addiction have exhibited impairment of these functions (Matochik et al., 2003). Two frontal regions in particular have been implicated in addiction: the orbitofrontal cortex and the cingulate gyrus. These structures are connected with subcortical limbic structures and systems (Goldstein & Volkow, 2002). Bolla et al. (2003) proposed that the orbitofrontal cortex plays an important role in decision making and assessed whether cocaine-dependent individuals who were abstinent for 25 days would show altered cerebral blood flow in the orbitofrontal cortex. Using PET, the researchers found that cocaine abusers did evidence greater activation than controls in this region and reduced activation in other regions (e.g., left prefrontal cortex). The authors interpreted the findings as supporting *persistent* functional abnormalities in neural networks involved in decision making in individuals who are cocaine-dependent.

In related work, Nutt, Lingford-Hughes, and Daglish (2003) recently noted that the anterior cingulate appears to play a critical role in the emotional salience associated with addictive drugs, and the orbitofrontal pathways are more involved in impulse control and higher-order thinking. The frontal regions also have been implicated in motivation, craving, and withdrawal symptoms characteristic of addiction (Goldstein & Volkow, 2002). Interestingly, Small, Zatorre, Dagher, Evans, and Jones-Gotman (2001) reported that blood flow increased signficantly in the orbitofrontal cortex and striatum in volunteers while they ate chocolate and rated eating the chocolate as "very pleasant." Other regions of the brain, however, increased in activity when the subjects ate chocolate but were satiated and and indicated that they did not find the experience pleasurable. O'Doherty and colleagues (2002) found similar results using fMRI to measure brain regions involved in anticipation of a pleasant taste. These results support the hypothesis that separate motivational systems exist in the brain and that those involved with pleasure and reward involve pathways and circuitry extending from the midbrain to the frontal cortex.

The mesolimbic pathways are rich in dopamine neurons. As Gardner (2002) recently noted, addictive drugs commonly influence such pathways in that: (1) they activate the neurons in the mesolimbic and projecting systems, (2) they result in an increase in firing of dopamine-releasing neurons, (3) they are associated with increased dopamine levels in the extracellular space, (4) they are self-administered, and (5) relapse is common after detoxification. Studies from the early 1960s found that amphetamines (dopamine agonists) increased lever-pressing behavior in rats while dopamine antagonists decreased lever-pressing behavior (Stein, 1962). Subsequent studies have substantiated that dopamine antagonists block the rewarding effects of stimulants (e.g., cocaine, amphetamines) and that these stimulants have a primary affinity for the dopamine transporter (DAT) rather than other neurotransmitter systems (e.g., Ritz et al., 1987). Wise et al. (1995) observed that dopamine levels in the nucleus accumbens increased during self-administered intravenous cocaine administration in rats. Humans suffering from Parkinson's disease have a compromised level of dopamine in the nucleus accumbens and mesolimbic pathways, and research has found that these patients report blunted effects of stimulants, further supporting the role of dopamine in the rewarding effects of drugs of abuse (Persico, Reich, Henningfield, Kuhar, & Uhl, 1998). Recently, Volkow, Fowler, and Wang (2002) studied subjects who were cocaine-dependent and reported that during drug intoxication, the rapid increase of dopamine levels in the striatum was associated with the rewarding effects of the drug. Additionally, they found that alterations of the dopaminergic midbrain system are associated with reduced activity in the frontal regions and that during drug craving the frontal regions (i.e., orbitofrontal cortex) increase in activity.

Although the cellular events that trigger dopamine release are not fully understood, Leite-Morris and colleagues (2004) recently reported that when opioid receptors located on GABA neurons in the ventral tegmental area are activated, dopamine cell activity is enhanced and dopamine is released in the nucleus accumbens. Self (2004) reported that opiates increase dopamine in part by removing the inhibitory influence of GABA neurons on dopamine-releasing cells. The mesolimbic dopaminergic system has also been implicated in the rewarding effects of other drugs—nicotine, alcohol, barbituates, benzodiazepines, and cannabis (Clarke & Pert, 1985; Due, Huettel, Hall, & Rubin, 2002; Wise & Gardner, 2004). Based on studies that have consistently found that drugs such as alcohol, opiates, and stimulants increase dopamine levels in the nucleus accumbens, researchers have begun to explore methods that will interfere with dopamine release and perhaps the addiction process. Research with other animals has discovered that opiate antagonists injected into the nucleus accumbens can block the rewarding effects of opiates (Vaccarino, Bloom, & Koob, 1985). Indeed, a popular pharmacological treatment for human alcohol and opiate addiction is the daily administration of naltrexone—an opioid, mu receptor antagonist (Mason et al., 2002). Di Ciano and Everitt (2003) recently reported that the mesolimbic system, in conjunction with GABA pathways throughout the limbic system, is involved when stimuli paired with drugs of abuse become capable of inducing drug-seeking behavior and relapse. The researchers found that a GABA receptor agonist, baclofen, reduced the propensity of conditioned stimuli to induce drug-seeking behavior in rats and suggested that GABA agonists may reduce these motivational behaviors in human addicts as well. Recent baclofen trials with humans have produced mixed findings, with some studies supporting the efficacy of baclofen in reducing cocaine use (Shoptaw et al., 2003) and alcohol craving and consumption (Addolorato et al., 2002), while in other studies it has been ineffective (Lile et al., 2004).

Collectively, human and other animal studies indicate that dopamine plays an integral role in the rewarding effects of different types of drug addiction. Recently, Leyton and colleagues (2002) used PET to measure dopamine levels in the striatum (nucleus accumbens, caudate, and putamen) in healthy men during placebo and amphetamine administration. Results revealed significant increases in dopamine levels in the ventral but not dorsal striatum. Similar findings were reported by Boileau et al. (2003) using PET and alcohol administration in healthy human volunteers. Other studies, including de la Fuente-Fernandez et al. (2002), have demonstrated that dopamine release is also increased in the ventral striatum of humans in anticipation of drug administration. Collectively, these studies further reinforce that mesolimbic dopamine activation plays a critical role in the rewarding effects of drugs and that, over time, chronic drug use leads to neuronal adaptations. These cellular changes are complex and poorly understood but are believed to underlie the behavioral characteristics of drug addiction, namely tolerance, dependence, and withdrawal.

Cellular Adaptation

Although drug abuse initially induces changes at the level of the synapse—such as increased levels of dopamine in the intracellular fluid—continued use of drugs is associated with complex intracellular changes. Specifically, with repeated drug exposure, neurons adapt over time and these cellular changes are believed to be responsible for tolerance, addiction, and withdrawal. Withdrawal, for example, is associated with a number of extracellular and intracellular changes such as extracellular dopamine depletion, up- and down-regulation of receptors, and alteration of second messenger systems (Wise & Gardner, 2004). Liu and Anand (2001) reported that opioid tolerance and addiction are associated with a number of intracellular changes: up-regulation of the cyclic adenosine monophosphate (cAMP) pathway, supersensitization of adenylyl cyclase, coupling of opioid receptors to second and perhaps third messenger systems, and activation and interactions of various intracellular proteins. These same intracellular changes are associated with other drugs of abuse such as cocaine and methamphetamine.

The cAMP pathway is part of a complex second messenger system that is activated when addictive drugs are administered. For example, when the mu receptor is occupied by opiates, the conductance of the K+ channels is increased and second messenger systems are activated. When the second messenger system is activated, a cascade of events occur, the details of which are not fully understood. Research with other animals suggests that K+ channels are coupled to intracellular Gproteins that inhibit the enzyme adenylyl cyclase, which in turn reduces cAMP levels (Smart, Smith, & Lambert, 1994). Reduction in these enzymes results in a series of intracellular changes. One such change is the reduced phosphorylation of the protein CREB (cyclic adenosine monophosphate response element binding protein), thought to initiate additional intracellular events such as altered gene expression that lead to long-term changes in cellular function (Fig. 8.1; see also Color Plate 4).

One example is the increased production of the transcription factors, dynorphin and delta FosB. Dynorphin levels have been found to increase with chronic drug use and are associated with the decreased rewarding effects of drugs and tolerance. Another intracellular protein, delta FosB, also increases with chronic drug use and levels remain elevated after prolonged abstinence. According to Nestler, Barrot, and Self (2001) and Kelz et al. (1999), these prolonged changes in delta FosB activity are associated with increased sensitivity to environmental cues and the rewarding effects of drugs and likely contribute to drug craving and relapse. Interestingly, research has also found that cAMP levels change over time. For example, initially exposure to opiates decreases cAMP levels and cellular inhibition is increased, but chronic exposure results in increased levels of cAMP (Nestler, 2002). This up-regulation of cAMP is thought to increase the firing of neurons in certain regions of the brain (i.e., locus coeruleus) to the previously normal level, and according to Monteggia and Nestler (2003), can be viewed as the brain's effort to establish homeostasis in response to the increased opiate induced cellular inhibition.

An additional effect of chronic exposure to opioids is a decreased sensitivity of neuron receptors to opioids, which means larger amounts of the drug are required to achieve a desired effect (tolerance). Although the physiological basis of tolerance is not well understood, long-lasting intracellular, enzymatic, and genetic changes modulated by CREB and other transcription factors such as delta FosB may account for drug tolerance (Nestler, 2002). For example, Hyman (1996) proposed that opiate receptors in the locus coeruleus are especially involved in addiction and withdrawal. As mentioned previously, opiates initially decrease the firing rate (i.e., increases inhibition) of neurons in the locus coeruleus, but if an opiate is administered chronically, neurons return to a normal firing rate. If an opioid antagonist is administered following chronic opioid use, withdrawal occurs and the firing rate of neurons in the locus

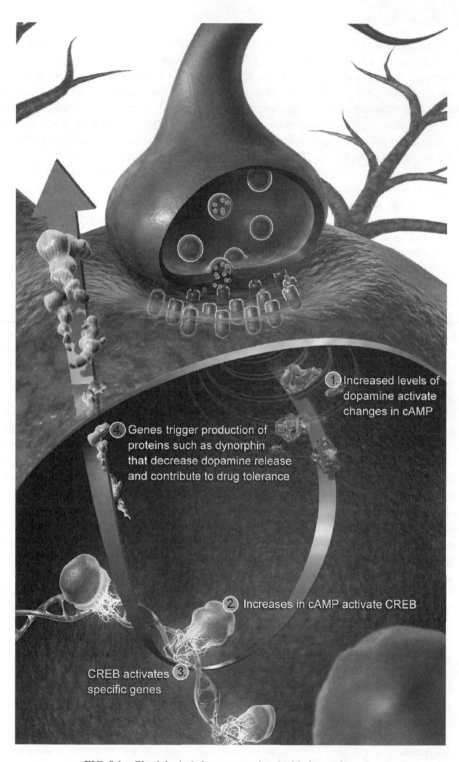

FIG. 8.1. Physiological changes associated with drug tolerance.
Copyright Blausen Medical Communications. Reproduced by permission. (See Color Plate 4.)

coeruleus increases significantly. Studies by Aghajanian and colleagues (1994) have found that during antagonist-precipitated withdrawal, the levels of a number of neurotransmitters are increased in the locus coeruleus (e.g., aspartate, glutamate, norepinephrine) and are correlated with behavioral effects of withdrawal. Thus, addictive drugs such as opioids produce complex, long-lasting intracellular changes that are associated with drug tolerance, dependence, and withdrawal.

Monteggia and Nestler (2003) reported that the chronic use of opiates that leads to up-regulation of the cAMP pathway and increases tolerance also makes an animal less sensitive to natural rewards. This decreased state of sensitivity likely contributes to the blunted and depressed emotional state characteristic of opiate withdrawal in humans and often leads to relapse, they suggested. According to Koenig and Edwardson (1997), desensitization is partially explained by the uncoupling of receptors from the cell membrane due to a series of intracellular changes and altered gene expression. Several studies also suggest that chronic opiate abuse leads to a reduction in the synthesis of receptors and hence decreases the total number of binding sites. Structural changes have also been documented after chronic drug abuse.

Structural Changes

Several studies have found structural changes in neurons with chronic use of drugs, such as smaller dendrites and cell bodies of dopaminergic neurons (Sklair-Tavron et al., 1996), cell membrane damage, alterations in brain metabolism (Sharma et al., 2003), reduced synaptic plasticity of hippocampal neurons (Pu et al., 2002), and genetic alterations associated with neuronal death (Fan, Zhang, Zhang, & Ma, 2003). A study by Sklair-Tavron and colleagues (1996) found chronic opiate (morphine) use resulted in a 25% reduction of dopamine neurons located in the ventral tegmental area (VTA) of mice but did not alter the size of other types of neurons in this area. This study suggests that structural changes may occur specifically in dopamine neurons of the VTA, and it is likely that these changes affect functioning of the mesolimbic system. Postmortem brain studies of humans with a history of substance abuse have also found evidence of functional and structural changes relating to brain metabolism, synaptic function and plasticity, and intracellular cytoskeleton abnormalities (Lehrmann et al., 2003). Garcia-Sevilla and colleagues (1997) found a significant decrease in the amount of neurofilament proteins in the postmortem brains of chronic opiate addicts. Neurofilament proteins are the major components of the neuronal cytoskelton and are important in maintaining the structure of the cell and the transport of substances from the soma to the terminal button. Robinson, Gorny, Mitton, and Kolb (2001) also found structural changes in neurons located in the prefrontal cortex of rats that self-administered cocaine. Specifically, they reported that the dendrites of cells were misshapen, with large, bulbous structures at their tips. The authors speculated that these morphological changes may effect the compromised decision making and judgment typical of cocaine abusers.

With respect to alcohol, Pfefferbaum and Sullivan (2002) reported that a significant loss of cerebral white matter was found postmortem in individuals who had suffered from alcoholism. Fein et al. (2002) measured total brain volume and cortical gray and white matter volumes in alcohol-dependent males who had not received treatment. Relative to control subjects, those with alcohol dependency showed reduced total brain volume and reduced prefrontal and parietal cortical gray matter based on MRI scans. Harper, Dixon, Sheedy, and Garrick (2003) recently reported that the reduced brain volume often found in postmortem samples of humans who were alcohol-dependent is largely accounted for by loss of white matter. White matter loss has also been found in the cerebral cortex, hypothalamus, and cerebellum of alcoholics relative to control subjects (Harper, Dixon, Sheedy & Garrick, 2003). But, when Schweinsburg et al. (2001)

used magnetic resonance spectroscopy (MRS) to measure concentrations of neurotransmitter metabolites in several regions of the brain in recently detoxified alcoholics, results showed lower levels (14.7%) of metabolites in the frontal regions and, surprisingly, *higher* levels of white matter (11.8%) than in healthy controls. The authors speculated that the lower levels of metabolites in the frontal regions reflected neuronal loss or damage and the higher levels of white matter proliferation of glial cells in response to neuronal changes. De Bellis and colleagues (2001) measured hippocampal volumes in adolescents with alcohol use disorders compared to control subjects and found that those who abused alcohol had significantly smaller hippocamal volumes, which correlated with age of onset and duration of alcohol use.

Brooks (2000) proposed that chronic alcohol abuse leads to intracellular changes that damage DNA; consequently, gene expression is inhibited followed by neuronal death. Bjork, Grant, and Hommer (2003) recently investigated whether differences in alcohol consumption history and comorbid cocaine use were related to differential patterns of brain atrophy. The researchers used MRI to compared whole-brain gray and white matter images in 134 male subjects ages 30–50 who were exclusively alcohol-dependent or abused alcohol and cocaine. Results indicated that level of brain atrophy was associated with individual differences in exposure to alcohol and that cocaine use may exacerbate white matter loss. Netrakom, Krasuski, Miller, and O'Tuama (1999) reported that the frontal lobes and limbic structures are particularly vulnerable to the effects of alcohol, but that with continued abstinence, brain metabolism and brain size can improve to near-normal levels. Recently, Wang et al. (2004) used PET to measure brain glucose metabolism in two groups: methamphetamine abusers who were abstinent for 6 months and for a longer period of 12–17 months. Results indicated that significantly greater metabolism was found in the thalamus following protracted abstinence, finding that was associated with improvement in cognitive tasks. Compared to control subjects, however, cocaine-dependent individuals showed persistent lower levels of metabolism in the striatum, which the authors suggested may reflect long-lasting changes in the dopaminergic system. Thus, while structural improvement may occur in some regions of the brain following detoxification and abstinence, other drug-induced changes may persist. These long-lasting structural and neurochemical changes are likely related to the high relapse rate associated with addictive drugs. In other words, structural changes may persist over time and individuals return to drug use despite detoxification and dire consequences of their drug use behavior.

Neuroimaging studies have also found brain functioning differences in individuals with alcohol dependence relative to control subjects. For example, Desmond et al. (2003) used fMRI and found that although subjects with alcoholism performed similarly to controls on a verbal working memory task, they exhibited greater activation in regions of the cerebellum. These findings suggest individuals with alcoholism may require greater cellular activation to maintain the same level of performance as those without alcoholism. Using fMRI, Pfefferbaum and colleagues (2001) also found that individuals who were alcohol-dependent demonstrated different patterns of brain activation while performing a verbal memory task relative to controls. Their behavioral performance was similar. The researchers speculated that chronic exposure to alcoholism may result in functional reorganization of brain systems in an effort to compensate for the effects of chronic alcohol abuse. Hietala et al. (1994), Volkow et al. (2002), and Tupala et al. (2003a) employed PET to study dopamine receptor availability (D2) in individuals with and without alcoholism. Results from all three studies indicated that alcoholics had lower D2 receptor levels in the striatum (caudate and putamen) relative to controls. Furthermore, Volkow et al. reported that this level remained unchanged even after a significant period of detoxification and recovery. The authors suggested that low D2 receptor levels in alcoholics are not due to abuse or withdrawal but instead may be a predisposing factor for the development of alcoholism.

In an earlier PET study, Volkow and colleagues (1996) found decreased D2 receptors in individuals with alcoholism relative to controls but no differences in dopamine transporter levels. Recently, Tupala and colleagues (2003b) investigated the effects of age on dopamine transporters in the striatum of individuals who were alcohol-dependent and control subjects. Postmortem findings indicated that the mean densities of the dopamine transporter declined with age in control subjects but not in a subgroup of alcoholic individuals with late-onset alcoholism (Type 1 alcoholism). The researchers suggested the results may reflect a preexisting dopamine deficit in individuals with alcoholism. Tiihonen et al. (1995) reported that dopamine transporter density was lower in alcoholics who were nonviolent relative to control subjects, while dopamine transporter levels were significantly higher in alcoholics with a history of violence compared to controls. In a later study, Tiihonen et al. (1998) measured dopamine reuptake in individuals with late-onset alcoholism relative to control subjects. Based on PET findings, the striatal uptake values were significantly higher in those with alcoholism. In addition, higher rates of dopamine reuptake were associated with poorer performance on a behavioral task (Wisconsin Card Sorting Test). The researchers speculated that higher rates of reuptake may compensate for reduced levels of postsynaptic dopamine receptors. Collectively, these studies implicate the D2 receptor in the pathophysiology of alcoholism. Recently, Davies et al. (2003) identified the gene (SLO-1) that controls cellular potassium channels responsible for the acute intoxicating effects of alcohol (ethanol) in worms. Specifically, the researchers established that gene variants of the SLO-1 gene cause worms to be resistant to the intoxicating effects of ethanol, but if the potassium channels regulated by the SLO-1 gene are caused to artificially open (without alcohol), worms behave as if they are intoxicated. Although not yet applicable to humans, these results may one day help researchers to develop medications or other interventions to successfully treat alcohol addiction.

Heritability Studies

Genetic factors that influence the metabolism, sensitivity, and effects of drugs play a role in the risk of addiction but are not deterministic, as environmental factors also contribute to addiction (Crabbe, 2002). Jacob et al. (2001) noted that the addiction literature has primarily focused on either genetic or psychosocial approaches, but not both. They offered an integrative approach to studying the etiology of addiction and emphasized the importance of twin and family studies. In 1996, Tsuang and colleagues studied 3,372 twin pairs and found that 10.1% of the sample had been addicted to at least one illicit drug. The concordance rate for monozygotic twins was 26.2% as compared to 16.5% of dizygotic twins, supporting a genetic influence in addiction. The heritability estimates for specific drugs were .33 for marijuana, .43 for opiates, .44 for stimulants, and .34 for general drug use. More recently, Fu and colleagues (2002) interviewed 3,360 pairs of twins and reported that the heritability estimate for alcohol dependence was .56 and .50 for marijuana dependence. Furthermore, they found that the heritability estimate for antisocial personality disorder was .69 and that presence of the disorder increased the risk of substance dependence. Xian et al. (2003) studied the heritability of failed smoking cessation in twins and reported that genetic influences accounted for 54% of the variance in risk for failed smoking cessation. Recently, Kendler, Jacobson, Prescott, and Neale (2003) investigated illicit substance use and misuse in male twin pairs and reported that genetic factors had a strong influence on risk for illicit drug use. A high degree of comorbidity occurred across the six illicit substance classes investigated in the study (cannabis, cocaine, hallucinogens, sedatives, stimulants, and opiates).

With respect to alcohol dependence, according to the DSM IV-TR (2000), 40 to 60% of the variance of risk of alcoholism is explained by genetic influences, and this applies to both males and females (Enoch & Goldman, 2001). Jacob and colleagues (2003) found that offspring of monozygotic and dizygotic twins with a history of alcoholism were significantly more likely to exhibit alcohol abuse or dependence than offspring of nonalcoholic fathers. In addition, offspring of an alcohol-abusing monozygotic twin whose twin was also alcohol-dependent were more likely to develop alcoholism than offspring of nonalcoholic twins. The authors interpreted the findings as evidence that environmental factors contribute to alcohol dependence and that a low-risk environment can help to offset high genetic risk for alcohol dependence. Collectively, findings from twin studies indicate that genetic factors contribute to the development of addiction, although their interplay with environmental factors is not well understood. It is plausible that individuals with a genetic history in combination with certain personality traits may be more likely to take drugs or drink alcohol. It is also plausible that genetic factors alter the brain's sensitivity to drugs and alcohol, making an individual more prone to addiction. Cloninger (1999) proposed that personality characteristics such as novelty seeking and impulsivity are associated with early-onset substance abuse and recommended more studies to clarify the nonlinear interactions among genetic and environmental risk factors that contribute to substance dependency.

Genetic, Neurotransmitter, and Neuroimaging Studies

Alcohol

Although scientists have identified genes that are *linked* to alcoholism and other addictions, a specific gene or genes responsible for substance dependence has not been found. Most genetic research concerning addiction has been conducted with alcohol. Approaches have included altering susceptible genes in other animals (i.e., "knockout mice"), mapping human genes and identifying gene variants correlated with alcohol dependence, and locating reliable chromosomal markers. In terms of specific chromosomal regions that may contain genes associated with increased risk of alcohol dependence, research suggests that chromosomes 1, 2, 3, and 7 may all be implicated in alcoholism but the findings are inconclusive (Foroud et al., 2000). A large number of genes have been identified as candidate genes for alcoholism and most have been studied in other animals. In many studies, different genes have been identified for the rewarding, craving, and withdrawal effects of alcohol. Cunningham and Phillips (2003) summarized the genetic–animal research concerning the rewarding effects of alcohol and organized the studies in terms of the neurobiological systems affected by genetic manipulation methods: serotonin, dopamine, opioid, GABA, protein kinase pathways, neuropeptide Y, and additional systems. Within these systems, multiple genes have been studied. A robust finding is that genetically bred mice that do not have the mu-opioid receptor (i.e., opioid receptor knockout mice) do not self-administer alcohol, which indicates that this receptor—and the gene that regulates it—play an important role in the rewarding effects of alcohol (Roberts et al., 2000). Bencherif et al. (2004) recently used PET to measure degree of mu receptor binding in men who were undergoing alcohol withdrawal and control subjects. Subjects were administered a tracer that attaches to mu receptors and asked to report their level of craving, withdrawal symptoms, and mood. Results indicated that alcoholics showed lower levels of mu receptor binding in several brain regions (right frontal, parietal, and dorsal lateral precortex), which was correlated with higher craving and depressive symptoms. Although the mu receptor appears to play a critical role in alcohol dependence, studies have also supported the role of dopamine, opioid, serotonin, and other systems in the rewarding effects of alcohol. For example, dopamine receptor antagonists and opioid receptor antagonists injected in the nucleus accumbens reduce animal responding and drinking of alcohol (Hodge, Samson, & Chappelle,

1997; Krystal, Cramer, Krol, Kirk, & Rosenheck, 2001). As Cunningham and Phillips (2003) suggested, alcoholism is likely influenced by "a relatively large number of genes acting through several different biological systems" (p. 282). Recently, Heinz et al. (2004) used fMRI and PET to compare dopamine receptor binding in the striatum of detoxified male alcoholics and healthy men during the presentation of alcohol cues. Results indicated that males with a history of alcoholism had fewer dopamine receptors in the striatum, which significantly correlated with alcohol craving severity.

Spanagel (2003) examined animal studies that have attempted to identify the molecular basis of alcohol craving and relapse, and concluded that different molecular mechanisms can induce craving and lead to relapse. Similar to the reinforcing properties of alcohol use, numerous neurotransmitter systems have been implicated in craving and relapse. These systems include the dopamine, glutamate, GABA, and opioid systems as well as the endocrine system. In general, research suggests that chronic alcohol intake leads to changes in the glutamate and corticotropin-releasing hormone (CRH) systems. During withdrawal, these systems become overactivated, leading to a state of autonomic dysregulation that is manifested as anxiety and craving (Tsai & Coyle, 1998). Quertemont and colleagues (1998) discovered that following exposure to alcohol-conditioned stimuli, animals had an increase in extracellular glutamate in the area of the amygdala. Spanagel (2003) suggested that alcohol increases GABA release, which in turn inhibits the release of glutamate. Over time, glutamate receptors likely change in function. Glutamate acts on two types of post-synaptic receptors: N-methyl-D-aspartate (NMDA) and alpha-amino-3-hydroxy-5methylisoazole-4-proprionic acid (AMPA). As Spanagel reported, the structure and functioning of the NMDA receptor changes during chronic alcohol consumption and these changes persist over time. These changes and increased sensitivity of the NMDA receptor are thought to relate to the hyperexcitability of glutamate-releasing neurons during withdrawal. Researchers have just begun to study the potential role of the AMPA receptor in alcoholism as well as the interactive effects of other neurotransmitter receptors. For example, one hypothesis is that the cannabinoid receptor may influence the functioning of the GABA receptor (the receptor to which alcohol attaches). Preuss, Koller, Zill, Bondy, and Soyka (2003) explored whether a polymorphism of the cannabionoid receptor gene was associated with alcohol dependence but did not find evidence of such an association.

Fewer human studies have been conducted, but overall the results support a genetic involvement in alcohol dependence. Recently, Noble (2003) conducted a meta-analyis of studies investigating the Dopamine2 receptor gene and reported that variants of the gene occur more frequently in Caucasians with a variety of addictive disorders including alcoholism and cocaine, nicotine, and opioid dependence. Lappalainen and colleagues (2002) explored whether a variation within the neuropeptide Y gene (Pro7 allele) was associated with increased alcohol consumption in alcohol-dependent individuals compared to those without the addiction. Results indicated that the frequency of the Pro7 allele was significantly higher in the alcohol-dependent subjects than controls, leading the authors to conclude that the NPY Pro7 allele is a risk factor for alcohol dependence. Soyka and colleagues (2004) recently reported that a lower frequency of a different allele associated with serotonin receptors, the 5HT1B 861C allele, was found in subjects with alcohol dependence and antisocial personality traits relative to controls. Further implicating the serotonergic system in alcohol dependency was a study by Johnson et al. (2000), who found that a serotonin receptor (5-HT3) antagonist (ondansetron) reduced the desire to drink and hence alcohol consumptom. Alternatively, Dick et al. (2004) suggested that a predisposition to alcohol dependence may be due to an inherited disinhibition of the central nervous system as a result of alterations of the GABA receptor. Specifically, they explored whether a relationship existed between alcohol dependence and three GABA receptor genes located on chromosome 15q. Results were significant for one of the genes (GABRG3), and the authors concluded that GABRG3 may be involved in the risk for alcohol dependence. Kumar and colleagues (2003) reported that chronic alcohol consumption alters the structure of a particular subunit (alpha4) of the GABA receptor that in turn may alter functioning of GABA neurons. Recently, Petrakis et al. (2004) found that healthy subjects with a family history of alcohol dependence showed an attenuated response to Ketamine, an NMDA receptor antagonist, compared to healthy subjects without such family history. The authors suggested that an alteration in the NMDA receptor may contribute to a differential response to alcohol and therefore increase the risk of developing alcoholism.

Not only may genes be involved in increasing risk of alcoholism, but they may also help to prevent individuals from developing alcoholism. Chen et al. (1999) identified a polymorphism in a gene (ALDH) that metabolizes alcohol and discovered that the presence of this variant allele leads to an accumulation of the metabolite acetaldehyde. When carriers of this gene drink alcohol, the buildup of acetaldehyde causes unpleasant effects such as nausea, dizziness, and skin flushing, and therefore the likelihood of using alcohol is greatly diminished. Yu, Li, Chen, and Yue (2002) discovered additional gene variants that play a protective role against alcoholism—ADH2*2, ADH3*1, and ALDH2*2—as well as two that appear to increase the susceptibility for liver disease attributed to alcohol (ADH2*2 and ALDH2X2).

Opioids

Opium extracted from poppy seeds is a highly effective but addictive pain reliever. Opioids include endogenous opioids (enkephalins and endorphins), morphine, and synthetic opioids such as heroin, Darvon (propoxyphene), Demerol (meperidine), Talwin (pentazocine), Dilaudid (hydromorphone), Oxycontin (oxycodone), and Vicodin (hydrocodone). Oxycodone has become one of the most frequently prescribed opioids in the United States (Davis et al., 2003). Miller and Greenfeld (2004) recently described the substantial increase and problematic use of hydrocodone and oxycodone, especially in the addiction treatment population. In a sample of 534 detoxification patients, 27% were addicted to prescription opiate medications. Most of the patients (53%) were dependent on hydrocone and 19% were addicted to oxycodone (medications were prescribed by physicians in 75% of the cases). Research indicates that there are large individual differences in clinical response to opiates and not everyone who uses opiates becomes addicted (Lotsch et al., 2002).

The endogenous opioid system consists of several complex pathways that are distributed throughout the central nervous system. Opioids occupy and activate opioid receptors (mu, delta, kappa) that in turn stimulate a number of interacting neurotransmitter pathways including the mesolimbic pathway (Inturrisi, 2002). As with all drugs prone to abuse, the mesolimbic pathway plays a critical role in the rewarding effects of opioids. Most genetic research concerning opioid addiction has been conducted with other animals (i.e., "knockout mice"). For example, three opioid receptor genes have been studied including the MOR gene that regulates the mu receptor; DOR, which regulates the delta receptor; and the KOR gene that regulates the kappa receptor. Collectively, studies with mice unequivocally demonstrate that the mu receptor is necessary for the rewarding and addicitive effects of opioids (morphine). Kieffer and Simonin (2003) referred to the mu receptor as the "molecular gate for opioid addiction" (p. 12). With regards to humans, several studies have implicated a variation (S268P) in the mu-opioid receptor gene (hMOR) with alterations in receptor density and signaling (e.g., Befort et al., 2001; Koch et al., 2000). Other studies have not found evidence of mu receptor gene variants in humans with and without opioid addiction (e.g., Compton, Geschwind, & Alarcon, 2003). Meana and colleagues (2000), however, did not find evidence that the mu-opioid receptor functioned differently in postmortem brains of opioid addicts compared to controls. This study did find a difference in the density of noradrenergic receptors that, according to the researchers could represent an adaptive response to the chronic presence of opiates. In general, however, according to Mayer and Hollt (2001), human studies have found only a weak association between variants of the mu receptor and opiate and alcohol addiction.

As mentioned previously, Bencherif et al. (2004) recently reported that alcoholics showed lower levels of mu receptor binding in several brain regions (right frontal, parietal, and dorsal lateral precortex) which was correlated with higher craving and depressive symptoms. In a similar study, Zubieta and colleagues (2000) measured mu receptor binding in three males addicted to heroin and found that during withdrawal, mu receptor binding increased compared to controls. Sell et al. (1999) used PET to measure the effects of heroin versus a video depicting an individual preparing and injecting heroin in ten male subjects who were inpatients at a detoxification hospital. Results revealed that both heroin and heroin-related visual cues activated similar midbrain regions rich in dopamine and opiate receptors (ventral tegmental area, mesolimbic system). Age and gender may have influenced the findings of these studies, however, as Zubieta, Dannals, and Frost (1999) also used PET and found that mu receptor binding increased with age in healthy individuals and that women had higher mu binding in cortical and subcortical areas. Recently, Daglish et al. (2003) used PET and autobiographical scripts to induce opiate craving to investigate brain regions activated in 12 subjects who were opiate-dependent but no longer using opiates. The study also compared patterns of brain activity with drug-related and nondrug-related stimuli. Results indicated that two distinct neural circuits were activated: anterior cingulate with drug-craving memories and the orbitofrontal cortex with opiate-craving states. In addition, drug-related stimuli activated similar brain regions as nondrug stimuli but to a significantly lesser degree. Daglish and colleagues suggested that craving and addiction are "normal" brain circuits but are activated to a greater degree in addicts. Collectively, these studies provide evidence that particular brain regions become more activated during drug use and that salient environmental cues also activate these same regions. These neuroimaging findings help to explain how cues can elicit cravings and conditioned emotional reactions that increase the risk of relapse (O'Brien, Childress, McLellan, & Ehrman, 1992).

The complexities of the opioid system are not fully understood, but homeostasis is thought to occur by interactions with other peptides and neurotransmitter systems (Berthele et al., 2003; Przewlocki & Przewlocka, 2001). Noble and Roques (2003) recently demonstrated that the opioid system is influenced by the peptide cholecystokinin (CCK), perhaps through regulatory loops. Hu and colleagues (2003) genetically altered mice to generate an overexpression of the GABA transporter I to investigate whether the GABA system and transporter were involved in the rewarding and withdrawal effects of the opioid morphine. Results revealed that the rewarding effects of morphine were significantly reduced in these genetically altered mice and that rewarding effects were increased with the administration of a GABA transporter I inhibitor. Because the dopaminergic system plays an integral role in rewarding effects of addictive drugs, dopamine receptors have also been a focus of etiologic studies of addiction, including opioid addiction. For example, Li et al. (1997) reported that two variants of a dopamine receptor gene (DRD4) occurred more frequently in 121 heroin-dependent subjects than control subjects. In a later study, however, Li et al. (2000) did not find a significant difference between subjects addicted to heroin and controls with respect to polymorphisms of the DRD4 gene. Recently, Li et al. (2002) investigated five candidate genes and specific polymorphisms for dopamine, serotonin, and GABA receptors (DRD2, DRD3, HTR2A, GABA(A), 5-HTT) to determine whether there was an association between these polymorphisms and heroin addiction. Based on their findings, the authors concluded that there is a possible association between the DRD2 gene and heroin addiction but that the remaining polymorphisms studied were not likely risk factors for opiate addiction.

Noble (2003) conducted a meta-analysis of studies investigating the D2 dopamine receptor gene and concluded that variants of the gene are associated with a number of addiction disorders including alcoholism and cocaine, nicotine, and opioid dependence. Compton, Geschwind, and Alarcon (2003) explored the role of the miro-opioid receptor gene (OPRM) in opioid addiction in 50 opioid addicts in methadone treatment and normal controls and hypothesized that a polymorphism (C17T) would be present in the addicts relative to the control group. Results failed to support the hypothesis as the polymorphism was found in only 3 (two addicts, one control) of the 109 subjects. The authors concluded that the role of the opioid receptor in opioid reward response remain uncertain.

Detoxification and Pharmacological Interventions

Chronic use of opiates results in cellular adaptation. As the opiate receptors become less sensitive to the drug, tolerance occurs, followed by withdrawal symptoms. Withdrawal symptoms are usually severe (e.g., nausea, vomiting, chills, insomnia, depression), can last several weeks, and are among the most distressing and hence highly problematic to successful detoxification treatment. Detoxification options include abrupt cessation of the opiate ("cold turkey"), tapering with other drugs used to minimize withdrawal symptoms, pharmacological substitution (e.g., methadone), or a procedure known as rapid detox (McCabe, 2000). Rapid detox is reportedly gaining in popularity and involves treating the opioid addiction at the level of the opioid receptor. Specifically, rapid detox requires hospitialization and the administration of general anesthesia. An opioid antagonist (e.g., naltrexone, naloxone) administered to the patient removes opiates that are attached to opioid receptors and then occupies the receptors. Rapid detox programs vary with respect to length of hospital stay, safety, cost, pre-evaluation measures, follow-up interventions, and the actual detox procedure. According to McCabe (2000), the detox procedure typically lasts from 4 to 6 hours and after the procedure, patients are technically detoxified from the opiate. To reduce cravings and the likelihood of relapse, an opiate antagonist is prescribed for several weeks to a year post-detox. Although rapid detox is a method to avoid the distressing effects of withdrawal, it is an invasive procedure with all the attendant risks associated with general anesthesia. In addition, rapid detox is a medical procedure and follow-up treatment is needed to address the psychological aspects of addiction (Brewer, Catalano, Haggerty, Gainey, & Fleming, 1998). Unfortunately, there is currently no standard for follow-up care and patients can not be forced to receive appropriate treatment. Perhaps most disconcerting is the limited research concerning the long-term safety and efficacy of rapid detox relative to other treatment methods for opioid addiction (McCabe, 2000). Rabinowitz, Cohen, and Atias (2002) recently compared the relapse rates of 30 opiate-dependent individuals who underwent rapid detox and a 9-month follow-up course of naltrexone and a similar group of opiate-dependent individuals who detoxified in a 30-day inpatient program and did not receive naltrexone. Result indicated that 34% of the subjects overall relapsed within 13 months of detox and there was no significant difference in relapse rates between the two groups. Clearly, more research is needed to understand the benefits and limitations of rapid detoxification.

Researchers are actively seeking to develop other pharmacological treatments for opioid addiction. For example, studies have recently begun to explore whether inhibitors of enzymes that break down naturally occurring opioids (enkephalins) in the brain are useful in decreasing craving and relapse. In addition to modulating pain, enkephalins are believed to help regulate the dopaminergic system, particularly within the mesolimbic pathways. Preliminary studies have found that enkephalin-degrading-enzyme inhibitors reduce the severity of withdrawal symptoms in rats and produce antidepressantlike effects (Noble et al., 1994; Baamonde et al., 1992). In October 2002, the FDA approved an opioid agonist, buprenorphine, for the treatment of opioid dependence and preliminary studies support its effectiveness in reducing opiate craving and use. For example, Greenwald et al. (2002) studied whether high versus low doses of buprenorphine influenced opiate craving and use and reported that high-dose buprenorphine was associated with opioid drug seeking and craving. Jaffe and O'Keeffe (2003) noted, however, that although buprenorphine is likely to assist in the treatment process, it has reinforcing properties and therefore the potential for abuse.

Stimulants

The most well-studied stimulants are cocaine and amphetamines. Although both drugs increase extracellular dopamine concentrations, cocaine does so by binding to the dopamine transporter and thereby inhibiting dopamine reuptake. Amphetamines cause a reversal of the transporter so that more dopamine is released into the extracellular fluid (White & Kalivas, 1998). Given that drugs that inhibit other types of neurotransmitter transporters such as serotonin (e.g. SSRIs) do not have reinforcing or addictive properties, the dopamine transporter and gene that governs the transporter have been a focus of research. For example, Giros and colleagues (1996) genetically altered mice so that the dopamine transporter was deleted. Results indicated that extracellular dopamine levels were dramatically elevated and dopamine remained in the cleft 100 times longer than in the control mice. Removal of the transporter has additional physiological effects, however, and the way in which the brain's compensatory mechanisms may alter dopaminergic functioning is poorly understood. Other transporter genes have been altered in mice including those that regulate serotonin or norepinephrine transporters (SERT, NET). According to Spielewoy and Giros (2003), removal of SERT and NET increases the reinforcing effects of cocaine and amphetamines, suggesting that both the serotonin and norepinephrine neurotransmitter systems are involved in dopaminergic and homeostasis functions. However, dopamine appears to be the primary neurotransmitter involved in the rewarding effects of addictive drugs.

Transporters within the cell have also been investigated with respect to their role in stimulant drug addiction. As discussed in chapter 2, neurotransmitters are packaged in vesicles contained in the presynaptic terminal button, and located on the membrane of the vesicle is the vesicular monoamine transporter (VMAT). The VMAT is comprised of proteins and uses a pump to collect neurotransmitters from the nearby cytoplasm. When mice have been genetically altered to remove the VMAT, neurotransmitter production remains normal and drugs maintain their reinforcing properties, but dopamine release is also severely compromised (Jones et al., 1998; Takahashi et al., 1997). Spielewoy and Giros (2003) reviewed the literature concerning a variety of dopamine receptors and genes that regulate these receptors in knockout mice. In general, research suggests that various dopamine receptors may be differentially involved in stimulant addiction. Overall, genetic findings with other animals suggest that dopamine plays an integral role in stimulant addiction but the underlying mechanisms are complex and are likely mediated by other neurotransmitter systems.

In terms of intracellular functioning, McClung and Nestler (2003) studied the effects of cocaine on two intracellular transcription factors—delta FosB and CREB—in mice in an effort to understand how these factors regulate gene expression. Results indicated that after a short period of cocaine administration, genetic alteration was more influenced by CREB, while gene expression after a longer period of cocaine administration was dependent on delta FosB. Thus, short- and long-term exposure to cocaine appear to have differential effects on the intracellular functioning of neurons. The specific manner in which genetic expression is altered remains unclear. Walters, Kuo, and Blendy (2003) noted that CREB is expressed in many cells throughout the brain, but little information is available concerning the relative contributions of this protein in various brain regions. Walters and colleagues therefore explored CREB levels in two regions of the mesolimbic pathway: the nucleus accumbens and ventral tegmental (VTA) area. Findings indicated that the nucleus accumbens had higher CREB levels than the VTA. The authors suggested that these findings may help us to understand the complex cellular reactions to chronic exposure to addictive substances in humans.

Amphetamines and cocaine are known to activate dopaminergic receptors and, over time, induce intracellular changes that lead to gene expression. The mechanisms by which gene expression is altered have not been fully elucidated. Dudman et al. (2003) proposed that stimulation of dopamine receptors (D1) leads to an increase in intracellular cyclic AMP that in turn facilitates glutamate activity at the level of the NMDA receptor. In other words, gene regulation may result from an interaction of the dopamine and glutamate systems. Deroche-Gamonet and colleagues (2003) suggested that glucocorticoid hormones (i.e., stress hormones) modulate the propensity of an individual to abuse cocaine. Specifically, they genetically altered the glucocorticoid receptor gene and found that self-administered levels of cocaine were significantly reduced in mice, and that administration of a glucocorticoid receptor antagonist reduced the motivation to self-administer cocaine. The authors suggested that the glucocorticoid receptor can modulate cocaine addiction and could be helpful in the treatment of cocaine addiction in humans. Recently, Yao and colleagues (2004) suggested that genes that regulate the glutamate system and are important in learning and memory may contribute to the structural changes observed after chronic cocaine abuse. Specifically, the researchers found that deletion of the PSD-95 gene in mice resulted in enhanced sensitivity to cocaine that was chronically administered, particularly in the mesolimbic region.

Albertson et al. (2004) recently reported that chronic cocaine abuse affects gene expression and results in a reduction of myelin-associated proteins. Specifically, they reported that gene expression of cocaine- and amphetamine-regulated transcript (CART) was increased in the nucleus accumbens of cocaine abusers as well as a decrease in the expression of a number of myelin-related genes, including myelin basic protein (MBP), proteolipid protein (PLP), and myelin-associated oligodendrocyte basic protein (MOBP). In addition, the researchers found a decrease in the number of glial cells (oligodendrocytes) present in the nucleus accumbens and surrounding white matter of cocaine abusers. The authors interpreted these findings as evidence of a dysregulation of myelin in human cocaine abusers.

Similar to other drugs of abuse, magnetic resonance imaging and neuroimaging studies have suggested that cocaine dependence is associated with structural brain changes and decreased glucose metabolism and blood flow of the frontal lobes. For example, Matochik et al. (2003) compared MRI scans of cocaine abusers abstinent for 20 days and a control group in terms of gray and white matter tissue volumes. Results revealed that cocaine abusers had significantly lower gray matter tissue in several brain regions, particularly frontal areas, relative to controls. However, no differences were found with respect to white matter. Lim, Choi, Pomarad, Wolkin, and Rotrosen (2002) suggested that cocaine dependence alters the functioning of the connections between the frontal lobes and other brain regions, and speculated that this altered connectivity may underlie the decision-making deficits often observed in cocaine abusers. Adinoff and colleagues (2003) investigated cerebral blood flow in female cocaine addicts using SPECT. Compared to control subjects, females addicted to cocaine demonstrated a distinctly different pattern of response to the cocainelike substance procaine. Kilts, Gross, Ely, and Drexler (2004) compared the PET results of cocaine-dependent males and females and found that environmental cues produced less activation in several brain regions (e.g., orbitofrontal cortex, amygdala, cingulate cortex) in females. These findings suggest that sex differences may exist with respect to the effect of cocaine on brain metabolism and conditioned associations that may trigger cocaine use.

Ernst and colleagues (2000) used SPECT to investigate glucose metabolism in cocaine addicts and controls and reported widespread reductions in cerebral glucose metabolism in the brains of cocaine abusers even after a period of abstinence. Paulus et al. (2002) reported similar findings with methamphetamine-dependent individuals and noted significant prefrontal lobe dysfunction in those addicted to cocaine. Upon administration of cocaine, human PET studies have revealed that cocaine blocks the dopamine transporter and level of binding is associated with the pleasurable effects of cocaine. For example, Volkow et al. (1997) reported that at least 50% occupancy of the dopamine transporter was required to induce a "high," and Schlaepfer et al. (1997) corroborated these findings using PET. Laruelle et al. (1995) used SPECT to locate areas of dopamine release with amphetamine and, similar to cocaine, found increased levels of dopamine in the striatum. Leyton et al. (2002) used PET to measure dopamine release in the striatum of eight healthy men who were administered amphetamine and placebo. Results supported that extracellular dopamine levels increase in the striatum following administration of amphetamine, and furthermore, greater levels of dopamine release were strongly correlated with the personality trait of novelty seeking. Recently, Volkow et al. (2002) investigated the effects of methylphenidate on brain glucose metabolism in 25 cocaine abusers using PET. Results indicated that increases in metabolism were 50% greater when methylphenidate was expected than when it was unexpected, and these changes were most notable in the thalamus and the cerebellum. When methylphenidate was unexpected, however, significant increases in glucose metabolism were found in the left orbitofrontal cortex. The authors suggested that the reinforcing effects of drugs may be mediated by different brain regions.

In addition to dopamine receptors, opioid receptors are involved in cocaine addiction and craving. Zubieta et al. (1996), for example, found that mu receptor binding was increased in several brain regions of cocaine-dependent men 1 to 4 days after abstaining from cocaine use. Furthermore, binding level was positively correlated with the severity of cocaine craving, providing strong evidence that the opioid system is involved in cocaine craving in human subjects. Chen et al. (2002) reported that the endogenous opioid peptide, dynorphin, increases in the caudate and putamen after chronic abuse of cocaine and therefore hypothesized that a variant of the gene for dynorphin may contribute to a *decreased* vulnerability to develop cocaine dependence. Based on their findings with cocaine-dependent human subjects and controls, the researchers concluded that presence of the allelic variation was indeed associated with decreased cocaine dependence.

SUMMARY

Substance dependence is a major health problem in the United States and around the world and is characterized by tolerance, withdrawal, and dependence. Research with other animals, genetic studies, and, more recently, neuroimaging studies with humans implicate several brain regions and systems in addiction. Prominently involved in addiction is the dopaminergic system, including the mesolimbic system and associated ascending and descending pathways and connecting circuits to the frontal regions. In addition to dopamine, other neurotransmitter systems such as the endogenous opioid, GABA, serotonin, and glutamate systems appear to play a modulating role in addiction although the mechanisms are poorly understood. Research has begun to unravel the structural and cellular changes that occur in response to chronic drug use, and intracellular transcription factors such as CREB and delta FosB appear to play an integral role in altering gene expression that ultimately may underlie the many facets of drug addiction. Heritability studies clearly implicate genetic and environmental factors in the risk of addiction, but the particular genes involved in addiction as well as the complex relationship between biological and environmental factors in the development and maintenance of addiction are poorly understood.

EATING DISORDERS

Prevalence and Background Information

According to the DSM IV-TR (2000), two specific eating disorders are anorexia nervosa and bulimia nervosa. *Anorexia* is characterized by refusal to maintain normal body weight, whereas *bulimia* is characterized by recurrent episodes of binge eating followed by inappropriate compensatory behavior in an effort to avoid weight gain. Both disorders are characterized by perceptual distortions with respect to body shape and weight (see Tables 8.2 and 8.3). Anorexia and bulimia occur more frequently in females than males (90% of cases). The onset of anorexia is usually during mid- to late adolescence, bulimia during adolescence or young adulthood (APA, 2000). Hoek and Van Hoeken (2003) recently conducted a review of the prevalence of eating disorders and reported that the average rate of anorexia for young females was .3% while the prevalence rates for bulimia were 1% for young women and .1% for young men. The incidence of anorexia was reported as 8 cases per 100,000 per year and 12 cases per 100,000 population per year for bulimia. The DSM IV-TR describes the lifetime prevalence of anorexia nervosa and bulimia nervosa are approximately .5% and 1–3%, respectively. Recovery rates vary, although bulimia is often associated with a better prognosis, especially if anorexia begins prior to adolescence. Herzog et al. (1999) conducted a prospective longitudinal study of 246 women who had a history of anorexia or bulimia and found 74% of women with bulimia reached full recovery compared to only 33% of those with anorexia. Results also indicated, however, that nearly 33% of both groups relapsed after full recovery.

Eating disorders commonly co-occur with anxiety and mood disorders such as obsessive compulsive disorder and depression (Vitousek & Manke, 1994; Rosenvinge, Matinussen, &

TABLE 8.2

Diagnostic Criteria for 307.1 Anorexia Nervosa (DSM IV-TR, 2000)

A. Refusal to maintain body weight at or above normal weight for age and height (e.g., weight loss leading to maintenance of body weight less than 85% of that expected; or failure to make expected weight gain during period of growth, leading to body weight less than 85% of that expected).

B. Intense fear of gaining weight or becoming fat, even though underweight.

C. Disturbance in the way in which one's body weight or shape is experienced, undue influence of body weight or shape on self-evaluation, or denial of the seriousness of the current low body weight.

D. In postmenarcheal females, amenorrhea, i.e., the absence of at least three consecutive menstrual cycles. (A woman is considered to have amenorrhea if her periods occur only following hormone, e.g., estrogen, administration.)

Specify type:

Restricting Type: during the current episode of Anorexia Nervosa, the person has not regularly engaged in binge-eating or purging behavior (i.e., self-induced vomiting or the misuse of laxatives, diuretics, or enemas)

Binge-Eating/ Purging Type: during the current episode of Anorexia Nervosa, the person has regularly engaged in binge-eating or purging behavior (i.e., self-induced vomiting or the misuse of laxatives, diuretics, or enemas)

TABLE 8.3

Diagnostic Criteria for 307.51 Bulimia Nervosa (DSM IV-TR, 2000)

A. Recurrent episodes of binge-eating. An episode of binge-eating is characterized by both of the following:
    (1) eating, in a discrete period of time (e.g., within any 2-hour period), an amount of food that is definitely larger than most people would eat during a similar period of time and under similar circumstances
    (2) a sense of lack of control over eating during the episode (e.g., a feeling that one cannot stop eating or control what or how much one is eating)
B. Recurrent inappropriate compensatory behavior in order to prevent weight gain, such as self-induced vomiting; misuse of laxatives, diuretics, enemas, or other medications; or excessive exercise.
C. The binge eating and inappropriate compensatory behaviors both occur, on average, at least twice a week for 3 months.
D. Self-evaluation is unduly influenced by body shape and weight.
E. The disturbance does not occur exclusively during episodes of Anorexia Nervosa.

Specify type:
   Purging Type: during the current episode of Bulimia Nervosa, the person has regularly engaged in self-induced vomiting or the misuse of laxatives, diuretics, or enemas
   Nonpurging Type: during the current episode of Bulimia Nervosa, the person has used other inappropriate compensatory behaviors, such as fasting or excessive exercise, but has not regularly engaged in self-induced vomiting or the misuse of laxatives, diuretics, or enemas.

Ostensen, 2000). Research also indicates that individuals suffering from bulimia and anorexia are at greater risk for substance use and dependency as well as personality disorders (Holderness, Brooks-Gunn, & Warren, 1994; O'Brien & Vincent, 2003). Halmi and colleagues (2000) studied a sample of 322 women with a history of anorexia and found that perfectionism was a robust discriminating characteristic of the disorder relative to control subjects. Recently, Stein et al. (2002) compared self-report ratings of women who were recovered from bulimia for longer than a year to women with no history of eating disorders. Results indicated that women with a history of bulimia had significantly higher ratings with respect to perfectionism, depression, anxiety, and body dissatisfaction. The researchers interpreted these findings as supporting persistent eating-related concerns and mood disturbances despite behavioral recovery from bulimia. Srinivasagam and colleagues (1995) also found that perfectionistic traits persisted in a group of women who recovered from anorexia, leading the authors to propose that these traits may actually contribute to the pathogenesis of the disorder.

Physiological and Anatomical Findings

According to the DSM IV-TR (2000), a number of physiological changes may accompany eating disorders such as fluid and electrolyte disturbances. Anemia, dehydration, elevated liver enzymes, low metabolic rate, and abnormal hormone levels are often characteristic of anorexia, and complications from vomiting such as esophageal tears, gastric rupture, and dental problems may accompany bulimia. Research also indicates that eating disorders can lead to structural brain changes. For example, Drevelengas and colleagues (2001) reported enlarged ventricles and sulci in females suffering from anorexia, although these changes were found to remit following recovery from the disorder. Katzman, Zipursky, Lambe, and Mikulis (1997) assessed cerebral gray and white matter volumes in adolescent females with anorexia (13 were low weight, 6 recovered, and controls) using MRI. Results revealed that white matter and ventricular cerebrospinal fluid volumes increased significantly on weight recovery from anorexia. However, the weight-recovered patients had significant gray matter volume deficits and elevated cerebrospinal fluid volumes compared with those of the age-matched controls. These results suggest that some structural brain changes that accompany anorexia (i.e., white matter reduction) are reversible while other changes (i.e., persistent gray matter volume deficits) may be irreversible in patients who have recovered weight after anorexia nervosa. Recently, Swayze et al. (2003) examined cerebral spinal fluid (CSF) levels as well as white and gray matter volumes in patients with anorexia relative to control subjects. Results revealed increased CSF levels in subjects with anorexia nervosa as well as reduced white matter volumes relative to control subjects, and after weight normalization, both white and gray matter volumes increased in subects with anorexia nervosa.

Krieg, Backmund, and Pirke (1987) reported patients suffering from bulimia often display enlarged external cerebrospinal fluid spaces based on cranial computed tomography (CT), regardless of whether or not they had a past history of anorexia nervosa. The authors noted that patients with bulimia are of near normal body weight and therefore the observed structural changes cannot be attributed to underweight, as is commonly assumed to be the case in anorexia. The results imply, therefore, that other factors may be contributing to the morphological brain alterations present in individual with eating disorders. Krieg, Lauer, and Pirke (1987) suggested that the structural changes observed in eating disorders are similar to the brain changes observed in individuals suffering from alcoholism and proposed that these similarities may help to elucidate the physiological basis of both disorders.

Stamatakis and Hetherington (2003) recently conducted a review of the neuroimaging studies on anorexia and bulimia. They concluded that anorexia nervosa is associated with enlargement of cerebral spinal fluid spaces which generally reduce as a function of weight gain, but that reduced serotonin receptor binding may be fundamental to the pathophysiology of the disorder as it is unaffected by long-term weight restoration. With respect to bulimia, structural studies provide evidence of brain atrophy that in the absence of significant weight loss may be related to chronic dietary restriction. In addition, functional investigations revealed reduced thalamic and hypothalamic serotonin transporter availability in bulimia which increases with longer illness duration. Several PET studies conducted with individuals with anorexia have revealed reduced global brain metabolism (Delvenne et al., 1996), significantly higher metabolism in the temporal cortex and caudate nucleus (Herholz et al., 1987), and reduced activity in the temporal lobe (Gordon et al., 1997). Recently, Tauscher et al. (2001) used PET to measure serotonin transporter availibility in females with bulimia nervosa. Relative to control subjects, results indicated reduced hypothalamic and thalamic serotonin transporter availability in individuals with bulimia, and the availability deficit was more pronounced with a longer duration of the illness. Thus, neuroimaging studies suggest that both anorexia and bulimia are associated with substantial structural and functional brain alterations (Barbarich, Kaye, & Jimerson, 2003).

Neurotransmitter Findings

There is no single etiologic theory of eating disorders. Current models focus on multidimensional causes including neurotransmitter, genetic, psychological, and social factors (Steiger, 2004). Neurotransmitter studies have focused primarily on the role of the serotonergic system in eating disorders. Research with other animals has discovered that elevated serotonin levels are associated with reduced eating behavior and significantly decreased levels with binge eating (Blundell, 1986). Studies have also found that prolonged caloric restriction results in a reduction in activity of the serotonin transporter (SERT) (Huether, Zhou, Schmidt, Wiltfang, & Ruther, 1997). As mentioned in chapter 2, the precursor to serotonin is tryptophan, which is found in food. Studies that have lowered tryptophan dietary intake have found that bulimia symptoms worsen in patients with bulimia and can trigger symptoms in individuals who are in recovery (Kaye et al., 2000; Smith, Fairburn, & Cowen, 1999). Women suffering from anorexia have also been found to have reduced levels of serotonin metabolites (Kaye, Ebert, Gwirtsman, & Weiss, 1984), abnormal hormonal (cortisol and prolactin) responses to serotonin agonists (Monteleone, Brambilla, Bortolototti, LaRocca, & Maj, 1998), lower monoamine oxidase activity, and disturbances of peptide systems (e.g., vasopressin, oxytocin) relative to women without a history of eating disorders (Barbarich, Kaye, & Jimerson, 2003). Neuropeptides are important in eating behavior as they help to regulate cortisol, thyroid and growth hormones, and gonadal hormones (Bailer & Kaye, 2003). Similar metabolite and peptide findings have been reported for women suffering from bulimia, as well as lower resting metabolic rates compared to control subjects (e.g., Jimerson, Lesem, Kaye, & Brewerton, 1992; Steiger et al., 2000; Obarzanek et al., 1991).

Jimerson et al. (1990) proposed that impairment in functionally distinct serotonin pathways may result in impulsivity, binge eating, and depression. It is important to note, however, that lower levels of serotonin metabolites in the cerebral spinal fluid and low serotonin blood platelet binding are not unique to eating disorders but have been associated as well with aggressive and impulsive behavior, suicide, and borderline personality disorder (Coccaro et al., 1998). Furthermore, elevated serotonin metabolites have been implicated in anxiety disorders including generalized anxiety disorder and obsessive compulsive disorder (Garvey, Noyes, Woodman, & Laukes, 1995). Steiger (2004) has proposed that bulimia may be driven by mood and impulse regulation problems while anorexia may be driven by compulsive, restrictive tendencies. Unfortunately, studies have not yielded serotonergic findings consistent with a simple "underactive serotonin system" for bulimia and "overactive serotonin system" for anorexia, and it is more likely that many neurotransmitter systems are involved in these disorders. Petty and colleagues (1996) argued that neurotransmitters such as dopamine, GABA, and norepinephrine modulate cognition, mood, and anxiety levels and that serotonin acts as a stabilizing agent to help maintain homeostasis. It is therefore likely that a complex interactive relationships exists between different neurotransmitter systems and that several transmitter systems are involved in eating disorders.

Individuals who have recovered from eating disorders have also been the focus of neurotransmitter research. Frank et al. (2002), for example, reported that women recovered from anorexia had elevated serotonin receptor binding and elevated serotonin metabolites in the cerebral spinal fluid. These finding suggest that women with anorexia may have an increased level of serotonin metabolism during the active periods of anorexia and that this dysregulation may persist to some degree following recovery. Steiger (2004) has proposed that anorexia may be characterized by an overactive serotonergic system and that this dysregulation may result in a compensatory down-regulation of serotonin receptors in certain brain regions (cingulated, temporal lobe, and sensorimotor cortical regions). Studies with women who have recovered from bulimia suggest that the serotonergic system may be compromised in these individuals as well. Kaye et al. (2001), for example, used PET and found lower levels of serotonin receptor binding in women recovered from bulimia relative to controls. In addition, similar to findings with individuals with anorexia, Kaye et al. (1998a) reported that women recovered from bulimia had significantly higher levels of cerebral spinal serotonin metabolites relative to women without eating disorders. Recently, however, Goethals et al. (2004) used PET to compare degree of serotonin binding in individuals with bulima and healthy subjects and found that the serotonin binding index did *not* differ between the groups. Bailer and Kaye (2003) recently reported that although problems with the serotonergic system may persist after behavioral recovery from eating disorders, many of the peptide and hormone alterations characteristic of eating disorders tend to normalize after recovery. Frank, Kaye, Altemus, and Greeno (2000), however, found that although oxytocin levels were normal in the cerebral spinal fluid of women recovered from anorexia and bulimia, the peptide vasopressin was elevated in both disorders and this elevation was associated with a lifetime history of major depression. Wolfe et al. (2000) reported that women who recovered from bulimia showed an elevation in blood levels of prolactin following treatment with a serotonin reuptake inhibitor relative to women who were currently suffering from bulimia and controls. Women with bulimia also showed an elevated prolactin level relative to women without the disorder. According to the researchers, these findings suggest that an alteration in serotonin regulation characterizes bulimia nervosa and that this alteration may persist in recovered individuals.

As Steiger (2004) stated, serotonin dysregulation is implicated in both anorexia and bulimia but the findings "lend themselves to ambiguous interpretation" (p. 23). Kaye, Gendall, and Strober (1998b) suggested that a disturbance of serotonin activity may create a predisposition for the expression of symptoms that are common to both anorexia and bulimia such as disordered eating and distortions in the perception of body weight and shape. Other neurotransmitter systems are also being investigated for a possible role in eating disorders. For example, Van der Stelt and Di Marzo (2003) recently noted that the endogenous cannabinoid system modulates glutamate release, which in turn modulates dopaminergic functioning in several regions including the mesolimbic system. They suggested that given the mesolimbic system's primary role in rewarding effects of many behaviors such as eating, dysfunction of the cannabinoid system can alter the normal functioning of the mesolimbic system and thereby affect eating behavior. Although this hypothesis seems logical, empirical studies are needed to better understand the role of the cannibinoid and other neurotransmitter systems in the development of eating disorders. Kaye, Frank, and McConaha (1999) reported that dopamine metabolites were significantly lower in women recovered from anorexia compared to women without eating disorders and women who were recovered from bulimia. The researchers suggested that perhaps a disturbance of the dopaminergic system is characteristic of anorexia but not bulimia. Clearly, more research is needed to better understand the role of various neurotransmitter systems in the pathogenesis of eating disorders.

Genetic Studies

A number of genes have been identified as candidate genes for eating disorders. Those most frequently studied regulate serotonin postsynaptic receptors and serotonin transporters (SERT). Gorwood, Klipman, and Foulon (2003) recently reviewed familial and twin studies and reported that the heritability estimate for anorexia is around 70%. With regard to specific molecular genetic studies, Di Bella and colleagues (2000) explored a gene variant for the SERT (5-HTTLPR) and concluded that presence of this variant resulted in a sevenfold increased risk for bulimia. Steiger (2004) reported that this same gene variant is associated with impulsivity and lower binding levels of a serotonin reuptake inhibitor in women suffering from bulimia. Lauzurica et al. (2003) and Sundaramurthy, Pieri, Gape, Markham, and Campbell (2000), however, also studied polymorphisms of the serotonin transporter gene and found no differences with respect to the frequency of these variants in women with anorexia, bulimia, or control subjects. Recently, Shioe and colleagues (2003) used PET to study serotonin receptor binding in subjects with variations of the serotonin transporter gene and concluded that these genetic variations do not contribute to the regulation of serotonin binding at the level of the transporter.

According to Branson and colleagues (2003), several genes are involved in regulating appetite and play a critical role in the production of hormones linked to eating behavior. A mutation (MC4R) on a gene (proopiomelanocortin gene) that regulates eating-related hormones was found in every obese subject they studied who engaged in binge-eating behavior, while none of the nonbinging control subjects carried this mutation. The authors concluded that binge eating is a major phenotypic characteristic of subjects with the MC4R mutation and, therefore, warrants exploration in the etiology of bulimia. Clearly, additional studies are needed to further explore genetic polymorphisms and the risk for eating disorders. Strober and colleagues (2001) conducted one of the few studies to investigate anorexia and bulimia in first-degree relatives of males suffering from anorexia. Based on a study of 210 males with anorexia and 747 relatives, results indicated that the relative risk of anorexia was 20.3 among females but the risk of bulimia was exceedingly rare. The authors concluded that a pattern of familial aggregation exists for anorexia and that genetic factors do not appear to distinguish the occurrence of the disorder in males and females.

Steiger (2004) suggested that "environmental stressors (e.g., child abuse) might act upon genetic predispositions, whereas sequelae of dieting might activate genetic (or developmental) predispositions" (p. 26). In other words, it is possible that early childhood and adolescent experiences such as trauma and dieting or binge eating affect brain development in such a way that gene expression is altered and neurotransmitter systems are dysregulated. This dysregulation in combination with heritability and ongoing environmental stressors increase the likelihood that an individual will develop an eating disorder. Indeed, studies have found that women who were victims of childhood sexual abuse often developed binge-eating disorders and other forms of self-destructive behavior in adolescence and adulthood (e.g., Wonderlich et al., 2001). In a study by Steiger et al. (2001), childhood abuse was reported by 76% of women with bulimia compared to 52% of nonbulimic women. Jacobi et al. (2004) recently reported that in addition to sexual abuse, a number of other risk factors are also associated with eating disorders: gender, ethnicity, early childhood eating problems, elevated weight gain and shape concerns, negative self evaluation, and psychiatric problems. Results of the McKnight longitudinal study (2003) found that thin body preoccupation and social pressure predicted the onset of eating disorders in 1,103 adolescent girls. Taken together, these findings suggest that a number of genetic and environmental factors can increase the risk of eating disorders. The brain mechanisms underlying the development and progression of eating disorders are not well understood but appear to involve multiple neurotransmitter systems and structural brain changes.

Pharmacological Interventions

A variety of pharmacological treatments have been used to treat anorexia and bulimia. Their overall effectiveness further implicates neurotransmitter systems in the pathophysiology of eating disorders. For example, a large number of studies have used SSRIs in the treatment of bulimia and have found significant improvement in binge-eating frequency and decreased likelihood of relapse (e.g., Arnold et al., 2002; Romano et al., 2002; Walsh, Hadigan, Devlin, Gladis, & Roose, 1991). Studies have also reported improvement in the reduction of symptoms of obsessive compulsive symptoms and depression in patients with anorexia (Kim, 2003). According to Kaye, Gendall, and Strober (1998b), SSRIs are not useful when women with anorexia are malnourished and underweight. After weight restoration, however, SSRIs may significantly reduce the extremely high rate of relapse normally seen in anorexia. Sodersten, Bergh, and Ammar (2003) recently warned that SSRIs can have undesirable side effects, especially for those suffering from anorexia, such as decreased body temperature. Collectively, however, studies with SSRIs suggest that the serotonergic system is altered in individuals with anorexia and bulimia but the details of these alterations are not well understood.

Other types of medications have also been used to treat bulimia with some success. Hoopes et al. (2003), for example, reported that the antiseizure medication topiramate (topamax) significantly reduced the frequency of binging and purging in a double-blind, placebo-controlled study with women suffering from bulimia. Sibutramine (merida), a drug used to treat obesity that inhibits reuptake of several neurotransmitters (serotonin, dopamine, norepinephrine), has also been found to decrease binge eating and depressive symptoms and may be useful in the treatment of bulimia (Appolinario et al., 2003). Interestingly, the opiate antagonist naltrexone that is used to treat alcohol and opioid addiction and restless leg syndrome has also been found to improve symptoms of anorexia and bulimia (Marrazzi, Bacon, Kinzie, & Luby, 1995). Other opioid antagonists (e.g., ketamine) have not been found to improve symptoms in women suffering from chronic eating disorders (Mills, Park, Manara, & Merriman, 1998). Cassanno (2003) recently explored the effectiveness of low doses of haloperidol, a dopamine antagonist, and concluded that the drug may be used as an adjunctive treatment for patients with severe anorexia. Given the improvement in symptoms using a variety of medications that target different transmitter systems, these findings suggest that the pathophysiology of eating disorders is complex and not simply the result of aberrant serotonin functioning.

SUMMARY

The lifetime prevalence rates of anorexia nervosa and bulimia nervosa are approximately .5% and 1–3%, respectively. Eating disorders affect females more often than males, although the incidence of eating disorders in males appears to be rising. Genetic, neurotransmitter, and neuroimaging studies implicate neurontransmitter systems in the pathophysiology of eating disorders, with most studies focusing on the serotonergic system. Other neurotransmitter systems appear to play a modulating role in eating disorders, but the mechanisms are poorly understood. Heritability studies implicate genetic and environmental factors in the risk of eating disorders, especially anorexia. The particular genes involved in eating disorders have yet to be identified as do the complex interactions between genetic, psychological, and environmental factors that contribute to the development of eating disorders.

Disorders of Childhood Origin

This chapter focuses on three disorders commonly diagnosed in childhood: ADHD, Tourette's disorder, and autistic disorder. Research regarding genetic, anatomical, neurochemical, and neuroimaging findings are presented for each disorder as well as information on both pharmacological and nonpharmacological interventions. The chapter concludes with a brief review of the physiological findings concerning learning disabilities.

BACKGROUND INFORMATION

A substantial number of developmental disorders originate during childhood: feeding and eating disorders, elimination disorders, anxiety disorders, motor skills disorder, communication disorders, mental retardation, learning disorders, pervasive developmental disorders, tic disorders, and behavior disorders (DSM IV-TR, 2000). Children also experience adult-associated disorders such as major depression, bipolar disorder, and schizophrenia, but their prevalence is lower in children than adults. Furthermore, prevalence estimates of childhood disorders vary depending on diagnostic methods and procedures (e.g., number of informants) as well as sampling differences. Overall, however, studies indicate that a significant percentage of children and adolescents in the United States and throughout the world have clinical disorders that cause impairment in daily living. For example, Roberts (1998) reviewed 52 child and adolescent prevalence studies and reported psychopatholgy estimates of 8% for preschoolers, 12% for preadolescents, and 15% for adolescents. Similar results (15%) were reported for adolescents from Scotland (West et al., 2003), and Ford, Goodman, and Meltzer (2003) recently reported that 1 in 10 British children have at least one DSM-IV disorder that warrants treatment. A recent cross-cultural study involving seven countries (Australia, China, Israel, Jamaica, Netherlands, Turkey, and United States) found that gender differences were similar across the seven cultures, with girls reporting significantly higher ratings with respect to internalizing disorders (e.g., anxiety) and boys higher ratings with respect to externalizing disorders (e.g., behavior disorders) (Verhulst et al., 2003).

Research also indicates that psychotropic medication use in children and adolescents has increased dramatically in the last decade, with stimulants and antidepressants prescribed most frequently (Zito et al., 2003). For example, Delate et al. (2004) reported that 2.4% of children were prescribed antidepressants in 2002, and a 2004 annual report by Medco Health Solutions, Inc. indicated that 3.4% of children were prescribed medications specifically for ADHD. A review of each of the childhood disorders is obviously beyond the scope of this chapter, and instead the primary focus will be on three disorders that are commonly diagnosed in childhood— attention-deficit/hyperactivity disorder (ADHD), Tourette's disorder, and autistic disorder.

ATTENTION-DEFICIT/HYPERACTIVITY DISORDER (ADHD)

ADHD is characterized by a persistent pattern of inattention and/or hyperactivity and impulsivity that causes impairment in multiple settings such as school and work, and whose symptoms are atypical for the individual's level of development (see Table 9.1). According to current diagnostic criteria, there are three subtypes of ADHD: combined type, predominately inattentive type, and predominately hyperactive–impulsive type. ADHD is estimated to affect 3 to 7% of the school age population, with the majority continuing to display significant symptoms in adulthood (Barkley, Fischer, Smallish, & Fletcher, 2004). The disorder is diagnosed more frequently in males than females with a male to female ratio ranging from 2:1 to 9:1 depending on subtype and evaluation setting (DSM IV-TR, 2000). ADHD occurs in countries and cultures throughout the world although prevalence rates are sometimes higher or lower than the 3 to 7% reported for American schoolchildren (e.g., Andres, Catala, & Gomez-Beneyto, 1999; DuPaul et al., 2001; Luk, Leung, & Lee, 1988; Magnusson, Smari, Gretarsdottir, & Prandardottir, 1999). According to Rowland, Lesesne, and Abramowitz (2002), not only is ADHD the most common neurodevelopmental disorder of childhood, but it is also the most commonly studied.

Disorders such as conduct disorder, oppositional defiant disorder, Tourette's disorder, mood disorders, and learning disabilities often co-occur with ADHD. Developmentally, children and adolescents with ADHD are at greater risk for academic deficits, school-related problems, social skill deficits, and peer rejection (Fischer, Barkley, Edelbrock, & Smallish, 1990). Adolescents with ADHD are at greater risk for antisocial behavior and school dropout (Barkley, Fischer, Edelbrock, & Smallish, 1990), although a small percentage pursue a college education (Heiligenstein, Guenther, Levy, Savino, & Fulwiler, 1999). Preliminary studies suggest that college students with ADHD do not differ with respect to intelligence compared to control subjects (Weyandt, 2001; Weyandt, Mitzlaff, & Thomas, 2002), but are more likely to have a lower GPA and report greater difficulty paying attention in lectures compared to college students without ADHD (Healy, 2000). As young adults, individuals with ADHD are more likely to suffer from depression or a personality disorder compared to control subjects (Fischer, Barkley, Smallish, & Fletcher, 2002), and many experience problems with employment, sexual relationships, driving, and illegal activities (Barkley, 2002; Barkley, Fischer, Smallish, & Fletcher, 2004). Rasmussen, Almvik, and Levander (2001) reported that ADHD is common among Norwegian prison inmates. According to Wilens (2004), ADHD is a risk factor for substance abuse in adults, and individuals with ADHD tend to become addicted more rapidly and severely than individuals without the disorder. Kodl and Wakschlag (2004) recently reported that persistent cigarette smokers are more likely to have a history of ADHD than spontaneous quitters or nonsmokers. Cognitively, young adults with ADHD have reported greater degrees of internal restlessness compared to control subjects (Weyandt et al., 2003), and both children and adults with ADHD are more likely than control subjects to have executive function deficits (Weyandt, 2005). It is important to note, however, that executive function deficits are not unique to ADHD (Weyandt, 2005). Despite the popularized myth that it is advantageous to have ADHD, preliminary studies do not support that young adults with ADHD have superior

TABLE 9.1

Diagnostic Criteria for Attention-Deficit/Hyperactivity Disorder (DSM IV-TR, 2000)

A. Either (1) or (2):
   (1) six (or more) of the following symptoms of inattention have persisted for at least six months to a degree that is maladaptive and inconsistent with developmental level:

Inattention
   (a) often fails to give close attention to details or makes careless mistakes in schoolwork, work, or other activities
   (b) often has difficulty sustaining attention in tasks or play activities
   (c) often does not seem to listen when spoken to directly
   (d) often does not follow through on instructions and fails to finish schoolwork, chores, or duties in the workplace (not due to oppositional behavior or failure to understand instructions)
   (e) often has difficulty organizing tasks and activities
   (f) often avoids, dislikes, or is reluctant to engage in tasks that require sustained mental effort (such as schoolwork or homework)
   (g) often loses things necessary for tasks or activities (e.g., toys, school assignments, pencils, books, or tools)
   (h) is often easily distracted by extraneous stimuli
   (i) is often forgetful in daily activities
   (2) six (or more) of the following symptoms of hyperactivity–impulsivity have persisted for at least 6 months to a degree that is maladaptive and inconsistent with developmental level:

Hyperactivity
   (a) often fidgets with hands or feet or squirms in seat
   (b) often leaves seat in classroom or in other situations in which remaining seated is expected
   (c) often runs about or climbs excessively in situations in which it is inappropriate (in adolescents or adults, may be limited to subjective feelings of restlessness)
   (d) often has difficulty playing or engaging in leisure activities quietly
   (e) is often "on the go" or often acts as if "driven by a motor"
   (f) often talks excessively

Impulsivity
   (g) often blurts out answers before questions have been completed
   (h) often has difficulty awaiting turn
   (i) often interrupts or intrudes on others (e.g., butts into conversations or games)
B. Some hyperactive–impulsive or inattentive symptoms that caused impairment were present before age 7 years
C. Some impairment from the symptoms is present in two or more settings (e.g., at school [or work] and at home)
D. There must be clear evidence of clinically significant impairment in social, academic, or occupational functioning
E. The symptoms do not occur exclusively during the course of a Pervasive Developmental Disorder, Schizophrenia, or other Psychotic Disorder and are not better accounted for by another mental disorder (e.g., Mood Disorder, Anxiety Disorder, Dissociative Disorder, or a Personality Disorder)

Code based on type:

314.01 Attention-Deficit/Hyperactivity Disorder, Combined Type: if both Criteria A1 and A2 are met for the past 6 months

314.00 Attention-Deficit/Hyperactivity Disorder, Predominantly Inattentive Type: if Criterion A1 is met but Criterion A2 is not met for the past 6 months

314.01 Attention-Deficit/Hyperactivity Disorder, Predominantly Hyperactive–Impulsive Type: if Criterion A2 is met but Criterion A1 is not met for the past 6 months

Coding note: For individuals (especially adolescents and adults) who currently have symptoms that no longer meet full criteria, "In Partial Remission" should be specified.

divided attention skills relative to young adults without the disorder (Linterman & Weyandt, 2001). Collectively, these studies indicate that ADHD is a chronic disorder that causes impairment in social, occupational, and academic functioning, and as the following sections attest, neurobiological studies strongly support a physiological basis for ADHD.

Genetic Studies

Within the past few years, interest in the genetic underpinnings of ADHD has grown enormously (Kent, 2004). Familial studies clearly support a heritability component of ADHD as the disorder is more common in first- and second-degree relatives (Biederman et al., 1986, 1991; Roizen et al., 1996). For example, Frick and colleagues (1991) studied 177 boys with ADHD and found that their mothers, fathers, and biological relatives were significantly more likely than control families to have a history of ADHD. Biederman et al. (1995) reported that individuals with ADHD are more likely to have siblings with ADHD relative to control subjects; and if one biological parent had ADHD, the likelihood that a child had ADHD was 57%. In an earlier study, Morrison and Stewart (1973) found that 20% of children with ADHD had a parent with the disorder (diagnosed retrospectively) compared to control families. Similar results were reported by Cantwell (1972), and Safer (1973) reported that ADHD occurred more frequently among siblings who shared the same mother and father than those who shared only one parent (i.e., half brothers and sisters). Studies also indicate that adoptive relatives of children with ADHD are less likely to have ADHD than biological relatives of children with the disorder (e.g., Alberts-Corush, Firestone, & Goodman, 1986). Faraone et al. (1991) evaluated family–genetic risk factors for girls with ADHD and reported that their relatives had a higher risk for ADHD as well as other psychiatric disorders. The higher risk for ADHD was not accounted for by factors such as social class, family intactness, or generation of the relative. Several studies have suggested that ADHD consists of two main subtypes—combined and inattentive—and that these subtypes may be influenced by different genetic factors (Neuman et al., 1999; Rasmussen et al., 2004; Todd et al., 2002). A recent report from the Third International Meeting of ADHD Molecular Genetics Network (2002), however, indicated that although DSM-IV ADHD subtypes are useful in clinical practice, molecular genetic studies have not yet determined that the subtypes represent distinct genetic conditions.

Twin studies indicate that ADHD occurs significantly more often in identical than fraternal twins. For example, Gjone, Stevenson, and Sundet (1996) reported a correlation of .78 between adolescent male monozygotic twins and .45 for dizygotic twins with respect to attention problems. Goodman and Stevenson (1989), Gillis, Gilger, Pennington, and DeFries (1992), Sherman, Iacono, and McGue (1997), Stevenson (1992), and many others have reported similar findings although some studies have reported larger or smaller concordance rates among twins with ADHD (Smalley, 1997). More recently, Willcutt, Pennington, and DeFries (2000) studied 373 8-to- 18-year-old twin pairs and found that monozygotic twins were significantly more likely than dizygotic twins to meet diagnostic criteria for ADHD (78% and 38%, respectively). Twin studies also suggest that although girls tend to display fewer behavioral problems than boys, heritability estimates for ADHD are similar for both (Rietveld et al., 2003). Burt, Krueger, McGue, and Iacono (2001) studied 1,506 twins from the Minnesota Twin Family Study and concluded that ADHD is primarily influenced by genetic factors. Tully and colleagues (2004) studied 2,232 twins and suggested that maternal warmth may decrease the likelihood of ADHD in twins who were low-birth-weight infants. However, this was a retrospective study and was based on ADHD symptoms, not an ADHD diagnosis. Sharp et al. (2003) noted that twins discordant for ADHD are rare but, recently, Castellanos et al. (2003) compared MRI scans of monozygotic twins *discordant* for ADHD and found that the affected twins had significantly smaller caudate volumes than unaffected co-twins. Recently, Larsson, Larsson, and Lichtenstein (2004) conducted a longitudinal study of 1,480 twin pairs born in Sweden and concluded that ADHD symptoms remain highly stable over time and attributed this stability in symptoms to genetic effects. Overall, twin studies indicate that the heritability component of ADHD is approximately .80, which is substantially higher than many psychiatric illnesses (Faraone, 2000).

Candidate Genes

Collaborative efforts such as that led by the International ADHD Genetics Consortium (Asherson et al., 2000) are currently taking place to search for and study susceptibility genes related to ADHD. Several genes have been targeted within the dopaminergic system including DRD4, DRD5, and DAT1. For example, McCracken et al. (2000) studied a polymorphism of the DRD4 gene (120bp repeat) in 371 children with ADHD and their parents, and results supported a significant preferential transmission of the polymorphism in ADHD. Tahir et al. (2000) also found evidence of increased transmission of a variant of the DRD4 gene (7-repeat allele) in a sample of Turkish children with ADHD, and Roman et al. (2001) reported similar findings in a sample of Brazilian children. Kirley et al. (2003) studied a sample of Irish children with ADHD and found a relationship between a polymorphism of the DAT1 gene (10-repeat VNTR) and a positive response methylphenidate. The authors speculated that this polymorphism may lead to overactivity of dopamine transporters in children with ADHD and helps to explain the effectiveness of methylphenidate in treating ADHD. More recently, Arcos-Burgos et al. (2004) studied two polymorphisms of the DRD4 Gene (a 120 bp tandem duplication at the promoter and a 48 bp-VNTR at exon 3) in ADHD in multigenerational families from Columbia. Results supported an association of the gene variants with ADHD. Langley et al. (2004) found that children with ADHD who had a specific gene variant of the DRD4 gene (7-repeat allele) performed significantly more poorly on neuropsychological tasks than children with ADHD without the gene variant. The authors suggested that the 7-repeat allele variant may be associated with an inaccurate, impulsive response style in children with ADHD. Many other studies have also found a relationship between polymorphisms of the DRD4 gene and ADHD (e.g., Cook, 1999; LaHoste et al., 1996; Swanson et al., 1998; Rowe et al., 1998).

Neuroimaging studies have found that adults and children with ADHD have increased density of the dopamine transporter, particularly in the striatum (Cheon et al., 2003; Krause et al., 2003), and this finding is consistent with abnormalities of the dopamine system. In addition, stimulants such as methylphenidate commonly used to treat ADHD are known to directly affect (i.e., block) the dopamine transporter (Volkow, Fowler, Wang, Ding, & Gatley, 2002). As a result, variants of the dopamine transporter gene (DAT1) have been explored in ADHD. Waldman and colleagues (1998) studied children with ADHD as well as their siblings and parents and concluded that variants of the DAT1 gene were associated with ADHD, especially with ADHD combined type. Similar results linking polymorphisms of the DAT1 gene to ADHD have been reported by other studies (e.g., Barr et al., 2001; Daly, Hawi, Fitzgerald, & Gill, 1999; Gill, Daly, Heron, Hawi, & Fitzgerald, 1997; Muglia et al., 2000; Payton et al., 2001).

Additional dopaminergic genes have been studied with respect to ADHD. For example, Smith et al. (2003) recently reported an association between the beta hydroxylase gene and ADHD. Beta hydroxylase is an enzyme that breaks down dopamine after its use, and inherited variants in the DNA sequence of the gene may increase risk of developing ADHD. Kustanovich et al. (2003) and Lowe et al. (2004) found an association between the DRD5 gene and ADHD, and other studies have explored the role of polymorphisms of the SNAP25, COMT, and DBH genes and ADHD (Kirley et al., 2002; Mill et al., 2002; Roman et al., 2002). Turic and colleagues

(2004) explored whether gene variants of second messenger systems (i.e., G proteins) that are known to affect functioning of dopamine postsynaptic receptors were associated with ADHD, but their findings did not suggest that polymorphisms of these genes were related to ADHD. Thus, although findings have been inconsistent across some studies, the general consensus is that polymorphisms of dopamine genes appear to alter dopamine transmission and consequently neural networks and circuitry in individuals with ADHD (Castellanos et al., 1998; Swanson et al., 2000). Based on a meta-analysis of the association between polymorphisms of the DRD4 gene and ADHD, Faraone and colleagues (2001) concluded that there is truly a relationship between ADHD and polymorphism of the DRD4 gene but that future studies are needed to clarify this relationship.

In addition to dopamine genes, many other genes have been studied in ADHD as well. For example, in a recent review, Willcutt (2005) noted that dopamine, serotonin, adrenergic, MAO, COMT, and nicotonic receptor genes have all been investigated in ADHD. Roman et al. (2003) reported that variants of adrenergic genes (e.g., ADRA2) may increase susceptibility for ADHD or modulate the severity of the disorder, while Jiang et al. (2001) suggested there may be a linkage between MAO genes and ADHD. As discussed in chapter 2, MAO in an enzyme that helps to metabolize norepinephrine and dopamine. Catechol-O-methyltransferase (COMT) is another enzyme that breaks down dopamine and norepinephrine, and Eisenberg et al. (1999) reported an association between polymorphisms of the COMT gene and ADHD. However, Barr et al. (1999) failed to find a relationship between variants of the COMT gene and ADHD. Others have suggested that variants of the serotonin transporter gene are linked to increased susceptibility to ADHD (Kent et al., 2002; Retz et al., 2002). Comings (2001) described ADHD as a polygenetic disorder that is due to the additive effects of several genes (dopamine, norepinephrine, GABA, serotonin) but noted that adrenergic genes play the largest role. As Willcutt (2005) described, research indicates that ADHD is caused by the combination of many genetic (and environmental) risk factors, and it is likely that complex interactions among these risk factors contribute to its development.

Neuroanatomical and Neuroimaging Studies

MRI

Numerous MRI, fMRI, and PET studies have been conducted with children and adults with ADHD and many, but not all, have found structural and functional differences between patients with and without ADHD. For example, using MRI, Castellanos and colleagues (1994) found that total brain volume was 5% smaller in boys with ADHD relative to children without the disorder, and the caudate nucleus was significantly larger in children with ADHD. More recently, Castellanos et al. (2002) found smaller total brain volumes in 152 children and adolescents with ADHD relative to control subjects as well as smaller cerebral volumes, white matter volumes, and cerebellar volumes. Group differences were not found with respect to the caudate nucleus. Hynd and colleagues (1993), however, found that 63.6% of a sample of children with ADHD had an abnormal pattern of asymmetry of the head of the caudate nucleus, in that the right side was larger than the left (72.7% of control subjects had the opposite pattern of asymmetry). Similar reversed asymmetry of the caudate was reported by Filipek et al. (1997). Aylward et al. (1996) also compared MRI scans of children with and without ADHD and reported smaller volumes of globus pallidus in children with ADHD but no group differences with respect to the caudate nucleus or putamen. Max et al. (2002) reported that lesions within the putamen increased the risk of ADHD in children who sustained focal strokes.

The cerebellum has also been found to be smaller in children with ADHD (Berquin et al., 1998; Castellanos et al., 2001; Mostofsky et al., 1998). Several MRI studies have found smaller corpus callosum volumes in children with ADHD as well (e.g., Giedd et al., 1994; Hill et al., 2003; Hynd et al., 1991; Semrud-Clikeman et al., 1994). Overmeyer and colleagues (2000), however, compared corpus callosum volumes of children with ADHD and their unaffected siblings and did not find a size difference. Durston et al. (2004) also reported that subjects with ADHD and their unaffected siblings both had volume reductions in right prefrontal and left occipital regions but that the right cerebellar volume was significantly smaller in subjects with ADHD. These findings may support a biological vulnerability to ADHD but do not explain why some siblings develop ADHD and others do not. Some studies have reported reductions in the frontal and prefrontal regions in individuals with ADHD (e.g., Mostofsky et al., 2002; Sowell et al., 2003). Recently, Pueyo et al. (2003) found adolescents with ADHD had a higher degree of myelination in the right frontal region compared to control subjects and speculated that this finding may reflect the brain's compensatory response for right frontal–striatal dysfunction.

Collectively, anatomical studies support reductions in volume of several regions and structures of the brain with preferential involvement of the frontal, striatum, and cerebellar regions in individuals with ADHD. These size reductions have been associated with poor response inhibition and impaired neuropsychological performance in several studies, reinforcing a role for these structures and regions in modulating ADHD symptomology. All of these regions are rich in dopaminergic-releasing neurons as well as other neurotransmitters and neuromodulators. It is important to note, however, that although some MRI studies have found smaller volumes of some structures (e.g., corpus callosum), these same studies often do not find volume differences in other structures (e.g., cerebellum). Inconsistencies also exist across studies, with some reporting structural differences between subjects with and without ADHD while other studies do not find these anatomical differences (e.g., caudate nucleus). It is also important to emphasize that the source of the structural brain differences is unclear and these structural differences are not necessarily directly related to ADHD symptomology.

PET and fMRI Studies

Overall, functional MRI and PET studies support dysfunction of frontal–striatal neural circuitry in ADHD. For example, Lou, Henriksen, and Bruhn (1984) were among the first to use PET to measure rCBF in children with ADHD and found reduced blood flow in the frontal lobes and caudate region. In a later study, reduced blood flow was also found in the right striatum in subjects with ADHD (Lou et al., 1989). Lorberboym and colleagues (2004) recently reported that subjects with ADHD had decreased blood flow in the basal ganglia and frontal regions based on SPECT scans. Lou et al. (1984) noted that following administration of methylphenidate, blood flow increased in the frontal lobes as well as the basal ganglia. Research has also found that methylphenidate has different physiological effects in children with ADHD compared to healthy controls. Vaidya et al. (1998) for example, found that based on fMRI scans both children with and without ADHD showed increased activation in the frontal lobes following methylphenidate treatment, but methylphenidate increased activity in the striatum with children with ADHD and decreased activity in this region in healthy control children. These results further support abnormal striatal–frontal circuitry in children with ADHD.

Recently, Lou and colleagues (2004) found increased dopamine receptor availability in adolescents with ADHD who had low cerebral blood flow as neonates. They speculated that low blood flow (cerebral ischaemia) during infancy may increase susceptibility to ADHD later in life. Cheon et al. (2003) also reported that medication-free children with ADHD showed significantly increased DAT binding in the basal ganglia compared to control children. Degree of DAT binding was not, however, correlated with severity of ADHD symptoms. But, Van Dyck et al. (2002) did not find differences in dopamine transporter availability in the area of the striatum in subjects with and without ADHD.

Studies have been mixed with regard to glucose metabolism and ADHD. For example, some studies have found reductions in glucose metabolism in several areas of the brain including the striatum in adults with ADHD, particularly females (e.g., Ernst, Zametkin, Phillips, & Cohen, 1998; Zametkin et al., 1990). Zametkin et al. (1993), however, did not find global glucose metabolism differences in adolescents with and without ADHD, although lower metabolism in the left frontal lobe was inversely correlated with ADHD symptom severity. Teicher et al. (2000) reported increased blood flow in the striatum (caudate and putamen) of boys with ADHD, and subsequent administration of methylphenidate reduced the activity within these regions. Recent studies suggest that the neural substrates involved in decision making may differ in adults with and without ADHD. Ernst and colleagues (2003) for example, used PET to measures areas of increased activation while subjects performed a decision-making and control task. Results showed increased activation in the ventral and dorsolateral prefrontal cortices in both groups, but subjects with ADHD had a lesser degree and fewer areas of activation. Interestingly, abstinent cocaine abusers have also showed decreased activity in the dorsolateral prefrontal cortex while performing decision-making tasks that require planning and working memory. Spalletta et al. (2001) found decreased activation in the left dorsolateral prefrontal cortex in children with ADHD. Lower levels of activity in the left region and higher levels of activation in the right region were associated with greater neuropsychological task impairment and severity of ADHD symptoms. Durston and colleagues (2003) and Rubia et al. (1999) used fMRI and reported that children with ADHD showed significantly less activation of the frontal–striatal regions while performing a neuropsychological inhibition task compared to control children. Kim et al. (2002) found decreased cerebral blood flow in right and left orbitofrontal cortices as well as the cerebellum in children with ADHD relative to controls. Recently, Schulz et al. (2004) reported that adolescents with ADHD had greater activation in the left anterior cingulate gyrus, bilateral frontal regions, and bilateral ventrolateral prefrontal cortex based on fMRI images than adolescents without a history of ADHD while they performed a response inhibition task. The researchers suggested that enhanced activation in these regions may reflect deficits in inhibitory control or adapative mechanisms due to impairments in other brain regions not examined in the study.

Stimulants and Neuroimaging

Studies have consistently demonstrated that stimulants (methylphenidate) improve ADHD symptoms in children and adults, although the way in which they affect neural activity—and in turn behavior—is not well understood. Lou et al. (1984) for example, found increased blood flow in the striatum following methylphenidate administration, and clinical improvement is associated with occupancy of a majority of dopamine transporters (Volkow et al., 2002). Moll and colleagues (2000) reported that children with ADHD evidenced inhibitory deficits within the motor cortex, but following treatment with methylphenidate significant increases in inhibition skills were observed. Similarly, studies have found significant changes in EEG activity in the frontal lobes of children with ADHD before and after treatment with methylphenidate (Loo, Teale, & Reite, 1999). Schweitzer et al. (2003) reported increased rCBF in the cerebellum (vermis) and midbrain following methylphenidate treatment, and increased rCBF in these regions was associated with a decrease in ADHD symptoms. Langleben et al. (2002) assessed rCBF in adolescents with ADHD while they were taking and not taking methylphenidate.

Results indicated that rCBF was increased in the motor, premotor, and anterior cingulate cortices while subjects were not taking methylphenidate and decreased in these regions while subjects were taking the medication. Recently, Shafritz and colleagues (2004) used fMRI to study the neural correlates of attention while adolescents with ADHD and adolescents with ADHD and reading disorder were taking methylphenidate or placebo. Results revealed that during the attention task, those with ADHD had less activation in the left ventral basal ganglia compared to those without the disorder. Interestingly, methylphenidate was associated with increased activation ("normalization") in this region in adolescents with ADHD and ADHD with reading disorder, but this increased activation was not associated with improved task performance. The authors speculated that increased activation in the striatum with methylphenidate may reflect an increase in neural processing due to improved inhibition or may reflect increased motivational salience. Studies have also found that treatment with methylphenidate over time (e.g., 4 to 6 weeks) is associated with decreased DAT binding in the striatum but not with changes in global glucose metabolism (Krause et al., 2000; Matochik et al., 1994). Vles et al. (2003) studied the effects of chronic (3 months) methylphenidate administration in male children with ADHD and found a 20% down-regulation of postsynaptic dopamine receptors and a 74% reduction of the dopamine transporter in the striatal system. These reductions in receptors were associated with improved neuropsychological test performance and ADHD symptoms. Recent studies with other animals have found that small doses of stimulants administered for 2 weeks result in increases in dendritic length and branching of neurons in the frontal cortex but not in the striatum (Diaz-Heijtz, Kolb, & Forssberg, 2003). These findings suggest that stimulants, like antidepressants, may promote growth and expansion of neurons in certain regions of the brain. Additional studies are needed to further investigate this possibility.

In a review of neuroimaging studies in ADHD, Giedd et al. (2001) concluded that neuroimaging techniques do not currently have diagnostic utility but strongly implicate right frontal–striatal circuitry in ADHD. A recent study by Rohde and colleagues (2003) suggests that this faulty frontal–striatal circuitry may be modulated by gene variants of the dopaminergic system. Specifically, the researchers found significantly higher rCBF in the medial frontal and left basal ganglia following administration of methylphenidate in children with ADHD who had a specific polymorphism of the DAT1 gene compared to children with ADHD without the polymorphism. These preliminary results suggest that polymorphisms affecting the dopaminergic system are associated with abnormal functional circuitry of ADHD.

Pharmacological Interventions

Psychostimulant medications are the most widely used and effective medications for the treatment of ADHD (Kutcher et al., 2004). The FDA has approved four stimulant medications for the treatment of the disorder: methylphenidate, dextroamphetamine, pemoline, and adderall. Approximately 20–30% of children who are prescribed stimulants do not show improvement in their ADHD symptoms and, as a result, alternative medications such as antidepressants are sometimes used (DuPaul, & Stoner, 2003; Ullmann & Sleator, 1986; see Table 9.2). In 2002, the FDA approved the use of Strattera (atomoxetine) for the treatment of ADHD. Strattera is a nonstimulant medication that prevents the reuptake of norepinephrine, and recent studies support its safety and effectiveness for both children and adults (Caballero & Nahata, 2003; Simpson & Plosker, 2004). Currently, there are no physiological tests to determine who will and will not respond favorably to stimulant medications. Yu-Feng and colleagues (2004), however, recently reported that a polymorphism of the norepinephrine transporter gene (G1287A) was associated with a poor response to stimulant medication (methylphenidate) while other markers were associated with a good response to medication. Athough the relationship between

TABLE 9.2

Stimulant and Nonstimulant Medications Used in the Treatment of ADHD

Medication	Trade Name
Methylphenidate	Ritalin, Metadate, Methylin, Concerta
Dexmethylphenidate	Focalin
Dextroamphetamine	Dexedrine
Pemoline	Cylert
Amphetamine salts	Adderall
Other	
Atomoxetine	Strattera
Antidepressant Medications	
Tricyclics	
Imipramine	Tofranil
Desipramine	Norpramin
Nortriptyline	Pamelor
SSRIs	
Sertraline	Zoloft
Fluoxetine	Prozac
Paroxetine	Paxil
Fluvoxamine	Luvox
Other	
Buproion	Wellbutrin

genetics and medication response is likely complex, future genetic studies may help to better predict medication response.

It has been estimated that 3 million children and adolescents in the United States take stimulants daily, including 1.2% of the preschool population (Zito et al., 1999, 2000). A plethora of studies have supported the efficacy and safety of stimulants with preschoolers, children, adolescents, and, more recently, adults with ADHD (Charach, Ickowicz, & Schachar, 2004; Short, Manos, Findling, & Schubel, 2004; Spencer, 2004). Fischer and Barkley (2003) found that stimulant therapy for ADHD in childhood is *not* associated with increased risk of adolescent experimentation with substance use, frequency of such use, or the risk of developing psychoactive substance use disorders by young adulthood. As discussed in chapter 2, stimulants such as methylphenidate (ritalin) increase arousal level of the CNS primarily by blocking the dopamine transporter (DAT), thereby increasing the availability of dopamine in the extracellular fluid (Volkow et al., 2002). Although stimulants are considered a safe and effective treatment for ADHD, Schwartz and colleagues (2004) recently reported that stimulants can induce slight, but significant, sleep disturbances in children and adolescents treated with these medications. A common misconception is that stimulants produce a paradoxical effect—that is, calm a hyperactive system—but research has found that the CNS of individuals with ADHD is actually underaroused (Anderson et al., 2000; Hastings & Barkley, 1978). Stimulants, therefore, increase arousal and help to regulate frontal–striatal pathways believed to be dysfunctional in ADHD (Volkow et al., 2002). Konrad and colleagues (2004) recently discovered that methylphenidate differentially affects attentional functions (e.g., executive functions, selective attention) depending on dosage.

Antidepressants or other medications such as anticonvulsants are sometimes used to treat ADHD when individuals fail to respond to stimulants or when comorbid disorders are present such as depression and OCD. For example, research by Biederman et al. (1989) found that 68% of children who failed to show improvement with stimulants demonstrated significant improvement in ADHD symptoms while taking tricyclic antidepressants. Selective serotonin reuptake inhibitors are most effective for obsessive compulsive disorder and depression, and may be effective in children and adolescents with ADHD who also have coexisting mood problems (Spencer & Biederman, 2002). Bupropion differs in chemical structure from other antidepressants and in that sense is considered novel. Several studies have found bupropion to be effective at improving ADHD symptoms in children (Spencer, 2004). It is important to note that although most research indicates that stimulants are superior to antidepressants at improving ADHD symptoms, the FDA has not approved the use of antidepressants for the specific treatment of ADHD.

Nonpharmacological Interventions

In addition to medication, research has found that a variety of behavioral and psychosocial interventions as well can be effective at reducing the symptoms of ADHD (DuPaul & Weyandt, in press; Weyandt, 2001, 2004). But, several types of alternative interventions marketed for the treatment of ADHD have produced highly conflicting results in studies. Moreover, because these interventions have not received the same level of scientific scrutiny as medication and behavioral interventions, numerous questions remain about their effectiveness and safety. Examples of alternative interventions include dietary modifications, nutritional supplements, biofeedback, caffeine, and homeopathy (Brue & Oakland, 2002). Based on a survey of parents of 381 children with ADHD, Stubberfield and Parry (1999) found that 69% were using medication, but almost as many (64% of the sample) were using alternative therapies for ADHD. The most commonly used alternative method was dietary changes (60%), and there was no difference in the prevalence of the use of alternative interventions among families whose children were medicated or nonmedicated. Recently, Chan, Rappaport, and Kemper (2003) found that 54% of 114 parents of children with ADHD reported using alternative interventions with their children, with vitamins and dietary manipulations the most common. Interestingly, only 11% of the parents had discussed using these methods with their child's physician.

The effects of nutritional supplements and dietary restrictions on ADHD symptoms have been explored by a substantial number of studies, with several reporting a reduction in ADHD symptoms (e.g., Dykman and Dykman, 1998; Harding, Judah, and Grant, 2003; Kaplan, McNicol, Conte, & Moghadam, 1989; Richardson & Puri, 2002) and others no change (Adams, 1981; Mattes & Gittelman, 1981; Voigt et al., 2001; Wender, 1986). Caffeine studies have also produced mixed findings (e.g., Garfinkel, Webster, & Sloman, 1981; Huestis, Arnold, & Smeltzer, 1975). Comparison studies of the effectiveness of caffeine versus stimulants have generally found that stimulants are significantly more effective at reducing ADHD symptoms (Garfinckel, Webster, and Sloman, 1975; Leon, 2000). A few studies have reported that massage therapy (e.g., Field, Quintino, Hernandez-Reif, & Koslovsky, 1998; Khilnani, Field, Hernandez-Reif, & Schanberg, 2003) as well as acupuncture (Arnold, 2001) reduce symptoms in adolescents with ADHD, although more well-designed studies are needed to empirically investigate these alternative methods in the treatment of ADHD. Neurofeedback (or biofeedback) has also been reported to effectively reduce ADHD symptomology in some studies (e.g., Fuchs, Birbaumer, Lutzenberger, Gruzelier, & Kaiser, 2003; Monastra, Monastra, & George, 2002), whereas other studies have failed to support its efficacy (e.g., Heywood & Beale, 2003). In general, neurofeedback studies have been criticized for a lack of methodological rigor and potentially misleading findings (e.g., Loo, 2003). Given research that indicates many parents are already using these approaches with their children, studies are needed to explore the potential effectiveness or lack of effectiveness of alternative interventions for ADHD.

SUMMARY

In summary, familial and twin studies strongly support the heritability of ADHD. Molecular genetic studies have focused primarily on polymorphisms of dopaminergic genes (e.g., DRD5, DRD4, DAT1), and numerous studies have found linkages between variants of these genes and ADHD. Nevertheless, a specific gene or group of genes has not been determined to cause ADHD and it is likely that several interactive genes increase the susceptibility to ADHD. Neuroanatomical, neuroimaging, and medication studies implicate dysfunctional frontal–striatal circuitry in ADHD. Pharmacological interventions are the most effective method for acutely treating ADHD symptoms. Many behavioral interventions have also been shown to reduce ADHD symptoms in children and adolescents with the disorder. Alternative interventions have produced mixed findings and, in general, have not undergone the same level of scientific scrutiny as more traditional approaches.

TOURETTE'S DISORDER

Tourette's Disorder is characterized by multiple motor tics and one or more vocal tics (see Table 9.3). A *tic* is a sudden, recurrent, rapid, and stereotyped vocalization or movement that may be either simple or complex. Eye blinking, nose wrinkling, and shoulder shrugging are examples of *simple motor tics* while jumping, pressing, stomping, squatting, twirling, and hand gestures are examples of *complex motor tics*. Throat clearing, sniffing, chirping, and snorting are examples of *simple vocal tics* and sudden expression of a single word or phrase or echolalia are examples of *complex vocal tics*. Contrary to popular perception, coprolalia (sudden and inappropriate expression of obscenities or racial slurs) is not a diagnostic criterion for Tourette's disorder, as it is seen in only 10 to 50% of individuals with the disorder (DSM IV-TR, 2000; Kano, Ohta, & Nagai, 1998). The prevalence of Tourette's disorder is estimated to be 5 to 30 per 10,000 children and 1 to 2 per 10,000 adults (DSM IV-TR, 2000), although recent studies have reported that approximately 1% to 2% of children between the ages of 5 and 16 have Tourette's disorder (Faridi & Suchowersky, 2003; Hornsey, Banerjee, Zeitlin, & Robertson, 2001; Robertson, 2003). The disorder occurs more frequently in males than females with a ratio of 4:1

TABLE 9.3

Diagnostic Criteria for 307.23 Tourette's Disorder (DSM IV-TR, 2000)

A. Both multiple motor and one or more vocal tics have been present at some time during the illness although not necessarily concurrently. (A *tic* is a sudden rapid, recurrent, nonrhythmic, stereotyped, motor movement or vocalization.)

B. The tics occur many times a day (usually in bouts) nearly every day or intermittently throughout a period of more than 1 year, and during this period there was never a tic-free period of more than 3 consecutive months.

C. The disturbance is not due to the direct physiological effects of a substance (e.g., stimulants) or a general medical condition (e.g., Huntington's disease or postviral encephalitis).

(Freeman et al., 2000). Tourette's disorder is found throughout the world and the incidence is similar in Western and Eastern countries (Kano, Ohta, & Nagai, 1998). Mathews et al. (2001) studied 85 individuals with Tourette's disorder from Costa Rica and found that the clinical characteristics in their sample were similar to studies from other countries. However, the researchers reported that many individuals acknowledged the presence and severity of their symptoms but denied that Tourette's disorder caused them impairment or distress. Recently, Wang and Kuo (2003) studied the prevalence of Tourette's disorder in Taiwan and found that less than 1% of children had the disorder (.56%). The male–female ratio was higher than expected (9:2), and 36% comorbid ADHD and 18% comorbid OCD.

The age of onset is usually during childhood or adolescence, and the mean age of onset of tics is 6.4 years (Freeman et al., 2000). The course of Tourette's disorder is variable and in some cases is lifelong with periods of remission, or the symptoms may disappear by early adulthood (DSM IV-TR, 2000). Based on an international study of 3,500 individuals with the disorder, ADHD is the most commonly co-occurring disorder (Freeman et al., 2000), followed by OCD (Zelnik, Newfield, Silman-Stolar, & Goikhman, 2002). Tourette's disorder is frequently accompanied by social, academic, and occupational impairment, and occasionally self-injurious behavior. Sukhodolsky et al. (2003) recently compared 42 children with Tourette's disorder, 52 with ADHD, and 52 with comorbid Tourette's and ADHD. Results indicated that children with Tourette's disorder (only) did not differ from control subjects with respect to parent or teacher ratings of aggression or delinquent behavior. Children with both Tourette's and ADHD, however, were rated as having significant problems with aggressive and disruptive behavior. Studies have also found that children with Tourette's disorder and comorbid ADHD arc more likely to have sudden, explosive outbursts than children with Tourette's only (Budman, Bruun, Park, Lesser, & Olson, 2000). The impact of Tourette's disorder on the individual and the family is significantly greater when ADHD is comorbid with Tourette's and when symptoms are severe (Spencer et al., 1998; Wilkinson et al., 2002).

Tourette's disorder is sometimes accompanied by neuropsychological impairments (Channon et al., 2003) as well as sleep disturbances and inappropriate sexual behavior (Nee et al., 1980). Zelnik and colleagues (2002) reported that individuals with Tourette's disorder tend to be lower in height and birth weight than individuals without the disorder and suggested that these findings may be due to dysfunctional neurotransmitter systems that interact with endocrine systems. Similarly, Kessler (2002) reported that 38% of a sample of patients with Tourette's disorder had body temperature dysregulation, which led him to suggest that the hypothalamus may be dysfunctional. Individuals with Tourette's disorder are also more likely to suffer migraine headaches than the general population (25% versus 10–13%, respectively). Interestingly, of patients with Tourette's disorder, 56% reported a family history of migraines. Wood and colleagues (2003) recently reported that the tics of children with Tourette's disorder tend to worsen with emotionally charged visual stimuli (i.e., video images), but tic severity does not appear to be related to heart or respiratory rate and therefore is not mediated by the autonomic nervous system.

Genetic Studies

Familial and twin studies support a genetic component of Tourette's disorder, although twin studies suggest that environmental factors likely play a role as well. McMahon and colleagues (2003), for example, reported that the rates of Tourette's disorder in children were three times higher if both parents had the disorder than if only one parent did. Walkup et al. (1996) found that 19% of a sample of 53 children and adolescents with Tourette's disorder had two parents who also had the disorder or chronic tic disorder or OCD. The concordance rate of Tourette's disorder in twins has been reported as 53% for monozygotic and 8% for dizygotic twins (Price, Kidd, Cohen, Pauls, & Leckman, 1985). Hyde et al. (1992) suggested that events affecting the developing fetus likely interact with genetic factors and lead to the phenotypic expression of Tourette's disorder. Goetz and Taner (1990) conducted a case study of monozygotic twins who were discordant for Tourette's disorder, and found that cerebral spinal fluid dopamine and serotonin metabolites did not differ between the twins and did not correlate with presence or severity of Tourette's disorder symptoms. Similar findings were reported by Cath et al. (2001). A postmortem analysis of frontal, temporal, and occipital regions of brains of adults with Tourette's disorder also did not find altered levels of dopamine, norepinephrine, or serotonin metabolites (Singer, Hahn, Krowiak, Nelson, & Moran, 1990). Kurup and Kurup (2002) have suggested that increased levels of dopamine can lead to tics characteristic of Tourette's disorder, but collectively studies do not support a one-to-one relationship between dopamine and symptoms of Tourette's syndrome. Segawa (2003) suggested that dopamine receptors may be "supersensitive" in patients with Tourette's disorder due to abnormal development of the neurotransmitter system early in life.

Candidate Genes

Similar to ADHD, a number of dopaminergic genes have been investigated in Tourette's disorder as well as genes of the serotonergic and adrenergic neurotransmitter systems. Price and colleagues (1986) were among the first to report that stimulants worsened tics in 24% of individuals with Tourette's disorder, thus implicating the dopaminergic system in the disorder. Nomura and Segawa (2003) as well as others have hypothesized that Tourette's disorder is a disorder of the dopaminergic system, and many studies have attempted to identify the genetic source of this dysregulation. For example, Diaz-Anzaldua et al. (2004a) studied 110 patients with Tourette's disorder and their families in a sample of French Canadians, and explored whether variants of several dopamine genes (e.g., DRD2, DRD3, and DRD4) and a monoamine oxidase genes (MAOA) were associated with Tourette's disorder. Results supported a linkage between the MAOA and DRD4 genes and Tourette's disorder but not the remaining dopamine genes.

A recent postmortem study examined tissue samples from the caudate, putamen, ventral striatum, and prefrontal cortex of three individuals of varying ages with Tourette's disorder. Results revealed substantial increased density of the dopamine transporter (DAT), dopamine receptor (D2), and several proteins important in neural communication in the area of the prefrontal cortex (not the striatum) compared to control subjects (Minzer, Lee, Hong, & Singer, 2004). Singer, Hahn, and Moran (1991) also reported significantly higher DAT binding in the caudate (37%) and putamen (50%) of postmortem brain tissue of individuals with Tourette's disorder relative to controls. The researchers hypothesized that the dopamine system within the striatum is hyperactive in patients with Tourette's disorder. Wolf and colleagues (1996) studied monozygotic living twins who were discordant for Tourette's disorder and also found significantly greater (17%) dopamine receptor binding (D2), but only in the head of the caudate nucleus of twins affected with the disorder. Wolf et al. noted that projections extend from the caudate to the orbitofrontal cortices and suggested that disruptions in these pathways may be responsible for the symptoms observed in patients with Tourette's.

In addition to the D2 receptor, polymorphisms of the DRD4 gene have also been linked to Tourette's disorder (Grice et al., 1996) as well as OCD (Millet et al., 2003). In fact, some authors have suggested that OCD may represent an alternative expression of genetic factors that underlie Tourette's disorder (Pauls, Towbin, Leckman, Zahner, & Cohen, 1986). Comings et al. (1996) reported that polymorphisms of three dopamine genes (DAT, DRD2, DBH) were associated with Tourette's disorder and suggested that inheritance of Tourette's or ADHD may be due to a contribution of each of these genes. Many studies have not, however, found evidence of linkage between dopaminergic genes and Tourette's disorder (e.g., Barr et al., 1996, 1997; Brett, Curtis, Robertson, & Gurling, 1995b; Gelernter et al., 1990). Serotonin genes have also been investigated and, based on a genetic analysis of 52 individuals with Tourette's disorder, Cavallini and colleagues (2000) concluded that the serotonin transporter gene (5-HTTLPR) does not appear to play a significant role in the etiology of Tourette's disorder. Brett, Curtis, Robertson, and Gurling (1995a) also reported a lack of relationship between polymorphisms of serotonin genes and the presence of Tourette's disorder. Glutamate has been implicated in Tourette's disorder, and McGrath and colleagues (2000) and Nordstrom and Burton (2002) proposed that hyperactivity of glutamate-releasing neurons within various cortical–limbic–striatal pathways underlies its symptoms.

Other studies have focused on broad chromosomal regions to determine whether a genetic linkage exists between chromosomal markers and Tourette's disorder. The findings have been inconsistent. For example, a number of studies have reported an association between chromosome 7 (7q31) and Tourette's disorder (e.g., Diaz-Anzaldua et al., 2004b; Kroisel et al., 2001; Petek et al., 2001) although Heutink et al. (1990) did not find evidence for genetic linkage on chromosomes 7 and 18 and Tourette's. Matsumoto et al. (2000) studied chromosome 8 and also failed to find abnormalities linked to the disorder. Barr et al. (1999) conducted a genome scan for Tourette's disorder linkage but, despite the use of 386 chromosomal markers, was unable to find any significant linkage. Recently, however, Verkerk et al. (2003) found an insertion on chromosome 7 that interfered with the functioning of a specific gene (CNTNAP2) that encodes a protein on part of the neuron's membrane at the nodes of Ranvier. They hypothesized that this disruption could interfere with action potentials and thus cause the unwanted movements characteristic of Tourette's disorder. Given the effectiveness of adrenergic antagonists (e.g., clonidine) at reducing symptoms of Tourette's disorder, Xu and colleagues (2003) explored whether variants of two adrenergic genes were associated with the disorder. Based on analysis of 113 families, concluded that adrenergic genes do not appear to contribute to susceptibility.

Neuroanatomical and Neuroimaging Studies

MRI Studies

Although a number of anatomical differences have been reported between subjects with and without Tourette's disorder, the findings are inconsistent. At least one study, for example, found evidence of ventricular enlargement in boys with Tourette's (Harcherik et al., 1985), but others have not reported ventricular differences between children with and without the disorder (e.g., Singer et al., 1993). In addition, reduced—rather than enlarged—ventricular size has been reported in girls with Tourette's disorder (Zimmerman, Abrams, Giuliano, Denckla, & Singer, 2000). Peterson et al. (1993) were among the first to report basal ganglia differences in patients with and without Tourette's disorder. For example, the researchers found that the caudate and globus pallidus were smaller in adults with Tourette's disorder and that these patients lacked the normal symmetry (left larger than right) of the basal ganglia. Recently, Peterson et al. (2003) used MRI to measure basal ganglia volumes in children and adults with Tourette's disorder compared to control subjects and reported that the caudate nucleus volumes were smaller in both children and adults with the disorder. Research has also documented that strokes that affect the basal ganglia often result in subsequent tics and other symptoms of Tourette's (Kwak & Jankovic, 2002). Groenewegen and colleagues (2003) have emphasized that different parts of the basal ganglia are functionally segregated and form separate circuits that likely influence the motor and cognitive symptoms of Tourette's disorder. Comings (1987) proposed that an imbalance of the dopamine pathways in the mesolimbic region leads to disinhibition of circuits within the striatum, causing unwanted motor and vocal tics. Interestingly, Lombroso (1999) described three cases in which children who took an antiseizure medication (lamotrigine) developed Tourettelike symptoms. He speculated that the medication interfered with dopamine release and reuptake in the striatum, thereby inducing symptoms characteristic of the disorder. Chemali and Bromfield (2003) recently described a case of a woman with intractable seizures who developed Tourette's disorder with complex vocal and motor tics as well as severe OCD following a right temporal lobectomy.

Size differences in additional anatomical structures have also been reported between subjects with Tourette's disorder and control subjects. For example, Peterson et al. (2001) reported that children and adults with Tourette's had larger volumes in the prefrontal and parietal regions and smaller volumes in the occipital regions, a finding which significantly correlated with severity of symptoms. Fredericksen et al. (2002) also reported increased volume of the right frontal region in children with Tourette's relative to control subjects. Several studies have reported that the corpus callosum is significantly smaller in subjects with Tourette's disorder (Peterson et al., 1994), and other studies that it is larger (e.g., Baumgardner et al., 1996). Mostofsky and colleagues (1999) studied girls with Tourette's disorder and found no differences in the size of the corpus callosum compared to control subjects and girls with ADHD. Kim and Peterson (2003) recently reported that the cavum septum pellucidum (CSP), an area near the corpus callosum that fuses early in development, was significantly smaller in children with Tourette's compared to normal control subjects, which supports the view of early disturbances in brain development in patients with Tourette's disorder. As Gerard and Peterson (2003) recently noted, however, structural differences in Tourette's disorder may be indicative of etiologic factors or simply represent compensatory changes in response to some unknown factor in the brain. Alternatively, Plessen et al. (2004) recently suggested that smaller corpus callosum size may reflect a compensatory, neuroplastic response in reaction to the presence of tics. Specifically, the researchers compared corpus callosum size in children and adults with and without Tourette's disorder and found that children with the disorder had significantly smaller corpus callosum size that was positively correlated with tic severity. Plessen et al. speculated that a smaller corpus callosum may limit neuronal communication across the hemispheres and thereby reduce inhibitory input to the prefrontal regions. Decreased inhibition to this region would theoretically enhance prefrontal excitation and possibly be involved in the expression of tics. It is important to note that these findings are purely correlational in nature and do not reveal whether the reduced size of the corpus callosum is associated with the expression of Tourette's disorder or whether verbal and motor tics contribute to the reduced size of the corpus callosum. Furthermore, as is true of all anatomical findings, reduced size reflects secondary effects of disturbances (neurochemical or genetic) elsewhere in the brain.

fMRI and PET Studies

Functional abnormalities of the basal ganglia and associated pathways extending to and from the striatum have been strongly implicated in Tourette's disorder (Segawa, 2003). For example, Wolf et al. (1996) were among the first to use PET to study monozygotic twins discordant for Tourette's and found increased binding to postsynaptic dopamine receptors (D2) in the caudate nucleus in all five twins affected with Tourette's relative to twins without the disorder (no differences were found with respect to the putamen). Minzer and colleagues (2004) examined postmortem tissue of three individuals with Tourette's disorder and found an approximate 140% increase in prefrontal D2 receptors in individuals with the disorder relative to controls. Increases were also found with respect to dopamine transporters and metabolite concentration of dopamine and norepinephrine in prefrontal and striatum regions of individuals with Tourette's. Additionally, studies have reported functional differences in the putamen and right ventral striatum in subjects with Tourette's disorder (e.g., Albin et al., 2003). Singer and colleagues (2002), for example, compared dopamine release in subjects with and without Tourette's following an intravenous injection of amphetamine. Results revealed that those with Tourette's disorder had significant increased dopamine release (21%) in the putamen compared to control subjects. Dopamine release was not significantly different between groups in the caudate. The researchers speculated that these findings may reflect an overactive dopamine transporter system, which would result in an increase in stimulant-dependent (amphetamine) dopamine release. Indeed, environmental factors such as stress and dopamine agonists (stimulants) have been found to exacerbate Tourette symptoms in some individuals. Research by Ernst et al. (1999) using PET supported heightened activity of the dopaminergic system in children with Tourette's disorder as indicated by increased presynaptic dopamine activity in the left caudate nucleus and right midbrain region.

Cheon and colleagues (2004) also studied children with Tourette's disorder and, using SPECT, found increased dopamine transporter (DAT) densities in the basal ganglia compared to control children. Similar elevated DAT findings have been reported in adults with Tourette's (e.g., Malison et al., 1995). Albin et al. (2003) reported slightly higher binding levels in the dorsal caudate and putamen in patients with Tourette's disorder relative to control subjects based on PET scans. Several studies however, have reported that dopamine uptake and binding potential in the caudate and putamen did not differ in subjects with Tourette's disorder and controls (e.g., Meyer et al., 1999; Stamenkovic et al., 2001; Turjanski et al., 1994). In addition, increased DAT binding has been observed in other disorders such as ADHD and is therefore not unique to Tourette's disorder (Cheon et al., 2003).

Studies have also reported differences in rCBF and glucose metabolism in individuals with and without Tourette's. Braun et al. (1993), for example, reported decreased glucose metabolism in prefrontal cortices, orbitofrontal regions, and hippocampal regions and striatum in 16 medication-free subjects with Tourette's disorder relative to control subjects. Stern and colleagues (2000), however, reported increased activity in the premotor cortices, anterior cingulate cortex, putamen, caudate, and primary motor cortex that was significantly correlated with the presence of tics as determined by PET and synchronized audio- and videotaping of subjects. Eidelberg et al. (1997) found increased glucose metabolism in the premotor and motor cortex and decreased activity in the caudate, thalamus, and hippocampal regions in subjects with Tourette's disorder. No differences were found with respect to global glucose metabolism between subjects with and without Tourette's. Similar glucose metabolism findings were reported by Jeffries and colleagues (2002).

Hershey et al. (2004) found that during a working memory task, subjects with Tourette's disorder showed excessive activity in the thalamus, medial frontal cortex, and parietal cortex. This level of neuronal activity was significantly decreased following administration of a dopamine agonist (Levodopa). With respect to rCBF, studies have also been inconsistent, with some reporting elevated rCBF in the frontal regions (George et al., 1992) and others reduced rCBF in frontal and striatal regions (e.g., Moriarty et al., 1997). Recently, Gates et al. (2004) used fMRI to study a patient with Tourette's disorder during coprolalia and found increased activity in the caudate nucleus, cingulate gyrus, occipital, and frontal regions relative to a control subject. Peterson et al. (1998) used fMRI to study voluntary suppression of tics compared to expression of tics in 22 adults with Tourette's disorder. Results indicated increased activation in the frontal cortex and right caudate nucleus, and decreased activation in the globus pallidus during tic expression compared to suppression. These findings make theoretical sense as excitatory projections extend from the frontal regions to the caudate nucleus and inhibitory projections extend from the caudate to the globus pallidus. Furthermore, lesions of the globus pallidus have also been associated with the disorder (Demirkol, Erdem, Inan, Yigit, & Guney, 1999). Groenewegen et al. (2003) hypothesized that Tourette's disorder symptoms may be due to a disturbance in the dopaminergic pathways that extend from the ventral striatum via the substantia nigra to the dorsal striatum. Recently, Nomura and Segawa (2003) proposed that Tourette's disorder is due to a developmentally underactive dopaminergic system, particularly in the striatum. According to Nomura and Segawa, normally the striatum is six times more active in early childhood to help foster maturation of brain circuitry and this level of activity decreases with age. In children with Tourette's disorder, however, the dopaminergic system is hypoactive, which is associated with supersensitivity of dopamine receptors. According to Nomura and Segawa, given that that brain is still developing in children and adolescents, dopamine agonists rather than antagonists should be used to treat Tourette's disorder.

Pharmacological and Additional Interventions

Several types of medication are available to treat Tourette's disorder. According to Kossoff and Singer (2001), first-line agents include adrenergic alpha-2 agonists such as clonidine (catapres) and guanfacine (tenex), which decrease the release of norpeinphrine as well as dopamine and glutamate (Leckman et al., 1991). Leckman and colleagues (1982) reported that approximately 50% of individuals with Tourette's disorder experience substantial improvement with clonidine, but common side effects such as fatigue and sedation are reported by nearly 90% of patients. Guanfacine reportedly has a less sedating effect than clonidine, but some studies have reported it has a propensity to induce mania in individuals with a family history of mania (Horrigan & Barnhill, 1999). A study by Cummings and colleagues (2002) reported that guanfacine was not more effective than placebo at reducing tic severity and parental ratings of the tics of children with Tourette's disorder. Chappell et al. (1995), however, found that guanfacine was effective at decreasing motor and vocal tics and improving neuropsychological performance of children with Tourette's disorder and comorbid ADHD.

Antipsychotic medications that block postsynaptic dopamine receptors (e.g., haloperidol/ haldol, thioridazine/mellaril, thiothixene/navane, pimozide/orap) and atypical antipsychotic medications that block serotonin and to a lesser extent dopamine receptors (e.g., clozapine/ clozaril, risperidone/risperdol, olanzapine/ zyprexa, quetiapine/seroquel, and ziprasidone/ geodon) are recommended as second-line agents for Tourette's disorder (Kossoff & Singer, 2001; Schotte et al., 1996). According to Dion and colleagues (2002), haloperidol is the most commonly used medication for treating Tourette's disorder in children, improving symptoms by 43 to 66% (Sallee et al., 1997). The most frequently studied atypical antipsychotic, risperidone, reportedly reduces symptoms by 21 to 61% (Dion et al., 2002; Scahill, Leckman, Schultz, Katsovich, & Peterson, 2003). Gaffney et al. (2002) found that risperidone and clonidine were equally effective at reducing tic symptoms in children and adolescents with Tourette's disorder but that fewer side effects were associated with risperidone. Pimozide (orap) has been found to have fewer side effects and is more effective at reducing tics in children and adolescents than haloperidol, according to Sallee and colleagues (1997). However, Bruggeman et al. (2001) reported that pimozide and risperidone were equally effective at reducing tics in children and adults but fewer side effects were associated with risperidone.

A few studies have reported that dopamine agonists such as pergolide reduce tics in individuals with Tourette's (Gilbert et al., 2004; Lipinski, Sallee, Jackson, & Sethuraman, 1997). The mechanisms by which a dopamine agonist could improve Tourette symptoms is poorly understood although it is possible that pergolide helps to normalize dopamine transmission in dysfunctional striatal–frontal pathways. For example, Linazasoro et al. (1999) found a reduction in dopamine reuptake in the striatum (14% reduction in putamen, 9% caudate) in patients with Parkinson's disease following 6 months of pergolide treatment. Additional studies are needed to clarify the mode of action and effects of pergolide in patients with Tourette's disorder. Alternatively, other dopamine agonists such as cocaine (Daniels, Baker, & Norman, 1996; Pascual-Leone & Dhuna, 1990) and methylphenidate (Gadow, Nolan, Sprafkin, & Sverd, 1995) have been found to induce or worsen symptoms in some patients with Tourette's. Clearly, the relationship between dopamine and Tourette's disorder is complex and warrants further investigation.

Studies investigating the use of antidepressants with Tourette's disorder indicate that, in general, these medications are significantly less effective than antipsychotic medications. The tricyclic antidepressant clomipramine has been found by a few studies to improve tics (e.g., Donahoe, Meador, Fortune, & Llorena, 1991; Ratzoni, Hermesh, Brandt, Lauffer, & Munitz, 1990). However, at least one study reported that clomipramine induced Tourette-like symptoms in a patient with OCD (Moshe, Iulian, Seth, Eli, & Joseph, 1994). SSRIs are also reportedly ineffective at reducing symptoms of Tourette's disorder (Scahill et al., 1997), but have been found to improve OCD symptoms with comorbid Tourette's disorder (Miguel et al., 2003; Riddle, Hardin, King, Scahill, & Woolston, 2001).

In addition to medications, preliminary studies suggest that marijuana, nicotine, and botulinum toxin injections may improve symptoms of Tourette's disorder (Kossoff & Singer, 2001; Mihailescu & Drucker-Colin, 2000; McConville et al., 1991; Mueller-Vahl et al., 2002). For example, Mueller-Vahl et al. (2003) recently conducted a 6-week study of 24 patients with Tourette's who were treated with 10 mg per day of delta-9-tetrahydrocannabinol marijuana (THC). Results revealed a significant decline in symptoms relative to placebo and no serious side effects. Other studies have produced similar results, suggesting that THC is a safe and effective treatment for tics. Given the therapeutic effects of THC in Tourette's disorder, Gadzicki et al. (2004) explored whether polymorphisms of the cannabinoid receptor gene (CNR1) were associated with the disorder. Based on genetic analyses of a large sample of patients with Tourette's, the researchers concluded there was no genetic linkage.

With respect to nicotine, numerous studies have reported that transdermal nicotine patch application reduces tics in patients with Tourette's disorder both short- and long-term (e.g., Dursun & Reveley, 1997; Dursun, Reveley, Bird, & Stirton, 1994; Sanberg et al., 1997; Silver et al., 2001). According to Zhou, Wilson, and Dani (2003), the striatum contains a dense mingling of dopamine receptors as well as other types of receptors including nicotinic receptors. Research indicates that these diverse neurotransmitter systems work together to coordinate functioning of the striatum and hence may help to explain the improvement of tics following application of the nicotine patch. Because botulinum toxin A injections have proven to be an effective treatment for several disorders characterized by abnormal muscle contractions, Kwak, Hanna, and Jankovic (2000) assessed whether these injections would improve motor tics in patients with Tourette's disorder. Thirty-five individuals with the disorder participated in the study and received botulinum toxin injections in the areas of their most severe tics (most frequently, the upper thoracic region and the upper face). Results indicated that 84% of the subjects experienced a reduction in premonitary sensations (i.e., urges to tic), and the majority showed a substantial improvement in tics within 3.8 days. Porta and colleagues (2004) recently reported that botulinum toxin injections in both vocal cords of 30 patients with Tourette's disorder resulted in improvement in 93% of patients; 50% became completely tic-free. The researchers also noted a significant reduction in premonitary experiences.

Behavioral interventions such as habit reversal, self-monitoring, and relaxation training have been found to reduce vocal and motor tics in a number of studies. Peterson and Azrin

(1992), for example, used behavioral interventions with six individuals with Tourette's disorder and reported that on the average, tics were reduced by 55% with habit reversal, 44% with self-monitoring, and 32% with relaxation training. Woods and colleagues (2003) also reported that habit reversal substantially reduced tics in four out of five children. Roane and colleagues (2002) have emphasized that behavioral interventions should be individually tailored depending on the child or adult's symptoms. Recently, Wilhelm and colleagues (2003) compared the effectiveness of habit reversal versus psychotherapy for Tourette's disorder and found that only the former was associated with tic improvement.

Psychosurgery and Deep Brain Stimulation (DBS)

According to Temel and Visser-Vandewalle (2004), the first ablative procedure for intractable Tourette's disorder was performed in 1962. Since that time, the target sites for psychosurgery for the disorder have been diverse and have included such areas as the frontal lobes, limbic system, thalamus, and cerebullum. For example, Kurlan and colleagues (1990) described the outcome of an anterior cingulotomy performed on two individuals with Tourette's disorder and comorbid OCD. Results indicated short- and long-term improvement in tics. In 2001, Babel, Warnke, and Ostertag followed up 11 patients with Tourette's disorder who underwent surgical treatment in Germany (lesioning of the thalamus) between 1970 and 1998. Results revealed that motor and vocal tics were substantially reduced, as were premonitory urges. Nearly 68% of the patients, however, experienced transient side effects of the surgery such as confusion, attention problems, numbness, and loss of muscle control. Since 1999, deep brain stimulation has been used as an alternative to lesioning surgery, and according to Temel and Visser-Vandewalle (2004), preliminary results look promising for the use of DBS in the treatment of Tourette's disorder. For example, Visser-Vandewalle and colleagues (2003) recently implanted chronic pulse generators in the region of the thalamus in three male patients who had manifested symptoms of intractable Tourette's disorder since childhood. Follow-up assessments (8 months to 5 years) indicated that major vocal and motor tics had disappeared and only minor serious side effects were observed (fatigue and changes in sexual behavior). Additional studies are needed to further explore the effectiveness and safety of both psychosurgery and DBS in the treatment of Tourette's syndrome.

PANDAS

Similar to OCD, studies have linked the development of Tourette's disorder in some children to an autoimmune response to streptococcal infections, known as PANDAS (Hoekstra, Kallenberg, Korf, & Minderaa, 2002; Loisell, Wendlandt, Rohde, & Singer, 2003). Specifically, children who have had streptococcal infections and subsequently developed Tourette's syndrome (or OCD) often have increased basal ganglia volumes, presumably due to increased antibodies within the basal ganglia. Mueller and colleagues (2000) examined titers of two different antistreptococcal antibodies (antistreptolysin and antiDNase B) in 13 children with Tourette's disorder, 23 adults with Tourette's disorder, 17 adults with schizophrenia, and control subjects. Results revealed that the titers were significantly higher in subjects with Tourette's syndrome compared to patients with schizophrenia and control subjects. These findings suggest that streptococcal infections can sometimes play a critical role in the development of Tourette's disorder, but specifically how this occurs is unclear. Hallett et al. (2000) determined that certain types of antibodies can cross the blood–brain barrier of other animals (rats) and selectively bind to neurons in the striatum, inducing stereotypic movements similar to Tourette's syndrome. The researchers suggested that antineuronal bodies may bind to neurons in the striatum of children and induce functional changes in cells within this region, leading to Tourette's. As with OCD, however, not everyone who is exposed to the streptococcal virus develops Tourette's syndrome and not everyone with the disorder had necessarily developed a strep infection. In a recent review of the PANDAS literature, Hoekstra, Kallenberg, Korf, and Minderaa (2002) stated that the "significance and validity of PANDAS remains to be established since we lack direct comparisons between Tourette Syndrome subjects who do and Tourette Syndrome subjects who do not meet criteria for PANDAS" (p. 442).

SUMMARY

Collectively, studies support dysfunction and disinhibition of dopaminergic systems between the prefrontal and striatal regions in Tourette's disorder. The findings are far from conclusive, however, and many questions remain concerning the physiological underpinnings of this disorder. Based on familial and twin studies, Tourette's disorder appears to have a genetic component and likely involves abnormalities of genes that are involved in dopamine regulation. Structural and functional imaging studies also support an underlying physiological basis for Tourette's involving the basal ganglia, caudate, thalamus, and frontal regions, although many of these studies have produced conflicting results. The striatum contains a diversity of neurotransmitter receptors, however, and given the effectiveness of THC and nicotine at reducing vocal and motor tics, symptoms of Tourette's disorder are likely mediated by a number of neurotransmitter systems. Dopamine antagonists such as antipsychotic medications are often effective at decreasing symptoms of Tourette's, as are medications that affect the noradrenergic system. Behavioral interventions, psychosurgery, and deep brain stimulation are also promising interventions for Tourette's disorder.

AUTISTIC DISORDER

Autistic disorder is a clinically and genetically heterogenous disorder and one of a broad spectrum of pervasive developmental disorders that include Rett's disorder, childhood disintegrative disorder, and Asperger's syndrome (DSM IV-TR, 2000). Pervasive developmental disorders are characterized by impairment in several areas of development such as communication and social skills, and these impairments are present in all settings. Stereotyped behavior, interests, and activities are also characteristic of the spectrum of pervasive developmental disorders. Constantino and Todd (2003) recently measured social deficits characteristic of the spectrum of pervasive developmental disorders in 788 twin pairs and reported that autistic traits were continuously distributed (i.e., common) and moderately to highly heritable. Pervasive developmental disorders are estimated to affect approximately 60 of 10,000 births (Merrick, Kandel, & Morad, 2004), and given the tremendous amount of information that is available concerning each of these disorders, the following section will focus on autistic disorder only.

According to DSM IV-TR diagnostic criteria, the essential features of autistic disorder include gross impairments in communication and social interactions as well as severely limited activities and interests (see Table 9.4). The degree of impairment is highly variable among individuals, but the disturbances in communication and social interactions are evident prior to age 3. Autistic disorder occurs four to five times more often in boys than girls, and approximately 5 out of 10,000 individuals are diagnosed with the disorder (DSM IV-TR, 2000). A recent epidemiological survey involving 32 studies from 13 countries, however, found the prevalence of autistic disorder ranged from 9 to 11 out of 10,000 (Fombonne, 2003). Prevalence rates

TABLE 9.4

Diagnostic Criteria for 299.00 Autistic Disorder (DSM IV-TR, 2000)

A. A total of six (or more) items from (1), (2), and (3), with at least two from (1), and one each from (2) and (3):
  (1) qualitative impairment in social interaction, as manifested by at least two of the following:
    (a) marked impairment in the use of multiple nonverbal behaviors such as eye-to-eye gaze, facial expression, body postures, and gestures to regulate social interaction
    (b) failure to develop peer relationships appropriate to developmental level
    (c) a lack of spontaneous seeking to share enjoyment, interests, or achievements with other people (e.g., by a lack of showing, bringing, or pointing out objects of interest)
    (d) lack of social or emotional reciprocity
  (2) qualitative impairments in communication as manifested by at least one of the following:
    (a) delay in, or total lack of, the development of spoken language (not accompanied by an attempt to compensate through alternative modes of communication such as gestures or mime)
    (b) in individuals with adequate speech, marked impairment in the ability to initiate or sustain a conversation with others
    (c) stereotyped and repetitive use of language or idiosyncratic language
    (d) lack of varied, spontaneous make-believe play or social imitative play appropriate to developmental level
  (3) restricted repetitive and stereotyped patterns of behavior, interests, and activities, as manifested by at least one of the following:
    (a) encompassing preoccupation with one or more stereotyped and restricted patterns of interest that is abnormal either in intensity or focus
    (b) apparently inflexible adherence to specific, nonfunctional routines or rituals
    (c) stereotyped and repetitive motor mannerisms (e.g., hand or finger flapping or twisting, or complex whole-body movements)
    (d) persistent preoccupation with parts of objects
B. Delays or abnormal functioning in at least one of the following areas, with onset prior to age 3 years: (1) social interaction, (2) language as used in social communication, or (3) symbolic or imaginative play.
C. The disturbance is not better accounted for by Rett's Disorder or Childhood Disintegrative Disorder.

---

are fairly similar throughout the world although some studies have reported higher rates than others. For example, Chakrabarti and Fombonne (2001) reported a prevalence rate of 16.8 per 10,000 for autistic disorder in Staffordshire, England, and Honda and colleagues (1996) reported a rate of 21 per 10,000 in children in Japan. Gillberg, Schaumann, and Gillberg (1995) reported that the rate of autistic disorder among boys born to mothers from Uganda was 200 times higher than the general population of children—but this study was later criticized for methodological problems such as small sample size and lack of an appropriate comparison group. Rates of autistic disorder in Norway are similar to those reported in the United States (4 to 5 per 10,000; Sponheim & Skjeldal, 1998). According to Fombonne (2003), despite previous reports, the available epidemiological studies do *not* suggest that the incidence of autism has increased, nor do the data support an association between social class or race and autistic disorder.

In approximately 70% of cases, individuals with autistic disorder also have mental retardation and medical disorders such as epilepsy, fragile X syndrome, and tuberous sclerosis (Fombonne, 2003; La Malfa et al., 2004). Behavioral problems are also common in autistic disorder and may include aggressiveness, hyperactivity, impulsivity, attention problems, and self-injurious behavior (DSM IV-TR, 2000). The communication impairments associated with autistic disorder appear to emerge early in life. Sheinkopf and colleagues (2000), for example, reported that preverbal young children with autistic disorder displayed significant impairments in vocal quality (e.g., atypical vocalizations). Usually, individuals with autistic disorder show marked and sustained nonverbal and verbal communication deficits, although in a minority of cases, children may show a period of normal development during the first 2 years of life (DSM IV-TR, 2000). If children with autistic disorder do acquire language, it is often characterized by stereotyped or repetitive use or an inability to sustain a conversation with others (see Table 9.4). In general, autistic disorder follows a continuous course but, depending on intelligence level and language skills, developmental gains are possible during the school-age years (DSM IV-TR, 2000; Szatmari et al., 2000). Outcome studies have revealed that approximately one third of individuals with the disorder gain partial independence, but most continue to struggle with communication and social interactions (DSM IV-TR, 2000). In a recent study, Howlin, Goode, Hutton, and Rutter (2004) followed into adulthood 68 children with autistic disorder who had IQs over 50. Based on social, communication, and behavioral measures, results indicated that the majority (46%) were rated as having a poor outcome and 12% a very poor outcome. The remaining individuals were rated as having a fair, good, or very good outcome in adulthood (19%, 10%, and 10%, respectively). Overall, very few individuals with autistic disorder lived alone or had close friends or consistent employment, and most remained dependent on their families or social support services. Masi and colleagues (2003) reported that preschool children who were treated with risperidone functioned better socially and behaviorally than children with autistic disorder not treated with the medication. A number of studies have reported that early intervention and structured education and behavioral support programs can enhance the functioning of children in later life (e.g., Howlin, 1997).

In addition to general impairments on social interactions, studies have also found children with autistic disorder often lack social referencing, that is, the tendency to turn toward an adult in the presence of an ambiguous (or unfamiliar) stimulus. For example, Bacon et al. (1998) found that both high-functioning and low-functioning children with autistic disorder failed to look to an adult for social cues when placed in a situation where another person was distressed. Maestro et al. (2002) studied home movies from the first 6 months of life of children with autism compared to movies of children without the disorder and concluded that children with autism exhibit a clear preference for nonsocial stimuli. The researchers speculated that these children may have a specific problem with orienting to people and human voices which may serve as a precursor to difficulties in other social behaviors later in childhood. In addition to social deficits, individuals with autistic disorder may also display odd responses to stimuli such as exaggerated responses to sounds or objects. Recent studies suggest these exaggerated responses are likely associated with physiological differences in processing information. For example, several studies have reported that individuals with autistic disorder showed an abnormal response (event-related potentials) to auditory stimulation compared to control subjects (Ferri et al., 2003; Gomot et al., 2002). In addition to communication and social skill impairments, individuals with autistic disorder may have feeding problems such as food refusal or selectivity based on type or texture (Field, Garland, & Williams, 2003) as well as sleeping problems such as early morning or recurrent night awakening (Hering et al., 1999).

Although most individuals with autistic disorder also have varying degrees of mental retardation, in rare cases they may have exceptional skills known as savant talents. Savant talents typically include music, memory, mathematics, specific knowledge, and drawing (Kehrer, 1992) and are also characteristic of disabilities other than autistic disorder—most commonly mental retardation. O'Connor and Hermelin (1991) argued that preoccupations and repetitive behaviors are closely associated with savant talents, and were among the first to demonstrate that memory skills alone did not sufficiently explain the exceptional calculating performance of individuals with savant talents (O'Connor & Hermelin, 1984). Shah and Frith (1983) found that children with autism and superior memory skills performed significantly better on a visual memory task than children without the disorder. In a later study, Shah and Frith (1993) reported that individuals with autistic disorder performed significantly better than control subjects on the Block Design Task of the Wechsler scales, regardless of overall intelligence. Thaut (1988) found that children with autistic disorder performed similarly to control children with respect to music responsiveness (rhythm, restriction, originality) and significantly better than children with mental retardation. In 1999, Miller reviewed the savant literature and concluded that (a) the skills displayed by savants share many characteristics with the same skills displayed by people without a disability such as autism, and (b) savant talents are usually accompanied by at least average levels of some aspects of intelligence. Recently, the incidence of savant syndrome was evaluated in Finland and it was reported that the incidence was 1.4 per 1,000 people with mental retardation. The most commonly reported savant talent was calendar calculation followed by memory skills. Currently, there is no physiological explanation that adequately addresses the rare but documented exceptional skills of a minority of individuals with autistic disorder.

General Cognitive Theories

A number of theories exist concerning the etiology of autistic disorder—cognitive, genetic, and physiologic. For example, a great deal of attention has been devoted to "theory of mind," which essentially is the ability to infer mental states (e.g., desires, beliefs, intentions, emotions) in one's self and in others (Perner, Frith, Leslie, & Leekam, 1989). A number of studies have found that children with autistic disorder perform substantially more poorly on tasks designed to assess theory of mind than children without the disorder (e.g., Sparrevohn & Howie, 1995), but other studies have not found impairments on theory of mind tasks with children with autistic disorder (e.g., Russell & Hill, 2001). Recently, Downs and Smith (2004) found that high-functioning children with autistic disorder actually performed better than children with ADHD with regard to cooperative behavior and level of emotional understanding, and no differences were found between control children and children with autistic disorder on Social-Emotional tasks.

Additional cognitive explanations of autistic disorder have been proposed such as disturbance in intersubjectivity (Trevarthen & Aitken, 2001) and deficits in central coherence (e.g., Morgan, Maybery, & Durkin, 2003). In addition, some researchers argue that theory of mind and central coherence impairments are interrelated and that it is highly unlikely that a single psychological impairment underlies the varied cognitive and behavioral features of autistic disorder (e.g., Jarrold, Butler, Cottington, & Jimenez, 2000). Brock, Brown, Boucher, and Rippon (2002) recently hypothesized that the central coherence deficits often observed in autistic disorder are due to impaired communication between localized and diffuse neural networks (i.e., temporal binding deficits). Although these theories contribute significantly to the description and our understanding of the clinical features of autistic disorder, the remainder of this chapter focuses on the physiological basis of the disorder.

Genetic Studies

In 1976, Hanson and Gottesman reported that genetic factors contributed very little, if at all, to childhood autism and schizophrenia. Nearly 30 years later, experts consistently report that autistic disorder is in fact predominately genetically based. Twin studies, for example, strongly support that autistic disorder is genetically determined. For example, Bailey et al. (1995) reported that 92% of a sample of monozygotic twins were concordant for autism compared to 0% of dizygotic twins. When a broader spectrum of autistic behaviors were considered, 60%

of monozygotic twins were concordant for the disorder versus 10% of the dizygotic pairs. In a twin study involving five Nordic countries (Denmark, Finland, Iceland, Norway, and Sweden), the concordance rate for autistic disorder was 91% for monozygotic twins and 0% for dizygotic twins (Steffenburg et al., 1989). Some researchers have speculated that twinning may be a risk factor in the etiology of autistic disorder, but Hallmayer et al. (2002) recently analyzed the rate of autistic disorder in twin births versus nontwin births and concluded that twinning itself is not an important risk factor in the development of the disorder. A number of chromosomes, chromosomal regions, and candidate genes, however, have been linked to autistic disorder, although no specific gene or group of genes has been identified as causing the disorder. Given the phenotypic variability of autistic disorder (and other pervasive developmental disorders), many researchers have suggested that autistic disorder has a complex inheritance and may involve anywhere from 10 to 100 genes (e.g., Bespalova and Buxbaum, 2003).

To date, chromosomes 1, 4, 2, 3, 6, 7, 13, 15, 16, 17, 19, 22, and X have been potentially linked to autistic disorder and, within each of the chromosomal regions, numerous candidate genes are currently under investigation as well (Auranen et al., 2000; IMGSAC, 2001). For example, on chromosome 7, candidate genes that have been linked in some studies to autistic disorder include FOXP2, RAY1/ST7, IMMP2L, and RELN, and on chromosome 15, genes UBE3A and GABRB3 (Muhle, Trentacoste, & Rapin, 2004). In general, findings have been inconsistent, with some studies reporting associations between polymorphisms of these genes and autistic disorder, while other studies have failed to find such associations. For example, the serotonin transporter gene is also located on chromosome 15 and polymorphisms of this gene have been linked to autistic disorder in several studies (e.g., Yirmiya et al., 2001) but not in others (e.g., Maestrini et al., 1999). Yirmiya et al. (2001) speculated that variants of the serotonin transporter gene may lead to enhanced serotonin reuptake, thereby accounting for the elevated serotonin levels found in many individuals with autistic disorder. Tordjman et al. (2001), however, reported that polymorphisms of the serotonin transporter gene did not differ between individuals with autistic disorder and their siblings and therefore may not convey risk for the disorder but instead may modify behaviors associated with the disorder. Similarly, Auranen and colleagues (2000) investigated ten chromosomal regions on several different chromosomes and reported that only one region on one chromosome (1p) increased susceptibility to autistic disorder. Shao et al. (2002), however, studied 52 families in which 2 or more family members had autistic disorder, and concluded that regions on chromosomes X, 2, 3, 7, 15, 18, and 19 were linked to the disorder.

Fragile X syndrome has also been associated with autistic disorder as some patients with the syndrome also develop autistic disorder (Petit et al., 1996). Shinahara and colleagues (2004) recently reported that a rare mutation in the gene usually associated with fragile X (FMR1) was present in a small percentage of individuals with autistic disorder but not in the control subjects. However, apparently only a very small percentage of autistic disorder, cases overall are associated with fragile X syndrome (Muhle, Trentacoste, & Rapin, 2004). The WNT2 gene, involved in cell growth and differentiation and located on chromosome 7, has received attention within the past few years since Wassink et al. (2001) reported that rare mutations of this gene significantly increased the susceptibility to autism. Subesquent studies, however, failed to find an association between variants of the WNT2 gene and autistic disorder (Buxbaum et al., 2002; Li et al., 2004; McCoy et al., 2002). Two additional genes on chromosome 7, the RELN and the HOXA1 gene that encode proteins critical in cell migration and connectivity, have also been implicated in autistic disorder. Persico et al. (2001), for example, reported that a specific polymorphism (i.e., longer triplet repeats) of the RELN was associated with increased vulnerability to autistic disorder in subjects from the United States and Italy. Similarly, Ingram et al. (2000) suggested that variants of the HOXA1 and HOXB1 genes increased susceptibility to autistic disorder. Other studies, however, have failed to support these associations (e.g., Bonora et al., 2003; Devlin et al., 2002; Krebs et al., 2002; Li et al., 2004). Additional candidate genes for autistic disorder such as the GABA receptor gene GABRB3 and genes on chromosome 2 have also been investigated, with conflicting results (Maestrini et al., 1999; Ramoz et al., 2004). Nurmi et al. (2003) recently suggested that chromosome 15 was linked to a subset of individuals with autistic disorder, namely those with savant talents.

In summary, familial and twin studies strongly support a genetic basis for autistic disorder. Although several chromosomal regions and candidate genes have been associated with the disorder, studies have produced conflicting results. To date, no single gene or group of genes has been identified as playing a definitive role in the etiology of autistic disorder. Part of the difficulty in identify genetic factors is that autistic disorder is a clinically heterogenous disorder. Goussè and colleagues (2002) have argued that progress in identifying genes implicated in autistic disorder will depend on more accurate descriptions of the various phenotypes associated with the disorder.

Neuroanatomical and Neuroimaging Studies

Postmortem and MRI

Various brain structures have been examined in both living individuals with autism and post-mortem samples. In general, postmortem studies have not found gross structural abnormalities in individuals with autistic disorder relative to control subjects. Williams and colleagues (1980) were among the first to examine postmortem tissue of four individuals with autism and mental retardation (ages 4, 14, 27, and 33 at death) and did not find evidence of cell loss or specific abnormalities. Similarly, Coleman, Romano, Lapham, and Simon (1985) counted the numbers of neurons and glial cells in the postmortem cerebral cortex of an individual with autistic disorder and found no differences in cell density relative to a control subject. Ritvo and colleagues (1986), however, examined brains of four individuals with autistic disorder and found that individuals with the disorder had significantly fewer neurons (Purkinje cells) in the cerebellum compared to control subjects. Likewise, Lee and colleagues (2002) compared nicotinic receptor densities in postmortem tissue of individuals with and without autistic disorder and found a near 50% reduction in the cerebellum of those with the disorder as well as substantial loss of Purkinje cells in the cerebellum. Interestingly, Fatemi et al. (2002) did not find a difference in cell density in postmortem cerebellum samples of five individuals with autistic disorder relative to control subjects but did find evidence that the size of these cells was reduced in individuals with the disorder. Specifically, the researchers reported that the average cross-sectional areas of Purkinje cells in the cerebellum of patients with autistic disorder were 24% smaller than control subjects, and the authors speculated that Purkinje cell atrophy may be characteristic of autistic disorder. Fatemi, Stary, Halt, and Realmuto (2001) hypothesized that cell migration problems and disturbances in proteins that help to regulate programmed cell death may be responsible for Purkinje cell abnormalities in the cerebellum. The researchers measured two proteins that are important in the process of cell migration and in reducing cellular death, known as Reelin and Bcl-2. Postmortem analysis of brain tissue revealed greater than 40% reductions of the protein Reelin and similar reductions of Bcl-2 levels in the cerebellum of individuals with autistic disorder. Fatemi et al. speculated that decreased levels of these two proteins may make the cerebellum particularly vulnerable to neuronal death and atrophy, and in turn affect cognitive and behavioral functioning.

Cellular abnormalities have also been found in cortical regions in individuals with autistic disorder. For example, Casanova and colleagues (2002) examined the arrangement of cells in the layers of the frontal and temporal cortex of postmortem tissue of individuals with and without autistic disorder and reported that individuals with autistic disorder had greater dispersion of cells and fewer cells per column than control subjects. Casanova, Buxhoeveden, and Gomez (2003) have proposed that a defect in these columns will affect excitatory input as well as inhibitory input to the cortex and subcortical structures, which could help to explain the increased prevalence of seizure disorders among individuals with autistic disorder. The reason for these structural cellular differences is unclear, but some researchers have suggested that neural cell adhesion molecules that contribute to cell migration and connectivity may be altered in individuals with autistic disorder and consequently interfere with normal brain development (Chih, Afridi, Clark, & Scheiffele, 2004). For example, Purcell et al. (2001) examined postmortem samples and found that one type of cell adhesion molecule (neural cell adhesion molecule, NCAM-180) was significantly decreased in brains of individuals with autistic disorder. Blood serum studies of living patients with autistic disorder have also reported decreased levels of neural cell adhesion molecules in individuals with autistic disorder relative to control subjects (e.g., Plioplys, Hemmens, & Regan, 1990). Nelson et al. (2001) reported that neonatal concentrations of several neurotrophins and neuropeptides (e.g., nerve growth factor, brain-derived neurotrophic factor, neuropeptide substance P) that are important in brain development were elevated in children with autistic spectrum disorders relative to children with mental retardation and control children. Although the relevance of these cellular abnormalities to the development and expression of autistic disorder remains to be determined, the findings support early neurodevelopmental dysfunction in patients with autistic disorder.

MRI

A number of MRI studies have reported enlarged brain volume (i.e., macroencephaly) in individuals with autistic disorder relative to subjects without the disorder (e.g., Gillberg & de Souza, 2002; Piven, Arndt, Bailey, & Andreasen, 1996). Fombonne et al. (1999) reported that approximately 20% of individuals with autistic disorder have unusually large head circumference (>97th percentile). Hardan and colleagues (2001) compared 16 high-functioning (i.e., nonmentally retarded) individuals with autistic disorder and control subjects and found that those with the disorder had increased brain volume including enlarged third ventricle volumes. It should be noted, however, that not all studies have found evidence of macrocephaly in autistic disorder—in fact, nearly 15% of individuals with autistic disorder have unusually small head circumference (<3rd percentile) (Fombonne et al, 1999). In a landmark study, Courchesne et al. (2001) studied 60 boys ages 2 to 16 with autistic disorder using MRI. Neonatal head circumferences indicated that overall brain volume was normal at birth; however, by ages 2 to 4 years, 90% of boys with the disorder had greater than average brain size and 37% were macroencephalic. With regard to the cerebellum, those with autistic disorder had reduced size, less gray matter, and smaller gray-to-white-matter ratios. Older children with autistic disorder had significantly less gray and white matter, however, which suggests that autistic disorder may be characterized by abnormal overgrowth of brain development during the first few years of life followed by disruptions in brain growth in later childhood. Overall, studies suggest that brain size is increased approximately 5% to 10% in individuals with autistic disorder (Schultz & Klin, 2002).

Studies have also found reduced cerebellar size (Murakami et al., 1989; Weber et al., 2000), reduced thalamic volume (Tsatsanis et al., 2003), reduced corpus callosum size (Egaas, Courchesne, & Saitoh, 1995; Hardan, Minshew, & Keshavan, 2000; Piven, Bailey, Ranson, & Arndt, 1997), and smaller as well as larger subcortical structures (Abell et al., 1999; Sparks et al., 2002). For example, Kates et al. (1998) compared MRI scans of twins discordant for autistic disorder and found that the twin with the disorder had a significantly smaller amygdala, caudate, hippocampus, and cerebellar lobes compared to the unaffected twin. Both twins, however, had significantly smaller frontal lobes than the control twins. More recently, Kates et al. (2004) compared seven twin pairs concordant for autistic disorder and nine twin pairs disconcordant for the disorder using MRI. Results revealed that twins concordant for autistic disorder had similar gray and white matter volumes. Both types of twins, however, had frontal, temporal, and occipital volumes that were significantly smaller compared to control subjects. Recently, a few studies have found a relationship between structural abnormalities and severity of impairment in autistic disorder. For example, using MRI, Elia and colleagues (2000) found a significant negative correlation between structural abnormalities and impaired performance on the Childhood Autism Rating Scale and the Psychoeducational Profile—Revised in a group of low-functioning boys with autistic disorder compared to control subjects.

According to a recent review by Schultz and Klin (2002), structural abnormalities of the limbic system appear to be particularly involved in autistic disorder and most notably include abnormalities in size, density, and connectivity of cells in this region. Given the importance of the limbic system in social and emotional regulation, in conjunction with the social and emotional deficits characteristic of autistic disorder, the limbic system and projecting systems have received a great deal of attention in the autism literature. Shaw and colleagues (2004) recently found that individuals without autistic disorder who acquired lesions of the amygdala congenitally or early in life, displayed significant impairments on tasks that involved theory of mind reasoning compared to subjects who acquired such lesions later in life. The researchers hypothesized that the amygdala plays a critical role in neural systems supporting theory of mind reasoning and is therefore implicated in autistic disorder. Aylward et al. (1999) found that the amygdala and hippocampus were significantly smaller compared to control subjects, and suggested that the reduction was likely due to underdevelopment of the limbic structures and neural connections to other brain regions. Recently, Rojas and colleagues (2004) used MRI to measure the hippocampus and amygdala in parents of children with autistic disorder and discovered that the hippocampal volume was significantly larger in these parents compared to adults who did not have children with the disorder. The researchers speculated that these findings support a potential genetic basis for hippocampal abnormalities in autism. However, it is important to note that this study did not measure hippocampal volume in the children with autistic disorder. Mundy (2003) proposed that neurodevelopmental disturbances of the pathways leading from limbic structures, especially the anterior cingulate, to the dorsal–medial–frontal cortex may interfere with attention and social interactions during infancy that are later manifested as disturbances in intersubjectivity and social cognition.

In a recent review of MRI studies in autistic disorder, Brambilla et al. (2003) also suggested that abnormalities of the cerebellum, limbic system, and pathways projecting from the frontal, parietal, and temporal cortices may underlie its pathophysiology. However, the researchers noted that MRI studies are often conflicting and many have reported no structural differences between subjects with and without autistic disorder. For example, Piven et al. (1998) studied MRI scans of 35 individuals with autistic disorder and 36 control subjects and found that the volume of the hippocampus did not differ between these groups. Similarly, Manes and colleagues (1999) found evidence of a smaller corpus callosum in individuals with autistic disorder, but no evidence of cerebellar abnormalities relative to control subjects. In addition, the amygdala is a highly complex structure and the manner in which the amygdala may be involved in autistic disorder is likely equally complex. Furthermore, reductions of amygdala volume have been found in individuals with other disorders such as bipolar disorder (Blumberg et al., 2003) and are therefore not unique to autistic disorder. In addition, Herbert et al. (2004)

reported that individuals with developmental language disorder had increased brain volume patterns that were similar to those of subjects with autistic disorder.

In summary, postmortem and MRI studies suggest that individuals with autistic disorder tend to have enlarged white matter volumes and reduced limbic system structures relative to comparison subjects. In addition, cell density and arrangement are often abnormal in the cerebellum of subjects with the disorder although the reason for these cellular changes is poorly understood. These structural and cellular differences are not reported by all studies, however, and additional research is needed to understand the origin of these differences as well as their relationship to the clinical symptoms of autistic disorder. It is also critical to emphasize that the anatomical studies are correlational in nature and do not reveal whether the anatomical differences are related to the expression of the disorder or whether the symptoms of autism influence the development of anatomical structures. In addition, it is possible that the anatomical findings are unrelated to the behavioral symptoms and reflect disturbances elsewhere in the brain.

PET, SPECT, and fMRI Studies

A plethora of neuroimaging studies have been conducted with individuals with autistic disorder and, similar to other disorders, the results have been conflicting. For example, George and colleagues (1992) reported that overall blood perfusion was significantly decreased in subjects with autistic disorder relative to control subjects, whereas Rumsey et al. (1985) reported that subjects with autistic disorder had significantly elevated glucose metabolism in widespread regions of the brain. Furthermore, according to Rumsey et al., no specific brain region showed reduced glucose metabolism in individuals with autistic disorder relative to control subjects. Hazlett et al. (2004), however, recently reported that glucose metabolism was significantly lower in the medial frontal lobes (but not the lateral regions) and significantly higher in occipital and parietal regions in individuals with autistic disorder relative to control subjects. Siegel and colleagues (1995) also reported that adults with a history of infantile autism had lower glucose metabolism in the medial frontal lobes while performing an attention task relative to control subjects. Zilbovicius et al. (1992) measured rCBF in 21 children with autistic disorder and control children and reported no differences between these groups. In a later study, however, Zilbovicius et al. (1995) measured rCBF in a group of children with autistic disorder when they were between 3 and 4 years of age and 3 years later. Results revealed that children with the disorder initially had decreased rCBF in the frontal regions but this attained normal values by ages 6 to 7 compared to control subjects. Recently, Zilbovicius et al. (2000) reported that 76% of children with autistic disorder showed increased rCBF in the temporal lobes relative to control children.

Hashimoto et al. (2000) found that individuals with autistic disorder had higher rCBF in the right temporal and right parietal lobes compared to their left temporal and parietal lobes, but subjects without the disorder did not show a lateralized difference in rCBF. Compared to the control group, subjects with autistic disorder exhibited reduced blood flow in the dorso–medio–lateral frontal areas as well as the temporal lobes. Ohnishi et al. (2000) reported reduced rCBF in the left prefrontal cortex, bilateral insula, and superior temporal gyri in children with autistic disorder relative to control children. Horwitz and colleagues (1988) also reported that individuals with autistic disorder displayed an activation pattern that differed from control subjects with respect to cortical and subcortical regions, and suggested that functional impairments exist between systems that subserve directed attention and social interactions.

With regard to rCBF and specific structures, Heh et al. (1989) were among the first to explore whether individuals with autistic disorder had reduced blood flow in the cerebellum given the previous findings of reduced Purkinje cells. Contrary to expectations, the results showed no significant difference between individuals with and without the disorder. Allen and Courchesne (2003) used fMRI to study activation patterns of the cerebellum while eight subjects with autistic disorder and comparison subjects performed a visual attention task and a motor function (pressing a button). Results revealed that subjects with autistic disorder showed significantly greater activation of the cerebellum during the motor task than control subjects and significantly less cerebellar activation than control subjects during the attention task. Haznedar et al. (2000) compared the glucose metabolism of 17 individuals with autism spectrum disorders relative to control subjects. Results revealed those with autism spectrum disorders had significantly reduced glucose metabolism in the anterior and posterior cingulate gyrus but not in the amygdala or hippocampus. Wilcox et al. (2002) found significantly reduced blood flow in the prefrontal areas of individuals with autistic disorder compared to control subjects, and this hypoperfusion increased in the left temporal lobe with age in individuals with the disorder. The researchers hypothesized that the prefrontal and language related regions are dysfunctional in individuals with autistic disorder at an early age, which interferes with the subsequent normal development of language. Recent studies also suggest that the pattern of brain activation is different in individuals with autistic disorder when presented with facial stimuli depicting emotions. For example, Hall, Szechtman, and Nahmias (2003) compared rCBF in eight high-functioning males with autistic disorder and eight control subjects during an emotion-recognition task. Results indicated individuals with autistic disorder had lower rCBF in the inferior frontal regions and higher rCBF in the anterior cingulate and thalamus than the control subjects.

In summary, functional imaging studies have found evidence of both decreased and increased glucose metabolism and blood flow in individuals with autistic disorder relative to control subjects, and overall these findings support the theory of functional brain differences in autistic disorder. Similar to structural findings, functional disturbances of limbic regions and projecting cortical pathways as well as the cerebellum are most often implicated in autistic disorder. It is important to note, however, that studies with other disorders such as Alzheimer's disease and schizophrenia have also found decreased glucose metabolism and rCBF in regions similar to those with autistic disorder (e.g., Paradiso et al., 2003).

Additional Theories

Prenatal Factors, Viruses, Vaccines, Dietary Deficiencies

In addition to genetic, structural, and functional studies of autistic disorder, researchers have explored other potential causes of autistic disorder. For example, a number of studies have reported a higher incidence of pregnancy and delivery complications (e.g., maternal vaginal infection and uterine bleeding) in mothers of children with autistic disorder (Juul-Dam, Townsend, & Courchesne, 2001) compared to the general population. Yamashita and colleagues (2003) suggested that cytomegalovirus infection during the third trimester may increase risk of autistic disorder, and Barak et al. (1999) suggested that viral encephalitis and viral meningitis also increase the risk. In addition to prenatal factors, there is an ongoing debate as to whether postnatal vaccinations (e.g., measles mumps rubella, or MMR) can cause autistic disorder. According to numerous studies, however, epidemiological evidence does *not* support an association between MMR vaccination and autistic disorder (e.g., Hviid, Stellfeld, Wohlfahrt, & Melbye, 2003; Miller, 2003; Phelan, 2002; Takahashi, 2003). Others have suggested that immunological abnormalities such as decreased T and B cells, macrophages, and natural killer cells are implicated in the pathogenesis of autistic disorder (e.g., Gupta, 2000). Torres (2003) hypothesized that medications used to control infectious fevers (e.g., acetaminophen) in pregnant women or in young children may interfere with normal immunological development and lead to neurodevelopmental disorders including autistic disorder. Exposure to mercury through vaccines containing a mercury-based preservative or during prenatal development has also been hypothesized to play a role in autistic disorder, although research indicates that most infants who were immunized with mercury-tainted vaccines do not develop neurodevelopmental side effects (Holmes, Blaxill, & Haley, 2003). Biotin deficiency, phenylketonuria, choline, and creatine abormalities have also been implicated in autistic disorder in rare cases but are not associated with the majority of individuals with the disorder (Baieli, Pavone, Meli, Fiumara, & Coleman, 2003; Sokol et al., 2002; Zaffanello, Zamboni, Fontana, Zoccante, & Tato, 2003). Overall, evidence suggests that a variety of prenatal and postnatal factors have been implicated in some individuals with autistic disorder but none of these factors are regarded as causal agents. Empirical studies are needed to further explore these and other etiologic hypotheses of autistic disorder.

Serotonin Dysregulation

According to Sodhi and Sanders-Bush (2004), serotonin facilitates prenatal brain development and interacts with other neurotransmitters systems and brain growth factors that contribute to normal brain development. Therefore, dysregulation of the serotonergic system early in life may lead to structural and functional impairments and contribute to CNS disorders such as autistic disorder. A number of studies have found that brain serotonin synthesis is higher in individuals with autistic disorder than control subjects (Posey & McDougle, 2001). Cohen et al. (1977), for example, found higher levels of serotonin metabolites but not dopamine metabolites in the cerebral spinal fluid of children with autistic disorder relative to control children. Leckman et al. (1980), however, did not find serotonin or dopamine cerebral spinal fluid metabolite differences among children with autism, schizophrenia, or controls. Chugani et al. (1999) compared serotonin synthesis in children with autism to children without the disorder. Results indicated that children with autistic disorder had higher serotonin levels than children without the disorder and this level of synthesis increased to a level one and a half times normal by age 15. The synthesis of serotonin depends on a number of factors including the number of serotonergic synapses. The findings by Chugani and colleagues suggest that children with autistic disorder do not undergo the normal pruning of serotonergic synapses as do children without the disorder. Coutinho et al. (2004) reported polymorphisms of the serotonin transporter gene (SLC6A4) were associated with high levels of platelet serotonin in patients with autistic disorder and suggested that this gene may interact with other genes (or possibly environmental factors) to produce abnormally high serotonin levels.

Pharmacological and Additional Interventions

Nonpharmacological behavioral interventions that target communication and social behaviors while reducing problem behavior are considered primary and potentially effective forms of intervention of autistic disorder, and excellent reviews of this literature are available (Campbell, 2003; Goldstein, 2002; Horner et al., 2002; McConnell, 2002). Alternative interventions such as dietary restrictions, supplements, and immune therapies are highly controversial; studies have produced conflicting results. Levy and colleagues (2003) reviewed 284 charts of children with autistic disorder treated at a hospital in Pennsylvania and found that greater than 30% were using some type of complementary alternative medicine. In a recent review, Kidd (2002) reported that omega-3 fatty acids, vitamins, nutrient supplements, and detoxification of heavy metals can have marked benefits in individuals with autistic disorder. Other studies have reported improvement in autistic behavior following adherence to special diets (e.g., ketogenic diet) (Evangeliou et al., 2003; Knivsberg, Reichelt, Høien, & Nødland, 2002). As Millward and colleagues (2004) noted, however, many of these studies are characterized by serious methodological problems such as small sample sizes and lack of randomized, controlled trials. The hormone secretin has also been studied in the treatment of autistic disorder and, again, results have been conflicting with some studies reporting beneficial effects (e.g., Chez et al., 2000) while other well-designed studies have found secretin is no more effective than placebo (Owley et al., 2001).

A number of medications are used as adjunctive treatments for autistic disorder, and most are used to reduce behavioral problems associated with the disorder such as aggressiveness, agitation, hyperactivity, stereotypies (repetitive behavior) and self-injurious behavior. Antipsychotic medications such as haloperidol and risperidone have been found to reduce hyperactive, aggressive, and self-injurious behavior in individuals with autistic disorder, including preschoolers (e.g., Masi, Cosenza, Mucci, & Brovedani, 2003; McCracken et al., 2002). Side effects of antipsychotic medications are similar in children and adults: increased appetite and weight gain, extrapyramidal symptoms, and loss of strength (Kemner et al., 2002). In addition, stimulants such as methylphenidate have been found to decrease hyperactivity, inappropriate speech, and stereotypies in some children with autistic disorder (Handen, Johnson, & Lubetsky, 2000), although side effects such as irritability and social withdrawal were observed in some children. Opiate antagonists such as naltrexone are often used to reduce sterotyped and ritualistic behaviors in individuals with autistic disorder although less is known about their effectiveness and safety (Chabane, Leboyer, & Mouren-Simeoni, 2000). Feldman, Kolmen, and Gonzaga (1999) evaluated the effects of naltrexone on the communication skills of 24 children with autistic disorder and concluded that the drug did not lead to improvement in communication skills. Clomipramine and other antidepressant drugs such as SSRIs have also been investigated, and several studies have reported decreased stereotypies, repetitive behavior, and hyperactive behavior in children with autistic disorder (McDougle & Posey, 2002; Strauss, Unis, Cowan, Dawson, & Dager, 2002).

Aman and Langworthy (2000) recently reviewed 41 pharmacological studies aimed at reducing symptoms such as hyperactivity in children with autistic disorder and other pervasive developmental disorders. The researchers concluded that empirical evidence supported the use of antipsychotic medications, serotonin reuptake inhibitors, and naltrexone to decrease hyperactivity symptoms in this population but that questions remained concerning the effectiveness of opiate blockers, psychostimulants, antianxiety drugs, and alpha adrenergic agonists. In another review, McDougle and Posey (2002) emphasized the need for larger, placebo-controlled trials as well as longitudinal studies of medications commonly used in the treatment of autistic disorder. In light of research that found that 55% of children, adolescents, and adults with autistic disorder and other pervasive developmental disorders were taking antipsychotics, antidepressants, or stimulants, and 29% were taking two or more types of medications, additional studies are sorely needed to understand the safety and effectiveness of these medications with individuals with autistic disorder (Martin, Scahill, Klin, & Volkmar, 1999).

SUMMARY

Autistic disorder is characterized by significant impairments in communication and social relationships as well as a restricted repertoire of interests and activities. Research strongly supports a genetic basis for the disorder although other variables such as prenatal factors may also play a role in its development. Postmortem and anatomical studies have produced conflicting results but generally indicate abnormal cellular development, particularly in the cerebellum, subcortical, and frontal regions. Functional studies such as PET, fMRI, and SPECT also support glucose and blood flow differences in individuals with autistic disorder although the cause of these differences remains to be determined. Pharmacological interventions play a secondary role to behavioral interventions in the treatment of autistic disorder, and more research is needed to better understand the effects and safety of medications used to treat the aggressive, repetitive, and self-injurious behaviors characteristic of some individuals with autistic disorder.

LEARNING DISABILITIES

Learning disabilities can be defined in both a broad and narrow sense and various definitions of learning disabilities exist (Sattler & Weyandt, 2002). In general, learning disabilities involve a disorder in learning that cannot be attributed to medical, emotional, or environmental causes, despite at least average intellectual abilities. The DSM IV-TR (2000) includes four main types of learning disorders: reading disorder, mathematics disorder, disorder of written expression, and learning disorder not otherwise specified (see Table 9.5). Given the complexity and breadth of knowledge available concerning learning disabilities, broad coverage of learning disabilities is beyond the scope of this chapter. A brief general discussion follows.

Learning disabilities are estimated to affect 2 to 10% of the general population and approximately 5% of the school-age population (DSM IV-TR, 2000). The most common type of learning disability, reading disability, was described by Orton in 1928. Reading disability affects approximately 4% of school-age children and is significantly more common in boys than girls (DSM IV-TR, 2000; Rutter et al., 2004). Learning disabilities are chronic in nature although specific skills and academic performance can be significantly improved with appropriate interventions (Kronenberger & Dunn, 2003). Developmental studies suggest that reading disability can be predicted with moderate accuracy by age 5 (Pennington & Lefly, 2001) and perhaps as early as infancy. Molfese (2000), for example, found that auditory event-related potentials in newborn infants could reliably identify those children who 8 years later were characterized as normal, poor, or disabled readers. A number of studies have documented that deficits in phonemic awareness in early childhood are associated with reading disability (e.g. Betourne & Friel-Patti, 2003; Torgesen, Wagner, & Rashotte, 1994).

Genetic Studies

Similar to other disorders of childhood origin, twin and familial studies suggest that learning disabilities have a strong genetic component. For example, concordance rates for monozygotic and dizygotic twins consistently indicate that learning disabilities are more common in monozygotic twins, with rates varying from .91 to 1 and .45 to .52, respectively (Alarcón & DeFries, 1997; Brooks, Fulker, & DeFries, 1990; DeFries & Light, 1996). Wadsworth, Olson, Pennington, and DeFries (2000) suggested that genetic influences may be more prominent in children with a reading disability and higher IQs than children with lower IQs. Willcutt, Pennington, and DeFries (2000) reported substantial overlap between inattention symptoms and reading disability they suggested was due to the same genetic factors. With respect to specific chromosomes and genes, a number of candidate genes have been investigated that vary according to the type of learning disability investigated. Pennington (1999) emphasized that specific genes for dyslexia or reading skill are unlikely to be identified but, instead, genes

TABLE 9.5

Diagnostic Criteria for Learning Disabilities (DSM IV-TR, 2000)

Diagnostic Criteria for 315.00 Reading Disorder

A. Reading achievement, as measured by individually administered standardized tests of reading accuracy or comprehension, is substantially below that expected given the person's chronological age, measured intelligence, and age-appropriate education.

B. The disturbance in Criterion A significantly interferes with academic achievement or activities of daily living that require reading skills.

C. If a sensory deficit is present, the reading difficulties are in excess of those usually associated with it.

Coding note: If a general medical (e.g., neurological) condition or sensory deficit is present, code the condition on Axis III.

Diagnostic Criteria for 315.1 Mathematics Disorder

A. Mathematical ability, as measured by individually administered standardized tests, is substantially below that expected given the person's chronological age, measured intelligence, and age-appropriate education.

B. The disturbance in Criterion A significantly interferes with academic achievement or activities of daily living that require mathematical ability.

C. If a sensory deficit is present, the difficulties in mathematic ability are in excess of those usually associated with it.

Coding note: If a general medical (e.g., neurological) condition or sensory deficit is present, code the condition on Axis III.

Diagnostic Criteria for 315.2 Disorder of Written Expression

A. Writing skills, as measured by individually administered standardized tests (or functional assessments of writing skills), are substantially below that expected given the person's chronological age, measured intelligence, and age-appropriate education.

B. The disturbance in Criterion A significantly interferes with academic achievement or activities of daily living that require the composition of written texts (e.g., writing grammatically correct sentences and organized paragraphs).

C. If a sensory deficit is present, the difficulties in writing skills are in excess of those usually associated with it.

Coding note: If a general medical (e.g., neurological) condition or sensory deficit is present, code the condition on Axis III.

315.9 Learning Disorder Not Otherwise Specified

---

that lead to abnormal development of brain regions and networks critical for reading. In this regard, chromosomes 2, 6, 15, and 18 have all received a great deal of attention and various regions and genes on these chromosomes have been linked to reading disability (Fisher et al., 2002; Francks et al., 2002; Grigorenko et al., 1997; Kaplan et al., 2002). Gilger and Kaplan (2001) suggested that genetic in conjunction with environmental factors may contribute to atypical brain development which may be manifested as disorders in learning.

Postmortem, MRI, PET Studies

Postmortem, anatomical, and functional imaging studies of subjects with learning disabilities have produced mixed findings, and most of the studies have been conducted with individuals with reading disabilities. For example, Galaburda and colleagues (1985) examined the brains of four individuals who had developmental dyslexia (ages 14, 20, 20, and 32). Results revealed that all four patients had alterations in brain asymmetry, with the right hemisphere larger than the left in the region of the planum temporale. The planum temporale is a triangular-shaped area located on the superior temporal gyrus, and in most individuals this area in the left hemisphere is larger than the right. Given the location of the planum temporale and its connection with Wernicke's area and the auditory cortex, the planum temporale is believed to play a critical role in language functions (Shapleske, Rossell, Woodruff, & David, 1999). Results of the Galaburda study also revealed that all four patients had cellular abnormalities at the level of the cortex including neuronal ectopias (abnormal positioning of neurons). Two patients had an area of the cortex that had only four layers instead of six (i.e., micropolygyria). Additional postmortem studies of patients with dyslexia have reported significantly smaller neurons in the left hemisphere (medial geniculate nuclei), abnormal arrangement of neurons, and lack of normal asymmetry of neuronal size (Galaburda, Menard, & Rosen, 1994; Jenner, Rosen, & Galaburda, 1999; Livingstone, Rosen, Drislane, & Galaburda, 1991). Pennington et al. (1999) also reported cortical abnormalities in individuals with reading disability compared to control subjects.

Recent MRI studies have also found structural differences between subjects with and without reading problems. For example, Casanova, Araque, Giedd, and Rumsey (2004) reported significantly smaller total cerebral volume and a reduction in gyri volume in 16 individuals with dyslexia compared to control subjects. Larsen and colleagues (1990) reported that 70% of subjects with dyslexia had an abnormal symmetry of the planum temporale while only 30% of control subjects had this pattern of symmetry (i.e., in most subjects the left was larger than right). In a later study, however, Larsen, Hoien, Lundberg, and Odegaard (1992) did not find structural or symmetry differences between subjects with and without dyslexia, nor did the size of the corpus callosum differ between these groups. Schultz et al. (1994) used MRI to study 17 children with dyslexia and also reported no significant differences between children with and without dyslexia with respect to the size and symmetry of the planum temporale. In a review of the literature on dyslexia and the planum temporale, Eckert and Leonard (2000) noted the inconsistencies across imaging studies and suggested that these inconsistencies may be due to sex differences, cognitive ability, differences in imaging techniques, and diagnostic criteria. It is also important to note that size reductions of the planum temporale have been found in patients with schizophrenia (Kwon et al., 1999) as well as Down's syndrome (Frangou et al., 1997).

Functional studies including fMRI, PET, and SPECT have found that individuals without reading disabilities show increased blood flow in the left temporal lobe (superior posterotemporal regions) while subjects with reading disability tend to activate different regions (temporoparietal region; Flowers, Wood, & Naylor, 1991). Gross-Glenn and colleagues (1991) studied glucose metabolism patterns in adults with a history of childhood dyslexia and found different areas of activation as well as more bilateral activation in subjects with dyslexia relative to control subjects. Brunswick et al. (1999) compared PET scans of adults with and without dyslexia during a reading-aloud experiment and found that those with dyslexia showed less activation in the regions associated with language (left posterior inferior temporal cortex, left thalamus, and left cerebellum). Similarly, Paulesu et al. (1996) compared PET scans of adults with and without dyslexia during a rhyming and visual short-term memory task and found that those with dyslexia had substantially different patterns of brain activation. The researchers suggested that individuals with dyslexia have defective phonological systems due to connectivity aberrations between anterior and posterior language areas. A similar study was conducted by Temple et al. (2001) with children with dyslexia and results were consistent with Paulesu et al. (2001). Collectively, these studies suggest that areas associated with language processing are compromised in individuals with reading disability and may reflect abnormal connectivity between these regions due to genetic or neurodevelopmental factors (Démonet, Taylor, & Chaix, 2004; Semrud-Clikeman, 1997).

Although learning disabilities are generally considered chronic conditions (DSM IV-TR, 2000), recent studies suggest that partial remediation of deficits may be possible and these improvements may be due to changes in brain activation patterns. For example, Merzenich et al. (1996) studied the effects of adaptive training exercises (i.e., audiovisual games) with children ages 5 to 10 who had been diagnosed with language-based learning impairments. The training exercises were conducted over a 4-week period and designed to improve temporal processing skills. Results indicated markedly improvements in the children's abilities to recognize fast and brief squences of speech and nonspeech sounds. Small and colleagues (1998) used fMRI to study brain activation patterns in a female who had acquired a reading disorder subsequent to a stroke. fMRI scans taken before and after a reading therapy program showed a shift in activation from the left angular gyrus to the left lingual gyrus. The researchers interpreted the findings as evidence that brain physiology can be altered with specific interventions that target regions typically involved in language and reading. Recently, Temple et al. (2003) conducted a landmark study in which fMRI scans were conducted with 20 children with dyslexia before and after a remediation program designed to target auditory processing and oral language skills. Prior to the training, children with dyslexia had reduced activity in a number of brain regions compared to normal reading children, and these regions increased in activation after remediation (left temporoparietal coretx, inferior frontal gyrus). Increased activity also observed in a number of additional regions was associated with improved reading and language performance. Overall, these findings suggest that physiological changes are possible with behavioral remediation techniques and these changes are associated with improved reading performance. Additional fMRI or PET studies are needed that compare scans and the performance of individuals with reading disabilities who receive and do not receive remediation training with repeated scans over time, as well as a comparison of different types of interventions.

SUMMARY

Collectively, twin, molecular genetics, anatomical, and neuroimaging studies support a physiological basis for learning disabilities, particularly reading disability. Similar to other disorders of childhood, a gene or group of genes has not been conclusively linked to the etiology of learning disabilities although several candidate genes are currently under study. Anatomical and functional studies suggest that the brain regions involved in language are compromised in individuals with reading disability, particularly areas of the left temporal lobe, and consequently individuals with reading disability process language-related information differently than those without the disorder. Recent studies suggest that it may be possible to partially remediate language and reading deficits in children with specially designed training programs, but additional research is needed to further explore this hypothesis.

References

Aarsland, D., Larsen, J. P., Lim, N. G., Janvin, C., Karlsen, K., Tandberg, E., et al. (1999). Range of neuropsychiatric disturbances in patients with Parkinson's disease. *Journal of Neurology, Neurosurgery, and Psychiatry, 67*, 492–496.

Aarsland, D., Larsen, P. J., Lim, N. G., Janvin, C., Karlsen, K., Tandberg, E., & Cummings, J. L. (1999). Range of neuropsychiatric disturbances in patients with Parkinson's disease. *Journal of Neurology, Neurosurgery, and Psychiatry, 67*, 492–496.

Aarsland, D., Larsen, J. P., Waage, O., & Langeveld, J. H. (1997). Maintenance electroconvulsive therapy for Parkinson's disease. *Convulsive Therapy, 13*, 274–277.

Abbott, A. (2003). British panel bans use of antidepressant to treat children. *Nature, 423*, 792.

Abbott, R. D., Petrovitch, H., White, L. R., Masaki, K. H., Tanner, C. M., Curb, J. D., et al. (2001). Frequency of bowel movements and the future risk of Parkinson's disease. *Neurology, 57*, 456–462.

Abbott, R. D., Ross, G. W., White, L. R., Nelson, J. S., Masaki, K. H., Tanner, C. M., et al. (2002). Midlife adiposity and the future risk of Parkinson's disease. *Neurology, 59*, 1051–1057.

Abbott, R. D., Ross, G. W., White, L. R., Sanderson, W. T., Burchfiel, C. M., Kashon, M., et al. (2003). Environmental, life-style, and physical precursors of clinical Parkinson's disease: Recent findings from the Honolulu–Asia Aging Study. *Journal of Neurology, 250*, 30–39.

Abe, Y., Kachi, T., Kato, T., Arahata, Y., Yamada, T., Washimi, Y., et al. (2003). Occipital hypoperfusion in Parkinson's disease without dementia: Correlation to impaired cortical visual processing. *Journal of Neurology, Neurosurgery, and Psychiatry, 74*, 419–422.

Abell, F., Krams, M., Ashburner, J., Passingham, R., Friston, K., Frackowiak, R., et al. (1999). The neuroanatomy of autism: A voxel-based whole brain analysis of structural scans. *NeuroReport, 10*, 1647–1651.

Abi-Dargham, A., Krystal, J. H., Anjilvel, S., Scanley, B. E., Zoghbi, S., Baldwin, R. M., et al. (1998). Alterations of benzodiazepine receptors in type II alcoholic subjects measured with SPECT and [123I]iomazenil. *American Journal of Psychiatry, 155*, 1550–1555.

Abi-Dargham, A., Rodenhiser, J., Printz, D., Zea-Ponce, Y., Gil, R., Kegeles, L. S., et al. (2000). Increased baseline occupancy of D2 receptors by dopamine in schizophrenia. *Proceedings of the National Academy of Sciences, 97*, 8104–8109.

Abramowitz, J. S., Franklin, M. E., Schwartz, S. A., & Furr, J. M. (2003). Symptom presentation and outcome of cognitive-behavioral therapy for obsessive-compulsive disorder. *Journal of Consulting and Clinical Psychology, 71*, 1049–1057.

Abramowitz, J. S., Huppert, J. D., Cohen, A. B., Tolin, D. F., & Cahill, S. P. (2002). Religious obsessions and compulsions in a non-clinical sample: The Penn Inventory of Scrupulosity (PIOS). *Behaviour Research and Therapy, 40*, 825–838.

Abramowitz, J. S., Schwartz, S. A., Moore, K. M., & Luenzmann, K. R. (2003). Obsessive-compulsive symptoms in pregnancy and the puerperium: A review of the literature. *Journal of Anxiety Disorders, 17*, 461–478.

Abrams, R. (2000). Electroconvulsive therapy requires higher dosage levels: Food and Drug Administration action is required. *Archives of General Psychiatry, 57*, 445–446.

Acosta, M. T., & Pearl, R. L. (2003). The neurobiology of autism: New pieces of the puzzle. *Current Neurology and Neuroscience Reports, 3*, 149–156.

Adams, W. (1981). Lack of behavioral effects from Feingold diet violations. *Perception and Motor Skills, 52*, 307–313.

Addolorato, G., Caputo, F., Capristo, E., Domenicali, M., Bernardi, M., Janiri, L., et al. (2002). Baclofen efficacy in reducing alcohol craving and intake: A preliminary double-blind randomized controlled study. *Alcohol and Alcoholism, 37*, 504–508.

ADHD Molecular Genetics Network. (2002). Report from the third international meeting of the Attention-Deficit Hyperactivity Disorder Molecular Genetics Network. *American Journal of Medical Genetics, 114*, 272–276.

Adinoff, B., Devous, M. D., Best, S. E., Harris, T. S., Chandler, P., Frock, S. D., et al. (2003). Regional cerebral blood flow in female cocaine-addicted subjects following limbic activation. *Drug and Alcohol Dependence, 71*, 255–268.

Adler, C. M., McDonough-Ryan, P., Sax, K. W., Holland, S. K., Arndt, S., & Strakowski, S. M. (2000). fMRI of neuronal activation with symptom provocation in unmedicated patients with obsessive compulsive disorder. *Journal of Psychiatric Research, 34*, 317–324.

Agargün, M. Y., Algün, E., Sekeroglu, R., Kara, H., & Tarakçioglu, M. (1998). Low cholesterol level in patients with panic disorder: The association with major depression. *Journal of Affective Disorders, 50*, 29–32.

Aghajanian, G. K., Kogan, J. H., & Moghaddam, B. (1994). Opiate withdrawal increases glutamate and aspartate efflux in the locus coerleus: An in vivo microdialysis study. *Brain Research, 636*, 126–130.

Aisen, P. S., & Davis, K. L. (1994). Inflammatory mechanisms in Alzheimer's disease: Implications for therapy. *American Journal of Psychiatry, 151*, 1105–1113.

Aisen, P. S., Davis, K. L., Berg, J. D., Schefer, K., Campell, K., Thomas, R. G., et al. (2000). A randomized controlled trial of prednisone in Alzheimer's disease. *Neurology, 54*, 588–593.

Akbarian, S., Huntsman, M. M., Kim, J. J., Tafazzoli, A., Potkin, S. G., Bunney, W. E. Jr., et al. (1995). GABAA receptor subunit gene expression in human prefrontal cortex: Comparison of schizophrenics and controls. *Cerebral Cortex, 5*, 550–560.

Akiyoshi, J., Hieda, K., Aoki, Y., & Nagayama, H. (2003). Frontal brain hypoactivity as a biological substrate of anxiety in patients with panic disorders. *Neuropsychobiology, 47*, 165–170.

Alarcón, M., & DeFries, J. C. (1997). Reading performance and general cognitive ability in twins with reading difficulties and control pairs. *Personality and Individual Differences, 22*, 793–803.

Alberts-Corush, J., Firestone, P., & Goodman, J. T. (1986). Attention and impulsivity characteristics of the biological and adoptive parents of hyperactive and normal control children. *American Journal of Orthopsychiatry, 56*, 413–423.

Albertson, D. N., Pruetz, B., Schmidt, C. J., Kuhn, D. M., Kapatos, G., & Bannon, M. J. (2004). Gene expression profile of the nucleus accumbens of human cocaine abusers: Evidence for dysregulation of myelin. *Journal of Neurochemistry, 88*, 1211–1219.

Albin, R. L., Koeppe, R. A., Bohnen, N. I., Nichols, T. E., Meyer, P., Wernette, K., et al. (2003). Increased ventral striatal monoaminergic innervation in Tourette syndrome. *Neurology, 61*, 310–315.

Alegret, M., Junqué, C., Valldeoriola, F., Vendrell, P., Martí, M. J., & Tolosa, E. (2001). Obsessive-compulsive symptoms in Parkinson's disease. *Journal of Neurology, Neurosurgery, and Psychiatry, 70*, 394–396.

Alevizos, B., Lykouras, L., Zervas, I. M., & Christodoulou, G. N. (2002). Risperidone-induced obsessive-compulsive symptoms: A series of six cases. *Journal of Clinical Psychopharmacology, 22*, 461–467.

Ali, S., & Milev, R. (2003). Switch to mania upon discontinuation of antidepressants in patients with mood disorders: A review of the literature. *Canadian Journal of Psychiatry, 48*, 258–264.

Ali, S. O., Denicoff, K. D., Altshuler, L. L., Hauser, P., Li, X., Conrad, A. J., et al. (2001). Relationship between prior course of illness and neuroanatomic structures in bipolar disorder. *Neuropsychiatry, Neuropsychology, and Behavioral Neurology, 14*, 227–232.

Allen, G. & Courchesne, E. (2003). Differential effects of developmental cerebellar abnormality on cognitive and motor functions in the cerebellum: An fMRI study of autism. *American Journal of Psychiatry, 160*, 262–273.

Almeida, O. P., Burton, E. J., McKeith, I., Gholkar, A., Burn, D., & O'Brien, J. T. (2003). MRI study of caudate nucleus volume in Parkinson's disease with and without dementia with Lewy bodies and Alzheimer's disease. *Dementia and Geriatric Cognitive Disorders, 16*, 57–63.

Al-Mousawi, A. H., Evans, N., Ebmeier, K. P., Roeda, D., Chaloner, F., & Ashcroft, G. W. (1996). Limbic dysfunction in schizophrenia and mania. A study using 18F-labelled fluorodeoxyglucose and positron emission tomography. *British Journal of Psychiatry, 169*, 509–516.

Alsobrook, J. P. II, Zohar, A. H., Leboyer, M., Chabane, N., Ebstein, R. P., & Pauls, D. L. (2002). Association between the COMT locus and obsessive-compulsive disorder in females but not males. *American Journal of Medical Genetics, 114*, 116–120.

Altar, C. A., Cai, N., Bliven, T., Juhasz, M., Conner, J. M., Acheson, A. L., et al. (1997). Anterograde transport of brain-derived neurotrophic factor and its role in the brain. *Nature, 389*, 85–860.

Altar, C. A., Whitehead, R. E., Chen, R., Wortwein, G., & Madsen, T. M. (2003). Effects of electroconvulsive seizures and antidepressant drugs on brain-derived neurotrophic factor protein in rat brain. *Biological Psychiatry, 54*, 703–709.

Altemus, M., Swedo, S. E., Leonard, H. L., Richter, D., Rubinow, D. R., Potter, W. Z., et al. (1994). Changes in cerebrospinal fluid neurochemistry during treatment of obsessive-compulsive disorder with clomipramine. *Archives of General Psychiatry, 51*, 794–803.

Altshuler, L. L. (1993). Bipolar disorder: Are repeated episodes associated with neuroanatomic and cognitive changes? *Biological Psychiatry, 33*, 563–565.

Altshuler, L. L., Bartzokis, G., Grieder, T., Curran, J., & Mintz, J. (1998). Amygdala enlargement in bipolar disorder and hippocampal reduction in schizophrenia: An MRI study demonstrating neuroanatomic specificity. *Archives of General Psychiatry, 55*, 663–664.

Aman, M. G., & Langworthy, K. S. (2000). Pharmacotherapy for hyperactivity in children with autism and other pervasive developmental disorders. *Journal of Autism and Developmental Disorders, 30*, 451–459.

American Psychiatric Association (1994). *Diagnostic and statistical manual of mental disorders* (4th ed.). Washington, DC: author.

American Psychiatric Association (2000). *Diagnostic and statistical manual of mental disorders* (4th ed. text revision). Washington, DC: Author.

American Psychiatric Association (2001). *The practice of electroconvulsive therapy: Recommendations for treatment, training, and privileging, 2nd edition.* A task force report of the American Psychiatric Association. Washington, DC: American Psychiatric Association.

Anand, A., & Shekhar, A. (2003). Brain imaging studies in mood and anxiety disorders: Special emphasis on the amygdala. *Annals of the New York Academy of Sciences, 985*, 370–388.

Anand, A., Verhoeff, P., Seneca, N., Zoghbi, S. S., Seibyl, J. P., Charney, D. S., et al. (2000). Brain SPECT imaging of amphetamine-induced dopamine release in euthymic bipolar patients. *American Journal of Psychiatry, 157*, 1108–1114.

Andersen, G., Vestergaard, K., Riis, J., & Lauritzen, L. (1994). Incidence of post-stroke depression during the first year in a large unselected stroke population determined using a valid standardized rating scale. *Acta Psychiatrica Scandinavica, 90*, 190–195.

Andersen, K., Balldin, J., Gottfries, C. G., Granerus, A. K., Modigh, K., Svennerholm, L., et al. (1987). A double-blind evaluation of electroconvulsive therapy in Parkinson's disease with "on–off" phenomena. *Acta Neurologica Scandinivica, 76*, 191–199.

Anderson, D., & Ahmed, A. (2003). Treatment of patients with intractable obsessive-compulsive disorder with anterior capsular stimulation. Case report. *Journal of Neurosurgery, 98*, 1104–1108.

Anderson, G. M., Dover, M. A., Yang, B. P., Holahan, J. M., Shaywitz, S. E., Marchione, K. E., et al. (2000). Adrenomedullary function during cognitive testing in attention-deficit/hyperactivity disorder. *Journal of the American Academy of Child and Adolescent Psychiatry, 39*, 635–643.

Anderson, K. E., & Mullins, J. (2003). Behavioral changes associated with deep brain stimulation surgery for Parkinson's disease. *Current Neurology and Neuroscience Reports, 3*, 306–313.

Andrade, C., Srinivasamurthy, G. M., Vishwasenani, A., Prakash, G. S., Srihari, B. S., & Chandra, J. S. (2002). High but not low ECS stimulus intensity augments apomorphine-stimulated dopamine postsynaptic receptor functioning in rats. *Journal of ECT, 18*, 80–83.

Andreasen, N. C., Arndt, S., Swayze, V., Cizadlo, T., Flaum, M., O'Leary, D., et al. (1994). Thalamic abnormalities in schizophrenia visualized through magnetic resonance image averaging. *Science, 266*, 294–298.

Andreasen, N. C., O'Leary, D. S., Cizadlo, T., Arndt, S., Rezai, K., Boles Ponto, L. L., et al. (1996). Schizophrenia and cognitive dysmetria: A positron-emission tomography study of dysfunctional prefrontal-thalamic-cerebellar circuitry. *Proceedings of the National Academy of Sciences, 93*, 9985–9990.

Andreasen, N. C., O'Leary, D. S., Flaum, M., Nopoulos, P., Watkins, G. L., Ponto, L. L. B., et al. (1997). Hypofrontality in schizophrenia: Distributed dysfunctional circuits in neuroleptic-naïve patients. *Lancet, 349*, 1730–1734.

Andreasen, N. C., Rezai, K., Alliger, R., Swayze, V. W., II, Flaum, M., Kirchner, P., et al. (1992). Hypofrontality in neuroleptic-naïve patients and in patients with chronic schizophrenia. Assessment with xenon 133 single-photon emission computed tomography and the Tower of London. *Archives of General Psychiatry, 49*, 943–958.

Andreasen, N. C., Swayze, V., II, Flaum, M., Alliger, R., & Cohen, G. (1990). Ventricular abnormalities in affective disorder: Clinical and demographic correlates. *American Journal of Psychiatry, 147*, 893–900.

Andres, M. A., Catala, M. A., & Gomez-Beneyto, M. (1999). Prevalence, comorbidity, risk factors and service utilization of disruptive behavior disorders in a community sample of children in Valencia (Spain). *Social Psychiatry and Psychiatric Epidemiology, 34*, 175–179.

Andrews, J. A., Tildesley, E., Hops, H., Duncan, S. C., & Severson, H. H. (2003). Elementary school age children's future intentions and use of substances. *Journal of Clinical Child and Adolescent Psychology, 32*, 556–567.

Anfinson, T. J. (2002). Akathisia, panic, agoraphobia, and major depression following brief exposure to metoclopramide. *Psychopharmacology Bulletin, 36*, 82–93.

Angst, J. (1985). Switch from depression to mania: A record survey over decades between 1920 and 1982. *Psychopathology, 18*, 140–154.

Anguelova, M., Benkelfat, C., & Turecki, G. (2003). A systematic review of association studies investigating genes coding for serotonin receptors and the serotonin transporter: I. Affective disorders. *Molecular Psychiatry, 8*, 574–591.

Appolinario, J. C., Bacaltchuk, J., Sichieri, R., Claudino, A. M., Godoy-Matos, A., Morgan, C., et al. (2003). A randomized, double-blind, placebo-controlled study of sibutramine in the treatment of binge-eating disorder. *Archives of General Psychiatry, 60*, 1109–1116.

Arai, Y., Yamazaki, M., Mori, O., Muramatsu, H., Asano, G., & Katayama, Y. (2001). Alpha-synuclein-positive structures in cases with sporadic Alzheimer's disease: Morphology and its relationship to tau aggregation. *Brain Research, 888*, 287–296.

Arango, C., Breier, A., McMahon, R., Carptenter, W. T., & Buchanan, R. W. (2003). The relationship of clozapine and haloperidol treatment response to prefrontal, hippocampal and caudate brain volumes. *American Journal of Psychiatry, 160*, 1421–1427.

Arango, V., Underwood, M. D., Boldrini, M., Tamir, H., Kassir, S. A., Hsiung, S., et al. (2001). Serotonin 1A receptors, serotonin transporter binding and serotonin transporter mRNA expression in the brainstem of depressed suicide victims. *Neuropsychopharmacology, 25*, 892–903.

Arborelius, L., Owens, M. J., Plotsky, P. M., & Nemeroff, C. B. (1999). The role of corticotropin-releasing factor in depression and anxiety disorders. *Journal of Endocrinology, 160*, 1–12.

Arcos-Burgos, M., Castellanos, F. X., Konecki, D., Lopera, F., Pineda, D., Palacio, J. D., et al. (2004). Pedigree disequilibrium test (PDT) replicates association and linkage between DRD4 and ADHD in multigenerational and extended pedigrees from a genetic isolate. *Molecular Psychiatry, 9*, 252–259.

Armstrong, D., Dunn, J. K., Antalffi, B., & Trivetti, R. (1995). Selective dendritic alterations in the cortex of Rett syndrome. *Journal of Neuropathology and Experimental Neurology, 54*, 195–201.

Arnold, L. E. (2001). Alternative treatments for adults with attention-deficit hyperactivity disorder. *Annals of the New York Academy of Sciences, 931*, 310–341.

Arnold, L. M. (1999). A case series of women with postpartum-onset obsessive-compulsive disorder. *Primary Care Companion to the Journal of Clinical Psychiatry, 1*, 103–108.

Arnold, L. M., McElroy, S. L., Hudson, J. I., Welge, J. A., Bennett, A. J., & Keck, P. E. (2002). A placebo-controlled, randomized trial of fluoxetine in the treatment of binge-eating disorder. *Journal of Clinical Psychiatry, 63*, 1028–1033.

Arnold, P. D., & Richter, M. A. (2001). Is obsessive-compulsive disorder an autoimmune disease? *Canadian Medical Association Journal, 165*, 1353–1358.

Arnold, P., Banerjee, S. P., Bhandari, R., Lorch, E., Ivey, J., Rose, M., et al. (2003). Childhood anxiety disorders and developmental issues in anxiety. *Current Psychiatry Reports, 5*, 252–265.

Asada, T., Motonaga, T., Yamagata, Z., Uno, M., & Takahashi, K. (2000). Associations between retrospectively recalled napping behavior and later development of Alzheimer's disease: Association with APOE genotypes. *Sleep, 23*, 629–634.

Aschenbrand, S. G., Kendall, P. C, Webb, A., Safford, S. M., & Flannery-Schroeder, E. (2003). Is childhood separation anxiety disorder a predictor of adult panic disorder and agoraphobia? A seven-year longitudinal study. *Journal of the American Academy of Child and Adolescent Psychiatry, 42*, 1478–1485.

Ascherio, A., Zhang, S. M., Hernan, M. A., Kawachi, I., Colditz, G. A., Speizer, F. E., et al. (2001). Prospective study of caffeine consumption and risk of Parkinson's disease in men and women. *Annals of Neurology, 50*, 56–63.

Asherson, P., Barkley, R., Barr, C., Berg, K., Biederman, J., Castellanos, X., et al. (2000). Collaborative possibilities for molecular genetic studies of attention deficit hyperactivity disorder. *American Journal of Medical Genetics: Neuropsychiatric Genetics, 96*, 251–257.

Ashford, J. W., & Mortimer, J. A. (2002). Non-familial Alzheimer's disease is mainly due to genetic factors. *Journal of Alzheimer's Disease, 4*, 169–177.

Ashwell, K., Tancred, E., & Paxinos, G. (2000). The brain's anatomy. In E. Gordon (Ed.), *Integrative neuroscience: Bringing together biological, psychological, and clinical models of the human brain* (pp. 88–108). Amsterdam, Netherlands: Overseas Publishers Association.

Asnis, G. M., Hameedi, F. A., Goddard, A. W., Potkin, S. G., Black, D., Jameel, M., et al. (2001). Fluvoxamine in the treatment of panic disorder: A multi-center, double-blind, placebo-controlled study in outpatients. *Psychiatry Research, 103*, 1–14.

Asverg, M., Bertillsson, L., Martensson, B., Scalia-Tomba, G. P., Thoren, P., & Traskman-Bendz, L. (1984). CSF monoamine metabolites in melancholia. *Acta Psychiatrica Scandinavica, 69*, 201–219.

Atwood, C. S., Obrenovich, M. E., Liu, T., Chan, H., Perry, G., Smith, M. A., et al. (2003). Amyloid-beta: A chameleon walking in two worlds: A review of the trophic and toxic properties of amyloid-beta. *Brain Research, 43*, 1–16.

Auranen, M., Varilo, T., Alen, R., Vanhala, R., Ayers, K., Kempas, E. et al. (2000). Evidence for allelic association on chromosome 3q25-27 in families with autism spectrum disorders originating from a subisolate of Finland. *Molecular Psychiatry, 8*, 879–884.

Austen, B., Christodoulou, G., & Terry, J. E. (2002). Relation between cholesterol levels, statins and Alzheimer's disease in the human population. *Journal of Nutrition, Health & Aging, 6*, 377–382.

Aylward, E. H., Minshew, N. J., Field, K., Sparks, B. F., & Singh, N. (2002). Effects of age on brain volume and head circumference in autism. *Neurology, 59*, 175–183.

Aylward, E. H., Minshew, N. J., Goldstein, G., Honeycutt, N. A., Augustine, A. M., Yates, K. O., et al. (1999). MRI volumes of amygdala and hippocampus in non-mentally retarded autistic adolescents and adults. *Neurology, 53*, 2145–2150.

Aylward, E. H., Reiss, A. L., Reader, M. J., Singer, H. S., Brown, J. E., & Denckla, M. B. (1996). Basal ganglia volumes in children with attention-deficit hyperactivity disorder. *Journal of Child Neurology, 11*, 112–115.

Aylward, E. H., Roberts-Twillie, J. V., Barta, P. E., Kumar, A. J., Harris, G. J., Geer, M., et al. (1994). Basal ganglia volumes and white matter hyperintensities in patients with bipolar disorder. *American Journal of Psychiatry, 151*, 687–693.

Azari, N. P., & Seitz, R. J. (2000). Brain plasticity and recovery from stroke. *American Scientist, 88*, 426–431.

Baamonde, A., Dauge, V., Ruiz-Gayo, M., Fulga, I. G., Turcaud, S., Fournie-Zaluski, et al. (1992). Antidepressant-type effects of endogenous enkephalins protected by systemic RB 101 are mediated by opioid delta and dopamine D1 receptor stimulation. *European Journal of Pharmacology, 216*, 157–166.

Baba, M., Jakajo, S., Tu, P., Tomita, T., Nakaya, K., Lee V. M. Y., et al. (1998). Aggregation of alpha-synuclein in bodies of sporadic Parkinson's disease and dementia with Lewy bodies. *American Journal of Pathology, 152*, 879–884.

Babel, T. B., Warnke, P. C., & Ostertag, C. B. (2001). Immediate and long term outcome after infrathalamic and thalamic lesioning for intractable Tourette's syndrome. *Journal of Neurology, Neurosurgery and Psychiatry, 70*, 666–671.

Bacon, A. L., Fein, D., Morris, R., Waterhouse, L., & Allen, D. (1998). The responses of autistic children to the distress of others. *Journal of Autism and Developmental Disorders, 28*, 129–142.

Badner, J. A., & Gershon, E. S. (2002). Meta-analysis of whole-genome linkage scans of bipolar disorder and schizophrenia. *Molecular Psychiatry, 7*, 405–411.

Baer, L., Rauch, S. L., Ballantine, H. T. Jr., Martuza, R., Cosgrove, R., Cassem, E., et al. (1995). Cingulotomy for intractable obsessive-compulsive disorder. Prospective long-term follow-up of 18 patients. *Archives of General Psychiatry, 52*, 384–392.

Baieli, S., Pavone, L., Meli, C., Fiumara, A., & Coleman, M. (2003). Autism and phenylketonuria. *Journal of Autism and Developmetal Disorders, 33*, 201–204.

Bailer, U. F., & Kaye, W. H. (2003). A review of neuropeptide and neuroendocrine dysregulation in anorexia and bulimia nervosa. *Current Drug Target CNS Neurological Disorders, 2*, 53–59.

Bailey, A., Le Couteur, A., Gottesman, I., Bolton, P., Simonoff, E., Yuzda, E., et al. (1995). Autism as a strongly genetic disorder: Evidence from a British twin study. *Psychological Medicine, 25*, 63–77.

Bailey, J. E., Argyropoulos, S. V., Lightman, S. L., & Nutt, D. J. (2003). Does the brain noradrenaline network mediate the effects of the CO_2 challenge? *Journal of Psychopharmacology, 17*, 252–259.

Baiyewu, O., Adeyemi, J. D., & Ogunniyi, A. (1997). Psychiatric disorders in Nigerian nursing home residents. *International Journal of Geriatric Psychiatry, 12*, 1146–1150.

Bajwa, W. K., Asnis, G. M., Sanderson, W. C., Irfan, A., & van Praag, H. M. (1992). High cholesterol levels in patients with panic disorder. *American Journal of Psychiatry, 149*, 376–278.

Balbernie, R. (2001). Circuits and circumstances: The neurobiological consequences of early relationship experiences and how they shape later behaviour. *Journal of Child Psychotherapy, 27*, 237–255.

Baldereschi, M., Di Carlo, A., Vanni, P., Ghetti, A., Carbonin, P., Amaducci, L., et al. (2003). Lifestyle-related risk factors for Parkinson's disease: A population-based study. *Acta Neurologica Scandinavica, 108*, 239–244.

Baldessarini, R. J., Tondo, L., & Hennen, J. (2001). Treating the suicidal patient with bipolar disorder. Reducing suicide risk with lithium. *Annals of the New York Academy of Science, 932*, 24–38.

Baldwin, R., Jeffries, S., Jackson, A., Sutcliffe, C., Thacker, N., Scott, M., et al. (2004). Treatment response in late-onset depression: Relationship to neuropsychological, neuroradiological and vascular risk factors. *Psychological Medicine, 34*, 125–136.

Ballard, C. G., Jacoby, R., Del Ser, T., Khan, M. N., Munoz, D. G., Holmes, C., et al. (2004). Neuropathological substrates of psychiatric symptoms in prospectively studied patients with autopsy-confirmed dementia with Lewy bodies. *American Journal of Psychiatry, 161*, 843–849.

Balldin, J., Granerus, A. K., Lindstedt, G., Modigh, K., & Walinder, J. (1982). Neuroendocrine evidence for increased responsiveness of dopamine receptors in humans following electroconvulsive therapy. *Psychopharmacology, 76*, 371–376.

Balldin, J., Granerus, A. K., Lindstedt, G., Modigh, K., & Walinder, J. (1981). Predictors for improvement after electroconvulsive therapy in Parkinsonian patients with on-off symptoms. *Journal of Neural Transmission, 52*, 199–211.

Ballmaier, M., Toga, A. W., Blanton, R. E., Sowell, E. R., Lavretsky, H., Peterson, J., et al. (2004). Anterior cingulated, gyrus rectus, and orbitofrontal abnormalities in elderly depressed patients: An MRI-based parcellation of the prefrontal cortex. *American Journal of Psychiatry, 161*, 99–108.

Balon, R. (2003). Selective serotonin reuptake inhibitors and suicide: Is the evidence, as with beauty, in the eye of the beholder? *Psychotherapy and Psychosomatics, 72*, 293–299.

Banasr, M., Hery, M., Brezun, J., & Daszuta, A. (2001). Serotonin mediates oestrogen stimulation proliferation in the adult dentate gyrus. *European Journal of Neuroscience, 14*, 1417–1424.

Bandelow, B., Behnke, K., Lenoir, S., Hendriks, G. J., Alkin, T., Goebel, C., et al. (2004). Sertraline versus paroxetine in the treatment of panic disorder: An acute, double-blind noninferiority comparison. *Journal of Clinical Psychiatry, 65*, 405–413.

Bandelow, B., Späth, C., Tichauer, G. A., Broocks, A., Hajak, G., & Rüther, E. (2002). Early traumatic life events, parental attitudes, family history, and birth risk factors in patients with panic disorder. *Comprehensive Psychiatry, 43*, 269–278.

Banich, M. T. (1997). *Neuropsychology: The neural bases of mental function.* New York: Houghton Mifflin.

Bankier, B., Januzzi, J. L., & Littman, A. B. (2004). The high prevalence of multiple psychiatric disorders in stable outpatients with coronary heart disease. *Psychosomatic Medicine, 66*, 645–650.

Barak, Y., Kimhi, R., Stein, D., Gutman, J., & Weizman, A. (1999). Autistic subjects with comorbid epilepsy: A possible association with viral infections. *Child Psychiatry and Human Development, 29*, 245–251.

Barbarich, N. C., Kaye, W. H., & Jimerson, D. (2003). Neurotransmitter and imaging studies in anorexia nervosa: New targets for treatment. *Current Drug Target CNS Neurological Disorders, 2*, 61–72.

Barinaga, M. (2001). Olfaction: Smell's course is predetermined. *Science, 294*, 1269–1271.

Barkley, R. A. (2002). Major life activity and health outcomes associated with attention-deficit/hyperactivity disorder. *Journal of Clinical Psychiatry, 63*, 10–15.

Barkley, R. A., Fischer, M., Edelbrock, C. S., & Smallish, L. (1990). The adolescent outcome of hyperactive children diagnosed by research criteria: I. An 8-year prospective follow-up study. *Journal of the American Academy of Child and Adolescent Psychiatry, 29*, 546–557.

Barkley, R. A., Fischer, M., Smallish, L., & Fletcher, K. (2004). Young adult follow-up of hyperactive children: Antisocial activities and drug use. *Journal of Child Psychology and Psychiatry, 45*, 195–211.

Barnea, A., & Nottebohm, F. (1996). Recruitment and replacement of hippocampal neurons in young and adult chickadees: An addition to the theory of hippocampal learning. *Proceedings of the National Academy of the Sciences, USA, 93*, 714–718.

Barnes, L. L., Wilson, R. S., Schneider, J. A., Bienias, J. L., Evans, D. A., & Bennett, D. A. (2003). Gender, cognitive decline, and risk of AD in older persons. *Neurology, 60*, 1777–1781.

Barnhill, J., & Horrigan, J. P. (2002). Tourette's syndrome and autism: A search for common ground. *Mental Health Aspects of Developmental Disabilities, 5*, 7–15.

Baron-Cohen, S. (2002). The extreme male brain theory of autism. *Trends in Cognitive Sciences, 6*, 248–254.

Barr, C. L., Wigg, K. G., Pakstis, A. J., Kurlan, R., Pauls, D., Kidd, K. K., Tsui, L. C., & Sandor, P. (1999). Genome scan for linkage to Gilles de la Tourette syndrome. *American Journal of Medical Genetics, 88*, 437–445.

Barr, C. L., Wigg, K. G., Zovko, E., Sandor, P., & Tsui, L. C. (1996). No evidence for a major gene effects of the dopamine D4 receptor gene in the susceptibility to Gilles de la Tourette syndrome in five Canadian families. *American Journal of Medical Genetics, 67*, 301–305.

Barr, C. L., Wigg, K., Malone, M., Schachar, R., Tannock, R., Roberts, W., & Kennedy, J. L. (1999). Linkage study of catechol-o-methyltransferase and attention-deficit hyperactivity disorder. *American Journal of Medical Genetics, 88*, 710–713.

Barr, C. L., Wigg, K. G., Zovko, E., Sandor, P., & Tsui, L. C. (1997). Linkage study of the dopamine D5 receptor gene and Gilles de la Tourette syndrome. *American Journal of Medical Genetics, 74*, 58–61.

Barr, C. L., Xu, C., Kroft, J., Feng, Y., Wigg, K., Zai, G., et al. (2001). Haplotype study of three polymorphisms at the dopamine transporter locus confirm linkage to attention-deficit/hyperactivity disorder. *Biological Psychiatry, 49*, 333–339.

Barta, P. E., Pearlson, G. D., Powers, R. E., Richards, S. S., & Tune, L. E. (1990). Auditory hallucinations and smaller superior temporal gyral volume in schizophrenia. *American Journal of Psychiatry, 147,* 1457–1462.

Bartha, R., Stein, M. B., Williamson, P. C., Drost, D. J, Neufeld, R. W., Carr, T. J., et al. (1998). A short echo 1H spectroscopy and volumetric MRI study of the corpus striatum in patients with obsessive-compulsive disorder and comparison subjects. *American Journal of Psychiatry, 155,* 1584–1591.

Basser, L. S. (1962). Hemiplegia of early onset and the faculty of speed, with special reference to the effects of hemispherectomy. *Brain, 85,* 427–460.

Bassett, A. S., Chow, E. W. C., Waterworth, D. M., & Brzustowica, L. (2001). Genetic insights into schizophrenia. *Canadian Journal of Psychiatry, 46,* 131–137.

Bassett, A. S., Chow, E. W. C., AbdelMalik, P., Gheorghiu, M., Husten, J., & Weksberg, R. (2003). The schizophrenia phenotype in 22q11 deletion syndrome. *American Journal of Psychiatry, 160,* 1580–1586.

Basso, M. R., Lowery, N., Neel, J., Purdie, R., & Bornstein, R. A. (2002). Neuropsychological impairment among manic, depressed, and mixed-episode inpatients with bipolar disorder. *Neuropsychology, 16,* 84–91.

Bates, E. (1999a). Plasticity, localization and language development. In S. Broman & J. M. Fletcher (Eds.), *The changing nervous system: Neurobehavioral consequences of early brain disorders* (pp. 214–253). New York: Oxford University Press.

Bates, E. (1999b). Language and the infant brain. *Journal of Communication Disorders, 32,* 195–205.

Bauer, M. S., & Mitchner, L. (2004). What is a "mood stabilizer"? An evidence-based response. *American Journal of Psychiatry, 161,* 3–18.

Baumann, B., Bileau, H., Krell, D., Agelink, M. W., Diekmann, S., Wurthmann, C., et al. (2002). Circumscribed numerical deficit of dorsal raphe neurons in mood disorders. *Psychological Medicine, 32,* 93–103.

Baumgardner, T. L., Dinger, H. S., Denckla, M. B., Rubin, M. A., Abrams, M. T., Colli, M. J., et al. (1996). Corpus callosum morphology in children with Tourette syndrome and attention deficit hyperactivity disorder. *Neurology, 47,* 477–482.

Bauminger, N., & Shulman, C. (2003). The development and maintenance of friendship in high-functioning children with autism. *Autism, 7,* 81–97.

Baxter, L. R. Jr., Schwartz, J. M., Phelps, M. E., Mazziotta, J. C., Guze, B. H., Selin, C. E., et al. (1989). Reduction of prefrontal cortex glucose metabolism common to three types of depression. *Archives of General Psychiatry, 46,* 243–250.

Beal, M. F. (2003). Mitochondria, oxidative damage, and inflammation in Parkinson's disease. *Annals of the New York Academy of Sciences, 991,* 120–131.

Bearden, C. E., Hoffman, K. M., & Cannon, T. D. (2001). The neuropsychology and neuroanatomy of bipolar affective disorder: A critical review. *Bipolar Disorders, 3,* 106–150.

Beart, P. M. (2000). The brain's chemistry. In E. Gordon (Ed.), *Integrative neuroscience: Bringing together biological, psychological, and clinical models of the human brain* (pp. 75–85). Amsterdam, Netherlands: Overseas Publishers Association.

Beck, D. D. (in press). *The biology of Gila monsters and beaded lizards.* Berkeley: University of California Press.

Becker, K. G. (2004). The common variants/multiple disease hypothesis of common complex genetic disorders. *Medical Hypotheses, 62,* 309–317.

Befort, K., Filliol, D., Decaillot, F. M., Gaveriaux-Ruff, C., Hoehe, M. R., & Kieffer, B. L. (2001). A single nucleotide polymorphic mutation in the human mu-opioid receptor severely impairs receptor signaling. *Journal of Biological Chemistry, 276,* 3130–3137.

Begic, D., Hotujac, L., & Jokic-Bcgic, N. (2001). Elcctrocnccphalographic comparison of veterans with combat-related post-traumatic stress disorder and healthy subjects. *International Journal of Psychophysiology, 40,* 167–172.

Bell, C., Abrams, J., & Nutt, D. (2001). Tryptophan depletion and its implications for psychiatry. *British Journal of Psychiatry, 178,* 399–405.

Belsham, B. (2001). Glutamate and its role in psychiatric illness. *Human Psychopharmacology, 16,* 139–156.

Benazon, N. R., Ager, J., & Rosenberg, D. R. (2002). Cognitive behavior therapy in treatment-naive children and adolescents with obsessive-compulsive disorder: An open trial. *Behaviour Research and Therapy, 40,* 529–539.

Benazon, N. R., Moore, G. J., & Rosenberg, D. R. (2003). Neurochemical analyses in pediatric obsessive-compulsive disorder in patients treated with cognitive-behavioral therapy. *Journal of the American Academy of Child and Adolescent Psychiatry, 42,* 1279–1285.

Bencherif, B., Wand, G. S., McCaul, M. E., Kim, Y. K., Ilgin, N., Dannals, R. F., et al. (2004). Mu-opioid receptor binding measured by [11C]carfentanil positron emission tomography is related to craving and mood in alcohol dependence. *Biological Psychiatry, 55,* 255–262.

Benes, F. M., & Bird, E. D (1987). An analysis of the arrangement of neurons in the cingulate cortex of schizophrenic patients. *Archives of General Psychiatry, 44,* 608–616.

Benes, F. M., Davidson, J., & Bird, E. D. (1986). Quantitative cytoarchitectural studies of the cerebral cortex of schizophrenics. *Archives of General Psychiatry, 43*, 31–35.

Benes, F. M., Vincent, S. L., & Todtenkopf, M. (2001). The density of pyramidal and nonpyramidal neurons in anterior cingulate cortex of schizophenic and bipolar subjects. *Society of Biological Psychiatry, 50*, 395–406.

Beng-Choon, H., Alicata, D., Ward, J., Moser, D. J., O'Leary, D. S., Arndt, S., et al. (2003). Untreated initial psychosis: Relation to cognitive deficits and brain morphology in first-episode schizophenia. *American Journal of Psychiatry, 160*, 142–148.

Bengel, D., Greenberg, B. D., Corá-Locatelli, G., Altemus, M., Heils, A., Li, Q., et al. (1999). Association of the serotonin transporter promoter regulatory region polymorphism and obsessive-compulsive disorder. *Molecular Psychiatry, 4*, 463–466.

Benjamin, J., Levine, J., Fux, M., Aviv, A., Levy, D., & Belmaker, R. H. (1995). Double-blind, placebo-controlled, crossover trial of inositol treatment for panic disorder. *American Journal of Psychiatry, 152*, 1084–1086.

Benjamin, J., Osher, Y., Lichtenberg, P., Bachner-Melman, R., Gritsenko, I., Kotler, M. et al. (2000). An interaction between the catechol O-methyltransferase and serotonin transporter promoter region polymorphisms contributes to tridimensional personality questionnaire persistence scores in normal subjects. *Neuropsychobiology, 41*, 48–53.

Ben-Menachem, E., Hamberger, A., Hedner, T., Hammond, E. J., Uthman, B. M., Slater, J., et al. (1995). Effects of vagus nerve stimulation on amino acids and other metabolites in the CSF of patients with partial seizures. *Epilepsy Research, 20*, 221–227.

Bennett, J. P., Enna, S. J., Bylund, D. B., Gillin, J. C., Wyatt, R. J., & Synder, S. H. (1979). Neurotransmitter receptors in frontal cortex of schizphrenics. *Archives of General Psychiatry, 36*, 927–934.

Benton, A. L., Hannay, H. J., & Varney, N. R. (1975). Visual perception of line direction in patients with unilateral brain disease. *Neurology, 25*, 907–910.

Bergem, A. L., Engedal, K., & Kringlen, E. (1997). The role of heredity in late-onset Alzheimer's disease and vascular dementia: A twin study. *Archives of General Psychiatry, 54*, 264–270.

Bergem, A. L., & Lannfelt, L. (1997). Apolipoprotein E type epsilon4 allele, heritability and age at onset in twins with Alzheimer disease and vascular dementia. *Clinical Genetics, 52*, 408–413.

Berman, K. F., & Weinberger, D. R. (1991). Functional localization in the brain in schizophrenia. In A. Tasman & S. M. Goldfinger (Eds.), *American Psychiatric Press Review of Psychiatry*, 10 (pp. 24–59). Washington, DC: American Psychiatric Press.

Berquin, P. C., Giedd, J. N., Jacobsen, L. K., Hamburger, S. D., Krain, A. L., Rapoport, J. L., & Castellanos, F. X. (1998). Cerebellum in attention-deficit hyperactivity disorder: A morphometric MRI study. *Neurology, 4*, 1087–1093.

Berrettini, W. H., Ferraro, T. N., Goldin, L. R., Weeks, D. E., Detera-Wadleigh, S., Nurnberger, J. I. J., et al. (1994). Chromosome 18 DNA markers and manic-depressive illness: Evidence for a susceptibility gene. *Proclamations of the National Academy of Science, U.S.A., 91*, 5918–5921.

Bertelsen, A., Harvald, B., & Hauge, M. (1977). A Danish twin study of manic-depressive disorders. *British Journal of Psychiatry, 130*, 330–351.

Berthele, A., Platzer, S., Dworzak, D., Schadrack, J., Mahal, B., Buttner, A., et al. (2003). [3H]-nociceptin ligand-binding and nociceptin opioid receptor MRNA expression in the human brain. *Neuroscience, 12*, 629–640.

Berthier, M. L., Kulisevsky, J., Gironell, A., & Heras, J. A. (1996). Obsessive-compulsive disorder associated with brain lesions: Clinical phenomenology, cognitive function, and anatomic correlates. *Neurology, 47*, 353–361.

Berthier, M. L., Kulisevsky, J. J., Gironell, A., & López, O. L. (2001). Obsessive-compulsive disorder and traumatic brain injury: Behavioral, cognitive, and neuroimaging findings. *Neuropsychiatry, Neuropsychology, and Behavioral Neurology, 14*, 23–31.

Bertolino, A., Esposito, G., Callicott, J. H., Mattay, V. S., Van Horn, J. D., Frank, J. A., et al. (2000). Specific relationship between prefrontal neuronal N-Acetylaspartate and activation of the working memory cortical network in schizophrenia. *American Journal of Psychiatry, 157*, 26–33.

Bertschy, G., Ragama-Pardos, E., Ait-Ameur, A., Muscionico, M., Favre, S., & Roth, L. (2003). Lithium augmentation in venlafaxine non-responders: An open study. *European Psychiatry, 18*, 314–317.

Bespalova, I. N., & Buxbaum, J. D. (2003). Disease susceptibility genes for autism. *Annals of Medicine, 35*, 274–281.

Betourne, L. R., & Friel-Patti, S. (2003). Phonological processing and oral language abilities in fourth-grade poor readers. *Journal of Communication Disorders, 36*, 507–527.

Betz, W. J., Bewick, G. S., & Ridge, R. M. (1992). Intracellular movements of the fluorescently lableled synaptic vesicles in frog motor nerve terminals during nerve stimulation. *Neuron, 9*, 805–813.

Bezchlibnyk, Y., & Young, L. T. (2002). The neurobiology of bipolar disorder: Focus on signal transduction pathways and the regulation of gene expression. *Canadian Journal of Psychiatry, 47*, 135–148.

Bhagwagar, Z., Montgomery, A. J., Grasby, P. M., & Cowen, P. J. (2003). Lack of effect of a single dose of hydrocortisome on serotonin (IA) receptors in recovered depressed patients measured by positron emission tonography with [IIC] WAY-100635. *Biological Psychiatry, 54*, 890–895.

Bhagwagar, Z., Whale, R., & Cowen, P. J. (2002). State and trait abnormalities in serotonin function in major depression. *British Journal of Psychiatry, 180*, 24–28.

Bhalla, U. S., & Iyengar, R. (1999). Emergent properties of networks of biological signaling pathways. *Science, 283*, 381–387.

Bhanji, N. H., Margolese, H. C., Saint-Laurent, M., & Chouinard, G. (2002). Dysphoric mania induced by high-dose mirtazapine: A case for "norepinephrine syndrome"? *International Clinical Psychopharmacology, 17*, 319–322.

Bickford, P. C., Gould, T., Briederick, L., Chadman, K., Pollock, A., Young, D., et al. (2000). Antioxidant-rich diets improve cerebellar hysiology and motor learning in aged rats. *Brain Research, 866*, 211–217.

Biederman, J., & Fara ne, S. V. (2002). Current concepts on the neurobiology of Attention-Deficit/Hyperactivity Disorder. *Journal o, Attention Disorders, 1*, S7–16.

Biederman, J., Faraone, S. V., Keenan, K., Steingard, R., & Tsuang, M. T. (1991). Familial association between attention deficit disorder and anxiety disorders. *American Journal of Psychiatry, 148*, 251–256.

Biederman, J., Faraone, S. V., Mick, E., Spencer, T., Wilens, T., Kiely, K., et al. (1995). High risk for attention deficit hyperactivity disorder among children of parents with childhood onset of the disorder: A pilot study. *American Journal of Psychiatry, 152*, 431–435.

Biederman, J., Munir, K., Knee, D., Habelow, W., Armentano, M., Autor, S., et al. (1986). A family study of patients with attention deficit disorder and normal controls. *Journal of Psychiatry Research, 20*, 261–274.

Biederman, J., & Spencer, T. (1999). Attention-deficit/hyperactivity disorder (ADHD) as a noradrenergic disorder. *Biological Psychiatry, 46*, 1234–1242.

Billett, E. A., Richter, M. A., King, N., Heils, A., Lesch, K. P., & Kennedy, J. L. (1997). Obsessive compulsive disorder, response to serotonin reuptake inhibitors and the serotonin transporter gene. *Molecular Psychiatry, 2*, 403–406.

Birkenhager, T. K., van den Broek, W. W., Mulder, P. G., Bruijin, J. A., & Moleman, P. (2004). Comparison of two-phase treatment with imipramine or fluvoxamine, both followed by lithiuim addition in inpatients with major depressive disorder. *American Journal of Psychiatry, 161*, 2060–2065.

Birks, J., & Flicker, L. (2003). Selegiline for Alzheimer's disease. *Cochrane Database of Systematic Reviews*, CD000442.

Birmaher, B., Ryan, N. D., Williamson, B. A., Brent, D. A., Kaufman, J., Dahl, R. E., et al. (1996). Childhood and adolescent depression: A review of the past 10 years. Part I. *Journal of the American Academy of Child and Adolescent Psychiatry, 35*, 1427–1437.

Bisaga, A., Katz, J. L., Antonini, A., Wright, C. E., Margouleff, C., Gorman. J. M., et al. (1998). Cerebral glucose metabolism in women with panic disorder. *American Journal of Psychiatry, 155*, 1178–1183.

Biver, F., Goldman, S., Delvenne, V., Luxen, A., De Maertelaer, V., Hubain, P., et al. (1994). Fontal and parietal metabolic disturbances in unipolar depression. *Biological Psychiatry, 36*, 381–388.

Bjork, J. M., Grant, S. J., & Hommer, D. W. (2003). Cross-sectional volumetric analysis of brain atrophy in alcohol dependence: Effects of drinking history and comorbid substance use disorder. *American Journal of Psychiatry, 160*, 2038–2045.

Blackwell, A. D., Sahakian, B. J., Vesey, R., Semple, J. M., Robbins, T. W., & Hodges, J. R. (2004). Detecting dementia: Novel neuropsychological markers of preclinical Alzheimer's disease. *Dementia and Geriatric Cognitive Disorders, 17*, 42–48.

Blackwood, D. H. R., He, L., Morris, S. W., McLean, A., Whitton, C., Thomson, M., et al. (1996). A locus for bipolar affective disorder on chromosome 4p. *Nature Genetics, 4*, 427–430.

Blackwoord, J. J., IIoward, R. J., Bcntall, R. P., & Murray, R. M. (2001). Cognitive neuropsychiatric models of persecutory delusions. *American Journal of Psychiatry, 158*, 527–539.

Blair Simpson, H., Tenke, C. E., Towey, J. B., Liebowitz, M. R., & Bruder, G. E. (2000). Symptom provocation alters behavioral ratings and brain electrical activity in obsessive-compulsive disorder: A preliminary study. *Psychiatry Research, 95*, 149–155.

Blasi, V., Young, A. C., Tansy, A. P., Petersen, S. E., Snyder, A. Z., & Corbetta, M. (2002). Word retrieval learning modulates right frontal cortex in patients with left frontal damage. *Neuron, 36*, 159–170.

Blennow, K., & Vanmechelen, E. (2003). CSF markers for pathogeneic processes in Alzheimer's disease: Diagnostic implications and use in neurochemistry. *Brain Research Bulletin, 61*, 235–242.

Bligh-Glover, W., Kolli, T. N., Shapiro-Kulnane, L., Dilley, G. E., Friedman, L., Balraj, E., et al. (2000). The serotonin transporter in the midbrain of suicide victims with major depression. *Biological Psychiatry, 47*, 1015–1024.

Bloom, O., Evergren, E., Tomilin, N., Kjaerulff, O., Low, P., Brodin, L., et al. (2003). Colocalization of synapsin and actin during synaptic vesicle recycling. *Journal of Cell Biology, 161*, 737–747.

Blumberg, H. P., Kaufman, J., Martin, A., Whiteman, R., Zhang, J. H., Gore, J. C., et al. (2003). Amygdala and hippocampal volumes in adolescents and adults with bipolar disorder. *Archives of General Psychiatry, 60*, 1201–1208.

Blumberg, H. P., Martin, A., Kaufman, J., Leung, H. C., Skudlarski, P., Lacadie, C., et al. (2003). Frontostriatal abnormalities in adolescents with bipolar disorder: Preliminary observations from functional MRI. *American Journal of Psychiatry, 160*, 1345–1347.

Blumenfeld, H., McNally, K. A., Ostroff, R. B., & Zubal, I. G. (2003). Targeted prefrontal cortical activation with bifrontal ECT. *Psychiatry Research, 123*, 165–170.

Blumenthal, J. A., Babyak, M. A., Moore, K. A., Craighead, W. E., Herman, S., Khatri, P., et al. (1999). Effects of exercise training on older patients with major depression. *Archives of Internal Medicine, 159*, 2349–2356.

Blumer, D., & Benson, D. F. (1975). Personality changes with frontal and temporal lesions. In D. F. Benson & F. Blumer (Eds.), *Psychiatric aspects of neurologic disease.* New York: Grune & Stratton.

Blundell, J. E. (1986). Serotonin manipulations and the structure of feeding behavior. *Appetite, 7*, 39–56.

Bodner, S. M., Morshed, S. A., & Peterson, B. S. (2001). The question of PANDAS in adults. *Biological Psychiatry, 49*, 807–810.

Bogetto, F., Venturello, S., Albert, U., Maina, G., & Ravizza, L. (1999). Gender-related clinical differences in obsessive-compulsive disorder. *European Psychiatry, 14*, 434–441.

Boileau, I., Assadd, J. M., Pihl, R. O., Benkelfat, C., Leyton, M., Diksic, M., et al. (2003). Alcohol promotes dopamine release in human nucleus accumbens. *Synapse, 49*, 226–231.

Boksa, P., & El-Khodor, B. F. (2003). Birth insult interacts with stress at adulthood to alter dopaminergic function in animal models: Possible implications for schizophrenia. *Neuroscience and Biobehavioral Reviews, 27*, 91–101.

Bolla, K. I., Eldreth, D. A., London, E. D., Kiehl, K. A., Mouratidus, M., Contoreggi, C., et al. (2003). Orbitofrontal cortex dysfunction in abstinent cocaine abusers performing a decision-making task. *Neuroimage, 19*, 1085–1094.

Bolton, J., Moore, G. J., MacMillan, S., Stewart, C. M., & Rosenberg, D. R. (2001). Case study: Caudate glutamatergic changes with paroxetine persist after medication discontinuation in pediatric OCD. *Journal of the American Academy of Child and Adolescent Psychiatry, 40*, 903–906.

Bolwig, T. G. (2003). Putative common pathways in therapeutic brain stimulation for affective disorders. *CNS Spectrums, 8*, 490–495.

Bonari, L., Bennett, H., Einarson, A., & Koren, G. (2004). Risks of untreated depression during pregnancy. *Canadian Family Physician, 50*, 37–39.

Bondy, B., Baghai, T. C., Zill, P., Bottlender, R., Jaeger, M., Minov, C., et al. (2002). Combined action of the ACE D- and the G-protein β3 T-allele in major depression: A possible link to cardiovascular disease? *Molecular Psychiatry, 7*, 1120–1126.

Bonne, O., Gilboa, A., Louzoun, Y., Brandes, D., Yona, I., Lester, H., et al. (2003). Resting regional cerebral perfusion in recent posttraumatic stress disorder. *Biological Psychiatry, 54*, 1077–1086.

Bonne, O., Krausz, Y., Aharon, Y., Gelfin, Y., Chisin, R., & Lerer, B. (1999). Clinical doses of fluoxetine and cerebral blood flow in healthy volunteers. *Psychopharmacology, 143*, 24–28.

Bonne, O., Louzoun, Y., Aharon, I., Krausz, Y., Karger, H., Lerer, B., et al. (2003). Cerebral blood flow in depressed patients: A methodological comparison of statistical parametric mapping and region of interest analyses. *Psychiatry Research, 122*, 49–57.

Bonora, E., Beyer, K. S., Lamb, J. A., Parr, J. R., Klauck, S. M., Benner, A., et al. (2003). Analysis of reelin as a candidate gene for autism. *Molecular Psychiatry, 8*, 885–892.

Bookheimer, S. Y., Zeffiro, T. A., Blaxton, T., Gailard, W., & Theodore, W. (1995). Regional cerebral blood flow during object naming and word reading. *Human Brain Mapping, 3*, 93–106.

Bookstein, F. L., Sampson, P. D., Connor, P. D., & Streissguth, A. P. (2002). Midline corpus callosum is a neuroanatomical focus of fetal alcohol damage. *Anatomical Record, 269*, 162–174.

Borcherding, B. G., Keysor, C. S., Rapoport, J. L., Elia, J., & Amass, J. (1990). Motor/vocal tics and compulsive behaviors on stimulant drugs: Is there a common vulnerability? *Psychiatry Research, 33*, 83–94.

Borg, J., Andree, B., Soderstrom, H., & Farde, L. (2003). The serotonin system and spiritual experiences. *American Journal of Psychiatry, 160*, 1965–1969.

Bosboom, J. L. W., Stoffers, D., & Wolters, Ech. (2003). The role of acetylcholine and dopamine in dementia and psychosis in Parkinson's disease. *Journal of Neural Transmission, 65*, 185–195.

Bosch-Bayard, J., Baldes-Sosa, P., Virues-Alba, T., Aubert-Vazquez, E., John, E. R., Harmony, T., et al. (2001). 3D statistical parametric mapping of EEG source spectra by means of variable resolution electromagnetic tomographay (VARETA). *Clinical Electroencephalograph, 32*, 47–61.

Boshuisen, M. L., Ter Horst, G. J., Paans, A. M., Reinders, A. A., den Boer, J. A., et al. (2002). rCBF differences between panic disorder patients and control subjects during anticipatory anxiety and rest. *Biological Psychiatry, 52*, 126–135.

Bottiglieri, T., Laundy, M., Crellin, R., Toone, B. K., Carney, M. W. P., & Reynolds, E. H. (2000). Homocysteine, folate, methylation, and monoamine metabolism in depression. *Journal of Neurology, Neurosurgery, and Psychiatry, 69*, 228–232.

Bounds, T. A., Schoop, L., Johnstone, B., Unger, C., & Goldman, H. (2003). Gender differences in a sample of vocational rehabilitation clients with TBI. *NeuroRehabilitation, 18*, 189–196.

Bowden, C. L. (2000). The ability of lithium and other mood stabilizers to decrease suicide risk and prevent relapse. *Current Psychiatry Reports, 2*, 490–494.

Bowers, D., Bauer, R. M., Coslett, H. B., & Heilman, K. M. (1985). Processing of faces by patients with unilateral hemispheric lesions. I. Dissociations between judgements of facial affect and identity. *Brain and Cognition, 4*, 258–272.

Bown, C. D., Wang, J. F., & Young, L. T. (2003). Attenuation of N-methyl-D-aspartate-mediated cytoplasmic vacuolization in primary rat hippocampal neurons by mood stabilizers. *Neuroscience, 117*, 949–955.

Boyle, P. A. (2004). Assessing and predicting functional impairment in Alzheimer's disease: The emerging role of frontal system dysfunction. *Current Psychiatry Reports, 6*, 20–24.

Bradbury, T. N., & Miller, G. A. (1985). Season of birth in schizophrenia: A review of evidence, methodology, and etiology. *Psychological Bulletin, 98*, 569–594.

Bradwejn, J., & Koszycki, D. (1994). The cholecystokinin hypothesis of anxiety and panic disorder. *Annals of the New York Academy of Sciences, 713*, 273–282.

Bradwejn, J., & Koszycki, D. (2001). Cholecystokinin and panic disorder: Past and future clinical research strategies. *Scandinavian Journal of Clinical and Laboratory Investigation Supplementum, 234*, 19–27.

Brambilla, P., Barale, F., Caverzasi, E., & Soares, J. C. (2002). Anatomical MRI findings in mood and anxiety disorders. *Epidemiologia E Psichiatria Sociale, 11*, 88–99.

Brambilla, F., Biggio, G., Pisu, M. G., Bellodi, L., Perna, G., Bogdanovich-Djukic, V., et al. (2003). Neurosteroid secretion in panic disorder. *Psychiatry Research, 118*, 107–116.

Brambilla, P., Hardan, A., di Nemi, S. U., Perez, J., Soares, J. C., & Barale, F. (2003). Brain anatomy and development in autism: Review of structural MRI studies. *Brain Research Bulletin, 61*, 557–569.

Brambilla, P., Harenski, K., Nicoletti, M., Mallinger, A. G., Frank, E., Kupfer, D. J., et al. (2001). MRI study of posterior fossa structure and brain ventricles in bipolar patients. *Journal of Psychiatry Research, 35*, 313–322.

Brambilla, P., Harenski, K., Nicoletti, M., Sassi, R. B., Mallinger, A. G., Frank, E., et al. (2003). MRI investigation of temporal lobe structures in bipolar patients. *Journal of Psychiatry Research, 37*, 287–295.

Brand, N., Geenen, R., Oudenhoven, M., Lindenborn, B., van der Ree, A., Cohen-Kettenis, P., et al. (2002). Brief report: Cognitive functioning in children with Tourette's syndrome with and without comorbid ADHD. *Journal of Pediatric Psychology, 27*, 203–208.

Brandes, M., Soares, C. N., & Cohen, L. S. (2004). Postpartum onset obsessive-compulsive disorder: Diagnosis and management. *Archives of Women's Mental Health, 7*, 99–110.

Brandt, C. A., Meller, J., Keweloh, L., Höschel, K., Staedt, J., Munz, D., et al. (1998). Increased benzodiazepine receptor density in the prefrontal cortex in patients with panic disorder. *Journal of Neural Transmission, 105*, 1325–1333.

Branson, R., Potoczna, N., Kral, J. G., Lentes, K. U., Hoehe, M. R., & Horber, F. F. (2003). Binge eating as a major phenotype of melanocortin 4 receptor gene mutations. *New England Journal of Medicine, 348*, 1096–1103.

Braun, A. R., Stoetter, B., Randolph, C., Hsiao, J. K., Vladar, K., Gernert, J., et al. (1993). The functional neuroanatomy of Tourette's syndrome: An FDG-PET study. I. Regional changes in cerebral glucose metabolism differentiating patients and controls. *Neuropsychopharmacology, 9*, 277–291.

Breakey, W. R., & Dunn, G. J. (2004). Racial disparity in the use of ECT for affective disorders. *American Journal of Psychiatry, 161*, 1635–1641.

Breggin, P. R., & Breggin, G. R. (1994). *Talking back to Prozac.* New York: St. Martin's Press.

Breiter, H. C., Rauch, S. L., Kwong, K. K., Baker, J. R., Weisskoff, R. M., Kennedy, D. N., et al. (1996). Functional magnetic resonance imaging of symptom provocation in obsessive-compulsive disorder. *Archives of General Psychiatry, 53*, 595–606.

Bremmer, J. D., Innis, R. B., Southwick, S. M., Staib, L., Zoghbi, S., & Charney, D. S. (2000). Decreased benzodiazepine receptor binding in prefrontal cortex in combat-related posttraumatic stress disorder. *American Journal of Psychiatry, 157*, 1120–1126.

Bremner, J. D., Narayan, M., Anderson, E. R., Staib, L. H., Miller, H. L., & Charney, D. S. (2000). Hippocampal volume reduction in major depression. *American Journal of Psychiatry, 157*, 115–118.

Brent, D. A., Oquendo, M., Birmaher, B., Greenhill, L., Kolko, D., Stanley, B., et al. (2003). Peripubetal suicide attempts in offspring of suicide attempters with sibling concordant for suicidal behavior. *American Journal of Psychiatry, 160*, 1486–1493.

Bressan, R. A., Erlandsson, K., Jones, H. M., Flanagan, R. J., Ell, P. J., & Pilowsky, L. S. (2003). Is regionally selective D2/D3 dopamine receptor occupancy sufficient for atypical antipsychotic effect? An in vivo quantitative [123I] epidepride SPECT study of amisulpride-treated patients. *American Journal of Psychiatry, 160*, 1413–1420.

Brett, P. M., Curtis, D., Robertson, M. M., & Gurling, H. M. (1995a). Exclusion of the 5-HT1A serotonin neuroreceptor and tryptophan axygenase genes in a large British kindred multiply affected with Tourette's syndrome, chronic motor tics, and obsessive-compulsive behavior. *American Journal of Psychiatry, 152*, 427–440.

Brett, P. M., Curtis, D., Robertson, M. M., & Gurling, H. M. (1995b). The genetic susceptibility to Gilles de la Tourette syndrome in a large multiple affected British kindred: Linkage analysis excludes a role for the genes encoding for dopamine D1, D2, D3, D4, D5 receptors, dopamine beta hydroxylase, tyrosinase, and tyrosine hydroxylase. *Biological Psychiatry, 37*, 533–540.

Brewer, D. D., Cantalano, R. F., Haggerty, K., Gainey, R. R., & Fleming, C. B. (1998). A meta-analysis of predictors of continued drug use during and after treatment for opiate addiction. *Addiction, 93*, 73–92.

Brock, J., Brown, C. C., Boucher, J., & Rippon, G. (2002). The temporal binding deficit hypothesis of autism. *Development and Psychopathology, 14*, 209–224.

Broman-Fulks, J. J., Berman, M. E., Rabian, B. A., & Webster, M. J. (2004). Effects of aerobic exercise on anxiety sensitivity. *Behaviour Research and Therapy, 42*, 125–136.

Broocks, A., Bandelow, B., Pekrun, G., George, A., Meyer, T., Bartmann, U., et al. (1998). Comparison of aerobic exercise, clomipramine, and placebo in the treatment of panic disorder. *American Journal of Psychiatry, 155*, 603–609.

Brooks, A., Fulker, D. W., & DeFries, J. C. (1990). Reading performance and general cognitive ability: A multivariate genetic analysis of twin data. *Personality and Individual Differences, 11*, 141–146.

Brooks, P. J. (2000). Brain atrophy and neuronal loss in alcoholism: A role for DNA damage? *Neurochemistry International, 37*, 403–412.

Broytman, O., & Malter, J. S. (2004). Anti-Abeta: The food, the bad, and the unforseen. *Journal of Neurscience Research, 75*, 301–306.

Bruce, S. E., Vasile, R. G., Goisman, R. M., Salzman, C., Spencer, M., Machan, J. T., et al. (2003). Are benzodiazepines still the medication of choice for patients with panic disorder with or without agoraphobia? *American Journal of Psychiatry, 160*, 1432–1438.

Brue, A. W., & Oakland, T. D. (2002). Alternative treatments for attention-deficit/hyperactivity disorder: Does evidence support their use? *Alternative Therapy in Health and Medicine, 8*, 72–74.

Bruggeman, R., van der Linden, C., Buitelaar, J. K., Gericke, G. S., Hawkridge, S. M., & Temlett, J. A. (2001). Risperidone versus pimozide in Tourette's disorder: A comparative double-blind parallel-group study. *Journal of Clinical Psychiatry, 62*, 50–56.

Bruijn, J. A., Moleman, P., Milder, P. G. H., & van den Broek, W. W. (1999). Depressed in-patients respond differently to imipramine and mirtazapine. *Pharmacopsychiatry, 32*, 87–92.

Brunner, H. G., Breakefield, N. X. O., Ropers, H. H., & van Oost, B. A. (1993). Abnormal behavior associated with a point mutation in the structural gene for monoamine oxidase A. *Science, 262*, 578–580.

Brunswick, D. J., Amsterdam, J. D., Mozley, P. D., & Newberg, A. (2003). Greater availability of brain dopamine transporters in major depression shown by [99mTc]TRODAT-1 SPECT imaging. *American Journal of Psychiatry, 160*, 1836–1841.

Brunswick, N., McCrory, E., Price, C. J., Frith, C. D., & Frith, U. (1999). Explicit and implicit processing of words by adult developmental dyslexics. A search for Wernicke's Wortschatz? *Brain, 122*, 1901–1917.

Brzustowica, L. M., Hodgkinson, K. A., Chow, E. W. C., Honer, W. G., & Bassett, A. S. (2000). Location of a major susceptibility locus for familial schizophrenia on chromosome 1q21q22. *Science, 288*, 678–682.

Buchsbaum, M. S., Nuechterlein, K. H., Haier, R. J., Wu, J., Sicotte, N., Hazlett, E., et al. (1990). Glucose metabolic rate in normals and schizophrenics during the continuous performance test assessed by positron emission tomography. *British Journal of Psychiatry, 156*, 216–227.

Buckley, P. F., Hrouda, D. R., Friedman, L., Noffsinger, S. G., Resnick, P. J., & Camlin-Shingler, K. (2004). Insight and its relationship to violent behavior in patients with schizophrenia. *American Journal of Psychiatry, 161*, 1712–1714.

Budman, C. L., Brunn, R. D., Park, K. S., Lesser, M., & Olson, M. (2000). Explosive outbursts in children with Tourette's disorder. *Journal of the American Academy of Child and Adolescent Psychiatry, 39*, 1270–1276.

Buell, S. J., & Coleman, P. D. (1981). Quantitative evidence for selective dendritic growth in normal aging, but not in senile dementia. *Brain Research, 214*, 23–31.

Bugental, B. D., Martorell, G. A., & Barraza, V. (2003). The hormonal costs of subtle forms of infant maltreatment. *Hormones and Behavior, 43*, 237–244.

Bullido, M. J., Aldudo, J., Frank, A., Coria, F., Avila, J., & Valdivieso, F. (2000). A polymorphism in the tau gene associated with risk for Alzheimer's disease. *Neuroscience Letters, 278*, 49–52.

Bunney, W. E., & Garland, B. L. (1982). A second generation catecholamine hypothesis. *Pharmacopsychiatry, 15*, 111–115.

Burghaus, L., Schütz, U., Krempel, U., Lindstrom, J., & Schröder, H. (2003). Loss of nicotinic acetylcholine receptor subunits alpha4 and alpha7 in the cerebral cortex of Parkinson patients. *Parkinsonism & Related Disorders, 9*, 243–246.

Burns, B. J., Phillips, S. D., Wagner, H. R., Barth, R. P., Kolko, D. J., Campbell, Y., et al. (2004). Mental health need and access to mental health services by youth involved with child welfare: A national survey. *Journal of Child and Adolescent Psychiatry, 43*, 960–970.

Burruss, J. W., Hurley, R. A., Taber, K. H., Rauch, R. A., Norton, R. E., & Hayman, L. A. (2000). Functional neuroanatomy of the frontal lobe circuits. *Radiology, 214*, 227–230.

Burt, D. R., Creese, I., & Synder, S. S. (1977). Antischizophrenic drugs: Chronic treatment elevates dopamine receptor binding in brain. *Science, 196*, 326–328.

Burt, S. A., Krueger, R. F., McGue, M., & Iacono, W. G. (2001). Sources of covariation among attention-deficit/hyperactivity disorder, oppositional defiant disorder, and conduct disorder: The importance of shared environment. *Journal of Abnormal Psychology, 110*, 516–525.

Burt, T., Lisanby, S. H., & Sackeim, H. A. (2002). Neuropsychiatric applications of transcranial stimulation: A meta analysis. *International Journal of Neuropsychopharmacology, 5*, 73–103.

Burton, E. J., McKeith, I. G., Burn, D. J., Williams, E. D., & O'Brien, J. T. (2004). Cerebral atrophy in Parkinson's disease with and without dementia: A comparison with Alzheimer's disease, dementia with Lewy bodies and controls. *Brain, 127*, 791–800.

Burvill P. W., Johnson, G. A., Jamrozik, K. D., Anderson, C. S., Stewart-Wynne, E. G., & Chakera, T. M. (1995). Prevalence of depression after stroke: The Perth Community Stroke Study. *British Journal of Psychiatry, 166*, 320–327.

Busatto, G. F., Buchpiguel, C. A., Zamignani, D. R., Garrido, G. E., Glabus, M. F., Rosario-Campos, M. C., et al. (2001). Regional cerebral blood flow abnormalities in early-onset obsessive-compulsive disorder: An exploratory SPECT study. *Journal of the American Academy of Child and Adolescent Psychiatry, 40*, 347–354.

Busatto, G. F., Zamignani, D. R., Buchpiguel, C. A., Garrido, G. E., Glabus, M. F., Rocha, E. T., et al. (2000). A voxel-based investigation of regional cerebral blood flow abnormalities in obsessive-compulsive disorder using single photon emission computed tomography (SPECT). *Psychiatry Research, 99*, 15–27.

Bush, G., Frazier, J. A., Rauch, S. L., Seidman, L. J., Whalen, P. J., Jenike, M. A., et al. (1999). Anterior cingulated cortex dysfunction in attention-deficit/hyperactivity disorder revealed by f MRI and the Counting Stroop. *Biological Psychiatry, 45*, 1542–1552.

Bush, G., Luu, P., & Posner, M. I. (2000). Cognitive and emotional influences in anterior cingulate cortex. *Trends in Cognitive Sciences, 4*, 215–222.

Bush, G., Whalen, P. J., Rosen, B. R., Jenike, M. A., McInerney, S. C., & Rauch, S. L. (1998). The counting stoop: An interference task specialized for functional neuroimaging—validation study with functional MRI. *Human Brain Mapping, 6*, 270–282.

Butterfield, D. A., Howard, B., Yatin, S., Koppal, T., Drake, J., Hensley, K., et al. (1999). Elevated oxidative stress in models of normal brain aging and Alzheimer's disease. *Life Sciences, 65*, 1883–1892.

Butterweck, V. (2003). Mechanism of action of St John's wort in depression: What is known? *CNS Drugs, 17*, 539–562.

Buxbaum, J. D., Silverman, J. M., Smith, C. J., Greenberg, D. A., Kilifarski, M., Reichert, J., et al. (2002). Association between a GABRB3 polymorphism and autism. *Molecular Psychiatry, 7*, 311–316.

Buydens-Branchey, L., Branchey, M., Hudson, J., Rothman, M., Fergeson, P., & McKernin, C. (1999). Serotonerigic function in cocaine addicts: Prolactin responses to sequential D, L-fenfluaramine challenges. *Biological Psychiatry, 45*, 1300–1306.

Byne, W., Buchsbaum, M. S., Mattiace, L. A., Hazlett, E. A., Kemether, E., Elhakem, S. L., et al. (2002). Postmortem assessment of thalamic nuclear volumes in subjects with schizophrenia. *American Journal of Psychiatry, 159*, 59–65.

Byne, W., Kemether, E., Jones, L., Haroutunian, V., & Davis, K. L. (1999). The neurochemistry of schizophrenia. In *Neurobiology of mental illness* (pp. 236–245). D. S. Charney, E. J. Nesterl, & B. S. Bunney (Eds.), New York: Oxford University Press.

Bystritsky, A., Pontillo, D., Powers, M., Sabb, F. W., Craske, M. G., & Bookheimer, S. Y. (2001). Functional MRI changes during panic anticipation and imagery exposure. *Neuroreport, 12*, 3953–3957.

Caballero, J., & Nahata, M. C. (2003). Atomoxetine hydrochloride for the treatment of attention-deficit/hyperactivity disorder. *Clinical Therapy, 25*, 3056–3083.

Cabeza, R., & Nyberg, L. (1997). Imagining cognition: An empirical review of PET studies with normal subjects. *Journal of Cognitive Neuroscience, 9*, 1–26.

Caccia, S. (2000a). Biotransformation of post-clozapine antipsychotics: Pharmacological implications. *Clinical Pharmacokinetics, 38*, 393–414.

Caccia, S. (2000b). New antipsychotic agents for schizophrenia: Pharmacokinetics and metabolism update. *Current Opinion Investigational Drugs, 3*, 1073–1080.

Caetano, S. C., Sassi, R., Brambilla, P., Harenski, K., Nicoletti, M., Mallinger, A. G., et al. (2001). MRI study of thalamic volumes in bipolar and unipolar patients and healthy individuals. *Psychiatry Research: Neuroimaging Section, 108*, 161–168.

Cahn, W., Hulshoff Pol, H. E., Lems, E. B. T. E., van Haren, N. E. M., Schnack, H. G., Van der Linden, J. A., et al. (2002). Brain volume changes in first-episode schizophrenia: A one-year follow-up study. *Archives of General Psychiatry, 59*, 1002–1010.

Cahn-Weiner, D. A., Ready, R. E., & Malloy, P. F. (2003). Neuropsychological predictors of everyday memory and everyday functioning in patients with mild Alzheimer's disease. *Journal of Geriatric Psychiatry and Neurology, 16*, 84–89.

Caliguri, M. P., Brown, G. G., Meloy, M. J., Eberson, S. C., Kindermann, S. S., Frank, L. R., et al. (2003). An fMRI study of affective state and medication on cortical and subcortical brain regions during motor performance in bipolar disorder. *Psychiatry Research, 123*, 171–182.

Callicott, J. H., Egan, M. F., Mattay, V. S., Bertolino, A., Bone, A. D., Verchinski, B., et al. (2003). Abnormal fMRI response of the dorsolateral prefrontal cortex in cognitively intact siblings of patients with schizophrenia. *American Journal of Psychiatry, 160*, 709–719.

Calne, S. M. (2003). The psychosocial impact of late-stage Parkinson's disease. *Journal of Neuroscience Nursing, 35*, 306–313.

Camaioni, L., Perucchini, P., Muratori, F., Parrini, B., & Cesari, A. (2003). The communicative use of pointing in autism: Developmental profile and factors related to change. *European Psychiatry, 18*, 6–12.

Camarena, B., Rinetti, G., Cruz, C., Gómez, A., de La Fuente, J. R., & Nicolini, H. (2001a). Additional evidence that genetic variation of MAO-A gene supports a gender subtype in obsessive-compulsive disorder. *American Journal of Medical Genetics, 105*, 279–282.

Camarena, B., Rinetti, G., Cruz, C., Hernández, S., de la Fuente, J. R., & Nicolini, H. (2001b). Association study of the serotonin transporter gene polymorphism in obsessive-compulsive disorder. *International Journal of Neuropsychopharmacology, 4*, 269–272.

Cameron, O. G., Zubieta, J. K., Grunhaus, L., & Minoshima, S. (2000). Effects of yohimbine on cerebral blood flow, symptoms, and physiological functions in humans. *Psychosomatic Medicine, 62*, 549–559.

Cami, J., & Farre, M. (2003). Drug addiction. *New England Journal of Medicine, 349*, 975–986.

Camicioli, R., Moore, M. M., Kinney, A., Corbridge, E., Glassberg, K., & Kaye, J. A. (2003). Parkinson's disease is associated with hippocampal atrophy. *Movement Disorders, 18*, 784–790.

Campbell, F. A., & Ramey, C. T. (1994). Effects of early intervention on intellectual and academic achievement: A follow up study of children from low income families. *Child Development, 65*, 684–698.

Campbell, J. M. (2003). Efficacy of behavioral interventions for reducing problem behavior in persons with autism: A quantitative synthesis of single-subject research. *Research in Developmental Disabilities, 24*, 120–138.

Campbell, S., Marriott, M., Nhamias, C., & MacQueen, G. M. (2004). Lower hippocampal volume in patients suffering from depression: A meta-analysis. *American Journal of Psychiatry, 161*, 598–607.

Cannon, T. D., Rosso, I. M., Bearden, C. E., Sanchez, L. E., & Hadley, T. (1999). A prospective cohort study of neurodevelopmental processes in the genesis and epigenesis of schizophrenia. *Development and Psychopathology, 11*, 467–485.

Cannon, T. D., Thompson, P. M., van Erp, T. G. M., Toga, A. W., Poutanen, V., Huttunen, M., et al. (2002). Cortex mapping reveals regionally specific patterns of genetic and disease-specific gray-matter deficits in twins discordant for schizophrenia. *Proceedings of the National Academy of the Sciences, 99*, 3228–3233.

Cantor-Graae, E., Warkentin, S., Franzen, G., & Risberg, J. (1993). Frontal lobe challenge: A comparison of activation procedures during rCBF measurements in normal subjects. *Neuropsychiatry, Neuropsychology, and Behavioral Neurology, 6*, 83–92.

Cantwell, D. P. (1972). Psychiatric illness in the families of hyperactive children. *Archives of General Psychiatry, 27*, 414–417.

Caplan, L. R., Gomez Beldarrain, M., Bier, J. C., Vokaer, M., Bartholme, E. J., & Pandolfo, M. (2002). The cerebellum may be directly involved in cognitive functions. *Neurology, 59*, 790–791.

Caradoc-Davies, T. H., Weatherall, M., Dixon, G. S., Caradoc-Davies, G., & Hantz, P. (1992). Is the prevalence of Parkinson's disease in New Zealand really changing? *Acta Neurologica Scandinavica, 86*, 40–44.

Cardno, A. G., Marshall, E. J., Coid, B., Macdonald, A. M., Ribchester, T. R., Davies, M. J., et al. (1999). Heritability estimates for psychotic disorders: The Mudsley twin psychosis series. *Archives of General Psychiatry, 56*, 162–168.

Carlbring, P., Gustafsson, H., Ekselius, L., & Andersson, G. (2002). 12-month prevalence of panic disorder with or without agoraphobia in the Swedish general population. *Social Psychiatry and Psychiatric Epidemiology, 37*, 207–211.

Carlson, M., & Earls, F. (1997). Physiological and neuroendocrinological sequelae of early social deprivation in institutionalized children in Romania. *Annals of the New York Academy of the Sciences, 807*, 419–428.

Carlson, N. R. (2001). *Physiology of behavior* (7th ed.). Boston: Allyn & Bacon.

Carlsson, A., Lindqvist, M., & Magnusson, T. (1957). 3, 4-Dihydroxphenylalanine and 5-hydroxytyramine as resperpine antagonists. *Nature, 180*, 1200–1202.

Carlsson, A., Waters, N., Holm-Waters, S., Tedroff, J., Nilsson, M., & Carlsson, M. (2001). Interactions between monoamines, glutamate, and GABA in schizophrenia: New evidence. *Annual Review of Pharmacology and Toxicology, 41*, 237–260.

Carpenter, L. L., Friehs, G. M., & Price, L. H. (2003). Cervical vagus nerve stimulation for treatment-resistant depression. *Neurosurgery Clinics of North America, 14*, 275–282.

Carvey, P. M. (1998). *Drug action in the central nervous system.* New York: Oxford University Press.

Casanova, M. F., Araque, J., Giedd, J., & Rumsey, J. M. (2004). Reduced brain size and gyrification in the brains of dyslexic patients. *Journal of Child Neurology, 19*, 275–281.

Casanova, M. F., Buxhoeveden, D., & Gomez, J. (2003). Disruption in the inhibitory architecture of the cell minicolumn: Implications for autisim. *The Neuroscientist, 9*, 496–507.

Casanova, M. F., Buxhoeveden, D. P., Switala, A. E., & Roy, E. (2002). Asperger's syndrome and cortical neuropathology. *Journal of Child Neurology, 17*, 142–145.

Casanova, M. F., Buxhoeveden, D. P., Switala, A. E., & Roy, E. (2002). Neuronal density and architecture (Gray Level Index) in the brains of autistic patients. *Journal of Child Neurology, 17*, 515–521.

Caspi, A., Sugden, K., Moffitt, T. E., Taylor, A., Craig, I. W., Harrington, H., et al. (2003). Influence of life stress on depression: Moderation by a polymorphism in the 5-HTT gene. *Science, 301*, 386–389.

Cassano, G. B., Miniati, M., Pini, S., Rotondo, A., Banti, S., Borri, C., et al. (2003). Six month open trial of haloperidol as an adjunctive treatment for anorexia nervosa: A preliminary report. *International Journal of Eating Disorders, 33*, 172–177.

Castellanos, F. X., Giedd, J. N., Berquin, P. C., Walter, J. M., Sharp, W., Tran, T., et al. (2001). Quantitative brain magnetic resonance imaging in girls with attention-deficit/hyperactivity disorder. *Archives of General Psychiatry, 58*, 289–295.

Castellanos, F. X., Giedd, J. N., Eckburg, P., Marsh, W. L., Vaituzis, A. C., Kaysen, D., et al. (1994). Quantitative morphology of the caudate nucleus in attention deficit hyperactivity disorder. *American Journal of Psychiatry, 151*, 1791–1796.

Castellanos, F. X., Giedd, J. N., Hamburger, S. D., Marsh, W. L., & Rapoport, J. L. (1996). Brain morphometry in Tourette's syndrome: The influence of comorbid attention-deficit/hyperactivity disorder. *Neurology 47*, 1581–1583.

Castellanos, F. X., Lau, E., Tayebi, N., Lee, P., Long, R. E., Giedd, J. N., et al. (1998). Lack of an association between a dopamine-4 receptor polymorphism and attention-deficit/hyperactivity disorder: genetic and brain morphometric analyses. *Molecular Psychiatry, 3*, 431–434.

Castellanos, F. X., Lee, P. P., Sharp, W., Jeffries, N. O., Greenstein, D. K., Clasen, L. S., et al. (2002). Developmental trajectories of brain volume abnormalities in children and adolescents with attention-deficit/hyperactivity disorder. *Journal of the American Medical Association, 288*, 1740–1748.

Castellanos, F. X., Sharp, W. S., Gottesman, R. F., Greenstein, D. K., Giedd, J. N., & Rapoport, J. L. (2003). Anatomic brain abnormalities in monozygotic twins discordant for attention deficit. *American Journal of Psychiatry, 160*, 1693–1696.

Castillo, A. R., Buchpiguel, C. A., de Araujo, L. A., Castillo, J. C., Asbahr, F. R., Maia, A. K., et al. (2005). Brain SPECT imaging in children & adolescents with obsessive-compulsive disorder. *Journal of Neural Transmission*, 1435–1463.

Cath, D. C., Spinhiven, P., Landman, A. D., & van Kempen, G. M. J. (2001). Psychopathology and personality characteristics in relations to blood serotonin in Tourette's syndrome and obsessive-compulsive disorder. *Journal of Psychopharmacology, 15*, 111–119.

Cavallini, M. C., Di Bella, D., Catalano, M., & Bellodi, L. (2000). An association study between 5-HTTLPR polymorphism, COMT polymorphism, and Tourette's syndrome. *Psychiatry Research, 97*, 93–100.

Ceballos-Baumann, A. O., Boecker, H., Bartenstein, P., von Falkenhayn, I., Riescher, H., Conrad, B., et al. (1999). A positron emission tomography study of subthalamic nucleus stimulation in Parkinson disease: Enhanced movement-related activity of motor-association cortex and decreased motor cortex resting activity. *Archives of Neurology, 56*, 997–1003.

Cecil, K. M., BelBello, M. P., Sellars, M. C., & Strakowski, S. M. (2003). Proton magnetic resonance spectroscopy of the frontal lobe and cerebellar vermis in children with mood disorder and a familial risk for bipolar disorders. *Journal of Child and Adolescent Psychopharmacology, 13*, 545–555.

Chabane, N., Leboyer, M., & Mouren-Simeoni, M. C. (2000). Opiate antagonists in children and adolescents. *European Child & Adolescent Psychiatry, 9*, 44–50.

Chakrabarti, S., & Fombonne, E. (2001). Pervasive developmental disorders in preschool children. *Journal of the American Medical Association, 285*, 3093–3099.

Chan, D., Janssen, J. C., Whitwell, J. L., Watt, H. C., Jenkins, R., Frost, C., et al. (2003). Change in rates of cerebral atrophy over time in early-onset Alzheimer's disease: Longitudinal MRI study. *Lancet, 362*, 1121–1122.

Chan, E., Rappaport, L. A., & Kemper, K. J. (2003). Complementary and alternative therapies in childhood attention and hyperactivity problems. *Journal of Development in Behavioral Pediatrics, 24*, 4–8.

Chana, G., Landau, S., Beasley, C., Everall, I. P., & Cotter, D. (2003). Two-dimensional assessment of cytoarchitecture in the anterior cingulate cortex in major depressive disorder, bipolar disorder, and schizophrenia: Evidence for decreased neuronal somal size and increased neuronal density. *Biological Psychiatry, 53*, 1086–1098.

Chang, A., Li, P. P., & Warsh, J. J. (2003). cAMP-Dependent protein kinase (PKA) subunit mRNA levels in postmortem brain from patients with bipolar affective disorder (BD). *Molecular Brain Research, 116*, 27–37.

Channon, S., Crawford, S., Vakili, K., & Robertson, M. M. (2003). Real-life-type problem solving in Tourette syndrome. *Cognitive Behavioral Neurology, 16*, 3–15.

Chantarujikapong, S. I., Scherrer, J. F., Xian, H., Eisen, S. A., Lyons, M. J., Goldberg, J., et al. (2001). A twin study of generalized anxiety disorder symptoms, panic disorder symptoms and post-traumatic stress disorder in men. *Psychiatry Research, 103*, 133–145.

Chappell, P. B., Riddle, M. A., Scahill, L., Lynch, K. A., Schultz, R., Arnsten, A., et al. (1995). Guanfacine treatment of comorbid attention-deficit hyperactivity disorder and Tourette's syndrome: Preliminary clinical experience. *Journal of the American Academy of Child and Adolescent Psychiatry, 34*, 1140–1146.

Charach, A., Ickowicz, A., & Schachar, R. (2004). Stimulant treatment over five years: Adherence, effectiveness, and adverse effects. *Journal of the American Academy of Child and Adolescent Psychiatry, 43*, 559–567.

Charnay, D. S. (2003). Neuroanatomical circuits modulating fear and anxiety behaviors. *Acta Psychiatrica Scandanavica, 417*, 38–50.

Charnay, Y., Leger, L., Vallet, P. G., Hof, P. R., Jouvet, M., & Bouras, C. (1995), [3H] Nisoxetine binding sites in the cat brain: An autoradiographic study. *Neuroscience, 69*, 259–270.

Charney, D. S. (2003). Neuroanatomical circuits modulating fear and anxiety behaviors. *Acta Psychiatrica Scandinavica, Supplementum*, 38–50.

Charney, D. S., & Heninger, G. R. (1986). Abnormal regulation of noradrenergic function in panic disorders. Effects of clonidine in healthy subjects and patients with agoraphobia and panic disorder. *Archives of General Psychiatry, 43*, 1042–1054.

Charney, D. S., Woods, S. W., Goodman, W. K., & Heninger, G. R. (1987). Neurobiological mechanisms of panic anxiety: Biochemical and behavioral correlates of yohimbine-induced panic attacks. *American Journal of Psychiatry, 144*, 1030–1036.

Charney, D. S., Woods, S. W., & Heninger, G. R. (1989). Noradrenergic function in generalized anxiety disorder: Effects of yohimbine in healthy subjects and patients with generalized anxiety disorder. *Psychiatry Research, 27*, 173–182.

Checkoway, H., & Nelson, L. M. (1999). Epidemiologic approaches to the study of Parkinson's disease etiology. *Epidemiology, 10*, 327–336.

Checkoway, H., Powers, K., Smith-Weller, T., Franklin, G. M., Longstreth, W. T. Jr., & Swanson, P. D. (2002). Parkinson's disease risks associated with cigarette smoking, alcohol consumption, and caffeine intake. *American Journal of Epidemiology, 155*, 732–738.

Cheeta, S., Schifano, F., Oyefeso, A., Webb, L., & Ghodse, A. H. (2004). Antidepressant-related deaths and antidepressant prescriptions in England and Wales, 1998–2000. *British Journal of Psychiatry, 184*, 41–47.

Chemali, Z., & Bromfield, E. (2003). Tourette's syndrome following temporal lobectomy for seizure control. *Epilepsy Behavior, 4*, 564–566.

Chen, A. C., LaForge, K. S., Ho, A., McHugh, P. F., Kellogg, S., Bell, K., et al. (2002). Potentially functional polymorphism in the promoter region of prodynorphin gene may be associated with protection against cocaine dependence or abuse. *American Journal of Medical Genetics, 114*, 429–435.

Chen, C. C., Lu, R. B., Chen, Y. C., Wang, M. F., Chang, Y. C., Li, T. K., et al. (1999). Interaction between the functional polymorphisms of the alcohol-metabolism genes in protection against alcohol. *American Journal of Human Genetics, 6*, 795–807.

Chen, C. Y., Liu, C. Y., & Yang, Y. Y. (2001). Correlation of panic attacks and hostility in chronic schizophrenia. *Psychiatry and Clinical Neurosciences, 55*, 383–387.

Chen, G., Hasanat, K. A., Bebchuk, J. M., Moore, G. J., Glitz, D., & Manji, H. K. (1999). Regulation of signal transduction pathways and gene expression by mood stabilizers and antidepressants. *Psychosomatic Medicine, 61*, 599–617.

Chen, G., Huang, L. D., Zeng, W. Z., & Manji, H. (2001). Mood stabilizers regulate cytoprotective and mRNA-binding proteins in the brain: Long-term effects on cell survival and transcript stability. *International Journal of Neuropsychopharmacology, 4*, 47–64.

Chen, R., Wei, J., Fowler, S. C., & Wu, J. Y. (2003). Demonstration of functional coupling between dopamine synthesis and its packaging into synaptic vesicles. *Journal of Biomedical Science, 10*, 774–781.

Chen, Y. S., Akula, N., Detera-Wadleigh, S. D., Schulze, T. G., Thomas, J., Potash, J. B., et al. (2004). Findings in an independent sample support an association between bipolar affective disorder and the G72/G30 locus on chromosome 13q33. *Molecular Psychiatry, 9*, 87–92.

Cheng, F. C., Kuo, J. S., Chia, L. G., & Dryhurst, G. (1996). Elevated 5-S-cysteinyldopamine/homovanillic acid ratio and reduced homovanillis acid in cerebrospinal fluid: Possible markers for and potential insights into the pathoetiology of Parkinson's disease. *Journal of Neural Transmission, 103*, 433–446.

Cheon, K.-A., Ryu, Y. H., Kim, Y.-K., Namkoong, K., Kim, C. H., & Lee, J. D. (2003). Dopamine transporter density in the basal ganglia assessed with [123I]IPT SPET in children with attention deficit hyperactivity. *European Journal of Nuclear Medicine, 30*, 306–311.

Cheon, K. A., Ryu, Y. H., Namkoong, K., Kim, C.-H., Kim, J. J., & Lee, J. D. (2004). Dopamine transporter density of the basal ganglia assessed with [123I]IPT SPECT in drug-naïve children with Tourette's disorder. *Psychiatry Research, 130*, 85–95.

Chez, M. G., Buchanan, C. P., Bagan, B. T., Hammer, M. S., McCarthy, K. S., Ovrutskaya, I., et al. (2000). Secretin and autism: A two-part clinical investigation. *Journal of Autism and Developmental Disorders, 30*, 87–94.

Chia, L. G., Cheng, F. C., & Kuo, J. S. (1993). Monoamines and their metabolites in plasma and lumbar cerebrospinal fluid of Chinese patients with Parkinson's disease. *Journal of Neurological Science, 116*, 125–134.

Chih, B., Afridi, S. K., Clark, L., & Scheiffele, P. (2004). Disorder-associated mutations lead to functional inactivation of neuroligins. *Human Molecular Genetics, 13*, 1471–1477.

Christ, S. E., White, D. A., Mandernach, T., & Keys, B. A. (2001). Inhibitory control across the life span. *Developmental Neuropsychology, 20*, 653–669.

Chugani, D. C., Muzik, O., Behen, M., Rothermel, R., Janisse, J. J., Lee, J., et al. (1999). Developmental changes in brain serotonin synthesis capacity in autistic and nonautistic children. *Annals of Neurology, 45*, 287–295.

Chugani, H., & Phelps, M. (1991). Imaging human brain development with positron emission tomography. *Journal of Nuclear Medicine, 32*, 23–26.

Chugani, H. T. (1998). Biological basis of emotions: Brain systems and brain development. *Pediatrics, 102*, 1225–1229.

Chugani, H. T., Behen, M. E., Muzik, O., Juhasz, C., Nagy, F., & Chugani, C. D. (2001). Local brain functional activity following early deprivation: A study of postinstitutionalized Romanian orphans. *Neuroimage, 14*, 1290–1301.

Chumakov, I., Blumenfeld, M, Guerassimenko, O., Cavarec, L., Palicio, M., Aberrahim, H., et al. (2002). Genetic and physiological data implicating the new human gene G72 and the gene for D-amino acid oxidase in schizophrenia. *Proceedings of the National Academy of Sciences, 99*, 13365–13367.

Chung, T., Martin, C. S., Grella, C. E., Winters, K. C., Abrantes, A. M., & Brown, S. A. (2003). Course of alcohol problems in treated adolescents. *Alcoholism: Clinical and Experimental Research, 27*, 253–261.

Clarke, P. B. S., & Pert, A. (1985). Autoradiographic evidence for nicotine receptors on nigrostriatal and mesolimbic dopaminergic neurons. *Brain Research, 348*, 355–358.

Clarkson, E. D., & Freed, C. R. (1999). Development of fetal neural transplantation as a treatment for Parkinson's disease. *Life Sciences, 65*, 2427–2437.

Clavería, L. E., Duarte, J., Sevillano, M. D., Pérez-Sempere, A., Cabezas, C., Rodríguez, F., et al. (2002). Prevalence of Parkinson's disease in Cantalejo, Spain: A door-to-door survey. *Movement Disorders, 17*, 242–249.

Cleghorn, J. M., Franco, S., Szechtman, B., Kaplan, R. D., Szechtman, H., Brown, G. M., et al. (1992). Toward a brain map of auditory hallucinations. *American Journal of Psychiatry, 149*, 1062–1069.

Clinton, S. M., Haroutunian, V., Davis, K. L., Meador-Woodruff, J. H. (2003). Altered transcript expression of NMDA receptor-associated postsynaptic proteins in the thalamus of subjects with schizophrenia. *American Journal of Psychiatry, 160*, 1100–1109.

Cloninger, C. R. (1999). Genetics of substance abuse. In Galanter, M., & Kleber, H. (Eds.), *Textbook of substance abuse treatment* (2nd ed., pp. 59–66). Washington, DC: American Psychiatric Press, Inc.

Cloninger, R. C. (2003). The discovery of susceptibility genes for mental disorders. *Proceedings of the National Academy of the Sciences, 99*, 13365–13367.

Cobb, W. S., & Abercrombie, E. D. (2003). Relative involvement of globus pallidus and subthalamic nucleus in the regulation of somatodendritic dopamine release in substantia nigra is dopamine-dependent. *Neuroscience, 119*, 777–786.

Coccaro, E. F., Siever, L. J., Klar, H. M., Cochrane, K., Cooper, T. B., Mohs, R. C., et al. (1998). Serotonergic studies in patients with affective and personality disorders: Correlates with suicidal and impulsive aggressive behavior. *Archives of General Psychiatry, 46*, 587–599.

Coccaro, E. F., Siever, L. J., Klar, H. M., Maurer, G., Cochrane, K., Cooper, T. B., et al. (1989). Serotonergic studies in patients with affective and personality disorders: Correlates with suicidal and impulsive aggressive behavior. *Archives of General Psychiatry, 46*, 587–599.

Coelho, R., Rangel, R., Ramos, E., Martins, A., Prata, J., & Barros, H. (2000). Depression and severity of substance abuse. *Psychopathology, 33*, 103–109.

Coffey, C. E., Wilkinson, W. E., Weiner, R. D., Parashos, I. A., Djang, W. T., Webb, M. C., et al. (1993). Quantitative cerebral anatomy of depression: A controlled magnetic resonance imaging study. *Archives of General Psychiatry, 50*, 7–16.

Cohen, D. J., Caparulo, B. K., Shaywitz, B. A., & Bowers, M. B. (1977). Dopamine and serotonin metabolism in neuropsychiatrically disturbed children. *Archives of General Psychiatry, 34*, 545–550.

Cohen, D. J., Shaywitz, B. A., Caparulo, B., Young, J. G., & Bowers, M. B. Jr. (1978). Chronic, multiple tics of Gilles de la Tourette's disease. CSF acid monoamine metabolites after probenecid administration. *Archives of General Psychiatry, 35*, 245–250.

Cohen, I. L. (2003). Criterion-related validity of the PDD behavior inventory. *Journal of Autism and Developmental Disorders, 33*, 47–53.

Coleman, P. D., Romano, J., Lapham, L., & Simon, W. (1985). Cell counts in cerebral cortex of an autistic patient. *Journal of Autism and Developmental Disorders, 15*, 245–255.

Collier, D. A., Stober, G., Li, T., Heils, A., Catano, M., Di Bella, D., et al. (1996). A novel functional polymorphism within the promoter of the serotonin transporer gene: Possible role in susceptibility to affective disorders. *Molecular Psychiatry, 1*, 453–460.

Colohan, H., O'Callaghan, E., Larkin, C., & Waddington, J. L. (1989). An evaluation of cranial CT scanning in clinical psychiatry. *Irish Journal of Medical Science, 58*, 178–181.

Comings, D. E. (1987). A controlled study of Tourette syndrome. VII. Summary: A common genetic disorder causing disinhibition of the limbic system. *American Journal of Human Genetics, 41*, 839–866.

Comings, D. E. (2001). Clinical and molecular genetics of ADHD and Tourette syndrome. Two related polygenic disorders. *Annals of the New York Academy of Sciences, 931*, 50–83.

Comings, D. E., Gade-Andavolu, R., Gonzalez, N., Wu, S., Muhleman, D., Blake, H., et al. (2000). Comparison of the role of dopamine, serotonin, and noradrenaline genes in ADHD, ODD and conduct disorder: Multivariate regression analysis of 20 genes. *Clinical Genetics, 57*, 178–196.

Comings, D. E., Wu, S., Chiu, C., Ring, R. H., Gade, R., Ahn, C., MacMurray, J. P., Dietz, G., & Muhleman, D. (1996). Polygenic inheritance of Tourette syndrome, atuttering, attention deficit hyperactivity, conduct, and oppositional defiant disorder: The additive and subtractive effect of the three dopaminergic genes—DRD2, DβH, and DAT1. *American Journal of Medical Genetics, 67*, 264–288.

Compton, P., Geschwind, D. H., & Alarcon, M. (2003). Association between human mu-opiod receptor gene polymorphism, pain tolerance, and opioid addiction. *American Journal of Medical Genetics, 121*, 76–82.

Conley, R. R., & Kelly, D. L. (2001). Management of treatment resistance in schizophrenia. *Biological Psychiatry, 50*, 898–911.

Conley, R. R., & Mahmoud, R. (2001). A randomized double-blind study of risperidone and olanzapine in the treatment of schizophenia or schizoaffective disorder. *American Journal of Psychiatry, 158*, 765–774.

Constantino, J. N., & Todd, R. D. (2003). Autistic traits in the general population: A twin study. *Archives of General Psychiatry, 60*, 524–530.

Conti, L., Sipione, S., Magrassi, L., Bonfanti, L., Rigamont, D., Pettirossi, V., et al. (2001). Shc signaling in differentiating neural progenitor cells. *Nature Neuroscience, 4*, 579–586.

Convit, A., de Asis, J., de Leon, M. J., Tarshish, C. Y., De Santi, S., & Rusinek, H. (2000). Atrophy of the medial occipitotemporal, inferior, and middle temporal gyri in non-demented elderly predict decline to Alzheimer's disease. *Neurobiology of Aging, 21*, 19–26.

Convit, A., de Leon, M. J., Hoptman, M. J., Tarshish, C., De Santi, S., & Rusinek, H. (1995). Age-related changes in brain: I. Magnetic resonance imaging measures of temporal lobe volumes in normal subjects. *Psychiatric Quarterly, 66*, 343–355.

Cook, E. H. Jr. (1999). Genetics of attention-deficit hyperactivity disorder. *Mental Retardation and Developmental Disabilities Research Reviews, 5*, 191–198.

Cook, I. A., Leuchter, A. F., Morgan, M., Witte, E., Stubbeman, W. F., Abrams, M., et al. (2002). Early changes in prefrontal activity characterize clinical responders to antidepressants. *Neuropsychopharmacology, 27*, 120–131.

Cook, L. J., Ho, L. W., Taylor, A. E., Brayne, C., Evans, J. G., Xuereb, J., et al. (2004). Candidate gene association studies of the alpha 4 (CIIRNA4) and beta 2 (CIIRNB2) neuronal nicotinic acetylcholine receptor subunit genes in Alzheimer's disease. *Neuroscience Letters, 358*, 142–146.

Cooper, J. R., Bloom, F. E., & Roth, R. H. (2003). *The biochemical basis of neuropharmacology* (8th ed.). New York: Oxford University Press.

Cope, D. N. (1995). The effectiveness of traumatic brain injury rehabilitation: A review. *Brain Injury, 9*, 649–670.

Coplan, J. D., & Lydiard, R. B. (1998). Brain circuits in panic disorder. *Biological Psychiatry, 44*, 1264–1276.

Corbetta, M., Miezin, F. M., Dobmeyer, S., Shulman, G. L., & Petersen, S. E. (1991). Selective and divided attention during visual discriminations of shape, color, and speed: Functional anatomy by positron emission tomography. *Journal of Neuroscience, 11*, 2383–2402.

Cosgrove, G. R., & Rauch, S. L. (1995). Psychosurgery. *Neurosurgery Clinics in North America, 6*, 167–176.

Costa, P., Checkoway, H., Levy, D., Smith-Weller, T., Franklin, G. M., Swanson, P. D., et al. (1997). Association of a polymorphism in intron 13 of the monoamine oxidase B gene with Parkinson disease. *American Journal of Medical Genetics, 74*, 154–156.

Costello, E. J., & Angold, A. (1995). Developmental epidemilogy. In D. Ciccchetti & D. J. Cohen (Eds.), *Developmental psychopathology*. New York: Wiley.

Cotter, D., Mackay, D., Landau, S., Kerwin, R., & Everall, I. (2001). Reduced glial cell density and neuronal size in the anterior cingulate cortex in major depressive disorder. *Archives of General Psychiatry, 58*, 545–553.

Cottraux, J., Note, I., Yao, S. N., Lafont, S., Note, B., Mollard, E., et al. (2001). A randomized controlled trial of cognitive therapy versus intensive behavior therapy in obsessive compulsive disorder. *Psychotherapy and Psychosomatics, 70*, 288–297.

Courchesne, E., Carper, R., & Akshoomoff, N. (2003). Evidence of brain overgrowth in the first year of life in autism. *Journal of the American Medical Association, 290*, 337–344.

Courchesne, E., Karns, C. M., Davis, H. R., Ziccardi, R., Carper, R. A., Tigue, Z. D., et al. (2001). Unusual brain growth patterns in early life in patients with autistic disorder: An MRI study. *Neurology, 57*, 245–254.

Coutin-Churman, P., Anez, Y., Uzcategui, M., Alvarez, L., Vergara, F., Mendez, L., et al. (2003). Quantitative spectral analysis of EEG in psychiatry revisited: Drawing signs out of numbers in a clinical setting. *Clincal Neurophysiology, 114*, 2294–2306.

Coutinho, A. M., Oliveira, G., Morgadinho, T., Fesel, C., Macedo, T. R., & Bento, C. (2004). Variants of the serotonin transporter gene (SLC6A4) significantly contribute to hyperserotonemia in autism. *Molecular Psychiatry, 9*, 264–271.

Cowan, M. W., & Kandel, E. R. (2001). A brief history of synapses and synaptic transmission. In M. W. Cowan, T. C. Sudhof, & C. F. Stevens (Eds.), *Synapses* (pp. 1–88). Baltimore: Johns Hopkins University Press.

Cowan, M. W., Sudhof, T. C., & Stevens, C. F. (2001). *Synapses*. Baltimore: Johns Hopkins University Press.

Cowan, W. M. (1979). The development of the brain. *Scientific American, 241*, 113–133.

Cox, B. J., Norton, G. R., Dorward, J., & Fergusson, P. A. (1989). The relationship between panic attacks and chemical dependencies. *Addictive Behaviors, 14*, 53–60.

Cox, D. D., & Savoy, R. L. (2003). Functional magnetic resonance imaging (fMRI) brain reading: Detecting and classifying distributed patterns of fMRI activity in the human visual cortex. *Neuroimage, 19*, 261–270.

Coyle, J. T., & Duman, R. S. (2003). Finding the intracellular signaling pathways affected by mood disorder treatments. *Neuron, 38*, 157–160.

Crabbe, J. (2002). Genetic contributions to addiction. *Annual Review of Psychology, 53*, 435–462.

Craddock, N., & Jones, I. (2001). Molecular genetics of bipolar disorder. *British Journal of Psychiatry Supplement, 41*, 128–133.

Cragg, B. G. (1975). The density of synapses and neurons in normal, mentally defective and aging human brains. *Brain, 98*, 81–90.

Craig, A. M., & Lichtman, J. W. (2001). Getting a bead on receptor movements. *Nature Neuroscience, 4*, 219–220.

Cravchik, A., & Goldman, D. (2000) Neurochemical individuality: Genetic diversity among human dopamine and serotonin receptors and transporters. *Archives of General Psychiatry, 57*, 1105–1114.

Cravchik, A., & Goldman, D. (2000). Genetic diversity among human dopamine and serotonin receptors and transporters. *Archives of General Psychiatry, 57*, 1105–1114.

Crawford, F., Freeman, M., Town, T., Fallin, D., Gold, M., Duara, R., et al. (1999). No genetic association between polymorphisms in the tau gene and Alzheimer's disease in clinic or population based samples. *Neuroscience Letters, 266*, 193–196.

Crowe, M., Andel, R., Pedersen, N. L., Johansson, B., & Gatz, M. (2003). Does participation in leisure activities lead to reduced risk of Alzheimer's disease? A prospective study of Swedish twins. *Journals of Gerontology, 58*, 249–255.

Crowe, R. R. (2004). Molecular genetics of anxiety. In D. S. Charney and E. J. Nestler (Eds.), Neurobiology of mental illness (2nd ed., pp. 535–545). New York: Oxford University Press.

Crum, R. M., & Anthony, J. C. (1993). Cocaine use and other suspected risk factors for obsessive-compulsive disorder: A prospective study with data from the Epidemiologic Catchment Area surveys. *Drug and Alcohol Dependence, 31*, 281–295.

Cruz, D. A., Eggan, S. M., Azmitia, E. C., & Lewis, D. A. (2004). Serotonin1A receptors at the axon segment of prefrontal pyramidal neurons in schizophrenia. *American Journal of Psychiatry, 161*, 739–742.

Csernansky, J. G., Mahmoud, R., & Brenner, R. (2002). A comparison of risperidone and haloperidol for the prevention of relapse in patients with schizophrenia. *New England Journal of Medicine, 346*, 16–21.

Cummings, D. D., Singer, H. S., Krieger, M., Miller, T. L., & Mahone, E. M. (2002). Neuropsychiatric effects of guanfacine in children with mild Tourette syndrome: A pilot study. *Clinical Neuropharmacology, 25*, 325–332.

Cummings, J. L. (1992). Depression and Parkinson's disease: A review. *American Journal of Psychiatry, 149*, 443–454.

Cunningham, C. L., & Phillips, T. J. (2003). Genetic basis of ethanol reward. In R. Maldonado (Ed.), *Molecular biology of drug addiction* (pp. 263–294). Totowa, NJ: Humana Press.

Curtis, V. A., Bullmore, E. T., Brammer, M. J., Wright, L. C., Williams, S. C. R., Morris, R. G., et al. (1998). Attenuated frontal activation during verbal fluency in schizophrenia. *American Journal of Psychiatry, 155*, 1056–1063.

Curtis, V. A., Dixon, T. A., Morris, R. G., Bullmore, E. T., Brammer, M. J., Williams, S. C. R., et al. (2001). Differential frontal activation in schizophrenia and bipolar illness during verbal fluency. *Journal of Affective Disorders, 66*, 111–121.

Curtiss, S., & Schaeffer, J. (1997). Syntactic development in children with hemispherectomy: The Infl-system. In E. Hughes, M. Hughes, & Greenhill, A. (Eds.), *Proceedings of the 21st Annual Boston University Conference on Language Development*, Volume 2. Somerville, MA: Cascadilla Press.

Dager, S. R., Holland, J. P., Cowley, D. S., & Dunner, D. L. (1997). Panic disorder precipitated by exposure to organic solvents in the work place. *American Journal of Psychiatry, 144*, 1056–1058.

Daglish, M. R., Weinstein, A., Malizia, A. L., Wilson, S., Melichar, J. K., Lingford-Hughes, A., et al. (2003). Functional connectivity analysis of the neural circuits of opiate craving: "More" rather than "different"? *Neuroimage, 20*, 1964–1970.

Dahl, M. L. (2002). Cytochrome p450 phenotyping/genotyping in patients receiving antipsychotics: Useful aid to prescribing? *Clinical Pharmacokinetics, 41*, 453–470.

Dahlstrom, M., Ahonen, A., Ebeling, H., Torniainen, P., Heikkila, J., & Moilanen, I. (2000). Elevated hypothalamic/midbrain serotonin (monoamine) transporter availability in depressive drug-naïve children and adolescents. *Molecular Psychiatry, 5*, 514–522.

Dalman, C., Thomas, H. V., David, A. S., Gentz, J., & Lewis, G. (2001). Signs of asphyxia at birth and risk of schizophrenia. Population-based case-control study. *British Journal of Psychiatry, 179*, 403–408.

Daly, G., Hawi, Z., Fitzgerald, M., & Gill, M. (1999). Mapping susceptibility loci in attention deficit hyperactivity disorder: Preferential transmission of parental alleles at DAT1, DBH and DRD5 to affected children. *Molecular Psychiatry, 4*, 192–196.

Damadzic, R., Bigelow, L. B., Krimer, L. S., Goldenson, D. A., Saunders, R. C., Kleinman, J. E., et al. (2001). A quantitative immunohistochemical study of astrocytes in the entorhinal cortex in schizophrenia, bipolar disorder and major depression: Absence of significant astrocytosis. *Brain Research Bulletin, 55*, 611–618.

Damasio, H. C. (1991). Neuroanatomical correlates of the aphasias. In M. T. Sarno (Ed.), *Acquired aphasia* (2nd ed., pp. 45–70). New York: Academic Press.

D'Amico, G., Cedro, C., Muscatello, M. R., Pandolfo, G., Di Rosa, A. E., Zoccali, R., et al. (2003). Olanzapine augmentation of paroxetine-refractory obsessive-compulsive disorder. *Progress in Neuro-Psychopharmacology & Biological Psychiatry, 27*, 619–623.

Daniel, D. G., Weinberger, D. R., Jones, D. W., Zigon, J. R., Cippola, R., Handel, S., et al. (1991). The effect of amphetamine on regional cerebral blood flow during cognitive activation in schizophrenia. *Journal of Neuroscience, 11*, 1907–1917.

Daniels, J., Baker, D. G., & Norman, A. B. (1996). Cocaine-induced tics in untreated Tourette's syndrome. *American Journal of Psychiatry, 153*, 956.

Danos, P., Baumann, B., Kramer, A., Bernstein, H. G., Stauch, R., Krell, D., et al. (2003). Volumes of association thalamic nuclei in schizophrenia: A postmortem study. *Schizophrenia Research, 60*, 141–155.

Dantendorfer, K., Prayer, D., Kramer, J., Amering, M., Baischer, W., Berger, P., et al. (1996). High frequency of EEG and MRI brain abnormalities in panic disorder. *Psychiatry Research, 68*, 41–53.

Das, M., Barkataki, I., Kumari, V., & Sharma, T. (2002). Neuroimaging violence in the mentally ill: What can it tell us? *Hospital Medicine, 63*, 604–609.

Datto, C. J. (2000). Side effects of electroconvulsive therapy. *Depression and Anxiety, 12*, 130–134.

Davanzo, P., Thomas, M. A., Yue, K., Oshiro, T., Belin, T., Strober M., et al. (2001). Decreased anterior cingulated myo-insitol/creatine spectroscopy resonance with lithium treatment in children with bipolar disorder. *Neuropsychopharmacology, 24*, 359–369.

Davanzo, P., Yue, K., Thomas, M. A., Belin, T., Mintz, J., Venkatraman, T. N., et al. (2003). Proton magnetic resonance spectroscopy of bipolar disorder versus intermittent explosive disorder in children and adolescents. *American Journal of Psychiatry, 160*, 1442–1452.

David, A. S. (1999). Auditory hallucinations: Phenomenology, neuropsychology, and neuroimaging update. *Acta Psychiatrica Scandinavia, 99*, 95–104.

Davidson, R. J., Irwin, W., Anderle, M. J., & Kalin, N. H. (2003). The neural substrates of affective processing in depressed patients treated with venlafaxine. *American Journal of Psychiatry, 160*, 64–75.

Davies, A. G., Pierce-Shimomura, J. T., Kim, H., VanHoven, M. K., Thiele, T. R., Bonci, A., et al. (2003). A central role of the BK potassium channel in behavioral responses to ethanol in C. elegans. *Cell, 115*, 655–666.

Davies, G., Ahmad, F., Chant, D., Welhamd, J., & McGrath, J. (2000). Seasonality of first admissions for schizophrenia in the Southern Hemisphere. *Schizophrenia Research, 41*, 457–462.

Davies, J., Lloyd, K. R., Jones, I. K., Barnes, A., & Pilowsky, L. S. (2003). Changes in regional cerebral blood flow with venlafaxine in the treatment of major depression. *American Journal of Psychiatry, 160*, 374–376.

Davies, M. (2002). A few thoughts about the mind, the brain, and a child with early deprivation. *Journal of Analytical Psychology, 47*, 421–435.

Davis, J. M., Chen, N., & Glick, I. D. (2003). A meta-analysis of the efficacy of second-generation antipsychotics. *Archives of General Psychiatry, 60*, 553–564.

Davis, J. O., Phelps, J. A., & Bracha, H. S. (1995). Prenatal development of monozygotic twins and concordance rate for schizophrenia. *Schizophrenia Bulletin, 21*, 357–366.

Davis, K. L., Kahn, R. S., Ko, G., & Davidson, M. (1991). Dopamine in schizophrenia: A review and reconceptualization. *American Journal of Psychiatry, 148*, 1474–1486.

Davis, M. P., Varga, J., Dickerson, D., Walsh, D., LeGrand, S. B., & Lagman, R. (2003). Normal-release and controlled-release oxycodone: Pharmacokinetics, pharmacodynamics, and controversy. *Support Care Cancer, 11*, 84–92.

Davis, M. R., Votaw, J. R., Bremmer, J. D., Byas-Smith, M. G., Faber, T. L., Voll, R. J., et al. (2003). Initial human PET imaging studies with the dopamine transporter ligand 18F-FECNT. *Journal of Nuclear Medicine, 44*, 855–861.

Dawson, G., Klinger, L. G., Panagiotides, H., Lewy, A., & Castelloe, P. (1995). Subgroups of autistic children based on social behavior display distinct patterns of brain activity. *Journal of Abnormal Child Psychology, 23*, 569–583.

De Bellis, M. D. (2001). Developmental traumatology: The psychobiological development of maltreated children and its implication for research, treatment, and policy. *Development and Psychopathology, 13*, 539–564.

De Bellis, M. D., Clark, D. B., Beers, S. R., Soloff, P. H., Boring, A. M., Hall, J., et al. (2001). Hippocampal volume in adolescent-onset alcohol use disorders. *American Journal of Psychiatry, 157*, 737–744.

De Bellis, M. D., Geracioti, T. D., Altemus, M. Jr., & Kling, M. A. (1993). Cerebrospinal fluid monoamine metabolites in fluoxetine-treated patients with major depression and in healthy volunteers. *Biological Psychiatry, 33*, 636–641.

de Bode, S., & Curtiss, S. (2000). Language after hemispherectomy. *Brain and Cognition, 43*, 135–138.

De Camilli, P., Haucke, V., Takei, K., & Mugnaini, E. (2001). The structure of synapses. In M. W. Cowan, T. C. Sudhof, & C. F. Stevens (Eds.), *Synapses* (pp. 89–133). Baltimore: Johns Hopkins University Press.

De Camilli, P., Slepnev, V. I., Shupliakov, O., & Brodin, L. (2001). Synaptic vesicle endocytosis. In M. W. Cowan, T. C. Sudhof, & C. F. Stevens (Eds.), *Synapses* (pp. 217–274). Baltimore: Johns Hopkins University Press.

De Cristofaro, M. T., Sessarego, A., Pupi, A., Biondi, F., & Faravelli, C. (1993). Brain perfusion abnormalities in drug-naive, lactate-sensitive panic patients: A SPECT study. *Biological Psychiatry, 33*, 505–512.

De Deyn, P. P., Carrasco, M. M., Deberdt, W., Jeandel, C., Hay, D. P., Feldman, P. D., et al. (2004). Olanzapine versus placebo in the treatment of psychosis with or without associated behavioral disturbances in patients with Alzheimer's disease. *International Journal of Geriatric Psychiatry, 19*, 115–126.

de Haan, E., Hoogduin, K. A., Buitelaar, J. K., & Keijsers, G. P. (1998). Behavior therapy versus clomipramine for the treatment of obsessive-compulsive disorder in children and adolescents. *Journal of the American Academy of Child and Adolescent Psychiatry, 37*, 1022–1029.

De la Fuente-Fernandez, R., Phillips, A. G., Zamburlini, M., Sossie, V., Calne, D. B., Ruth, T. J., et al. (2002). Dopamine release in human ventral striatum and expectation of reward. *Behavioral Brain Research, 136*, 359–363.

De Silva, R., Hardy, J., Crook, J., Khan, N., Graham, E. A., Morris, C. M., et al. (2002). The tau locus is not significantly associated with pathologically confirmed sporadic Parkinson's disease. *Neuroscience Letters, 330*, 201–203.

DeBar, L. L., Lynch, F., Powell, J., & Gale, J. (2003). Use of psychotropic agents in preschool children. Associated symptoms, diagnoses, and health care services in a health maintenance organization. *Archives of Pediatrics and Adolescent Medicine, 157*, 121–123.

DeCarli, C., Grady, C. L., Clark, C. M., Katz, D. A., Brady, D. R., Murphy, D. G., et al. (1996). Comparison of positron emission tomography, cognition, and brain volume in Alzheimer's disease with and without severe abnormalities of white matter. *Journal of Neurology, Neurosurgery, and Psychiatry, 60*, 158–167.

DeFries, J. C., & Light, J. G. (1996). Twin studies of reading disability. In J. H. Beitchman, N. J. Cohen, M. M. Konstantareas, & R. Tannock (Eds.), *Language, learning, and behavior disorders*. (pp. 272–292). New York: Cambridge University Press.

Deisenhammer, E. A., Kramer-Reinstadler, K., Liensberger, D., Kemmler, G., Hinterhuber, H., & Fleischhacker, W. (2004). No evidence for an association between serum cholesterol and the course of depression and suicidality. *Psychiatry Research, 121*, 253–261.

Dekaban, A. S. (1978). Changes in brain weights during the span of human life: Relation of brain weights to body heights and body weights. *Annals of Neurology, 4*, 345–356.

Delate, T., Gelenberg, A. J., Simmons, V. A., & Motheral, B. R. (2004). Trends in the use of antidepressants in a national sample of commercially insured pediatric patients, 1998 to 2002. *Psychiatric Services, 55*, 387–391.

DelBello, M. P., Schwiers, M. L., Rosenberg, H. L., & Strakowski, S. M. (2002). A double-blind, randomized, placebo-controlled study of quetiapine as adjunctive treatment for adolescent mania. *Journal of the American Academy of Child and Adolescent Psychiatry, 41*, 1216–1230.

DelBello, M. P., Zimmerman, M. F., Mills, N. P., Getz, G. E., & Strakowski, S. M. (2004). Magnetic resonance imaging analysis of amygdala and other subcortical brain regions in adolescents with bipolar disorder. *Bipolar Disorder, 6*, 43–52.

Delgado, P. L. (2000). Depression: The case for a monoamine deficiency. *Journal of Clinical Psychiatry, 61*, 7–11.

Delgado, P. L., Price, L. H., Miller, H. L., Salomon, R. M., Aghajanian, G. K., Heninger, G. R., et al. (1991). Serotonin and the neurobiology of depression: Effects of tryptophan depletion in drug-free depressed patients. *Archives of General Psychiatry, 51*, 865–874.

DeLisi, L. E., Tew, W., Xie, S. H, Hoff, A. L., Sakuma, M., Kushner, M., et al. (1995). A prospective follow-up study of brain morphology and cognition in 1st episode schizophrenic patients: Preliminary findings. *Biological Psychiatry, 38*, 349–360.

Delsing, B. J., Catsman-Berrevoets, C. E., & Appel, I. M. (2001). Early prognostic indicators of outcome in ischemic childhood stroke. *Pediatric Neurology, 24*, 283–289.

Delvenne, V., Goldman, S., De Maertelaer, V., Simon, Y., Luxen, A., & Lotstra, F. (1996). Brain hypometabolism of glucose in anorexia nervosa: Normalization after weight gain. *Biological Psychiatry, 40*, 761–768.

Demirkol, A., Erdem, H., Inan, L., Yigit, A., & Guney, M. (1999). Bilateral globus pallidus in a patients with Tourette syndrome and related disorders. *Biological Psychiatry, 46*, 863–867.

Démonet, J. F., Price, C., Wise, R., & Frackowiak, R. S. J. (1994). A PET study of cognitive strategies in normal subjects during language tasks. *Brain, 117*, 671–682.

Démonet, J. F., Taylor, M. J., & Chaix, Y. (2004). Developmental dyslexia. *Lancet, 363*, 1451–1460.

Den Boer, J. A., & Westenberg, H. G. (1990). Serotonin function in panic disorder: A double blind placebo controlled study with fluvoxamine and ritanserin. *Psychopharmacology, 102*, 85–94.

Denckla, M. B. (1993). The child with developmental disabilities grown up: Adult residua of childhood disorders. *Neurologic Clinics, 11*, 105–125.

Derbyshire, S. W., Vogt, B. A., & Jones, A. K. (1998). Pain and stroop intereference tasks activate separate processing modules in anterior cingulate cortex. *Experimental Brain Research, 118*, 52–60.

Deroche-Gamonet, V., Sillaber, I., Aouizerate, B., Izawa, R., Jabber, M., Ghozland, S., et al. (2003). The glucocorticoid receptor as a potential target to reduce cocaine abuse. *Journal of Neuroscience, 23*, 4785–4790.

Desmond, J. E., Chen, S. H., DeRosa, E., Pryor, M. R., Pfefferbaum, A., & Sullivan, E. V. (2003). Increased fronto-cerebellar activation in alcoholics during verbal working memory: An fMRI study. *Neuroimage, 19*, 1510–1520.

Detera-Wadleigh, S. D., Badner, J. A., Berrettini, W. H., Yoshikawa, T., Goldin, L. R., Turner, G., et al. (1999). A high-density genome scan detects evidence for a bipolar-disorder susceptibility locus on 13q32 and other potential loci on 1q32 and 18p11.2. *Proclamations of the National Academy of Science, U.S.A., 96*, 5604–5609.

Detoledo-Morrell, L., Sullivan, M. P., Morrell, F., Wilson, R. S., Bennett, D. A., & Spencer, S. (1997). Alzheimer's disease: In vivo detection of differential vulnerability of brain regions. *Neurobiology of Aging, 18*, 463–468.

Devi, G., Ottman, R., Tang, M. X., Marder, K., Stern, Y., & Mayeux, R. (2000). Familial aggregation of Alzheimer disease among whites, African Americans, and Caribbean Hispanics in northern Manhattan. *Archives of Neurology, 57*, 72–77.

Devi, G., Williamson, J., Massoud, F., Anderson, K., Stern, Y., Devanand, D. P., et al. (2004). A comparison of family history of psychiatric disorders among patients with early- and late-onset Alzheimer's disease. *Journal of Neuropsychiatry and Clinical Neurosciences, 16*, 57–62.

Devlin, B., Bennett, P., Cook, E. H. Jr., Dawson, G., Gonen, D., Grigorenko, E. L., et al. (2002). No evidence for linkage of liability to autism to HOXA1 in a sample from the CPEA network. *American Journal of Medical Genetics, 114*, 667–672.

Dhossche, D., Ferdinand, R., van Der Ende, J., Hofstra, M. B., & Verhulst, F. (2002). Diagnostic outcome of self-reported hallucinations in a community sample of adolescents. *Psychological Medicine, 32*, 619–627.

Di Bella, D. D., Catalano, M., Cavallini, M. C., Riboldi, C., & Bellodi, I. (2000). Serotonin transporter linked polymorphic regions in anorexia nervosa and bulimia nervosa. *Molecular Psychiatry, 5*, 233–241.

Di Chiara, G. (1999). Drug addiction as dopamine-dependent associative learning disorder. *European Journal of Pharmacology, 375*, 13–30.

Di Ciano, P., & Everitt, B. J. (2003). The GABA(B) receptor agonist baclofen attenuates cocaine- and heroin-seeking behavior by rats. *Neuropsychopharmacology, 28*, 510–518.

Diamond, M. C., & Hopson, J. (1998). *Magic trees of the mind: How to nurture your child's intelligence, creativity, and healthy emotions from birth through adolescence.* New York: Dutton.

Diamond, M. C., Scheibel, A. B., Murphy, J. G. M., & Harvey, T. (1985). On the brain of a scientist: Albert Einstein. *Experimental Neurology, 88*, 198–204.

Diaz-Anzaldua, A., Joober, R., Riviere, J. B., Dion, Y., Lesperance, P., Chouinard, S., et al. (2004a). Assocation between 7q31 markers and Tourette syndrome. *American Journal of Medical Genetics, 127A*, 17–20.

Diaz-Anzaldua, A., Joober, R., Riviere, J. B., Dion, Y., Lesperance, P., Richer, F., Chouinard, S., & Rouleau, G. A., Montreal Tourette Syndrome Study Group. (2004b). Tourette syndrome and dopaminergic genes: A family-based association study in the French Canadian founder population. *Molecular Psychiatry, 9*, 272–277.

Diaz-Heijtz, R., Kolb, B., & Forssberg, H. (2003). Can a therapeutic dose of amphetamine during pre-adolescence modify the pattern of synaptic organization in the brain? *European Journal of Neuroscience, 18*, 3394–3399.

Dick, D. M., Edenberg, H. J., Xuei, X., Goate, A., Kuperaman, S., Schuckit, M., et al. (2004). Association of GABRG3 with alcohol dependence. *Alcoholism: Clinical and Experimental Research, 28*, 4–9.

Dickenson, A. H. (2001). Amino acids: Excitatory. In R. A. Webster (Ed.), *Neurotransmitters, drugs, and brain function* (pp. 211–223). New York: Wiley.

Dickerson, F. B., Boronow, J. J., Stallings, C., Origoni, A. E., Ruslanova, I., & Yolken, R. H. (2003). Association of serum antibodies to herpes simplex virus 1 with cognitive deficits in individuals with schizophrenia. *Archives of General Psychiatry, 60*, 466–472.

Diler, R. S., Kibar, M., & Avci, A. (2004). Pharmacotherapy and regional cerebral blood flow in children with obsessive compulsive disorder. *Yonsei Medical Journal, 29*, 90–99.

Dimeo, F., Bauer, M., Varahram, I., Proest, G., & Halter, U. (2001). Benefits from aerobic exercise in patients with major depression: A pilot study. *British Journal of Sports Medicine, 35*, 114–117.

Dion, Y., Annable, L., Sandor, P., & Chouinard, G. (2002). Risperidone in the treatment of tourette syndrome: A double-blind, placebo-controlled trial. *Journal of Clinical Psychopharmacology, 22*, 31–39.

Do, K. Q., Benz, B., Binns, K. E., Eaton, S. A., & Salt, T. E. (2004). Release of homocysteic acid from rat thalamus following stimulation of somatosensory afferents in vivo: Feasibilitiy of glial participation in synaptic transmission. *Neuroscience, 124*, 387–393.

Dobkin, B. H. (2003). *The clinical science of neurologic rehabilitation* (2nd (Ed.). New York: Oxford University Press.

Domschke, K., Freitag, C. M., Kuhlenbumer, G., Schirmacher, A., Sand, P., Nyhuis, P., et al. (2004). Association of the functional V158M catechol-O-methyl-transferase polymorphism with panic disorder in women. *International Journal of Neuropsychopharmacology, 7*, 183–188.

Donahoe, D. H., Meador, M., Fortune, T., & Llorena, R. (1991). Tourette's syndrome and treatment with clomipramine hydrochloride. *West Virginia Medical Journal, 87*, 468–470.

Donnelly, C. L. (2003). Pharmacological treatment approaches for children and adolescents with posttraumatic stress disorder. *Child and Adolescent Psychiatry Clinical North America, 12*, 251–269.

Dostrovsky, J. O., Levy, R., Wu, J. P., Hutchison, W. D., Tasker, R. R., & Lozano, A. M. (2000). Microstimulation-induced inhibition of firing in human globus pallidus. *Journal of Neurophysiology, 84*, 570–574.

Dougherty, D. D., Baer, L., Cosgrove, G. R., Cassem, E. H., Price, B. H., Nierenberg, A. A., et al. (2002). Prospective long-term follow-up of 44 patients who received cingulotomy for treatment-refractory obsessive-compulsive disorder. *American Journal of Psychiatry, 159*, 269–275.

Douyon, R., Serby, M., Klutchko, B., & Rotrosen, J. (1989). ECT and Parkinson's disease revisited: A "naturalistic" study. *American Journal of Psychiatry, 146*, 1451–1455.

Downs, A., & Smith, T. (2004). Emotional understanding, cooperation, and social behavior in high functioning children with autism. *Journal of Autism and Developmental Disorders, 34*, 625–635.

Doyle, A., & Pollack, M. H. (2004). Long-term management of panic disorder. *Journal of Clinical Psychiatry, 65, Supplement 5*, 24–28.

Drake, R. G., Davis, L. L., Cates, M. E., Jewell, M. E., Ambrose, S. M., & Lowe, J. S. (2003). Baclofen treatment for chronic posttraumatic stress disorder. *Annals of Pharmacotherapy, 37*, 1177–1181.

Dratcu, L. (2001). Physical exercise: An adjunctive treatment for panic disorder? *European Psychiatry, 16*, 372–374.

Drevelengas, A., Chourmouzi, D., Pitsavas, G., Charitandi, A., & Boulogianni, G. (2001). Reversible brain atrophy and subcortical high signal on MRI in a patient with anorexia nervosa. *Neuroradiology, 43*, 838–840.

Drevets, W. C. (1998). Functional neuroimaging studies of depression: The anatomy of melancholia. *Annual Review of Medicine, 49*, 341–361.

Drevets, W. C. (2000). Neuroimaging studies of mood disorder. *Biological Psychiatry, 48*, 813–829.

Drevets, W. C., Frank, E., Price, J. C., Kupfer, D. J., Greer, P. J., & Mathis, C. (2000). Serotonin type-1A receptor imaging in depression. *Nuclear Medicine and Biology, 27*, 499–507.

Drevets, W. C., Oengur, D., & Price, J. L. (1998). Reduced glucose metabolism in the subgenual prefrontal cortex in unipolar depression. *Molecular Psychiatry, 3*, 190–191.

Drevets, W. C., Price, J. L., Simpson, J. R., Todd, R. D., Reich, T., Vannier, M., et al. (1997). Subgenual prefrontal cortex abnormalities in mood disorders. *Nature, 386*, 824–827.

Drevets, W. C., Videen, T. O., Price, J. L., Preskorn, S. H., Carmichael, S. T., & Raichle, M. E. (1992). A functional anatomical study of unipolar depression. *The Journal of Neuroscience, 12*, 3628–3641.

D'Sa, C., & Duman, R. S. (2002). Antidepressants and neuroplasticity. *BiPolar Disorders, 4*, 183–194.

D'Souza, C., Gupta, A., Alldrick, M. D., & Sastry, B. S. (2003). Management of psychosis in Parkinson's disease. *International Journal of Clinical Practice, 57*, 295–300.

Dudman, J. T., Eaton, M. E., Rajadhyaksha, A., Macias, W., Taher, M., Barczak, A., et al. (2003). Dopamine D1 receptors mediate CREB phosphorylation of the NMDA receptor at Ser897-NR1. *Journal of Neurochemistry, 87*, 922–934.

Due, D. L., Huettel, S. A., Hall, W. G., & Rubin, D. C. (2002). Activation in mesolimbic and visuospatial neural circuits elicited by smoking cues: Evidence from functional magnetic resonance imaging. *American Journal of Psychiatry, 159*, 954–960.

Dujardin, K., Blairy, S., Defebvre, L., Duhem, S., Noël, Y., Hess, U., et al. (2004). Deficits in decoding emotional facial expressions in Parkinson's disease. *Neuropsychologia, 42*, 239–250.

Duke, P. J., Pantelis, C., McPhillips, M. A., & Barnes, T. R. E. (2001). Comorbid non-alcohol substance misuse among people with schizophrenia. *British Journal of Psychiatry, 179*, 509–513.

Duman, R. S. (1998). Novel therapeutic approaches beyond the serotonin receptor. *Biological Psychiatry, 44*, 324–335.

Duman, R. S. (2002). Pathophysiology of depression: The concept of synaptic plasticity. *European Psychiatry, 17*, 306–310.

Duman, R. S., Heninger, G. R., & Nestler, E. J. (1997). A molecular and cellular theory of depression. *Archives of General Psychiatry, 54*, 597–606.

Duman, R. S., Malberg, J., & Thome, J. (1999). Neural plasticity to stress and antidepressant treatment. *Biological Psychiatry, 46*, 1181–1191.

Duman, R. S., Nakagawa, S., & Malberg, J. (2001). Regulation of adult neurogenesis by antidepressant treatment. *Neuropsychopharmacology, 25*, 836–844.

Dunn, R. T., Kimbrell, T. A., Ketter, T. A., Frye, M. A., Willis, M. W., Luckenbaugh, D. A., et al. (2002). Principal components of the Beck Depression Inventory and regional cerebral metabolism in unipolar and bipolar depression. *Biological Psychiatry, 51*, 387–399.

DuPaul, G. J., Schaughency, E. A., Weyandt, L. L., Tripp, G., Kiesner, J., Ota, K., & Stanish, H. (2001). Self-report of ADHD symptoms in university students: Cross-gender and cross-national prevalence. *Journal of Learning Disabilities, 34*, 370–379.

DuPaul, G. J., & Stoner, G. (2003). ADHD in the schools (2nd. ed., pp. 190–226). New York: The Guilford Press.

Dupont, R. M., Jernigan, T. L., Heindel, W., Butters, N., Shafer, K., Wilson, T., et al. (1995). Magnetic resonance imaging and mood disorders. *Archives of General Psychiatry, 52*, 747–755.

Durston, S., Hulshoff, H. E., Casey, B. J., Gieed, J. N., Buitelaar, J. K., & van Engeland, H. (2001). Anatomical MRI of the developing human brain: What have we learned? *Journal of the American Academy of Child and Adolescent Psychiatry, 40*, 1012–1020.

Durston, S., Hulshoff Pol, H. E., Casey, B. J., Giedd, J. N., Buitelaar, J. K., & van Engeland, H. (2001). Anatomical MRI of the developing human brain: What have we learned? *Journal of the American Academy of Child and Adolescent Psychiatry, 40*, 1012–1020.

Durston, S., Hulshoff Pol, H. E., Schnack, H. G., Buitelaar, J. K., Steenhuis, J. K., Minderaa, R. B., et al. (2004). Magnetic resonance imaging of boys with attention-deficit/hyperactivity disorder and their unaffected siblings. *Journal of the American Academy of Child and Adolescent Psychiatry, 43*, 332–340.

Durston, S., Tottenham, N. T., Thomas, K. M., Davidson, M. C., Eigsti, I. M., Yang, Y., et al. (2003). Differential patterns of striatal activation in young children with and without ADHD. *Biological Psychiatry, 53*, 871–878.

Dursun, S. M., & Reveley, M. A. (1997). Differential effects of transdermal nicotine on microstructured analyses of tics in Tourette's syndrome: An open study. *Psychological Medicine, 27*, 483–487.

Dursun, S. M., Reveley, M. A., Bird, R., & Stirton, F. (1994). Longlasting improvement of Tourette's syndrome with transdermal nicotine. *Lancet, 344*, 1577.

Dykman, K. D., & Dykman, R. A. (1998). Effects of nutritional supplements on attention-deficit hyperactivity disorder. *Integration of Physiology and Behavioral Science, 33*, 49–60.

Eastwood, S. L., & Harrison, P. J. (2001). Synaptic pathology in the anterior cingulate cortex in schizophrenia and mood disorders. A review and a western blot study of synaptophysin, GAP-43 and the complexins. *Brain Research Bulletin, 55*, 569–578.

Ebersbach, G., Sojer, M, Müller, J., Heijmenberg, M., & Poewe, W. (2000). Sociocultural differences in gait. *Movement Disorders, 15*, 1145–1147.

Ebihara, M., Ohba, H., Hattori, E., Yamada, K., & Yoshikawa, T. (2003). Transcriptional activities of cholecystokinin promoter haplotypes and their relevance to panic disorder susceptibility. *American Journal of Medical Genetics, 118B*, 32–35.

Ebneth, A., Godemann, R., Stamer, K., Illenberger, S., Trinczek, B., Mandelkow, E. M., et al. (1998). Overexpression of tau protein inhibits kinesin-dependent trafficking of vesicles, mitochondria, and endoplasmic reticulum: Implications for Alzheimer's disease. *Journal of Cell Biology, 143*, 777–794.

Eckert, M. A., & Leonard, C. M. (2000). Structural imaging in dyslexia: The planum temporale. *Mental Retardation and Developmental Disabilities Research Reviews, 6*, 198–206.

Edelman, G. (1987). *Neural Darwinism*. New York: Basic Books.

Edland, S. D., Rocca, W. A., Petersen, R. C., Cha, R. H., & Kokmen, E. (2002). Dementia and Alzheimer disease incidence rates do not vary by sex in Rochester, Minn. *Archives of Neurology, 59*, 1589–1593.

Edland, S. D., Silverman, J. M., Peskind, E. R., Tsuang, D., Wijsman, E., & Morris, J. C. (1996). Increased risk of dementia in mothers of Alzheimer's disease cases: Evidence for maternal inheritance. *Neurology, 47*, 254–256.

Edwards, J. G., & Anderson, I. (1999). Systematic review and guide to selection of selective serotonin reuptake inhibitors. *Drugs, 57*, 507–533.

Egaas, B., Courchesne, E., & Saitoh, O. (1995). Reduced size of corpus callosum in autism. *Archives of Neurology, 52*, 794–801.

Egan, M. F., Weinberger, D. R., & Lu, B. (2003). Brain-derived neurotropic factor and genetic risk. *American Journal of Psychiatry, 160*, 1242.

Egeland, J. A., Gerhard, D. S., Pauls, D. L., Sussex, J. N., Kidd, K. K., Allen, C. R., et al. (1987). Bipolar affective disorders linked to DNA markers on chromosome 11. *Nature, 325*, 783–787.

Ehnvall, A., Sjögren, Zachrisson, O. C. G., & Ågren, H. (2003). Lifetime burden of mood swings and activation of brain norepinephrine turnover in patients with treatment-refractory depressive illness. *Journal of Affective Disorders, 74*, 185–189.

Ehrenkrantz, D., Silverman, J. M., Smith, C. J., Birstein, S., Marin, D., Mohs, R. C., et al. (1999). Genetic epidemiological study of maternal and paternal transmission of Alzheimer's disease. *American Journal of Medical Genetics, 88*, 378–382.

Eidelberg, D., Moeller, J. R., Antonini, A., Kazumata, K., Dhawan, V., Budman, C., et al. (1997). The metabolic anatomy of Tourette's syndrome. *Neurology, 48*, 927–934.

Eikelenboom, P., & van Gool, W. A. (2004). Neuroinflammatory perspectives on the two faces of Alzheimer's disease. *Journal of Neural Transmission, 111*, 281–294.

Einat, H., Manji, H. K., Gould, T. D., Du, J., & Chen, G. (2003). Possible involvement of ERK signaling cascade in bipolar disorder: Behavioral leads from the study of mutant mice. *Drug News and Perspectives, 16*, 453–463.

Eisenberg, J., Mei-Tal, G., Steinberg, A., Tartakovsky, E., Zohar, A., Gritsenko, I., et al. (1999). Haplotype relative risk study of catechol-o-methyltransferase (*COMT*) and attention deficit hyperactivity disorder (ADHD): Association of the high-enzyme activity val allele with ADHD impulsive-hyperactive phenotype. *American Journal of Medical Genetics, 88*, 497–502.

Elbert, T., Pantev, C., Wienbruch, C., Rockstroh, B., & Taub, E. (1995). Increased cortical representation of the fingers of the left hand in string players. *Science, 270*, 305–307.

Eldrup, E., Mogensen, P., Jacobsen., J., Pakkenberg, H., & Christensen, N. J. (1995). CSF and plasma concentrations of free norepinephrine, dopamine, 3,4–dihydroxyphenylacetic acid (DOPAC), 3,4–dihydroxyphenylalanine (DOPA), and epinephrine in Parkinson's disease. *Acta Neurologica Scandinavica, 92*, 116–121.

Eley, T. C., Bolton, D., O'Connor, T. G., Perrin, S., Smith, P., & Plomin, R. (2003). A twin study of anxiety-related behaviours in pre-school children. *Journal of Child Psychology and Psychiatry, and Allied Disciplines, 44*, 945–960.

Elia, M., Ferri, R., Musumeci, S. A., Panerai, S., Bottitta, M., & Scuderi, C. (2000). Clinical correlates of brain morphometric features of subjects with low-functioning autistic disorder. *Journal of Child Neurology, 15*, 504–508.

Eliez, S., & Reiss, A. L. (2000). Annotation: MRI neuroimaging of childhood psychiatric disorder: A selective review. *Journal of Child Psychology and Psychiatry, 41*, 679–694.

Elkis, H., Friedman, L., Wise, A., & Meltzer, H. Y. (1995). Meta-analyses of studies of ventricular enlargement and cortical sulcal prominence in mood disorders: Comparisons with controls or patients with schizophrenia. *Archives of General Psychiatry, 52*, 735–746.

Elliott, A. J., & Roy-Byrne, P. P. (1998). Major depressive disorder and HIV-1 infection: A review of treatment trials. *Seminars in Clinical Neuropsychiatry, 3*, 137–150.

El-Mallakh, R. S., Peters, C., & Waltrip, C. (2000). Antidepressant treatment and neural plasticity. *Journal of Child and Adolescent Psychopharmacology, 10*, 287–294.

Engelborghs, S., Marescau, B., & De Deyn, P. P. (2003). Amino acids and biogenic amines in cerebrospinal fluid of patients with Parkinson's disease. *Neurochemical Research, 28*, 1145–1150.

Engelhart, M. J., Geerlings, M. I., Ruitenberg. A., van Swieten, J. C., Hofman, A., Witteman, J. C., et al. (2002). Dietary intake of antioxidants and risk of Alzheimer disease. *JAMA, 287*, 3223–3229.

Engström, G., Alling, C., Blennow, K., Regnéll, G., & Träskman-Bendz, L. (1999). Reduced cerebrospinal HVA concentrations and HVA/5-HIAA ratios in suicide attempters: Monoamine metabolites in 120 suicide attempters and 47 controls. *European Neuropsychopharmacology, 9*, 399–405.

Enoch, R. J., & Goldman, D. (2001). The genetics of alcoholism and alcohol abuse. *Current Psychiatric Reports, 3*, 144–151.

Epstein, C. M., Lah, J. J., Meador, K., Weissman, J. D., Gaitan, L. E., & Dihenia, B. (1996). Optimum stimulus parameters for lateralized suppression of speech with magnetic brain stimulation. *Neurology, 47*, 1590–1593.

Erberich, S. G., Friedlich, P., Seri, I., Nelson, M. D., & Bluml, S. (2003). Functional MRI in neonates using neonatal head coil and MR compatible incubator. *Neuroimaging, 20*, 683–692.

Erdal, M. E., Tot, S., Yazici, K., Yazici, A., Herken, H., Erdem, P., et al. (2003). Lack of association of catechol-O-methyltransferase gene polymorphism in obsessive-compulsive disorder. *Depression and Anxiety, 18*, 41–45.

Eren, I., Tükel, R., Polat, A., Karaman, R., & Unal, S. (2003). Evaluation of regional cerebral blood flow changes in panic disorder with Tc99m-HMPAO SPECT. *Psychiatry Research, 123*, 135–143.

Eriksson, P., Perfilieva, E., Bjork-Eriksson, T., Albom, A. M., Nordborg, C., Peterson, D. A., et al. (1998). Neurogenesis in the adult human hippocampus. *Nature Medicine, 4*, 1313–1317.

Eriksson, P. S., Perfilieva, E. K., Bjoerk-Eriksson, T., Alborn, A.-M., Nordborg, C., Peterson, D. A., et al. (1998). Neurogenesis in the adult human hippocampus. *Nature Medicine, 4*, 1313–1317.

Ernst, M., Cohen, R. M., Liebenauer, L. L., Jons, P. H., & Zametkin, A. J. (1997). Cerebral glucose metabolism in adolescent girls with attention-deficit/hyperactivity disorder. *Journal of the American Academy of Child and Adolescent Psychiatry, 36*, 1399–1406.

Ernst, M., Kimes, A. S., London, E. D., Matochik, J. A., Eldreth, D., Tata, S., et al. (2003). Neural substrates of decision making in adults with attention deficit hyperactivity disorder. *American Journal of Psychiatry, 160*, 1061–1070.

Ernst, M., Zametkin, A. J., Phillips, R. L., & Cohen, R. M. (1998). Age-related changes in brain glucose metabolism in adults with attention-deficit/hyperactivity disorder and control subjects. *Journal of Neuropsychiatry and Clinical Neurosciences, 10*, 168–177.

Ernst, M., Zmetkin, A. J., Jons, P. H., Matochik, J. A., Pascualvaca, D., & Cohen, R. M. (1999). High presynaptic dopaminergic activity in children with Tourette's disorder. *Journal of the American Academy of Child and Adolescent Psychiatry, 38*, 86–94.

Ernst, T., Chang, L., Oropilla, G., Gustavson, S., & Speck, O. (2000). Cerebral perfusion abnormalities in abstinent cocaine abusers: a perfusion MRI and SPECT study. *Psychiatry Research, 99*, 63–74.

Eskandar, E. N., Flaherty, A., Cosgrove, G. R., Shinobu, L. A., & Barker, F. G. (2003). Surgery for Parkinson's disease in the United States, 1996 to 2000: Practice patterns, short-term outcomes, and hospital charges in a nationwide sample. *Journal of Neurosurgery, 99*, 863–871.

Eustache, F., Piolino, P., Giffard, B., Viader, F., Sayette Vde, L., Baron, J. C., et al. (2004). "In the course of time": A PET study of the cerebral substrates of autobiographical amnesia in Alzheimer's disease. *Brain, 127*, 1549–1560.

Evangeliou, A., Vlachonikolis, I., Mihalidou, H., Spilioti, M., Skarpalezou, A., Makaronas, N., et al. (2003). Application of a ketogenic diet in children with autistic behavior: Pilot study. *Journal of Child Neurology, 18*, 113–118.

Evans, R. M., Emsley, C. L., Gao, S., Sahota, A., Hall, K. S., Farlow, M. R., et al. (2000). Serum cholesterol, *APOE* genotype, and the risk of Alzheimer's disease: A population-based study of African Americans. *Neurology, 54*, 240–242.

Ewald, H., Mors, O., Flint, T., Koed, K., Eiberg, H., & Kruse, T. A. (1995). A possible locus for manic depressive illness on chromosome 16p13. *Psychiatric Genetics, 5*, 71–81.

Ezquerra, M., Lleó, A., Castellví, M., Queralt, R., Santacruz, P., Pastor, P., et al. (2003). A novel mutation in the PSEN2 gene (T430M) associated with variable expression in a family with early-onset Alzheimer disease. *Archives of Neurology, 60*, 1149–1151.

Factor, S. A., Feustel, P. J., Friedman, J. H., Comella, C. L., Goetz, C. G., Kurlan, R., et al. (2003). Longitudinal outcome of Parkinson's disease patients with psychosis. *Neurology, 60*, 1756–1761.

Fagiolini, A., Kupfer, D. J., Houck, P. R., Novick, D. M., & Frank, E. (2003). Obesity as a correlate of outcome in patients with bipolar disorder. *American Journal of Psychiatry, 160*, 112–117.

Fahnestock, M., Garzon, D., Holsinger, R. M., & Michalski, B. (2002). Neurotrophic factors and Alzheimer's disease: Are we focusing on the wrong molecule? *Journal of Neural Transmission Supplement, 62*, 241–252.

Fall, P. A., Ekman, R., Granerus, A. K., & Granerus, G. (2000). ECT in Parkinson's disease-dopamine transporter visualised by [123I]-beta-CIT SPECT. *Journal of Neural Transmission, 107*, 997–1008.

Fall, P. A., Ekman, R., Granerus, A. K., Thorell, L. H., & Walinder, J. (1995). ECT in Parkinson's disease. Changes in motor symptoms, monoamine metabolites and neuropeptides. *Journal of Neural Transmission, Parkinson's Disease and Dementia Section, 10*, 129–140.

Fall, P. A., & Granerus, A. K. (1999). Maintenance ECT in Parkinson's disease. *Journal of Neural Transmission, 106*, 737–741.

Fals-Stewart, W., & Angarano, K. (1994). Obsessive-compulsive disorder among patients entering substance abuse treatment. Prevalence and accuracy of diagnosis. *Journal of Nervous and Mental Disease, 182*, 715–719.

Fan, X. L., Zhang, J. S., Zhang, X. Q., & Ma, L. (2003). Chronic morphine treatment and withdrawal induce up-regulation of c-Jun N-terminal kinase 3 gene expression in rat brain. *Neuroscience, 122*, 997–1002.

Faraone, S. V. (2000). Genetics of childhood disorders: XX. ADHD, part 4: Is ADHD genetically heterogeneous? *Journal of the American Academy of Child and Adolescent Psychiatry, 39*, 1455–1457.

Faraone, S. V., Biederman, J., Keenan, K., & Tsuang, M. T. (1991). A family-genetic study of girls with DSM-III attention deficit disorder. *American Journal of Psychiatry, 148*, 112–117.

Faraone, S. V., Biederman, J., Mick, E., Williamson, S., Wilens, T., Spencer, T., et al. (2000). Family study of girls with attention deficit hyperactivity disorder. *American Journal of Psychiatry, 150*, 1077–1083.

Faraone, S. V., Doyle, A. E., Mick, E., & Biederman, J. (2001). Meta-analysis of the association between the 7-repeat allele of the dopamine (D4) receptor gene and attention deficit hyperactivity disorder. *American Journal of Psychiatry, 158*, 1052–1057.

Faraone, S. V., Glatt, S. J., & Tsuang, M. T. (2003). The genetics of pediatric-onset bipolar disorder. *Biological Psychiatry, 53*, 970–977.

Faraone, S. V., Tsuang, M. T., & Tsuang, D. W. (1999). *Genetics of mental disorders.* New York: Guilford.

Farde, L., Wiesel., F. A, Norstrom, A. L., & Sedvall, G. (1989). D1 and D2 dopamine receptor occupancy during treatment with conventional and atypical neuroleptics. *Psychopharmacology, 99*, 528–531.

Farde, L., Wiesel., F. A., Stone-Elander, S., Halldin, C., Nordstrom, A. L., Hall, H., et al. (1990). D2 Dopamine receptors in neuroleptic-naïve schizophrenic patients. *Archives of General Psychiatry, 47*, 213–219.

Faridi, K., & Suchowersky, O. (2003). Gilles de la Tourette's syndrome. *Canadian Journal of Neurological Science, 30*, 64–71.

Farrer, L. A., Myers, R. H., Cupples, L. A., St George-Hyslop, P. H., Bird, T. D., Rossor, M. N., et al. (1990). Transmission and age-at-onset patterns in familial Alzheimer's disease: Evidence for heterogeneity. *Neurology, 40*, 395–403.

Fatemi, S. H., Earle, J. A., Stary, J. M., Lee, S., & Sedgewich, J. (2001). Altered levels of the synaptosomal associated protein SNAP-25 in hippocampus of subjects with mood disorders and schizophrenia. *Clinical Neuroscience and Neuropathology, 12*, 3257–3262.

Fatemi, S. H., Halt, A. R., Realmuto, G., Earle, J., Kist, D. A., Thuras, P., et al. (2002). Purkinje cell size is reduced in cerebellum of patients with autism. *Cellular and Molecular Neurobiology, 22*, 171–175.

Fatemi, S. H., Stary, J. M., Halt, A. R., & Realmuto, G. R. (2001). Dysregulation of Reelin and Bcl-2 proteins in autistic cerebellum. *Journal of Autism and Developmental Disorders, 31*, 529–535.

Fava, M. (1997). Psychopharmacologic treatment of pathologic aggression. *Psychiatric Clinics of North America, 20*, 427–451.

Fava, M. (2003). The role of the serotonergic and noradrenergic neurotransmitter systems in the treatment of psychological and physical symptoms of depression. *Journal of Clinical Psychiatry, 64*, 26–29.

Fazekas, F., Alavi, A., Chawluk, J. B., Zimmerman, R. A., Hackney, D., Bilaniuk, L., et al. (1989). Comparison of CT, MR and PET in Alzheimer's dementia and normal aging. *Journal of Nuclear Medicine, 30*, 1607–1615.

Fein, G., Di Schlafani, V., Cardenas, V. A., Goldmann, H., Tolou-Shams, M., & Meyerhoff, D. J. (2002). Cortical gray matter loss in treatment-naïve alcohol dependent individuals. *Alcoholism: Clinical and Experimental Research, 26*, 558–564.

Feinberg, I. (1982). Schizophrenia: Caused by a fault in programmed synaptic elimination during adolescence. *Journal of Psychiatric Research, 17*, 319–334.

Feinstein, A., Roy, P., Lobaugh, N., Feinstein, K., O'Connor, P., & Black, S. (2004). Structural brain abnormalities in multiple sclerosis patients with major depression. *Neurology, 62*, 586–590.

Feldman, H. M., Kolmen, B. K., & Gonzaga, A. M. (1999). Naltrexone and communication skills in young children with autism. *Journal of the American Academy of Child and Adolescent Psychiatry, 38*, 587–593.

Felipo, V., Grau, E., Minana, M. D., & Grisolia, S. (1993). Hyperammonemia decreases protein-kinase-C-dependent phosphorylation of microtubule-associated protein 2 and increases its binding to tubulin. *European Journal of Biochemistry, 214*, 243–249.

Ferguson, J. M. (1993). The use of electroconvulsive therapy in patients with intractable anorexia nervosa. *International Journal of Eating Disorders, 13*, 195–201.

Ferrer, I., Boada Rovira, M., Sánchez Guerra, M. L, Rey, M. J., & Costa-Jussá, F. (2004). Neuropathology and pathogenesis of encephalitis following amyloid-beta immunization in Alzheimer's disease. *Brain Pathology, 14*, 11–20.

Ferri, R., Elia, M., Agarwal, N., Lanuzza, B., Musumeci, S. A., & Pennisi, G. (2003). The mismatch negativity and the P3a components of the auditory event-related potentials in autistic low-functioning subjects. *Clinical Neurophysiology, 114*, 1671–1680.

Feychting, M., Pedersen, N. L., Svedberg, P., Floderus, B., & Gatz, M. (1998). Dementia and occupational exposure to magnetic fields. *Scandinavian Journal of Work, Environment & Health, 24*, 46–53.

Field, D., Garland, M., & Williams, K. (2003). Correlates of specific childhood feeding problems. *Journal of Paediatric Child Health, 39*, 299–304.

Field, T. M., Quintino, O., Hernandez-Reif, M., & Koslovsky, G. (1998). Adolescents with attention deficit hyperactivity disorder benefit from massage therapy. *Adolescence, 33*, 103–108.

Figiel, G. S., Krishnan, K. R. R., Rao, V. P., Doraiswamy, M., Ellinwood, E. H., Nemeroff, C. B., et al. (1991). Subcortical hyperintensities on brain magnetic resonance imaging: A comparison of normal and bipolar subjects. *Journal of Neuropsychiatry and Clinical Neuroscience, 3*, 18–22.

Figueroa, Y., Rosenberg, D. R., Birmaher, B., & Keshavan, M. S. (1998). Combination treatment with clomipramine and selective serotonin reuptake inhibitors for obsessive-compulsive disorder in children and adolescents. *Journal of Child and Adolescent Psychopharmacology, 8*, 61–67.

Filiano, J. J., Goldenthal, M. J., Rhodes, H., & Marín-García, J. (2002). Mitochondrial dysfunction in patients with hypotonia, epilepsy, autism, and developmental delay: HEADD syndrome. *Journal of Child Neurology, 17*, 435–439.

Filipek, P. A. (1999). Neuroimaging in the developmental disorders: The state of the science. *Journal of Child Psychology and Psychiatry, 40*, 113–128.

Filipek, P. A., Semrud-Clikeman, M., Steingard, R. J., Renshaw, P. F., Kennedy, D. N., & Biederman, J. (1997). Volumetric MRI analysis comparing subjects having attention-deficit hyperactivity disorder with normal controls. *Neurology, 48*, 589–601.

Fillenbaum, G. G., Heyman, A., Huber, M. S., Woodbury, M. A., Leiss, J., Schmader, K. E., et al. (1998). The prevalence and 3–year incidence of dementia in older black and white community residents. *Journal of Clinical Epidemiology, 51*, 587–595.

Findley, D. B. (2002). Tourette syndrome: Information for educators. *NASP Communiqué, 31.*

Fink, M., & Coffey, C. E. (1998). ECT in pediatric neuropsychiatry. In C. E. Coffey & R. Brumback (Eds.), *Textbook of pediatric neuropsychiatry* (pp. 1389–1408). Washington, DC: American Psychiatric Press.

Fink, P., Hansen, M. S., Sondergaard, L., & Frydenberg, M. (2003). Mental illness in new neurological patients. *Journal of Neurology, Neurosurgery, and Psychiatry, 74*, 817–819.

Firbank, M. J., Colloby, S. J., Burn, D. J., McKeith, I. G., & O'Brien, J. T. (2003). Regional cerebral blood flow in Parkinson's disease with and without dementia. *Neuroimage, 20*, 1309–1319.

Fischer, H., Andersson, J. L., Furmark, T., & Fredrikson, M. (1998). Brain correlates of an unexpected panic attack: A human positron emission tomographic study. *Neuroscience Letters, 251*, 137–140.

Fischer, M., & Barkley, R. A. (2003). Childhood stimulant treatment and risk for later substance abuse. *Journal of Clinical Psychiatry, 64*, 19–23.

Fischer, M., Barkley, R. A., Edelbrock, C. S., & Smallish, L. (1990). The adolescent outcome of hyperactive children diagnosed by research criteria: II. Academic, attentional, and neuropsychological status. *Journal of Consultation in Clinical Psychology, 58*, 580–588.

Fischer, M., Barkley, R. A., Smallish, L., & Fletcher, K. (2002). Young adult follow-up of hyperactive children: Self-reported psychiatric disorders, comorbidity, and the role of childhood conduct problems and teen CD. *Journal of Abnormal Child Psychology, 30*, 463–475.

Fisher, S. E., Francks, C., Marlow, A. J., MacPhie, I. L., Newbury, D. F., Cardon, L. R., et al. (2002). Independent genome-wide scans identify a chromosome 18 quantitative-trait locus influencing dyslexia. *Nature Genetics, 30*, 86–91.

Fisman, M. (1991). Musical hallucinations: Report of two unusual cases. *Canadian Journal of Psychiatry, 36*, 609–611.

Fitzgerald, K. D., Moore, G. J., Paulson, L. A., Stewart, C. M., & Rosenberg, D. R. (2000). Proton spectroscopic imaging of the thalamus in treatment-naive pediatric obsessive-compulsive disorder. *Biological Psychiatry, 47*, 174–182.

Fitzmaurice, P. S., Ang, L., Guttman, M., Rajput, A. H., Furukawa, Y., & Kish, S. J. (2003). Nigral glutathione deficiency is not specific for idiopathic Parkinson's disease. *Movement Disorders, 18*, 969–976.

Fletcher, J. M. (1996). Executive functions in children: Introduction to the special series. *Developmental Neuropsychology, 12*, 1–3.

Flint, A., Bradwejn, J., Vaccarino, F., Gutkowska, J., Palmour, R., & Koszycki, D. (2002). Aging and panicogenic response to cholecystokinin tetrapeptide: An examination of the cholecystokinin system. *Neuropsychopharmacology, 27*, 663–671.

Flint, A. J. (1994). Epidemiology and comorbidity of anxiety disorders in the elderly. *American Journal of Psychiatry, 151*, 640–649.

Flowers, D. L., Wood, F. B., & Naylor, C. E. (1991). Regional cerebral blood flow correlates of language processes in reading disability. *Archives of Neurology, 48*, 637–643.

Foffani, G., Priori, A., Egidi, M., Rampini, P., Tamma, F., Caputo, E., et al. (2003). 300-Hz subthalamic oscillations in Parkinson's disease. *Brain, 126*, 2153–2163.

Fombonne, E. (2002). Prevalence of childhood disintegrative disorder. *Autism, 6*, 149–157.

Fombonne, E. (2003). Epidemiological surveys of autism and other pervasive developmental disorders: An update. *Journal of Autism and Developmental Disorders, 33*, 365–382.

Fombonne, E., Rogé, B., Claverie, J., Courty, S., & Frémolle, J. (1999). Microcephaly and macrocephaly in autism. *Journal of Autism and Developmental Disorders, 29*, 113–110.

Fontaine, R., Breton, G., Déry, R., Fontaine, S., & Elie, R. (1990). Temporal lobe abnormalities in panic disorder: An MRI study. *Biological Psychiatry, 27*, 304–310.

Ford, T., Goodman, R., & Meltzer, H. (2003). The British Child and Adolescent Mental Health Survey 1999: The prevalence of DSM-IV disorders. *Journal of the American Academy of Child and Adolescent Psychiatry, 42*, 1203–1211.

Foroud, T., Castelluccio, P. F., Koller, D. L., Edenberg, H. J., Miller, M., Bowman, E., et al. (2000). Suggestive evidence of a locus on chromosome 10p using the NIMH genetics initiative bipolar affective disorder pedigrees. *American Journal of Medical Genetics, 96*, 18–23.

Foroud, T., Edenberg, H. J., Goate, A., Rice, J., Flury, L., Koller, D. L., et al. (2000). Alcoholism susceptibility loci: Confirmation studies in a replicate sample and further mapping. *Alcoholism: Clinical and Experimental Research, 24*, 933–945.

Foster, P. S., & Eisler, R. M. (2001). An integrative approach to the treatment of obsessive-compulsive disorder. *Comprehensive Psychiatry, 42*, 24–31.

Fountoulakis, K. N., Nimatoudis, I., Iacovides, A., & Kaprinis, G. (2004). Off-label indications for atypical antipsychotics: A systematic review. *Annals of General Hospital Psychiatry, 18*, 4.

Fountoulakis, K. N., O'Hara, R., Iacovides, A., Camilleri, C. P., Kaprinis, S., Kaprinis, G., et al. (2003). Unipolar late-onset depression: A comprehensive review. *Annals of General Hospital Psychiatry, 2*, 11.

Francks, C., Fisher, S. E., Olson, R. K., Pennington, B. F., Smith, S. D., & DeFries, J. C. (2002). Fine mapping of the chromosome 2p12-16 dyslexia susceptibility locus: Quantitative association analysis and positional candidate genes SEMA4F and OTX1. *Psychiatric Genetics, 12*, 35–41.

Francobandiera, G. (2001). Olanzapine augmentation of serotonin uptake inhibitors in obsessive-compulsive disorder: An open study. *Canadian Journal of Psychiatry, 46*, 356–358.

Frangou, S., Aylward, E., Warren, A., Sharma, T., Barta, P., & Pearlson, G. (1997). Small planum temporale volume in Down's syndrome: A volumetric MRI study. *American Journal of Psychiatry, 154*, 1424–1429.

Frank, E., Kupfer, D. J., Perel, J. M., Cornes, C., Jarrett, D. B., Mallinger, A. G., et al. (1990). Three-year outcomes for maintenance therapies in recurrent depression. *Archives of Psychiatry, 47*, 1093–1099.

Frank, G. K., Kaye, W. H., Altemus, M., & Greeno, C. G. (2000). CSF oxytocin and vasopressin levels after recovery from bulimia nervosa and anorexia nervosa, bulimic subtype. *Biological Psychiatry, 48*, 315–318.

Frank, G. K., Kaye, W. H., Meltzer, C. C., Price, J. C., Greer, P., McConaha, C., et al. (2002). Reduced 5-HT2A receptor binding after recovery from anorexia nervosa. *Biological Psychiatry, 52*, 896–906.

Franklin, M. E., Kozak, M. J., Cashman, L. A, Coles, M. E., Rheingold, A. A., & Foa, E. B. (1998). Cognitive-behavioral treatment of pediatric obsessive-compulsive disorder: An open clinical trial. *Journal of the American Academy of Child and Adolescent Psychiatry, 37*, 412–419.

Fredericksen, K. A., Cutting, L. E., Kates, W. R., Mostofsky, S. H., Singer, H. S., Cooper, K. L., et al. (2002). Disproportionate increases of white matter in right frontal lobe in Tourette syndrome. *Neurology, 58*, 85–89.

Frederikse, M. E., Lu, A., Aylward, E., Barta, P., Sharma, T., & Pearlson, G. (2000). Sex differences in inferior parietal lobule volume in schizophrenia. *American Journal of Psychiatry, 157*, 422–427.

Frederikse, M. E., Lu, A., Aylward, E., Barta, P., Sharma, T., & Pearlson, G. (1999). Sex differences in inferior parietal lobule. *Cerebral Cortex, 9*, 896–901.

Freed, C. R., Breeze, R. E., Rosenberg, N. L., Schneck, S. A., Kriek, E., Qi, J. X., et al. (1992). Survival of implanted fetal dopamine cells and neurologic improvement 12 to 46 months after transplantation for Parkinson's disease. *The New England Journal of Medicine, 327*, 1549–1555.

Freed, C. R., Greene, P. E., Breeze, R. E., Tsai, W. Y., DuMouchel, W., Kao, R., et al. (2001). Transplantation of embryonic dopamine neurons for severe Parkinson's disease. *New England Journal of Medicine, 344*, 710–719.

Freed, C. R., Leehy, M. A., Zawada, M., Bjugstad, K., Thompson, L., & Breeze, R. E. (2003). Do patients with Parkinson's disease benefit from embryonic dopamine cell transplantation? *Journal of Neurology, 250*, 44–46.

Freeman, E. D., Fast, D. K., Burd, L., Kerbeshian, J., Robertson, M. M., & Sandor, P. (2000). An international perspective on Tourette syndrome: Selected findings from 3,500 individuals in 22 countries. *Development in Medicine and Child Neurology, 42*, 436–447.

Freeman, M. P., Freeman, S. A., & McElroy, S. L. (2002). The comorbidity of bipolar and anxiety disorders: Prevalence, psychobiology, and treatment issues. *Journal of Affective Disorders, 68*, 1–23.

Frick, P. J., Lahey, B. B., Christ, M. A. G., Loeber, R., & Green, S. (1991). History of childhood behavior problems in biological relatives of boys with attention-deficit hyperactivity disorder and conduct disorder. *Journal of Clinical Child Psychology, 20*, 445–451.

Friedland, R. P., Jagust, W. J., Huesman, R. H., Koss, E., Knittel, B., Mathis, C. A., et al. (1989). Regional cerebral glucose transport and utilization in Alzheimer's disease. *Neurology, 39*, 1427–1434.

Friedlander, A. H., Yagiela, J. A., Paterno, V. I., & Mahler, M. E. (2003). The pathophysiology, medical management, and dental implications of autism. *CDA Journal, 31*, 681–691.

Friedman, I., Dar, R., & Shilony, E. (2000). Compulsivity and obsessionality in opioid addiction. *Journal of Nervous and Mental Disease, 188*, 155–162.

Friedman, L., Findling, R. L., Kenny, J. T., Swales, T. P., Stuve, T. A., Jesberger, J. A., et al. (1999). An MRI study of adolescent patients with either schizophrenia or bipolar disorder as compared to healthy control subjects. *Biological Psychiatry, 46*, 78–88.

Friedman, L., Kenny, J. T., Wise, A. L., Wu, D., Stuve, T. A., Miller, D. A., et al. (1998). Brain activation during silent word generation evaluated with functional MRI. *Brain and Language, 64*, 231–256.

Friedman, S. D., Dager, S. R., Parow, A., Hirashima, F., Demopulos, C., Stoll, A. L., et al. (2004). Lithium and valproic acid treatment effects on brain chemistry in bipolar disorder. *Biological Psychiatry, 56*, 340–348.

Frisch, A., Laufer, N., Danziger, Y., Michaelovsky, E., Leor, S., Carel, C., et al. (2001). Association of anorexia nervosa with the high activity allele of the COMT gene: A family-based study in Israeli patients. *Molecular Psychiatry, 6*, 243–245.

Frisch, A., Postilnick, D., Rockah, R., Michaelovsky, E., Postilnick, S., Birman, E., et al. (1999). Association of unipolar major depressive disorder with genes of the serotonergic and dopaminergic pathways. *Molecular Psychiatry, 4*, 389–392.

Fritschy, J. M., & Grzanna, R. (1992). Degeneration of rat locus coeruleus neurons is not accompanied by an irreversible loss of ascending projections. *Annals of the New York Academy of Sciences, 648*, 275–278.

Frodl, T., Meisenzahl, E., Zetzsche, T., Bottlender, R., Born, C., Groll, C., et al. (2002b). Enlargement of the amygdala in patients with a first episode of major depression. *Biological Psychiatry, 51*, 708–714.

Frodl, T., Meisenzahl, E. M., Zetzsche, T., Born, C., Groll, C., Jäger, M., et al. (2002a). Hippocampal changes in patients with a first episode of major depression. *American Journal of Psychiatry, 159*, 1112–1118.

Frodl, T., Meisenzahl, E. M., Zetzsche, T., Born, C., Jäger, M., Groll, C., et al. (2003). Larger amygdala volumes in first depressive episode as compared to recurrent major depression and healthy control subjects. *Biological Psychiatry, 53*, 338–344.

Frodl, T., Meisenzahl, E. M., Zill, P., Baghai, T., Rujescu, D., Leinsinger, G., et al. (2004). Reduced hippocampal volumes associated with the long variant of the serotonin transporter polymorphism in major depression. *Archives of General Psychiatry, 61*, 117–183.

Frost, J. A., Binder, J. R., Springer, J. A., Hammeke, T. A., Bellgowan, P. S., Roa, S. M., et al. (1999). Language processing is strongly left lateralized in both sexes: Evidence from fMRI. *Brain, 122*, 199–208.

Frost, J. J. (1992). Receptor imaging by positron emission tomography and sing-photon emission computed tomography. *Investigative Radiology, 27*, 54–58.

Fu, Q., Heath, A. C., Bucholz, K. K., Nelson, E., Goldberg, J., Lyons, M. J., et al. (2002). Shared genetic risk of major depression, alcohol dependence, and marijuana dependence: Contribution of antisocial personality disorder in men. *Archives of General Psychiatry, 59*, 1125–1132.

Fuchs, E., Czeh, B., Michaelis, T., de Biurrun, G., Watanabe, T., & Frahm, J. (2002). Synaptic plasticity and tianeptine: Structural regulation. *European Journal of Psychiatry, 17*, 311–317.

Fuchs, T., Birbaumer, N., Lutzenberger, W., Gruzelier, J. H., & Kaiser, J. (2003). Neurofeedback treatment for attention-deficit/hyperactivity disorder in children: A comparison with methylphenidate. *Applied Psychophysiological Feedback, 28*, 1–12.

Fujioka, T., Fujioka, A., & Duman, R. S. (2004). Activation of camp signaling facilitates the morphological maturation of newborn neurons in adult hippocampus. *Journal of Neuroscience, 24*, 319–328.

Fullerton, C. S., Ursano, R. J., & Wang, L. (2004). Acute stress disorder, posttraumatic stress disorder, and depression in disaster or rescue workers. *American Journal of Psychiatry, 161*, 1370–1376.

Fundytus, M. E., & Coderre, T. J. (1994). Effect of activity at metabotropic, as well as ionotropic (NMDA), glutamate receptors on morphine dependence. *British Journal of Pharmacology, 113*, 1215–1220.

Furlong, R. A., Ho, L., Walsh, C., Rubinsztein, J. S., Jain, S., Paykel, E. S., et al. (1998). Analysis and meta-analysis of two serotonin transporter gene polymorphisms in bipolar and unipolar affective disorders. *American Journal of Medical Genetics, 81*, 58–73.

Fux, M., Benjamin, J., & Nemets, B. (2004). A placebo-controlled cross-over trial of adjunctive EPA in OCD. *Journal of Psychiatric Research, 38*, 323–325.

Gabriëls, L., Cosyns, P., Nuttin, B., Demeulemeester, H., & Gybels, J. (2003). Deep brain stimulation for treatment-refractory obsessive-compulsive disorder: Psychopathological and neuropsychological outcome in three cases. *Acta Psychiatrica Scandinavica, 107*, 275–282.

Gadow, K. D., Nolan, E., Sprafkin, J., & Sverd, J. (1995). School observations of children with attention-deficit hyperactivity disorder and comorbid tic disorder: Effects of mathylphenidate treatment. *Journal of Developmental Behavior and Pediatrics, 16*, 167–176.

Gadzicki, D., Muller-Vahl, K. R., Heller, D., Ossege, S., Nothen, M. M., Hebebrand, J., et al. (2004). Tourette syndrome is not caused by mutations in the central cannabinoid receptor (CNR1) gene. *American Journal of Medical Genetics, 127B*, 97–103.

Gaffney, G. R., Perry, P. J., Lund, B. C., Bever-Stille, K. A., Arndt, S., & Kuperman, S. (2002). Risperidone versus clonidine in the treatment of children and adolescents with Tourette's syndrome. *Journal of the American Academy of Child and Adolescent Psychiatry, 41*, 330–336.

Gagné, G. G., Furman, M. J., Carpenter, L. L., & Price, L. H. (2000). Efficacy of continuation ECT and antidepressant drugs compared to long-term antidepressants alone in depressed patients. *American Journal of Psychiatry, 157*, 1960–1965.

Galaburda, A. M., Menard, M. T., & Rosen, G. D. (1994). Evidence for aberrant auditory anatomy in developmental dyslexia. *Proceedings of the National Academy of Sciences of the United States of America, 91*, 8010–8013.

Galaburda, A. M., Sherman, G. F., Rosen, G. D., Aboitiz, F., & Geschwind, N. (1985). Developmental dyslexia: Four consecutive patients with cortical anomalies. *Annals of Neurology, 18*, 222–233.

Ganguli, M., Chandra, V., Kamboh, M. I., Johnston, J. M., Dodge, H. H., Thelma, B. K., et al. (2000). Apolipoprotein E polymorphism and Alzheimer disease: The Indo–US Cross-National Dementia Study. *Archives of Neurology, 57*, 824–830.

Garcia-Sevilla, J. A., Escriba, P. V., Ozaita, A., La Harpe, R., Walzer, C., Eytan, A., et al. (1999). Up-regulation of immunolabeled alpha2A-adrenoceptors, Gi coupling proteins, and regulatory receptor kinases in the prefrontal cortex of depressed suicides. *Journal of Neurochemistry, 72*, 282–291.

Garcia-Sevilla, J. A., Ventayol, P., Busquets, X., La Harpe, R., Walzer, C., & Guimon, J. (1997). Marked decrease of immunolabbelled 68 kDa neurofilament (NF-L) proteins in brains of opiate addicts. *Neuroreport, 6*, 1561–1565.

Garcia-Toro, M., Pascual-Leone, A., Romera, M., González, A., Micó, J., Ibarra, O., et al. (2001). Prefrontal repetitive transcranial magnetic stimulation as add on treatment in depression. *Journal of Neurology, Neurosurgery, and Psychiatry, 71*, 546–548.

Gardiner, S. J., Kristensen, J. H., Begg, E. J., Hackett, L. P., Wilson, D. A., Ilet, K. F., et al. (2003). Transfer of olanzapine into breast milk, calculation of infant drug dose, and effect on breast-fed infants. *American Journal of Psychiatry, 160*, 1428–1431.

Gardner, E. L. (2002). Addictive potential of cannabinoids: The underlying neurobiology. *Chemistry and Physics of Lipids, 121*, 267–290.

Garfinkel, B. D., Webster, C. D., & Sloman, L. (1975). Individual responses to methylphenidate and caffeine in children with minimal brain dysfunction. *Canadian Medical Association Journal, 113*, 729–732.

Garfinkel, B. D., Webster, C. D., & Sloman, L. (1981). Responses to methylphenidate and varied doses of caffeine in children with attention deficit disorder. *Canadian Journal of Psychiatry, 26*, 395–401.

Garre-Olmo, J., López-Pousa, S., Vilalta-Franch, J., Turon-Estrada, A., Lozano-Gallego, M., Hernández-Ferràndiz, M., et al. (2004). Neuropsychological profile of Alzheimer's disease in women: Moderate and moderately severe cognitive decline. *Archives of Women's Mental Health, 7*, 27–36.

Garvey, M. J., Noyes, R., Woodman, C., & Laukes, C. (1995). Relationship of generalized anxiety symptoms to urinary 5-hydroxyindoleacetic acid and vanillylmandelic acid. *Psychiatry Research, 57*, 1–5.

Garzon, D., Yu, G., & Fahnestock, M. (2002). A new brain-derived nerotrophic factor transcript and decrease in brain-derived neurotrophic factor transcripts 1, 2 and 3 in Alzheimer's disease parietal cortex. *Journal of Neurochemistry, 82*, 1058–1064.

Gaser, T. (2001). Genetics of Parkinson's disease. *Journal of Neurology, 248*, 833–840.

Gasser, T., Rousson, V., & Schreiter Gasser, U. (2003). EEG power and coherence in children with educational problems. *Journal of Clinical Neurophysilogy, 20*, 273–282.

Gater, R., Tansella, M., Korten, A., Tiemens, B. G., Mavreas, V. G., & Olatawura, M. O. (1998). Sex differences in the prevalence and detection of depressive and anxiety disorders in general health care settings: Report from the World Health Organization collaborative study on psychological problems in general health care. *Archives of General Psychiatry, 55*, 405–413.

Gates, L., Clarke, J. R., Stokes, A., Somarjai, R., Jarmasz, M., Vandorpe, R., et al. (2004). Neuroanatomy of corpolalia in Tourette syndrome using functional magnetic resonance imaging. *Progress in Neuropsychopharmacolgoy and Biological Psychiatry, 28*, 397–400.

Gatz, M., Pedersen, N. L., Berg, S., Johansson, B., Johansson, K., Mortimer J. A., et al. (1997). Heritability for Alzheimer's disease: The study of dementia in Swedish twins. *Journals of Gerontology, 52*, 117–125.

Gatz, M., Svedberg, P., Pedersen, N. L., Mortimer, J. A., Berg, S., & Johansson, B. (2001). Education and the risk of Alzheimer's disease: Findings from the study of dementia in Swedish twins. *Journals of Gerontology, 56*, 292–300.

Gelder, M. G. (1998). Combined pharmacotherapy and cognitive behavior therapy in the treatment of panic disorder. *Journal of Clinical Psychopharmacology, 18, Supplement 2*, 2S–5S.

Gelernter, J., Pakstis, A. J., Pauls, D. L., Kurlan, R., Gancher, S. T., Civelli, O., et al. (1990). Gilles de la Tourette syndrome is not linked to D2-dopamine receptor. *Archives of General Psychiatry, 47*, 1073–1077.

Gelfin, Y., Gorfine, M., & Lerer, B. (1998). Effect of clinical doses of fluoxetine on psychological variables in healthy volunteers. *American Journal of Psychiatry, 155*, 290–292.

Geller, B., Badner, J. A., Tillman, R., Christian, S. L., Bolhofner, K., & Cook, E. H. (2004). Linkage disequilibrium of the brain-derived neurotrophic factor Val66Met polymorphism in children with a prepubertal and early adolescent bipolar disorder phenotype. *American Journal of Psychiatry, 161*, 1698–1700.

Geller, B., Zimmerman, B., Williams, M., Bolhofner, K., Craney, J. L., Delbello, M. P., et al. (2000). Six-month stability and outcome of a prepubertal and early adolescent bipolar disorder phenotype. *Journal of Adolescent Psychopharmacology, 10*, 165–173.

Geller, D. A. (2004). Re-examining comorbidity of obsessive compulsive and attention-deficit hyperactivity disorder using an empirically derived taxonomy. *European Child & Adolescent Psychiatry, 13*, 83–91.

Geller, D. A., Biederman, J., Stewart, S. E., Mullin, B., Martin, A., Spencer, T., et al. (2003). Which SSRI? A meta-analysis of pharmacotherapy trials in pediatric obsessive-compulsive disorder. *American Journal of Psychiatry, 160*, 1919–1928.

George, M. S., & Belmaker, R. H. (2000). *Transcranial magnetic stimulation in neuropsychiatry*. Washington, DC: American Psychiatric Press.

George, M. S., Costa, D. C., Kouris, K., Ring, H. A., & Ell, P. J. (1992). Cerebral blood flow abnormalities in adults with infantile autism. *Journal of Nervous and Mental Disease, 180*, 413–417.

George, M. S., Nahas, Z., Kozel, A. F., Li, X., Yamanaka, K., Mishory, A., et al. (2003). Mechanisms and the current state of transcranial magnetic stimulation. *CNS Spectrums, 8*, 496–514.

George, M. S., Sallee, F. R., Nahas, Z., Oliver, N. C., & Wassermann, E. M. (2001). Transcranial magnetic stimulation (TMS) as a research tool in Tourette syndrome and related disorders. *Advances in Neurology, 85*, 225–235.

George, M. S., Trimble, M. R., Costa, D. C., Robertson, M. M., Ring, H. A., & Ell, P. J. (1992). Elevated frontal cerebral blood flow in Gilles de la Tourette syndrome: A 99Tcm-HMPAO SPECT study. *Psychiatry Research, 45*, 143–151.

George, M. S., Trimble, M. R., Ring, H. A., Sallee, F. R., & Robertson, M. M. (1993). Obsessions in obsessive-compulsive disorder with and without Gilles de la Tourette's syndrome. *American Journal of Psychiatry, 150*, 93–97.

Georgievska, B., Kirik, D., Rosen, C., Lundberg, C., & Bjoerklund, A. (2002). Neuroprotection in the rat Parkinson model by intrastriatal GDNF gene transfer using a lentibiral vector. *NeuroReport, 13*, 75–82.

Gerard, E., & Peterson, B. S. (2003). Developmental processes and brain imaging studies in Tourette syndrome. *Journal of Psychosomatic Research, 55*, 13–22.

Getz, K., Hermann, B., Seidenberg, M., Bell, B., Dow, C., Jones, J., et al. (2002). Negative symptoms in temporal lobe epilepsy. *American Journal of Psychiatry, 159*, 644–651.

Gevins, A. (1998). The future of electroencephalography in assessing neurocognitive functioning. *Electroencephalography and Clinical Neurophysiology, 106*, 165–172.

Ghadirian, A. M., Gauthier, S., & Bertrand, S. (1986). Anxiety attacks in a patient with a right temporal lobe meningioma. *Journal of Clinical Psychiatry, 47*, 270–271.

Ghaemi, S. N., Rosenquist, K. J., Ko, J. Y., Baldassano, C. F., Kontos, N. J., & Baldessarini, R. J. (2004). Antidepressant treatment in bipolar versus unipolar depression. *American Journal of Psychiatry, 161*, 163–165.

Ghaziuddin, M., Tsai, L. Y., Ghaziuddin, N., Eilers, L., Naylor, M., Alessi, N., et al. (1993). Utility of the head computerized tomography scan in child and adolescent psychiatry. *Journal of the American Academy of Child and Adolescent Psychiatry, 32*, 123–126.

Gibson, C. J., Logue, M., & Growdon, J. H. (1985). CSF monoamine metabolite levels in Alzheimer's and Parkinson's disease. *Archives of Neurology, 42*, 489–492.

Giedd, J. N., Blumenthal, J., Molloy, E., Castellanos, F. X. (2001). Brain imaging of attention deficit/hyperactivity disorder. *Annals of the New York Academy of Sciences, 931*, 33–49.

Giedd, J. N., Castellanos, F. X., Casey, B. J., Kozuch, P., King, A. C., Hamburger, S. D., et al. (1994). Quantitative morphology of the corpus callosum in attention deficit hyperactivity disorder. *American Journal of Psychiatry, 151*, 665–669.

Giedd, J., Snell, J., Lange, N., Rajapakse, J., Casey, B., Kozuch, P., et al. (1996). Quantitative magnetic resonance imaging of human brain development: Ages 4–18. *Cerebral Cortex, 6*, 551–560.

Giedd, J. N., Jefferies, N. O., Blumenthal, J., Castellanos, F. X., Vaituzis, A. C., Fernandez, T., et al. (1999). Childhood-onset schizophrenia: Progressive brain changes during adolescence. *Biological Psychiatry, 46*, 892–898.

Gilbert, A. R., Moore, G. J., Keshavan, M. S., Paulson, L. A., Narula, V., Mac Master, F. P., et al. (2000). Decrease in thalamic volumes of pediatric patients with obsessive-compulsive disorder who are taking paroxetine. *Archives of General Psychiatry, 57*, 449–456.

Gilbert, A. R., Rosenberg, D. R., Harenski, K., Spencer, S., Sweeney, J. A., & Keshavan, M. S. (2001). Thalamic volumes in patients with first-episode schizophrenia. *American Journal of Psychiatry, 158*, 618–624.

Gilbert, D. L., Bansal, A. S, Sethuraman, G., Sallee, F. R., Zhang, J., Lipps, T., et al. (2004). Association of cortical disinhibition with tic, ADHD, and OCD severity in Tourette syndrome. *Movement Disorders, 19*, 416–425.

Gilger, J. W., & Kaplan, B. J. (2001). Atypical brain development: A conceptual framework for understanding developmental learning disabilities. *Developmental Neuropsychology, 20*, 456–481.

Gill, A. R., & Rapin, I. (2001). Interventions for autism. *Journal of the American Medical Association, 286*, 670–671.

Gill, M., Daly, G., Heron, S., Hawi, Z., & Fitzgerald, M. (1997). Confirmation of association between attention deficit hyperactivity disorder and a dopamine transporter polymorphism. *Molecular Psychiatry, 2*, 311–313.

Gillberg, C., & de Souza, L. (2002). Head circumference in autism, Asperger syndrome, and ADHD: A comparative study. *Developmental Medicine and Child Neurology, 44–296.*

Gillberg, C., Schaumann, H., & Gillberg, I. C. (1995). Autism in immigrants: Children born in Sweden to mothers born in Uganda. *Journal of Intellectual Disabilities Research, 39*, 141–144.

Gilbert, D. L., Dure, L., Sethuraman, G., Raab, D., Lane, J., & Sallee, F. R. (2003). Tic reduction with perigolide in a randomized controlled trial in children. *Neurology, 60*, 606–611.

Gillis, J. J., Giliger, J. W., Pennington, B. F., & DeFries, J. C. (1992). Attention deficit disorder in reading-disabled twins: Evidence for genetic etiology. *Journal of Abnormal Child Psychology, 20*, 303–315.

Gillman, M. A., & Sandyk, R. (1986). The endogenous opioid system in Gilles de la Tourette syndrome. *Medical Hypotheses, 19*, 371–378.

Gilman, S., Koeppe, R. A., Little, R., An, H., Junck, L., Giordani, B., et al. (2004). Striatal monoamine terminals in Lewy body dementia and Alzheimer's disease. *Annals of Neurology, 55*, 774–780.

Gilmore, J. H., & Bouldin, T. W. (2002). Analysis of ependymal abnormalities in subjects with schizophrenia, bipolar disorder, and depression. *Schizophrenia Research, 57*, 267–271.

Gilotty, L., Kenworthy, L., Sirian, L., Black, D. O., & Wagner, A. E. (2002). Adaptive skills and executive function in autism spectrum disorders. *Child Neurology, 8*, 241–248.

Gironell, A., Kulievsky, J., Rami, L., Fortuny, N., Garcia-Sanchez, C., & Pascual-Sedano, B. (2003). Effects of pallidotomy and bilateral subthalamic stimulation on cognitive function in Parkinson's disease. A controlled comparative study. *Journal of Neurology, 250*, 917–923.

Giros, B., Jaber, M., Jones, S. R., Wightman, R. M., & Caron, M. G. (1996). Hyperlocomotion and indifference to cocaine and amphetamine in mice lacking the dopamine transporter. *Nature, 379*, 606–612.

Gjedde, A., & Wong, D. F. (2001). Quantification of neuroreceptors in living human brain. V. Endogenous neurotransmitter inhibition of haloperidol binding in psychosis. *Journal of Cerebral Blood Flow and Metabolism, 21*, 982–994.

Gjone, H., Stevenson, J., & Sundet, J. M. (1996). Genetic influence on parent-reported attention-related problems in a Norwegian general population twin sample. *Journal of the American Academy of Child and Adolescent Psychiatry, 35*, 588–598.

Glantz, L. A., & Lewis, D. A. (2000). Decreased dendritic spine density on prefrontal cortical pyramidal neurons in schizophrenia. *Archives of General Psychiatry, 57*, 65–73.

Glaser, D. (2000). Child abuse and neglect and the brain—A review. *Journal of Child Psychology and Psychiatry and Allied Disciplines, 41*, 97–116.

Glatt, C. E., Tampilic, M., Christie, C., DeYoung, J., & Freimer, N. B. (2004). Re-screening serotonin receptors for genetic variants identifies population and molecular genetic complexity. *American Journal of Medical Genetics, 124B,* 92–100.

Glatt, S. J., Faraone, S. V., & Tsuang, M. T. (2003). Association between a functional catechol O-methyltransferase gene polymorphism and schizophrenia: Meta-analysis of case-control and family-based studies. *American Journal of Psychiatry, 160,* 469–476.

Glenn, T. C., Kelly, D. F., Boscardin, W. J., McArthur, D. L., Vespa, P., Oetel, M., et al. (2003). Energy dysfunction as a predictor of outcome after moderate or severe head injury: Indices of oxygen, glucose, and lactate metabolism. *Journal of Cerebral Blood Flow Metabolism, 23,* 1239–1250.

Glosser, G. (2001). Neurobehavioral aspects of movement disorders. *Neurologic Clinics, 19,* 535–551.

Glowinski, A. L., Madden, P. A., Bucholz, K. K., Lynskey, M. T., & Heath, A. C. (2003). Genetic epidemiology of self-reported lifetime DSM-IV major depressive disorder in a population-based twin sample of female adolescents. *Journal of Child Psychology and Psychiatry, and Allied Disciplines, 44,* 988–996.

Goethals, I., Vervaet, M., Audenaert, K., Van de Wiele, C., Ham, H., Vandecapelle, M., et al. (2004). Comparison of cortical 5-HT2A receptor binding in bulimia nervosa patients and healthy volunteers. *American Journal of Psychiatry, 161,* 1916–1918.

Goetz, C. G. (1992). Tic disorders: Gilles de la Tourette syndrome. In H. L. Klawans, C. G. Goetz, & C. M. Tanner (Eds.), *Textbook of clinical neuropharmacology and therapeutics* (pp. 183–190). New York: Raven.

Goetz, C. G., & Tanner, C. M. (1990). Gilles de la Tourette's syndrome in twins: Clinical and neurochemical data. *Movement Disorders, 5,* 173–175.

Goff, D. C., Bottiglieri, T., Arning, E., Shih, V., Freudenreich, O., Evins, E., et al. (2004). Folate, homocysteine, and negative symptoms in schizophrenia. *American Journal of Psychiatry, 161,* 1705–1708.

Gold, L. H. (2003). Psychopharmacologic treatment of depression during pregnancy. *Current Womens Health Report, 3,* 236–41.

Goldberg, J. F., Burdick, K. E., & Endick, C. J. (2004). Preliminary randomized, double-blind, placebo-controlled trial of pramipexole added to mood stabilizers for treatment-resistant bipolar depression. *American Journal of Psychiatry, 161,* 564–566.

Goldstein, H. (2002). Communication intervention for children with autism: A review of treatment efficacy. *Journal of Autism and Developmental Disorders, 32,* 373–396.

Goldstein, R. Z., & Volkow, N. D. (2002). Drug addiction and its underlying neurobiological basis: Neuroimaging evidence for the involvement of the frontal cortex. *American Journal of Psychiatry, 159,* 1642–1652.

Gomez-Pinilla, F., Ying, Z., Roy, R. R., Molteni, R., & Edgerton, V. R. (2002). Voluntary exercise induces BDNF-mediated mechanism that promotes neuroplasticity. *Journal of Neurophysiology, 88,* 2187–2195.

Gomot, M., Giard, M. H., Adrien, J. L., Barthelemy, C., & Bruneau, N. (2002). Hypersensitivity to acoustic change in children with autism: Electrophysiological evidence of left frontal cortex dysfunctioning. *Psychophysiology, 39,* 577–584.

Gonzalez Castro, F., Barrington, E. H., Walton, M. A., & Rawson, R. A. (2000). *Psychology of Addictive Behaviors, 14,* 390–396.

Gonzalez-Rothi, L. J. (2001). Neurophysiologic basis of rehabilitation. *Journal of Medical Speech-Language Pathology, 9,* 117–127.

Goodman, R., & Stevenson, J. (1999). A twin study of hyperactivity—II. The aetiological role of genes, family relationships and perinatal adversity. *Journal of Child Psychology and Psychiatry, 30,* 691–709.

Goodman, W. K., McDougle, C. J., Price, L. H., Barr, L. C., Hills, O. F., Caplik, J. F., et al. (1995). m-Chlorophenylpiperazine in patients with obsessive-compulsive disorder: Absence of symptom exacerbation. *Biological Psychiatry, 38,* 138–149.

Goodnick, P. J., Rush, A. J., George, M. S., Marangell, L. B., & Sackeim, H. A. (2001). Vagus nerve stimulation in depression. *Expert Opinions in Pharmacotherapy, 2,* 1061–1063.

Goodwin, F. K., Fireman, B., Simon, G. E., Hunkeler, E. M., Lee, J., & Revicki, D. (2003). Suicide risk in bipolar disorder during treatment with lithium and divalproex. *Journal of the American Medical Association, 290,* 1467–1473.

Goodwin, R., Lyons, J. S., & McNally, R. J. (2002). Panic attacks in schizophrenia. *Schizophrenia Research, 58,* 213–220.

Goodwin, R. D., Fergusson, D. M., & Horwood, L. J. (2004). Panic attacks and psychoticism. *American Journal of Psychiatry, 161,* 88–92.

Goodwin, R. D., & Hoven, C. W. (2002). Bipolar-panic comorbidity in the general population: Prevalence and associated morbidity. *Journal of Affective Disorders, 70,* 27–33.

Goodwin, R. D., Pine, D. S., & Hoven, C. W. (2003). Asthma and panic attacks among youth in the community. *Journal of Asthma, 40,* 139–145.

Goodyer, I. M., Park, R. J., & Herbert, J. (2001). Psychosocial and endocrine features of chronic first-episode major depression in 8–16 year olds. *Society of Biological Psychiatry, 50*, 351–357.

Gordon, I., Lask, B., Bryant-Waugh, R., Christie, D., & Timimi, S. (1997). Childhood-onset anorexia nervosa: Towards identifying a biological substrate. *International Journal of Eating Disorders, 22*, 159–165.

Gordon, N. (1995). Apoptosis (programmed cell death) and other reasons for elimination of neurons and axons. *Brain and Development, 17*, 73–77.

Gorell, J. M., Peterson, E. L., Rybicki, B. A., & Johnson, C. C. (2004). Multiple risk factors for Parkinson's disease. *Journal of the Neurological Sciences, 217*, 169–174.

Gorman, J. M. (2003). New methods of brain stimulation: What they tell us about the old methods and about the brain. *CNS Spectrums, 8*, 475.

Gorman, J. M., Kent, J. M, Sullivan, G. M., & Coplan, J. D. (2000). Neuroanatomical hypothesis of panic disorder, revised. *American Journal of Psychiatry, 157*, 493–505.

Gorman, J. M., Liebowitz, M. R., Fyer, A. J., & Stein, J. (1989). A neuroanatoimical hypothesis for panic disorder. *American Journal of Psychiatry, 146*, 148–161.

Gorwood, P., Klipman, A., & Foulon, C. (2003). The human genetics of anorexia nervosa. *European Journal of Pharmacology, 480*, 163–170.

Gottesman, I. I. (1991). *Schizophrenia genesis*. New York: Freeman.

Gottesman, I. I., & Bertelsen, A. (1989). Confirming unexpressed genotypes for schizophrenia. *Archives of General Psychiatry, 46*, 867–872.

Goussé, V., Plumet, M. H., Chabane, N., Mouren-Siméoni, M. C., Ferradian, N., & Leboyer, M. (2002). Fringe phenotypes in autism: A review of clinical, biochemical and cognitive studies. *European Psychiatry, 17*, 120–128.

Grace, A. A. (2001). Psychostimulant actions on dopamine and limbic system function: Relevance to the pathophysiology and treatment of ADHD. In M. V. Solanto, A. F. T. Arnsten, & F. X. Castellanos (Eds.), *Stimulant drugs and ADHD: Basic and clinical neuroscience* (pp. 134–157). New York: Oxford University Press.

Grace, A. A., Bunney, B. S., Moore, H., & Todd, C. L. (1997). Dopamine-cell depolarization block as a model for the therapeutic actions of antipsychotic drugs. *Trends in Neuroscience, 20*, 31–73.

Grady, C. L. (1998). Brain imaging and age-related changes in cognition. *Experimental Gerontology, 33*, 661–673.

Grady, C. L., Furey, M. L., Pietrini, P., Horwitz, B., & Rapoport, S. I. (2001). Altered brain functional connectivity and impaired short-term memory in Alzheimer's disease. *Brain, 124*, 739–756.

Graf, M., Kantor, S., Anheuer, Z. E., Modos, E. A., & Bagdy, G. (2003). m-CPP-induced self-grooming is mediated by 5-HT2C receptors. *Behavioural Brain Research, 142*, 175–179.

GrandPre, T., Li, S., & Strittmatter, S. M. (2002). Nogo-66 receptor antagonist peptide promotes axonal regeneration. *Nature, 417*, 547–551.

Grant, J. E., & Kim, S. W. (2001). A case of kleptomania and compulsive sexual behavior treated with naltrexone. *Annals of Clinical Psychiatry, 13*, 229–231.

Grassian, S. (1983). Psychopathological effects of solitary confinement. *American Journal of Psychiatry, 140*, 1450–1454.

Gratacòs, M., Nadal, M., Martín-Santos, R., Pujana, M. A., Gago, J., Peral, B., et al. (2001). A polymorphic genomic duplication on human chromosome 15 is a susceptibility factor for panic and phobic disorders. *Cell, 106*, 367–379.

Graves, A. B., Bowen, J. D., Rajaram, L., McCormick, W. C., McCurry, S. M., Schellenberg, G. D., et al. (1999). Impaired olfaction as a marker for cognitive decline. *Neurology, 53*, 1480–1487.

Graves, A. B., Rosner, D., Echeverria, D., Mortimer, J. A., & Larson, E. B. (1998). Occupational exposures to solvents and aluminium and estimated risk of Alzheimer's disease. *Occupational and Environmental Medicine, 55*, 627–633.

Graves, A. B., Rosner, D., Echeverria, D., Yost, M., & Larson, E. B. (1999). Occupational exposure to electromagnetic fields and Alzheimer disease. *Alzheimer Disease and Associated Disorders, 13*, 165–170.

Green, M. S., Kaye, J. A., & Ball, M. J. (2000). The Oregon brain aging study: Neuropathology accompanying healthy aging in the oldest old. *Neurology, 54*, 105–113.

Greenberg, B. D. (2002). Update on deep brain stimulation. *Journal of ECT, 18*, 193–196.

Greenberg, B. D., George, M. S., Martin, J. D., Benjamin, J., Schlaepfer, T. E., Altemus, M., et al. (1997). Effect of prefrontal repetitive transcranial magnetic stimulation in obsessive-compulsive disorder: A preliminary study. *American Journal of Psychiatry, 154*, 867–869.

Greenberg, B. D., Price, L. H., Rauch, S. L., Friehs, G., Noren, G., Malone, D., et al. (2003). Neurosurgery for intractable obsessive-compulsive disorder and depression: Critical issues. *Neurosurgery Clinics of North America, 14*, 199–212.

Greenberg, B. D., & Rezai, A. R. (2003). Mechanisms and the current state of deep brain stimulation in neuropsychiatry. *CNS Spectrums, 8*, 522–526.

Greenberg, D., & Witztum, E. (1994). The influence of cultural factors on obsessive compulsive disorder: Religious symptoms in a religious society. *Israel Journal of Psychiatry and Related Sciences, 31*, 211–220.

Greenberg, P. E., Kessler, R. C., Birnbaum, H. G., Leong, S. A., Lowe, S. W., Berglund, P. A., et al. (2003). The economic burden of depression in the United States: How did it change between 1990 and 2000? *Journal of Clinical Psychiatry, 64*, 1465–1475.

Greenfield, S. F., Manwani, S. G., & Nargiso, J. E. (2003). Epidemiology of substance use disorders in women. *Obstetric and Gynecological Clinics in North America, 30*, 413–446.

Greengard, P. (2001). The neurobiology of slow synaptic transmission. *Science, 24*, 1024–1030.

Greengard, P., Valtorta, F., Czernik, A. J., & Benfenati, B. (1993). Synaptic vesicle phosphoproteins and regulation of synaptic function. *Science, 259*, 780–785.

Greenough, W. T., & Black, J. E. (1992). Induction of brain structure by experience: Substrates for cognitive development. In M. R. Gunnar & C. A. Nelson (Eds.), *Developmental behavioral neuroscience* (Minnesota symposia on child psychology, volume 24, pp. 155–200). Hillsdale, NJ: Lawrence Erlbaum Associates.

Greenough, W. T., Withers, G. S., & Anderson, B. J. (1992). Experience dependent synaptogenesis as a plausible memory mechanism. In I. Gormezano & E. A. Wasserman (Eds.), *Learning and memory: The behavioral and biological substrates* (pp. 209–299). Hillsdale, NJ: Lawrence Erlbaum Associates.

Greenwald, M. K., Schuh, K. J., Hopper, J. A., Schuster, C. R., & Johanson, C. E. (2002). Effects of buprenorphine sublingual tabler maintenance on opioid drug-seeking behavior in humans. *Psychopharmacology, 160*, 344–352.

Grice, D. E., Leckman, J. F., Pauls, D. L., Kurlan, R., Kidd, K. K., Pakstis, A. J., et al. (1996). Linkage disequilibrium between an allele at the dopamine D4 receptor locus and Tourette syndrome, by the transmission–disequilibrium test. *American Journal of Human Genetics, 59*, 644–652.

Griez, E., de Loof, C., Pols, H., Zandbergen, J., & Lousberg, H. (1990). Specific sensitivity of patients with panic attacks to carbon dioxide inhalation. *Psychiatry Research, 31*, 193–199.

Grigorenko, E. L., Wood, F. B., Meyer, M. S., Hart, L. A., Speed, W. C., Shuster, A., et al. (1997). Susceptibility loci for distinct components of developmental dyslexia on chromosomes 6 and 15. *American Journal of Human Genetics, 60*, 27–39.

Groenewegen, H. J., van den Heuvel, O. A., Cath, D. C., Voorn, P., & Veltman, D. J. (2003). Does an imbalance between the dorsal and ventral striatopallidal systems play a role in Tourette's syndrome? A neuronal circuit approach. *Brain Development, 25*, S3–S14.

Grossberg, S. (2000). How hallucinations may arise from brain mechanisms of learning, attention, and volition. *Journal of the International Neuropsychological Society, 6*, 583–592.

Gross-Glenn, K., Duara, R., Barker, W. W., Loewenstein, D., Chang, J.-Y., Yoshii, F., Apicellla, A. M., et al. (1991). Positron emission tomographic studies during serial word-reading by normal and dyslexic adults. *Journal of Clinical and Experimental Neuropsychology, 13*, 531–544.

Grossman, M. (1999). Sentence processing in Parkinson's disease. *Brain and Cognition, 40*, 387–413.

Grunder, G., Vernaleken I., Muller, M. J., Davids, E., Heydari, N., Buchholz, H. G., et al. (2003). Subchronic haloperidol downregulates dopamine synthesis capacity in the brain of schizophrenic patients in vivo. *Neuropsychopharmacology, 28*, 787–794.

Grupp-Phelan, J., Whitaker, R. C., & Naish, A. B. (2003). Depression in mothers of children presenting for emergency and primary care: Impact on mothers' perceptions of caring for their children. *Ambulatory Pediatrics, 3*, 142–146.

Gruzelier, J. H., Galderisi, S., & Strik, W. (2002). Neurophysiological research in psychiatry. In J. J. Lopez-Ibor, W. Gaebel, M. Maj, & N. Sartorius (Eds.), *Psychiatry as a neuroscience* (pp 125–180). New York: Wiley.

Guerrero, A. P., Hishinuma, E. S., Andrade, N. N., Bell, C. K., Kurahara, D. K., Lee, T. G., et al. (2003). Demographic and clinical characteristics of adolescents in Hawaii with obsessive-compulsive disorder. *Archives of Pediatrics & Adolescent Medicine, 157*, 665–670.

Guo, Z., Cupples, L. A., Kurz, A., Auerbach, S. H., Volicer, L., Chui, H., et al. (2000). Head injury and the risk of AD in the MIRAGE study. *Neurology, 54*, 1316–1323.

Gupta, S. (2000). Immunological treatments for autism. *Journal of Autism and Developmental Disorders, 30*, 475–479.

Gur, E., Dremencov, E., Garcia, F., Van de Kar, L. D., Lerer, B., & Newman, M. E. (2002). Functional effects of chronic electroconvulsive shock on serotonergic 5-HT(1A) and 5-HT(1B) receptor activity in rat hippocampus and hypothalamus. *Brain Research, 952*, 52–60.

Gur, E., Lerer, B., & Newman, M. E. (1997). Chronic electroconvulsive shock and 5-HT autoreceptor activity in rat brain: An in vivo microdialysis study. *Journal of Neural Transmission, 104*, 795–804.

Gur, R. C., Erwin, R. J., Gur, R. E., Zwil, A. S., Heimberg, C., & Kraemer, H. C. (1992). Facial emotion discrimination: II. Behavioral findings in depression. *Psychiatry Research, 42*, 241–251.

Gur, R. E., Cowell, P., Turetsky, B. I., Gallache, F., Cannon, T., Bilker, W., et al. (1998). A follow-up magnetic resonance imaging study of schizophrenia: Relationship of neuroanatomical changes to clinical and neurobehavioral measures. *Archives of General Psychiatry, 55*, 145–152.

Gur, R. E., Petty, R. G., Turetsky, B. I., & Gur, R. C. (1996). Schizophrenia throughout life: Sex differences in severity and profile of symptoms. *Schizophrenia Research, 2,* 1–12.

Gusnard, D. A., & Raichle, M. E. (2001). Searching for a baseline: Functional imaging and the resting human brain. *Nature Reviews, 2,* 685–694.

Gutiérrez, B., van Os, J., Vallés, V., Guillamat, R., Campillo, M., & Fañanás, L. (1998). Congenital dermatoglyphic malformations in severe bipolar depression. *Psychiatry Research, 78,* 133–140.

Guttman, M., Kish, S. J., & Furukawa, Y. (2003). Current concepts in the diagnosis and management of Parkinson's disease. *Canadian Medical Academy, 168,* 293–301.

Haan, L. D., Bruggen, M. V., Lavalaye, J., Booij, J., Dingemans, P. M. A. J., & Linszen, D. (2003). Subjective experience and D2 receptor occupancy in patients with recent-onset schizophrenia treated with low-dose olanzapine or haloperidol: A randomized, double-blind study. *American Journal of Psychiatry, 160,* 303–309.

Hagengimana, A., Hinton, D., Bird, B., Pollack, M., & Pitman, R. K. (2003). Somatic panic-attack equivalents in a community sample of Rwandan widows who survived the 1994 genocide. *Psychiatry Research, 117,* 1–9.

Haile, C. N., Brooks, A. I., Cunningham, L. C., Francis, J. S., Zuzga, D. S., & During, M. J. (2001). Gilatide: A novel nootropic peptide. *Society of Neuroscience, 27,* 78.

Hakkarainen, R., Partonen, T., Haukka, J., Virtamo, J., Albanes, D., & Lonnqvist, J. (2004). Is low dietary intake of omega-3 fatty acids associated with depression? *American Journal of Psychiatry, 161,* 567–569.

Halim, N. S. (1999). Neuronal migration: Researchers advance understanding of brain's wiring. *Scientist, 13,* 6–7.

Hall, G. B., Szechtman, H., & Nahmias, C. (2003). Enhanced salience and emotion recognition in autism: A PET study. *American Journal of Psychiatry, 160,* 1439–1441.

Hall, K. S., Gao, S., Unverzagt, F. W., & Hendrie, H. C. (2000). Low education and childhood rural residence. Risk for Alzheimer's disease in African Americans. *Neurology, 54,* 95–99.

Hall, W. D., Mant, A., Mitchell, P. B., Rendle, V. A., Hickie, I. B., & McManus, P. (2003). Association between antidepressant prescribing and suicide in Australia, 1991–2000: Trend analysis. *British Medical Journal, 326,* 1–5.

Hallett, J. J., Harling-Berg, C. J., Knopf, P. M., Stopa, E. G., & Kiessling, L. S. (2000). Anti-striatal antibodies in Tourette syndrome cause neuronal dysfunction. *Journal of Neuroimmunology, 111,* 195–202.

Hallett, M., & Dubinsky, R. M. (1993). Glucose metabolism in the brain of patients with essential tremor. *Journal of the Neurological Sciences, 114,* 45–48.

Halliday, J., Farrington, S., Macdonald, S., MacEwan, T., Sharkey, V., & McCreadie, R. (2002). Nithsdale schizophrenia surveys 23: movement disorders, 20 year review. *British Journal of Psychiatry, 181,* 422–427.

Hallmayer, J., Glasson, E. J., Bower, C., Petterson, B., Croen, L., Grether, J., et al. (2002). On the twin risk in autism. *American Journal of Human Genetics, 71,* 941–946.

Halmi, K. A., Sunday, S. R., Strober, M., Kaplan, A., Woodside, D. B., Fitcher, M., et al. (2000). Perfectionism in anorexia nervosa: Variation by clinical subtype, obsessionality, and pathological eating behavior. *American Journal of Psychiatry, 157,* 1799–1805.

Hamilton, S. P., Haghighi, F., Heiman, G. A., Klein, D. F., Hodge, S. E., Fyer, A. J., et al. (2000). Investigation of dopamine receptor (DRD4) and dopamine transporter (DAT) polymorphisms for genetic linkage or association to panic disorder. *American Journal of Medical Genetics, 96,* 324–330.

Hamilton, S. P., Slager, S. L., De Leon, A. B., Heiman, G. A., Klein, D. F., Hodge, S. E., et al. (2004). Evidence for genetic linkage between a polymorphism in the adenosine 2A receptor and panic disorder. *Neuropsychopharmacology, 29,* 558–565.

Hamilton, S. P., Slager, S. L., Heiman, G. A., Deng, Z., Haghighi, F., Klein, D. F., et al. (2002). Evidence for a susceptibility locus for panic disorder near the catechol-O-methyltransferase gene on chromosome 22. *Biological Psychiatry, 51,* 591–601.

Hamilton, S. P., Slager, S. L., Helleby, L., Heiman, G. A., Klein, D. F., Hodge, S. E., et al. (2001). No association or linkage between polymorphisms in the genes encoding cholecystokinin and the cholecystokinin B receptor and panic disorder. *Molecular Psychiatry, 6,* 59–65.

Hamilton, S. P., Slager, S. L., Mayo, D., Heiman, G. A., Klein, D. F., Hodge, S. E., et al. (2004). Investigation of polymorphisms in the CREM gene in panic disorder. *American Journal of Medical Genetics, 126B,* 111–115.

Hammond, E. J., Uthman, B. M., Wilder, B. J., Ben-Menachem, E., Hamberger, A., Hedner, T., et al. (1992). Neurochemical effects of vagus nerve stimulation in humans. *Brain Research, 583,* 300–303.

Handen, B. L., Johnson, C. R., & Lubetsky, M. (2000). Efficacy of methylphenidate among children with autism and symptoms of attention-deficit hyperactivity disorder. *Journal of Autism and Developmental Disorders, 30,* 245–255.

Hansen, E. S., Hasselbalch, S., Law, I., & Bolwig, T. G. (2002). The caudate nucleus in obsessive-compulsive disorder. Reduced metabolism following treatment with paroxetine: A PET study. *International Journal of Neuropsychopharmacology, 5,* 1–10.

Hanson, D. R., & Gottesman, I. I. (1976). The genetics, if any, of infantile autism and childhood schizophrenia. *Journal of Autism and Childhood Schizophrenia, 6*, 209–234.

Hanyu, H., Shimizu, T., Tanaka, Y., Takasaki, M., Koizumi, K., & Abe, K. (2003). Regional cerebral blood flow patterns and response to donepezil treatment in patients with Alzheimer's disease. *Dementia and Geriatric Cognitive Disorders, 15*, 177–182.

Harasty, J., Double, K. L., Halliday, G. M., Kril, J. J., & McRitchie, D. A. (1997). Language-associated cortical regions are proportionately larger in the female brain. *Archives of Neurology, 54*, 171–176.

Harcherik, D. F., Cohen, D. J., Ort, S., Paul, R., Shaywitz, B. A., Volkmar, F. R., et al. (1985). Computed tomographic brain scanning in four neuropsychiatric disorders of childhood. *American Journal of Psychiatry, 142*, 731–734.

Hardan, A. Y., Minshew, N. J., & Keshavan, M. S. (2000). Corpus callosum size in autism. *Neurology, 55*, 1033–1036.

Hardan, A. Y., Minshew, N. J., Mallikarjuhn, M., & Keshavan, M. S. (2001). Brain volume in autism. *Journal of Child Neurology, 16*, 421–424.

Harding, K. L., Judah, R. D., & Gant, C. (2003). Outcome-based comparison of Ritalin versus food supplement treated children with ADHD. *Alternative Medicine Review, 8*, 319–330.

Hargrave, R., Reed, B., & Mungas, D. (2000). Depressive syndromes and functional disability in dementia. *Journal of Geriatric Psychiatry and Neurology, 13*, 72–77.

Harmanci, H., Emre, M., Gurvit, H., Bilgic, B., Hanagasi, H., Gurol, E., et al. (2003). Risk factors for Alzheimer disease: A population-based case-control study in Istanbul, Turkey. *Alzheimer Disease and Associated Disorders, 17*, 139–145.

Harmer, C. J., Hill, S. A., Taylor, M. J., Cowen, P. J., & Goodwin, G. M. (2003). Toward a neuropsychological theory of antidepressant drug action: Increase in positive emotional bias after potentiation of norepinephrine activity. *American Journal of Psychiatry, 160*, 990–992.

Haroutunian, V., Perl, D. P., Purohit, D. P., Marin, D., Khan, K., Lantz, M., et al. (1998). Regional distribution of neuritic plaques in the nondemented elderly and subjects with very mild Alzheimer's disease. *Archives of Neurology, 55*, 1185–1191.

Harper, C., Dixon, G., Sheedy, D., & Garrick, T. (2003). Neuropathological alterations in alcoholic brains. Studies arising from the New South Wales Tissue Resource Centre. *Programs in Neuropsychopharmacology and Biological Psychiatry, 27*, 951–961.

Harper Mozley, L., Gur, R. C., Mozley, D. P., & Gur, R. E. (2001). Striatal dopamine transporters and cognitive functioning in healthy men and women. *American Journal of Psychiatry, 158*, 1492–1499.

Harris, A. W., Bahramali, H., Slewa-Younan, S., Gordon, E., Williams, L., & Li, W. M. (2001). The topography of quantified electroencephalography in three syndromes of schizophrenia. *International Journal of Neuroscience, 107*, 265–278.

Harris, T. W., Hartwieg, E., Horvitz, H. R., & Jorensen, E. M. (2000). Mutations in synaptojanin disrupt synaptic vesicle recycling. *Journal of Cell Biology, 150*, 589–600.

Harrison, D. W., Demaree, H. A., Shenal, B. V., & Everhart, D. E. (1998). QEEG assisted neuropsychological evaluation of autism. *International Journal of Neuroscience, 93*, 133–140.

Harsing, L. G., Prauda. I., Barkoczy, J., Matyus, P., & Juranyi, Z. (2004). A 5-HT7 heteroreceptor-mediated inhibition of [3H] serotonin release in raphe nuclei slices of the rat: Evidence for a serotonergic-glutamateric interaction. *Neurochemistry Research, 29*, 1487–1497.

Hart, D. J., Craig, D., Compton, S. A., Critchlow, S., Kerrigan, B. M., McIlroy, S. P., et al. (2003). A retrospective study of the behavioural and psychological symptoms of mid and late phase Alzheimer's disease. *International Journal of Geriatric Psychiatry, 18*, 1037–1042.

Harvey, I., Persaud, R., Ron, M. A., Baker, G., & Murray, R. M. (1994). Volumetric MRI measurements in bipolars compared with schizophrenics and healthy controls. *Psychological Medicine, 24*, 689–699.

Harwood, A. J. (2003). Neurodevelopment and mood stabilizers. *Current Molecular Medicine, 3*, 472–482.

Hasey, G. (2001). Transcranial magnetic stimulation in the treatment of mood disorder: A review and comparison with electroconvulsive therapy. *Canadian Journal of Psychiatry, 46*, 720–727.

Hashimoto, T., Sasaki, M., Fukumizu, M., Hanaoka, S., Sugai, K., & Matsuda, H. (2000). Single-photon emission computed tomography of the brain in autism: Effect of the developmental level. *Pediatric Neurology, 23*, 416–420.

Hastings, J. E., & Barkley, R. A. (1978). A review of psychophysiological research with hyperkinetic children. *Journal of Abnormal Child Psychology, 6*, 413–447.

Hatanpää, K., Isaac, K. R., Shirao, T., Brady, D., & Rapaport, S. I. (1999). Loss of protein regulating synaptic plasticity in normal aging of the human brain and in Alzheimer's disease. *Journal of Neuropathology and Experimental Neurology, 58*, 637–643.

Hattori, E., Yamada, K., Toyota, T., Yoshitsugu, K., Toru, M., Shibuya, H., et al. (2001). Association studies of the CT repeat polymorphism in the 5' upstream region of the cholecystokinin B receptor gene with panic disorder and schizophrenia in Japanese subjects. *American Journal of Medical Genetics, 105*, 779–782.

Haug, J. O. (1962). Pneumoencephalographic studies in mental disease. *Acta Psychiatrica Scandinavica, 38*, 1–114.

Hauser, R. A., Freeman, T. B., Snow, B. J., Nauert, M., Gauger, L., Kordower, J. H., et al. (1999). Long-term evaluation of bilateral fetal nigral transplantation in Parkinson disease. *Archives of Neurology, 56*, 179–187.

Hauser, R. A., Hubble, J. P., & Truong, D. D. (2003). Randomized trial of the adenosine A(2A) receptor antagonist istradefylline in advanced PD. *Neurology, 61*, 297–303.

Häusser, M., Spruston, N., & Stuart, G. J. (2000). Diversity and dynamics of dendritic signaling. *Science, 290*, 739–744.

Havassy, B. E., Alvidrez, J., & Owen, K. K. (2004). Comparisons of patients with comorbid psychiatric and substance use disorders: implications for treatment and service delivery. *American Journal of Psychiatry, 161*, 139–145.

Haxby, J. V., Horwitz, B., Ungerleider, L. G., Maisog, J. M., Pietrini, P., & Grady, C. L. (1994). The functional organization of human extrstriate cortex: a PET-rCBF study of selective attention to faces and locations. *Journal of Neuroscience, 14*, 6336–6353.

Hay, D. A., McStephen, M., Levy, F., & Pearsall-Jones, J. (2002). Recruitment and attrition in twin register studies of childhood behavior: The example of the Australian Twin ADHD Project. *Twin Research, 5*, 324–328.

Hay, D. F. (2001). Intellectual problems shown by 11-year-old children whose mothers had postnatal depression. *Journal of Child Psychology and Psychiatry, and Allied Disciplines*, 42, 871–889.

Hay, D. F., Pawlby, S., Angold, A., Harold, G. T., & Sharp, D. (2003). Pathways to violence in the children of mothers who were depressed postpartum. *Developmental Psychology*, 39, 1083–1094.

Hayward, C., Killen, J. D., & Taylor, C. B. (2003). The relationship between agoraphobia symptoms and panic disorder in a non-clinical sample of adolescents. *Psychological Medicine, 33*, 733–738.

Hazlett, E. A., Buchsbaum, M. S., Hsieh, P., Haznedar, M. M., Platholi, J., LiCalzi, E. M., et al. (2004). Regional glucose metabolism within cortical Brodmann areas in healthy individuals and autistic patients. *Neuropsychobiology, 49*, 115–125.

Haznedar, M. M., Buchsbaum, M. S., Wei, T. C., Hof, P. R., Cartwright, C., Bienstock, C. A., et al. (2000). Limbic circuitry in patients with autism spectrum disorders studied with positron emission tomography and magnetic resonance imaging. *American Journal of Psychiatry, 157*, 1994–2001.

Head, D., Buckner, R. L., Shimony, J. S., Williams, L. E., Akbudak, E., Conturo, T. E., et al. (2004). Differential vulnerability of anterior white matter in nondemented aging with minimal acceleration in dementia of the Alzheimer type: Evidence from diffusion tensor imaging. *Cerebral Cortex, 14*, 410–423.

Healy, D. (2003). Lines of evidence on the risk of suicide with selective serotonin reuptake inhibitors. *Psychotherapy and Psychosomatics, 72*, 71–79.

Healy, D. G., Abou-Sleiman, P. M., Ozawa, T., Lees, A. J., Bhatia, K., Ahmadi, K. R., et al. (2004). A functional polymorphism regulating dopamine beta-hydroxylase influences against Parkinson's disease. *Annals of Neurology, 55*, 443–446.

Healy, M. (2000). *The presenting profile of college students diagnosed with attention-deficit/hyperactivity disorder.* Unpublished master's thesis, Central Washington University, Department of Psychology, Ellensburg.

Hebb, D. (1949). *The organization of behavior.* New York: Wiley.

Hebert, M. A., Blanchard, D. C., & Blanchard, R. J. (1999). Intravenous cocaine precipitates panic-like flight responses and lasting hyperdefensiveness in laboratory rats. *Pharmacology, Biochemistry, and Behavior, 63*, 349–360.

Heckman, J. M., Low, W. C., de Villiers, C., Rutherfoord, S., Voster, A., Rao, H., et al. (2004). Novel presenilin 1 mutation with profound neurofibrillary pathology in an indigenous Southern African family with early-onset Alzheimer's disease. *Brain, 127*, 133–142.

Hegarty, K., Gunn, J., Chondros, P., & Small, R. (2004). Association between depression and abuse by partners of women attending general practice: Descriptive, cross sectional survey. *British Medical Journal, 328*, 621–624.

Heh, C. W., Smith, R., Wu, J., Hazlett, E., Russell, A., Asarnow, R., et al. (1989). Positron emission tomography of the cerebellum in autism. *American Journal of Psychiatry, 146*, 242–245.

Heiligenstein, E., Guenther, G., Levy, A., Savino, F., & Fulwiler, J. (1999). Psychological and academic functioning in college students with attention deficit hyperactivity disorder. *Journal of American College Health, 47*, 181–185.

Heimer, L. (2003). A new anatomical framework for neuropsychiatric disorders and drug abuse. *American Journal of Psychiatry, 160*, 1726–1739.

Heinz, A., Siessmeier, T., Wrase, J., Hermann, D., Klein, S., Gursser-Sinopoli, S. M., et al. (2004). Correlation between dopamine D2 receptors in the ventral striatum and central processing of alcohol cues and craving. *American Journal of Psychiatry, 161*, 1783–1789.

Heiske, A., Jesberg, J., Krieg, J. C., & Vedder, H. (2003). Differential effects of antidepressants on glucocorticoid receptors in human primary blood cells and human monocytic U-937 cells. *Neuropsychopharmacology, 28*, 807–817.

Helmuth, L. (2000). Further progress on a β-amyloid vaccine. *Science, 289*, 375.

Hemmings, S. M., Kinnear, C. J., Niehaus, D. J., Moolman-Smook, J. C., Lochner, C., Knowles, J. A., et al. (2003). Investigating the role of dopaminergic and serotonergic candidate genes in obsessive-compulsive disorder. *European Neuropsychopharmacology, 13*, 93–98.

Hemmingsen, R., Madsen, A., Glenthoj, B., & Rubin, P. (1999). Cortical brain dysfunction in early schizophrenia: Secondary pathogenetic hierarchy of neuroplasticity psychopathology and social impairment. *Acta Psychiatrica Scandinavica, 99*, 80–88.

Henderson, A. S., Korten, A. E., Jorm, A. F., Jacomb, P. A., Christensen, H., Rodgers, B., et al. (2000). COMT and DRD3 polymorphisms, environmental exposures, and personality traits related to common mental disorders. *American Journal of Medical Genetics, 96*, 102–107.

Henderson, V. W., Paganini-Hill, A., Miller, B. L., Elble, R. J., Reyes, P. F., Shoupe, D., et al. (2000). Estrogen for Alzheimer's disease in women. *Neurology, 54*, 295–301.

Hendrick, V., Smith, L. M., Hwang, S., Altshuler, L. L., & Haynes, D. (2003a). Weight gain in breastfed infants of mothers taking antidepressant medication. *Journal of Clinical Psychiatry, 64*, 410–412.

Hendrick, V., Stowe, Z. N., Altshuler, L. L., Hwang, S., Lee, E., & Haynes, D. (2003b). Placental passage of antidepressant medications. *American Journal of Psychiatry, 160*, 993–996.

Henricus, P., Van Domburg, H. J., & Donkelar, T. (1991). *The human substantia nigra and ventral tegmental area: A neuroanatomical study with notes on aging and aging diseases (advances in anatomy, embryolo).* New York: Springer-Verlag.

Henry, M. E., Schmidt, M. E., Matochik, J. A., Stoddard, E. P., & Potter, W. Z. (2001). The effects of ECT on brain glucose: A pilot FDG PET study. *Journal of ECT, 17*, 33–40.

Henry, T. R. (2003). *Vagus nerve stimulation for epilepsy: anatomical, experimental and mechanistic investigations.* In S. C. Schachter & D. Schmidt (Eds.), *Vagus nerve stimulation* (2nd ed., pp. 1–31). New York: Martin Dunitz, Taylor & Francis Group.

Henry, T. R., Bakay, R. A., Votaw, J. R., Pennell, P. B., Epstein, C. M., Faber, T. L., et al. (1998). Brain blood flow alterations induced by therapeutic vagus nerve stimulation in partial epilepsy: I. Acute effects at high and low levels of stimulation. *Epilepsia, 39*, 983–990.

Henry, T. R., Votaw, J. R., Pennell, P. B., Epstein, C. M., Bakay, R. A., Faber, T. L., et al. (1999). Acute blood flow changes and efficacy of vagus nerve stimulation in partial epilepsy. *Neurology, 52*, 1166–1173.

Herb, E., & Thyen, U. (1992). Mutism after cerebellar medulloblastoma surgery. *Neuropediatrics, 23*, 144–146.

Herbert, M. R., Ziegler, D. A., Deutsch, C. K., O'Brien, L. M., Lange, N., Bakardjiev, A., et al. (2003). Dissociations of cerebral cortex, subcortical and cerebral white matter volumes in autistic boys. *Brain, 126*, 1182–1192.

Herbert, M. R., Ziegler, D. A., Makris, N., Filipek, P. A., Kemper, T. L., Normandin, J. J., et al. (2004). Localization of white matter volume increase in autism and developmental language disorder. *Annals of Neurology, 55*, 530–540.

Herholz, K., Krieg, J. C., Emrich, H. M., Pawlik, G., Beil, C., Pirke, K. M., et al. (1987). Regional cerebral glucose metabolism in anorexia nervosa measured by positron emission tomography. *Biological Psychiatry, 22*, 43–51.

Hering, E., Epstein, R., Elroy, S., Iancu, D. R., & Zelnik, N. (1999). Sleep patterns in autistic children. *Journal of Autism and Developmental Disorders, 29*, 143–147.

Herman, R. C., Yang, D., Ettner, S. L., Marcus, S. C., Yoon, C., & Abraham, M. (2002). Prescription of antipsychotic drugs by office-based physicians in the United States, 1989–1997. *Psychiatry Services, 53*, 425–430.

Hernan, M. A., Takkouche, B., Caamano-Isorna, F., & Gestal-Otero, J. J. (2002). A meta-analysis of coffee drinking, cigarette smoking, and the risk of Parkinson's disease. *Annals of Neurology, 52*, 276–284.

Heron, W. (1957). The pathology of boredom. *Scientific American, 196*, 52–56.

Hershey, T., Black, K. J., Hartlein, J. M., Barch, D. M., Braver, T. S., Carl, J. L., et al. (2004). Cognitive-pharmacologic functional magnetic resonance imaging in tourette syndrome: A pilot study. *Biological Psychiatry, 55*, 916–925.

Hertz, L., Yu, A. C., Kala, G., & Schousboe, A. (2000). Neuronal-astrocytic and cytosolic-mitochondrial metabolite trafficking during brain activation, hyperammonemia and energy deprivation. *Neurochemistry International, 37*, 83–102.

Herzog, D. B., Dorer, D. J., Keel, P. K., Selwyn, S. E., Ekeblad, E. R., Flores, A. T., et al. (1999). *Journal of the American Academy of Child and Adolescent Psychiatry, 38*, 829–837.

Hettema, J. M., Neale, M. C., & Kendler, K. S. (2001). A review and meta-analysis of the genetic epidemiology of anxiety disorders. *American Journal of Psychiatry, 158*, 1568–1578.

Heutink, P., van de Wetering, B. J., Breedveld, G. J., Weber, J., Sandkuyl, L. A., Devor, E. J., et al. (1990). No evidence for genetic linkage of Gilles de la Tourette syndrome on chromosomes 7 and 18. *Journal of Medical Genetics, 27*, 433–436.

Heyman, I., Fombonne, E., Simmons, H., Ford, T., Meltzer, H., & Goodman, R. (2001). Prevalence of obsessive-compulsive disorder in the British nationwide survey of child mental health. *British Journal of Psychiatry, 179*, 324–329.

Heywood, C., & Beale, I. (2003). EEG biofeedback vs. placebo treatment for attention-deficit/hyperactivity disorder: A pilot study. *Journal of Attention Disorders, 7*, 43–55.

Hietala, J., Syvalahti, E., Vilkman, H., Vuorio, K., Rakkolamen, V., Bergman, J., et al. (1999). Depressive symptoms and presynaptic dopamine function in neuroleptic-naïve schizophrenia. *Schizophrenia Research, 35*, 41–50.

Hietala, J., Syvalahti, E., Vuorio, K., Rakkolamen, V., Bergman, J., Haaparanta, M., et al. (1995). Presynaptic dopamine function in striatum of neuroleptic-naïve schizophrenia patients. *Lancet, 346*, 1130–1131.

Hietala, J., West, C., Syvalahti, E., Nagren, K., Lehikoinen, P., Sonninen, P., et al. (1994). Striatal D2 dopamine receptor binding characteristics in vivo in patients with alcohol dependence. *Psychopharmacology, 116*, 285–290.

Higuchi, H., Kamata, M., Yoshimoto, M., Shimisu, T., & Hishikawa, Y. (1999). Panic attacks in patients with chronic schizophrenia: A complication of long-term neuroleptic treatment. *Psychiatry and Clinical Neurosciences, 53*, 91–94.

Hill, D. E., Yeo, R. A., Campbell, R. A., Hart, B., Vigil, J., & Brooks, W. (2003). Magnetic resonance imaging correlated of attention-deficit/hyperactivity disorder in children. *Neuropsychology, 17*, 496–506.

Hines, M. (2003). Sex steroids and human behavior: Prenatal androgen exposure and sex-typical play behavior in children. *Annals of the New York Academy of Sciences, 1007*, 272–282.

Hirschfeld, R. M. (2000). History and evolution of the monamine hypothesis of depression. *Journal of Clinical Psychiatry, 61*, 4–6.

Hirschfeld, R. M., & Schatzberg, A. F. (1994). Long-term management of depression. *American Journal of Medicine, 97*, 33–38.

Hoaken, P. C., & Schnurr, R. (1980). Genetic factors in obsessive-compulsive neurosis? A rare case of discordant monozygotic twins. *Canadian Journal of Psychiatry, 25*, 167–172.

Hodge, C. W., Samson, H. H., & Chappelle, A. M. (1997). Alcohol self-administration: Further examination of the role of dopamine receptors in the nucleus accumbens. *Alcoholism: Clinical and Experimental Research, 21*, 1083–1091.

Hoehn-Saric, R., Schlaepfer, T. E., Greenberg, B. D., McLeod, D. R., Pearlson, G. D., & Wong, S. H. (2001). Cerebral blood flow in obsessive-compulsive patients with major depression: Effect of treatment with sertraline or desipramine on treatment responders and non-responders. *Psychiatry Research, 108*, 89–100.

Hoek, H. W., & Van Hoenken, D. (2003). Review of the prevalence and incidence of eating disorders. *International Journal of Eating Disorders, 34*, 383–396.

Hoekstra, P. J., Kallenberg, C. G. M., Korf, J., & Minderaa, R. B. (2002). Is Tourette's syndrome an autoimmune disease? *Molecular Psychiatry, 7*, 437–445.

Hoffmann, G., Linkowski, P., Kerkhofs, M., Desmedt, D., & Mendlewicz, J. (1985). Effects of ECT on sleep and CSF biogenic amines in affective illness. *Psychiatry Research, 16*, 199–206.

Hogarty, G. E., Flesher, S., Ulrich, R., Carter, M., Greenwald, D., Pogue-Geile, M., et al. (2004). Cognitive enhancement therapy for schizophrenia: Effects of a 2-year randomized trial on cognition and behavior. *Archives of General Psychiatry, 61*, 866–876.

Hökfelt, T. (1991). Neuropeptides in perspective: The last ten years. *Neuron, 7*, 867–879.

Holderness, C., Brooks-Gunn, J., & Warren, M. (1994). Co-morbidity of eating disorders and substance abuse: Review of the literature. *International Journal of Eating Disorders, 16*, 1–34.

Hollander, E. (1999). Managing aggressive behavior in patients with obsessive-compulsive disorder and borderline personality disorder. *Journal of Clinical Psychiatry, 60*, 38–44.

Hollander, E., Bienstock, C. A., Koran, L. M., Pallanti, S., Marazziti, D., Rasmussen, S. A., et al. (2002). Refractory obsessive-compulsive disorder: State-of-the-art treatment. *Journal of Clinical Psychiatry, 63, Supplement 6*, 20–29.

Hollander, E., Kaplan, A., & Stahl, S. M. (2003). A double-blind, placebo-controlled trial of clonazepam in obsessive-compulsive disorder. *World Journal of Biological Psychiatry, 4*, 30–34.

Hollifield, M., Finley, M. R., & Skipper, B. (2003). Panic disorder phenomenology in urban self-identified Caucasian-Non-Hispanics and Caucasian-Hispanics. *Depression and Anxiety, 18*, 7–17.

Holloway, V., Gadian, D. G., Vargha-Khadem, F., Porter, D. A., Boyd, S. G., & Connelly, A. (2000). The reorganization of sensorimotor function in children after hemispherectomy: A functional MRI and somatosensory evoked potential study. *Brain, 123*, 2431–2444.

Holmes, A. S., Blaxill, M. F., & Haley, B. E. (2003). Reduced levels of mercury in first baby haircuts of autistic children. *International Journal of Toxicology, 22*, 277–285.

Holroyd, S., Currie, L., & Wooten, G. F. (2000). Prospective study of hallucinations and delusions in Parkinson's disease. *Journal of Neurology, Neurosurgery, and Psychiatry, 70*, 734–738.

Holtzham, P. S., & Matthysse, S. (1990). The genetics of schizophrenia: A review. *American Psychological Society, 1*, 279–286.

Holzer, J. C., Goodman, W. K., McDougle, C. J., Baer, L., Boyarsky, B. K., Leckman, J. F., et al. (1994). Obsessive-compulsive disorder with and without a chronic tic disorder. A comparison of symptoms in 70 patients. *British Journal of Psychiatry, 164*, 469–473.

Honda, H., Shimizu, Y., Misumi, K., Niimi, M., & Ohashi, Y. (1996). Cumulative incidence and prevalence of childhood autism in children in Japan. *British Journal of Psychiatry, 169*, 228–235.

Honer, W. G., Falkai, P., Young, C., Wang, T., Xie, J., Bonner, J., et al. (1997). Cingulate cortex synaptic terminal proteins and neural cell adhesion molecules in schizophrenia. *Neuroscience, 78*, 99–110.

Hoopes, S. P., Reimherr, F. W., Hedges, D. W., Rosenthal, N. R., Kamin, M., Karim, R., et al. (2003). Treatment of bulimia nervosa with topiramate in a randomized, double-blind, placebo-controlled trial, part 1: Improvement in binge and purge measures. *Journal of Clinical Psychiatry, 64*, 1335–1341.

Hoover, J. E., & Strick, P. L. (1993). Multiple output channels in the basal ganglia. *Science, 259*, 819–821.

Hoozemans, J. J., Rozemuller, A. J., Veerhuis, R., & Eikelenboom, P. (2001). Immunological aspects of Alzheimer's disease: Therapeutic implications. *BioDrugs, Clinical Immunotherapeutics, Biopharmaceuticals and Gene Therapy, 15*, 325–337.

Horiuchi, Y., Nakayama, J., Ishiguro, H., Ohtsuki, T., Detera-Wadleigh, S. D., Toyota, T., et al. (2004). Possible association between a haplotype of the GABA-A receptor alpha 1 subunit gene (GABRA1) and mood disorders. *Biological Psychiatry, 55*, 40–45.

Horner, R. H., Carr, E. G., Strain, P. S., Todd, A. W., & Reed, H. K. (2002). Problem behavior interventions for young children with autism: A research synthesis. *Journal of Autism and Developmental Disorders, 32*, 423–446.

Hornsey, H., Banerjee, S., Zeitlin, H., & Robertson, M. (2001). The prevalence of Tourette syndrome in 13–14-year-olds in mainstream schools. *Journal of Child Psychology and Psychiatry, 42*, 1035–1039.

Horrigan, J. P., & Barnhill, L. J. (1999). Guanfacine and secondary mania in children. *Journal of Affective Disorders, 54*, 309–314.

Horwitz, B., Rumsey, J. M., Grady, C. L., & Rapoport, S. I. (1988). The cerebral metabolic landscape in autism. Intercorrelations of regional glucose utilization. *Archives of Neurology, 45*, 749–755.

Howell, E. M., Heiser, N., & Harrington, M. (1999). A review of recent findings on substance abuse treatment for pregnant women. *Journal of Substance Abuse Treatment, 16*, 195–219.

Howells, D. W., Porritt, M. J., Wong, J. Y., Batchelor, P. E., Kalnins, R., Hughes, A. J., et al. (2000). Reduced BDNF mRNA expression in the Parkinson's disease substantia nigra. *Experimental Neurology, 166*, 127–135.

Howlin, P. (1997). Prognosis in autism: Do specialist treatments affect long-term outcome? *European Child and Adolescent Psychiatry, 6*, 55–72.

Howlin, P., Goode, S., Hutton, J., & Rutter, M. (2004). Adult outcome for children with autism. *Journal of Child Psychology and Psychiatry, 45*, 212–229.

Hu, J. H., Yang, N., Ma, Y. H., Zhou, X. G., Zhang, X. Y., Jiang, J., et al. (2003). Decrease of morphine-induced reward effects and withdrawal symptoms in mice overexpressing gamma-aminobutyric acid transporter I. *Journal of Neuroscience Research, 74*, 614–621.

Huang, W., Qiu, C., Winblad, B., & Fratiglioni, L. (2002). Alcohol consumption and incidence of dementia in a community sample aged 75 years and older. *Journal of Clinical Epidemiology, 55*, 959–964.

Huang, Y. Y., Oquendo, M. A., Friedman, J. M., Greenhill, L. L., Brodsky, B., Malone, K. M., et al. (2003). Substance abuse disorder and major depression are associated with the human 5-HT1B receptor gene (HTR1B) G861C Polymorphism. *Neuropsychopharmacology, 28*, 163–169.

Huestis, R. D., Arnold, L. E., & Smeltzer, D. J. (1975). Caffeine versus methylphenidate and d-amphetamine in minimal brain dysfunction: A double-blind comparison. *American Journal of Psychiatry, 132*, 868–870.

Huether, G., Zhou, D., Schmidt, S., Wiltfang, J., & Ruether, E. (1997). Long-term food restriction down regulates the density of serotonin transporters in the rat frontal cortex. *Biological Psychiatry, 41*, 1174–1180.

Hulshoff Pol, H. E., Schnack, G. H., Bertens, M.G.B.C., van Haren, N. E. M., van der Twell, I., Stall, W. G., et al. (2002). Volume changes in gray matter in patients with schizophrenia. *American Journal of Psychiatry, 159*, 244–250.

Humphreys, G., & Price, C. J. (2001). Cognitive neuropsychology and functional brain imaging: Implications for functional and anatomical models of cognition. *Acta Psychologica, 107*, 119–153.

Hunt, G. (2000). A cellular perspective of neural networks. In E. Gordon (Ed.), *Integrative neuroscience: Bringing together biological, psychological, and clinical models of the human brain* (pp. 65–73). Amsterdam, Netherlands: Overseas Publishers Association.

Huppi, P., Warfield, S., Kikinis, R., Barnes, P., Zientara, G., Jolesz, F., et al. (1998). Quantitative magnetic resonance imaging of brain development in premature and mature newborns. *Annals of Neurology, 43*, 224–235.

Hurley, M. J., Mash, D. C., & Jenner, P. (2003). Markers for dopaminergic neurotransmission in the cerebellum in normal individuals and patients with Parkinson's disease examined by RT-PCR. *European Journal of Neuroscience, 18*, 2668–2672.

Huttenlocher, J., Levine, S., & Vevea, J. (1998). Environmental input and cognitive growth: A study using time-period comparisons. *Child Development, 69*, 1012–1029.

Huttenlocher, P. R. (2002). *Neural plasticity: The effects of the environment on the development of the cerebral cortex.* Cambridge, MA: Harvard University Press.

Huttenlocher, P. R. (1979). Synaptic density in human frontal cortex—developmental changes and effects of aging. *Brain Research, 163*, 195–205.

Huttenlocher, P. R. (1994). Synaptogenesis in human cerebral cortex. In G. Dawson & K. W. Fischer (Eds.), *Human behavior and the developing brain* (pp. 137–152). New York: Guilford.

Huwig-Poppe, C., Voderholzer, U., Backhaus, J., Riemann, D., Konig, A., & Hohagen, F. (1999). The tryptophan depletion test. Impact on sleep in healthy subjects and patients with obsessive-compulsive disorder. *Advances in Experimental Medical Biology, 467*, 35–42.

Hviid, A., Stellfeld, M., Wohlfahrt, J., & Melbye, M. (2003). Association between thimerosal-containing vaccine and autism. *Journal of the American Medical Association, 290*, 1763–1766.

Hyde, T. M., Aaronson, B. A., Randolph, C., Ricker, K. C., & Weinberger, D. R. (1992). Relationship of birth weight to the phenotypic expression of Gilles de la Tourette's syndrome to monozygotic twins. *Neurology, 42*, 652–658.

Hyman, S. E. (1996). Shaking out the cause of addiction. *Science, 273*, 611–612.

Hyman, S. E. (2002). Neuroscience, genetics and the future of psychiatric diagnosis. *Psychopathology, 35*, 139–144.

Hyman, S. E., & Malenka, R. C. (2001). Addiction and the brain: The neurobiology of compulsion and its persistence. *Neuroscience, 2*, 695–703.

Hyman, S. E. (2003). Diagnosing disorders. *Scientific American, Special Issue*, 99.

Hyman, S. L., Rodier, P. M., & Davidson, P. (2001). Pervasive developmental disorders in young children. *Journal of the American Medical Association, 285*, 3141–3142.

Hynd, G. W., Hern, K. L., Novey, E. S., Eliopulos, D., Marshall, R., Gonzalez, J. J., et al. (1993). Attention-deficit-hyperactivity disorder and asymmetry of the caudate nucleus. *Journal of Child Neurology, 8*, 339–347.

Hynd, G. W., Semrud-Clikeman, M., Lorys, A. R., Novey, E. S., Eliopulos, D., & Lyytinen, H. (1991). Corpus callosum morphology in attention deficit-hyperactivity disorder: Morphometric analysis of MRI. *Journal of Learning Disabilities, 24*, 141–146.

Hynd, G. W., & Willis, W. G. (1988). *Pediatric neuropsychology.* Orlando, FL: Grune & Stratton.

Ibach, B., & Haen, E. (2004). Acetylcholinesterase inhibition in Alzheimer's disease. *Current Pharmaceutical Design, 10*, 231–251.

Ilani, T., Ben-Shachar, D., Strous, R. D., Mazor, M., Sheinkman, A., Kotler, M., et al. (2001). A peripheral marker for schizophrenia: Increased levels of D3 dopamine receptor in mRNA in blood lymphocytes. *Proceedings of the National Academy of Sciences, 98*, 625–628.

Imaizumi, Y. (1995). Geographical variations in mortality from Parkinson's disease in Japan, 1977–1985. *Acta Neurologica Scandinavica, 91*, 311–316.

Ingram, J. L., Stodgell, C. J., Hyman, S. L., Figlewicz, D. A., Weitkamp, L. R., & Rodier, P. M. (2000). Discovery of allelic variants of HOXA1 and HOXB1: Genetic susceptibility to autism spectrum disorders. *Teratology, 62*, 393–405.

Ingvar, D. H., & Franzen, G. (1974). Abnormalities of cerebral blood flow distribution in patients with chronic schizophrenia. *Acta Psychiatrica Scandinavica, 50*, 425–462.

Innis, R. B., Seibyl, J. P., Scanley, B. E., Laruelle, M., Abi-Dargham, A., Wallace, E., et al. (1993). Single photon emission computed tomography imaging demonstrates loss of striatal dopamine transporters in Parkinson disease. *Proclamations of the National Academy of Sciences, U. S. A., 90*, 11965–11969.

Insel, T. R., Mueller, E. A., Alterman, I., Linnoila, M., & Murphy, D. L. (1985). Obsessive-compulsive disorder and serotonin: Is there a connection? *Biological Psychiatry, 20*, 1174–1188.

International Molecular Genetic Study of Autism Consortium (2001). A genomewide screen for autism: Strong evidence for linkage to chromosomes 2q, 7q, and 16p. *American Journal of Human Genetics, 69*, 570–581.

Inturrisi, C. E. (2002). Clinical pharmacology of opioids for pain. *Clinical Journal of Pain, 18*, 3–13.

Iqbal, K., Alonso, A. C., El-Akkad, E., Gong, C. X., Haque, N., Khatoon, S., et al. (2002). Pharmacological targets to inhibit Alzheimer neurofibrillary degeneration. *Journal of Neural Transmission, Supplementum*, 309–319.

Iqbal, K., Alonso, A. C., Gong, C. X., Khatoon, S., Pei, J. J., & Wang, J. Z., et al. (1998). Mechanisms of neurofibrillary degeneration and the formation of neurofibrillary tangles. *Journal of Neural Transmission, 53*, 169–180.

Ise, K., Akiyoshi, J., Horinouchi, Y., Tsutsumi, T., Isogawa, K., & Nagayama, H. (2003). Association between the CCK-A receptor gene and panic disorder. *American Journal of Medical Genetics, 118B*, 29–31.

Iseki, E. (2004). Dementia with Lewy bodies: Reclassification of pathological subtypes and boundary with Parkinson's disease or Alzheimer's disease. *Neuropathology, 24*, 72–78.

Ishihara, K., & Sasa, M. (2001). Potentiation of 5–HT(3) receptor functions in the hippocampal CA1 region of rats following repeated electroconvulsive shock treatments. *Neuroscience Letters, 307*, 37–40.

Ishihara, K., Amano, T., Hayakawa, H., Yamawaki, S., & Sasa, M. (1999). Enhancement of serotonin(1A) receptor function following repeated electroconvulsive shock in young rat hippocampal neurons in vitro. *International Journal of Neuropsychopharmacology, 2*, 101–104.

Ishihara, T., Hong, M., Zhang, B., Nakagawa, Y., Lee, M. K., Trojanowski, J. Q., et al. (1999). Age-dependent emergence and progression of a tauopathy in transgenic mice overexpressing the shortest human tau isoform. *Neuron, 24*, 751–762.

Ishii, K., Sasaki, M., Kitagaki, H., Yamaji, S., Sakamoto, S., Matsuda, K., et al. (1997). Reduction of cerebellar glucose metabolism in advanced Alzheimer's disease. *Journal of Nuclear Medicine, 38*, 925–928.

Itil, T. M. (1977). Qualitative and quantitative EEG findings in schizophrenia. *Schizophrenia Bulletin, 3*, 61–79.

Ito, H., Kawashima, R., Awata, S., Ono, S., Sato, K., Goto, R., et al. (1996). Hypoperfusion in the limbic system and prefrontal cortex in depression: SPECT with anatomic standardization technique. *Journal of Nuclear Medicine, 37*, 410–414.

Ito, K., Yoshida, K., Sato, K., Takahashi, H., Kamata, M., Higuchi, H., et al. (2002). A variable number of tandem repeats in the serotonin transporter gene does not affect the antidepressant response to fluboxamine. *Psychiatry Research, 111*, 235–239.

Iwamoto, K., Kakiuchi, C., Bundo, M., Ikeda, K., & Kato, T. (2004). Molecular characterization of bipolar disorder by comparing gene expression profiles of postmortem brains of major mental disorders. *Molecular Psychiatry, 9*, 406–416.

Iwata, N., Cowley, D. S., Radel, M., Roy-Byrne, P. P., & Goldman, D. (1999). Relationship between a GABAZ alpha 6 Pro385Ser substitution and benzodiazepine sensitivity. *American Journal of Psychiatry, 159*, 1447–1449.

Jablensky, A. (1997). The 100-year epidemiology of schizophrenia. *Schizophrenia Research, 28*, 111–125.

Jacob, T., Sher, K. J., Bucholz, K. K., True, W. T., Sirevaag, E. J., Rohrbaugh, J., et al. (2001). An integrative approach for studying the etiology of alcoholism and other addictions. *Twin Research, 4*, 103–118.

Jacob, T., Waterman, B., Heath, A., True, W., Bucholz, K. K., Haber, R., et al. (2003). Genetic and environmental effects on offspring alcoholism: new insights using offspring-of-twins design. *Archives of General Psychiatry, 60*, 1265–1272.

Jacobi, C., Hayward, C., de Zwaan, M., Kraemer, H. C., & Agras, W. S. (2004). Coming to terms with risk factors for eating disorders: Application of risk terminology and suggestions for a general taxonomy. *Psychological Bulletin, 130*, 19–65.

Jacobsen, L. K., Staley, J. K., Malison, R. T., Zoghbi, S. S., Seibyl, J. P., Kosten, T. R., et al. (2000). Elevated central serotonin transporter binding availability in acutely abstinent cocaine-dependent patients. *American Journal of Psychiatry, 157*, 1134–1140.

Jaffe, J. H., & O'Keeffe, C. (2003). From morphine clinics to buprenorphine: Regulating opioid agonist treatment of addiction in the United States. *Drug and Alcohol Dependence, 70*, 3–11.

Janicak, P. G., Dowd, S. M., Martis, B., Alam, D., Beedle, D., Krasuski, J., et al. (2002). Repetitive transcranial magnetic stimulation versus electroconvulsive therapy for major depression: Results of a randomized trial. *Biological Psychiatry, 51*, 659–667.

Jankovic, J. (2001). Parkinson's disease therapy: Treatment of early and late disease. *Chinese Medical Journal, 114*, 227–234.

Jarrold, C., Butler, D. W., Cottington, E. M., & Jimenez, F. (2000). Linking theory of mind and central coherence bias in autism and in the general population. *Developmental Psychology, 36*, 126–138.

Jarvis, B., & Figgitt, D. P. (2003). Memantine. *Drugs & Aging, 20*, 465–478.

Javanmard, M., Shlik, J., Kennedy, S. H., Vaccarino, F. J., Houle, S., & Bradwejn, J. (1999). Neuroanatomic correlates of CCK-4-induced panic attacks in healthy humans: A comparison of two time points. *Biological Psychiatry, 45*, 872–882.

Järvenpää, T., Laakso, M. P., Rossi, R., Koskenvuo, M., Kaprio, J., Räihä, I., et al. (2004). Hippocampal MRI volumetry in cognitively discordant monozygotic twin pairs. *Journal of Neurology, Neurosurgery, and Psychiatry, 75*, 116–120.

Javitt, D., & Zukin, S. (1991). Recent advances in the phencyclidine mode of schizophrenia. *American Journal of Psychiatry, 148*, 1301–1308.

Jeffries, K. J., Schooler, C., Schoenbach, C., Herscovitch, P., Chase, T. N., & Braun, A. R. (2002). The functional neuroanatomy of Tourette's syndrome: An FDG PET study III: Functional coupling of regional cerebral metabolic rates. *Neuropsychopharmacology, 27*, 92–104.

Jenike, M. A., Baer, L., Ballentine, T., Martuza, R. L., Tynes, S., Giriunas, I., et al. (1991). Cingulotomy for refractory obsessive-compulsive disorder. A long-term follow-up of 33 patients. *Archives of General Psychiatry, 48*, 548–555.

Jenike, M. A., Breiter, H. C., Baer, L., Kennedy, D. N., Savage, C. R. Olivares, M. J, et al. (1996). Cerebral structural abnormalities in obsessive-compulsive disorder. A quantitative morphometric magnetic resonance imaging study. *Archives of General Psychiatry, 53*, 625–632.

Jenner, A. R., Rosen, G. D., & Galaburda, A. M. (1999). Neuronal asymmetries in primary visual cortex of dyslexic and nondyslexic brains. *Annals of Neurology, 46*, 189–196.

Jenner, P., Boyce, S., & Marsden, C. D. (1988). Receptor changes during chronic dopaminergic stimulation. *Journal of Neural Transmission, Supplementum*, 161–175.

Jessen, F., Scheef, L., Germeshausen, L., Tawo, Y., Kockler, M., Kuhn, K. U., et al. (2003). Reduced hippocampal activation during encoding and recognition of words in schizophrenia patients. *American Journal of Psychiatry, 160*, 1305–1312.

Jest, D. V., Jonathan, P. L., Bailey, A., Rockwell, E., Harris, M. J., & Caligiuri, M. P. (1999). Lower incidence of tardive dyskinesia with risperidone compared with haloperidol in older patients. *Journal of the American Geriatric Society, 47*, 716–719.

Jest, D. V., Lacro, J. P., Palmer, B., Rockwell, E., Harris, J., & Caligiuri, M. P. (1999). Incidence of tardive dyskinesia in early stages of low-dose treatment with typical neuroleptics in older patients. *American Journal of Psychiatry, 156*, 309–311.

Jiang, S., Xin, R., Lin, S., Qian, Y., Tang, G., Wang, D., et al. (2001). Linkage studies between attention-deficit hyperactivity disorder and the monoamine oxidase genes. *American Journal of Medical Genetics, 105*, 783–788.

Jimerson, D. C., Lesem, M. D., Kaye, W. H., & Brewerton, T. D. (1992). Low serotonin and dopamine metabolite concentrations in cerebrospinal fluid from bulimic patients with frequent binge episodes. *Archives of General Psychiatry, 49*, 132–138.

Jimerson, D. C., Lesem, M. D., Kaye, W. H., Hegg, A. P., & Brewerton, T. D. (1990). Eating disorders and depression: Is there a serotonin connection? *Biological Psychiatry, 28*, 443–454.

Joel, D., Avisar, A., & Doljansky, J. (2001). Enhancement of excessive lever-pressing after post-training signal attenuation in rats by repeated administration of the D1 antagonist SCH 23390 or the D2 agonist quinpirole, but not the D1 agonist SKF 38393 or the D2 antagonist haloperidol. *Behavioral Neuroscience, 115*, 1291–300.

Johns, L. C., & van Os, J. (2001). The continuity of psychotic experiences in the general population. *Clinical Psychology Review, 21*, 1125–1141.

Johnson, B. A. (2003). The role of serotonergic agents as treatments for alcoholism. *Drugs Today, 39*, 665–672.

Johnson, B. A., Roache, J. D., Javors, M. A., DiClemente, C. C., Cloninger, C. R., Prihoda, T. J., et al. (2000). Ondansetron for reduction of drinking among biologically predisposed alcoholic patients. A randomized controlled trial. *Journal of the American Medical Association, 284*, 963–971.

Johnson, L., El-Khoury, A., Aberg-Wistedt, A., Stain-Malmgren, R., & Mathe, A. A. (2001). Tryptophan depletion in lithium-stabilized patients with affective disorder. *International Journal of Neuropsychopharmacology, 4*, 329–336.

Johnstone, E. C., Crow, T. J., Frith, C. D., Husband, J., & Kreel, L. (1976). Cerebral ventricular size and cognitive impairment in chronic schizophrenia. *Lancet, 2*, 924–926.

Jokic-Begic, N., & Begic, D. (2003). Quantitative electroencephalogram (qEEG) in combat veterans with post-traumatic stress disorder (PTSD). *Nordic Journal of Psychiatry, 57*, 351– 355.

Jones, B. E. (1993). The organization of central cholinergic systems and their functional importance in sleep–waking states. *Progress in Brain Research, 98*, 61–71.

Jones, I., & Craddock, N. (2001). Familiarity of the puerperal trigger in bipolar disorder: Results of a family study. *American Journal of Psychiatry, 158*, 913–917.

Jones, N. A., & Field, T. (1999). Massage and music therapies attenuate frontal EEG asymmetry in depressed adolescents. *Adolescence, 34*, 529–534.

Jones, S. R., Gainetdinov, R. R., Wightman, R. M., & Caron, M. G. (1998). Mechanisms of amphetamine action revealed in mice lacking the dopamine transporter. *Journal of Neuroscience, 18*, 1979–1986.

Jonnal, A. H., Gardner, C. O., Prescott, C. A, & Kendler, K. S. (2000). Obsessive and compulsive symptoms in a general population sample of female twins. *American Journal of Medical Genetics, 96*, 791–796.

Jorge, R. E., Robinson, R. G., Moser, D., Tateno, A., Crespo-Facorro, B., & Arndt, S. (2004). Major depression following traumatic brain injury. *Archives of General Psychiatry, 61*, 42–50.

Josephs, K. A., Holton, J. L., Rossor, M. N., Braendgaard, H., Ozawa, T., Fox, N. C., et al. (2003). Neurofilament inclusion body disease: A new proteinopathy? *Brain, 126*, 2291–2303.

Joyce, J. N., Lexow, N., Brid, E., & Winokur, A. (1988). Organization of dopamine D1 and D2 receptors in human striatum: Receptor autoradiographic studies in Huntington's disease and Schizophrenia. *Synapse, 2*, 546–557.

Jozuka, H., Jozuka, E., Takeuchi, S., & Nishikaze, O. (2003). Comparison of immunological and endocrinological markers associated with major depression. *Journal of International Medical Research, 31*, 36–41.

Juan, D., Zhou, D. H., Li, J., Wang, J. Y., Gao, C., & Chen, M. (2004). A 2-year follow-up study of cigarette smoking and risk of dementia. *European Journal of Neurology, 11*, 277–282.

Just, M. A., Carpenter, P. A., Keller, T. A., Eddy, W. F., & Thulborn, K. R. (1996). Brain activation modulated by sentence comprehension. *Science, 274*, 114–116.

Juul-Dam, N., Townsend, J., & Courchesne, E. (2001). Prenatal, perinatal, and neonatal factors in autism, pervasive developmental disorder-not otherwise specified, and the general population. *Pediatrics, 107*, E63.

Kaasinen, V., Aalto, S., Nagren, K., & Rinne, J. O. (2004). Dopaminergic effects of caffeine in the human striatum and thalamus. *Neuroreport, 15*, 281–285.

Kahl, P. J., Jakowec, M., Teipel, S. J., Hampel, H., Petzinger, G. M., Di Monte, D. A., et al. (2000). Combined assessment of tau and neuronal thread protein in Alzheimer's disease CSF. *Neurology, 54*, 1498–1504.

Kahle, P. J., Jakowec, M., Teipel, S. J., Hampel, H., Petzinger, G. M., Di Monte, D. A., et al. (2000). Combined assessment of tau and neuronal thread protein in Alzheimer's disease CSF. *Neurology, 54*, 1498–1504.

Kajs-Wyllie, M. (2002). Ritalin revisited: Does it really help in neurological injury? *Journal of Neuroscience Nursing, 34*, 303–313.

Kampman, M., Keijsers, G. P., Hoogduin, C. A., & Verbraak, M. J. (2002). Addition of cognitive-behaviour therapy for obsessive-compulsive disorder patients non-responding to fluoxetine. *Acta Psychiatrica Scandinavica, 106*, 314–319.

Kanetaka, H., Matsuda, H., Asada, T., Ohnishi, T., Yamashita, F., Imabayashi, E. et al. (2004). Effects of partial volume correction on discrimination between very early Alzheimer's dementia and controls using brain perfusion SPECT. *European Journal of Nuclear Medicine and Molecular Imaging, 31*, 975–980.

Kang, D. H., Kwon, J. S., Kim, J. J., Youn, T., Park, H. J., Kim, M. S., et al. (2003). Brain glucose metabolic changes associated with neuropsychological improvements after 4 months of treatment in patients with obsessive-compulsive disorder. *Acta Psychiatrica Scandinavica, 107*, 291–297.

Kano, Y., Ohta, M., & Nagai, Y. (1998). Clinical characteristics of Tourette syndrome. *Psychiatry and Clinical Neuroscience, 52*, 51–57.

Kaplan, B. J., McNicol, J., Conte, R. A., & Moghadam, H. K. (1989). Dietary replacement in preschool-aged hyperactive boys. *Pediatrics, 83*, 7–17.

Kaplan, B. J., Simpson, J. S., Ferre, R. C., Gorman, C. P., McMullen, D. M., & Crawford, S. G. (2001). Effective mood stabilization with a chelated mineral supplement: An open-label trial in bipolar disorder. *Journal of Clinical Psychiatry, 62*, 936–944.

Kaplan, D. E., Gayán, J., Ahn, J., Won, T. W., Pauls, D., Olson, R. K., et al. (2002). Evidence for linkage and association with reading disability on 6p21.3-22. *American Journal of Human Genetics, 70*, 1287–1298.

Kaplan, R. D., Szechtman, H., Franco, S., Szechtman, B., Nahmias, C., Garnett, E. S., et al. (1993). Three clinical syndromes of schizophrenia in untreated subjects: Relation to brain glucose activity measured by positron emission tomography (PET). *Schizophrenia Research, 11*, 47–54.

Kapur, S. (2003). Psychosis as a state of aberrant salience: A framework for linking biology, phenomenology, and pharamcology in schizoprhenia. *American Journal of Psychiatry, 160*, 13–23.

Kapur, S., & Mann, J. J. (1993). Antidepressant action and the neurobiologic effects of ECT: Human studies. In C. E. Coffey (Ed.), *The clinical science of electroconvulsive therapy* (pp. 235–250). Washington, DC: American Psychiatric Press.

Kapur, S., & Seeman, P. (2001). Does fast dissociation from the dopamine D2 receptor explain the action of atypical antipsychotics?: A new hypothesis. *American Journal of Psychiatry, 158*, 360–369.

Kapur, S., Zipursky, R., Jones, C., Remington, G., & Hourle, S. (2000). Relationship between dopamine D2 occupancy, clinical response, and side effects: A double-blind PET study of first-episode schizophrenia. *American Journal of Psychiatry, 157*, 514–520.

Karajgi, B., Rifkin, A., Doddi, S., & Kolli, R. (1990). The prevalence of anxiety disorders in patients with chronic obstructive pulmonary disease. *American Journal of Psychiatry, 147*, 200–201.

Karamohamed, S., DeStefano, A. L., Wilk, J. B, Shoemaker, C. M., Golbe, L. I., Mark, M. H., et al. (2003). A haplotype at the PARK3 locus influences onset age for Parkinson's disease: The GenePD study. *Neurology, 61*, 1557–1561.

Karayiorgou, M., Altemus, M., Galke, B. L., Goldman, D., Murphy, D. L., Ott, J., et al. (1997). Genotype determining low catechol-O-methyltransferase activity as a risk factor for obsessive-compulsive disorder. *Proceedings of the National Academy of Sciences of the United States of America, 94*, 4572–4575.

Karayiorgou, M., Sobin, C., Blundell, M. L., Galke, B. L., Malinova, L., Goldberg, P., et al. (1999). Family-based association studies support a sexually dimorphic effect of COMT and MAOA on genetic susceptibility to obsessive-compulsive disorder. *Biological Psychiatry, 45*, 1178–1189.

Karlsson, H., Bachmann, S., Schroder, J., McArthur, J., Torrey, E. F., & Yolken, R. H. (2001). Retroviral RNA identified in the cerebral spinal fluids and brains of individuals with schizophrenia. *Proceedings of the National Academy of the Sciences, 98*, 4634–4639.

Kasai, K., Shenton, E. M., Salisbury, D. F., Hirayasu, Y., Lee, C., Ciszewski, A. A., et al. (2003). Progressive decrease of left superior temporal gyrus gray matter with first-episode schizophrenia. *American Journal of Psychiatry, 160*, 156–164.

Kaschka, W., Feistel, H., & Ebert, D. (1995). Reduced benzodiazepine receptor binding in panic disorders measured by iomazenil SPECT. *Journal of Psychiatric Research, 29*, 427–434.

Kassubek, J., Juengling, F. D., Hellwig, B., Knauff, M., Spreer, J., & Lücking, C. H. (2001). Hypermetabolism in the ventrolateral thalamus in unilateral Parkinsonian resting tremor: A positron emission tomography study. *Neuroscience Letters, 304*, 17–20.

Katerndahl, D. (2004). Panic plaques: Panic disorder and coronary artery disease in patients with chest pain. *Journal of the American Board of Family Practice, 17*, 114–126.

Kates, W. R., Burnette, C. P., Eliez, S., Strunge, L. A., Kaplan, D., Landa, R., et al. (2004). Neuroanatomic variation in monozygotic twin pairs discordant for the narrow phenotype for autism. *American Journal of Psychiatry, 161*, 539–546.

Kates, W. R., Mostofsky, S. H., Zimmerman, A. W., Mazzocco, M. M., Landa, R., Warsofsky, I. S., et al. (1998). Neuroanatomical and neurocognitive differences in a pair of monozygous twins discordant for strictly defined autism. *Annals of Neurology, 43*, 782–791.

Kato, T., Erhard, P., Takayama, Y., Strupp, J., Le, T. H., Ogawa, S., et al. (1998). Human hippocampal long-term sustained response during word memory processing. *NeuroReport, 9*, 1041–1047.

Katzan, I. L., Furlan, A. J., Lloyd, L. E., Frank, J. I., Harper, D. L., Hinchey, J. A., et al. (2000). Use of tissue-type plasminogen activator for acute ischemic stroke: The Cleveland area experience. *Journal of the American Medical Association, 283*, 1151–1158.

Katzman, D. K., Zipursky, R. B., Lambe, E. K., & Mikulis, D. J. (1997). A longitudinal magnetic resonance imaging study of brain in adolescents with anorexia nervosa. *Archives of Pediatrics and Adolescent Medicine, 151*, 793–797.

Kaufer, D., Friedman, A., Seidman, S., & Soreq, H. (1998). Acute stress facilitates long-lasting changes in cholinergic gene expresssion. *Nature, 393*, 373–377.

Kaufman, J., & Charney, D. (2001). Effects of early stress on brain structure and function: Implications for understanding the relationship between child maltreatment and depression. *Development and Psychopathology, 13*, 451–471.

Kawamata, J., & Shimohama, S. (2002). Association of novel and established polymorphisms in neuronal nicotinic acetylcholine receptors with sporadic Alzheimer's disease. *Journal of Alzheimer's Disease, 4*, 71–76.

Kaye, W. H., Lilenfeld, L. R., Berrettini, W. H., Strober, M., Devlin, B., Klump, K. L., et al. (2000). A search for susceptibility loci for anorexia nervosa: Methods and sample description. *Biological Psychiatry, 47*, 794–803.

Kaye, W., Gendall, K., & Strober, M. (1998b). Serotonin neuronal function and selective serotonin reuptake inhibitor treatment in anorexia and bulimia nervosa. *Biological Psychiatry, 44*, 825–838.

Kaye, W., Greeno, C. G., Moss, H., Fernstrom, J. D., Fernstrom, M. H., Lilenfeld, L. R., et al. (1998a). Alterations in serotonin activity and psychiatric symptoms after recovery from bulimia nervosa. *Archives of General Psychiatry, 55*, 927–935.

Kaye, W. H., Ebert, M. H., Gwirtsman, H. E., & Weiss, S. R. (1984). Differences in brain serotonergic metabolism between bulimic and nonbulimic patients with anorexia nervosa. *American Journal of Psychiatry, 141*, 1598–1601.

Kaye, W. H., Frank, G. K., & McConaha, C. (1999). Altered dopamine activity after recovery from restricting-type anorexia nervosa. *Neuropsychopharmacology, 21*, 503 506.

Kaye, W. H., Frank, G. K., Meltzer, C. M., Price, J. C., McConaha, C. W., Crossan, P. J., et al. (2001). Altered serotonin 2A receptor activity in women who have recovered from bulimia nervosa. *American Journal of Psychiatry, 158*, 1152–1155.

Kazdin, A. E., & Marciano, P. L. (1998). Childhood and adolescent depression. In E. J. Mash & R. A. Barkley (Eds.), *Treatment of childhood disorders* (2nd Ed.). New York: Guilford.

Kealey, C., Reynolds, A., Mynett-Johnson, L., Claffey, E., & McKeon, P. (2001). No evidence to support an association between the oestrogen receptor beta gene and bipolar disorder. *Psychiatric Genetics, 11*, 223–226.

Keep, M. F., Mastrofrancesco, L., Erdman, D., Murphy, B., & Ashby, L. S. (2002). Gamma knife subthalamotomy for Parkinson disease: The subthalamic nucleus as a new radiosurgical target. Case report. *Journal of Neurosurgery, 97*, 592–599.

Kegeles, L. S., Malone, K. M., Slifstein, M., Ellis, S. P., Xanthopoulos, E., Keilp, J. G., et al. (2003). Response of cortical metabolic deficits to serotonergic challenge in familial mood disorders. *American Journal of Psychiatry, 160*, 76–82.

Kehrer, H. E. (1992). Savant capabilities of autistic persons. *Acta Paedopsychiatrica, 55*, 151–155.

Keller, A., Castellanos, F. X., Jeffries, N. O., Giedd, J. N., & Rapoport, J. (2003). Progressive loss of cerebellar volume in childhood-onset schizophrenia. *American Journal of Psychiatry, 160*, 128–133.

Kelly, D. F., Martin, N. A, Kordestani, R., Counelis, G., Hovda, D. A., Bergsneider, M., et al. (1997). Cerebral blood flow as a predictor of outcome following traumatic brain injury. *Journal of Neurosurgery, 86*, 633–641.

Kelz, M. B., Chen, J., Carlezon, Jr., W. A., Whisler, K., Gilden, L., Beckmann, A. M., et al. (1999). Expression of the ΔFosB in the brain controls sensitivity to cocaine. *Nature, 401*, 272–276.

Kemeny, A. A. (2003). Surgical technique in vagus nerve stimulation. In S. C. Schachter & D. Schmidt (Eds.), *Vagus nerve stimulation* (2nd ed., pp. 33–48). New York: Martin Dunitz, Taylor & Francis Group.

Kemner, C., Oranje, B., Verbaten, M. N., & van Engeland, H. (2002). Normal P50 gating in children with autism. *Journal of Clinical Psychiatry, 63*, 214–217.

Kemner, C., Willemsen-Swinkels, S. H., de Jonge, M., Tuynman-Qua, H., & van Engeland, H. (2002). Open-label study of olanzapine in children with pervasive developmental disorder. *Journal of Clinical Psychopharmacology, 22*, 455–460.

Kendell, R., & Jablensky, A. (2003). Distinguishing between the validity and utility of psychiatric diagnoses. *American Journal of Psychiatry, 160*, 4–12.

Kendler, K. S. (1999). Molecular genetics of schizophrenia. In D. S. Charney, E. J. Nestler, & B. S. Bunney (Eds.), *Neurobiology of mental illness* (pp. 203–213). New York: Oxford University Press.

Kendler, K. S. (2004). Schizophrenia genetics and dysbindin: A corner turned? *American Journal of Psychiatry, 161*, 1533–1536.

Kendler, K. S., Gardner, C. O., & Prescott, C. A. (2001). Panic syndromes in a population-based sample of male and female twins. *Psychological Medicine, 31*, 989–1000.

Kendler, K. S., Jacobson, K. C., Prescott, C. A., & Neale, M. C. (2003). Specificity of genetic and environmental risk factors for use and abuse/dependence of cannabis, cocaine, hallucinogens, sedatives, stimulants, and opiates in male twins. *American Journal of Psychiatry, 160*, 687–695.

Kendler, K. S., Neale, M. C., Kessler, R. C., Heath, A. C., & Eaves, L. J. (1993). Panic disorder in women: A population-based twin study. *Psychological Medicine, 23*, 397–406.

Kendler, K. S., Pedersen, N., Johnson, L., Neale, M. C., & Mathe, A. A. (1995). A pilot Swedish twin study of affective illness, including hospital- and population-ascertained subsamples. *Archives of General Psychiatry, 25*, 217–232.

Kendler, K. S., Pedersen, N. L., Neale, M. C., & Mathe, A. A. (1995). A pilot Swedish twin study of affective illness including hospital- and population-ascertained subsamples: Results of model fitting. *Behavioral Genetics, 25*, 217–232.

Kendler, K. S., Prescott, C. A., Myers, J., & Neale, M. C. (2003). The structure of genetic and environmental risk factors for common psychiatric and substance use disorders in men and women. *Archives of General Psychiatry, 60*, 929–937.

Kennard, M. A. (1936). Age and other factors in motor recovery from precentral lesions in monkeys. *Journal of Neurophysiology, 1*, 477–496.

Kennedy, M. B. (2000). Signal-processing machines at the postsynaptic density. *Science, 290*, 750–754.

Kennedy, R., Mittal, D., & O'Jile, J. (2003). Electroconvulsive therapy in movement disorders: An update. *Journal of Neuropsychiatry and Clinical Neurosciences, 15*, 407–421.

Kennedy, S. H., Javanmard, M., & Vaccarino, F. J. (1997). A review of functional neuroimaging in mood disorders: Positron emission tomography and depression. *Canadian Journal of Psychiatry, 42*, 467–475.

Kent, L. (2004). Recent advances in the genetics of attention deficit hyperactivity disorder. *Current Psychiatry Reports, 6*, 143–148.

Kent, L., Doerry, U., Hardy, R., Parmar, R., Gingell, K., Hawi, Z., et al. (2002). Evidence that variation at the serotonin transporter gene influences susceptibility to attention deficit hyperactivity disorder (ADHD): Analysis and pooled analysis. *Molecular Psychiatry, 7*, 908–912.

Kerenyi, L., Ricaurte, G. A., Schretlen, D. J., McCann, U., Varga, J., Mathews, W. B., et al. (2003). Positron emission tomography of striatal serotonin transporters in Parkinson disease. *Archives of Neurology, 60*, 1223–1229.

Keshavan, M. S., Anderson, S., & Pettigrew, J. W. (1994). Is schizophrenia due to excessive synaptic pruning in the prefrontal cortex? The Feinberg hypothesis revisited. *Journal of Psychiatric Research, 28*, 239–265.

Kessler, A. R. (2002). Tourette syndrome associated with body temperature dysregulation: Possible involvement of an idiopathic hypothalamic disorder. *Journal of Child Neurology, 17*, 738–744.

Kessler, J., Mielke, R., Grond, M., Herholz, K., & Heiss, W. D. (2000). Frontal lobe tasks do not reflect frontal lobe function in patients with probable Alzheimer's disease. *International Journal of Neuroscience, 104*, 1–15.

Kessler, R. C., Berglund, P., Demler, O., Jin, R., Koretz, D., Merikangas, K. R., et al. (2003). The epidemiology of major depressive disorder: Results from the national comorbidity survey replication (NCS-R). *Journal of the American Medical Association, 289*, 3095–3105.

Kettenmann, H., & Ransom, B. R. (1995). *Neuroglia.* New York: Oxford University Press.

Ketter, T. A., Kimbrell, T. A., George, M. S., Dunn, R. T., Speer, A. M., Benson, B. E., et al. (2001). Effects of mood and subtype on cerebral glucose metabolism in treatment-resistant bipolar disorder. *Biological Psychiatry, 49*, 97–109.

Ketter, T. A., & Wang, P. W. (2002). Predictors of treatment response in bipolar disorders: Evidence from clinical and brain imaging studies. *Journal of Clinical Psychiatry, 63*, 21–25.

Ketter, T. A., & Wang, P. W. (2003). The emerging differential roles of GABAergic and antiglutamatergic agents in bipolar disorders. *Journal of Clinical Psychiatary, 64*, 15–20.

Kety, S. S., Wender, P. H., Jacobsen, B., Ingraham, L. J., Jansson, L., Faber, B., et al. (1994). Mental illness in the biological and adoptive relatives of schizophrenic adoptees: Replication of the Copenhagen Study in the rest of Denmark. *Archives of General Psychiatry, 51*, 442–455.

Khan, A., Khan, S., Kolts, R., & Brown, W. A. (2003). Suicide rates in clinical trials of SSRIs, other antidepressants, and placebo: Analysis of FDA reports. *American Journal of Psychiatry, 160*, 790–792.

Khanzode, S. D., Dakhale, G. N., Khanzode, S. S., Saoji, A., & Palasodkar, R. (2003). Oxidative damage and major depression: The potential antioxidant action of selective serotonin re-uptake inhibitors. *Redox Report, 8*, 365–370.

Khilnani, S., Field, T., Hernandez-Reif, M., & Schanberg, S. (2003). Massage therapy improves mood and behavior of students with attention-deficit/hyperactivity disorder. *Adolescence, 38*, 623–638.

Kidd, P. M. (2002). Autism, an extreme challenge to integrative medicine. Part 2: Medical management. *Alternative Medicine, 7*, 472–499.

Kieffer, B. L., & Simonin, F. (2003). Molecular mechanisms of opioid dependence by using knockout mice. In R. Maldonado (Ed.), *Molecular biology of drug addiction* (pp. 3–25). Totowa, NJ: Humana Press.

Kielinen, M., Linna, S. L., & Moilanen, I. (2002). Some aspects of treatment and habilitation of children and adolescent with autistic disorder in northern-Finland. *Internal Journal of Circumpolar Health, 61*, 69–79.

Kieseppa, T., Partonen, T., Haukka, J., Kaprio, J., & Lonnqvist, J. (2004). High concordance rate of bipolar I disorder in a nationwide sample of twins. *American Journal of Psychiatry, 161*, 1814–1821.

Kihara, T., Shimohama, S., Sawada, H., Honda, K., Nakamizo, T., Kanki, R., et al. (2002). Protective effect of dopamine D2 agonists in cortical neurons via the phosphatidylinositol 3 kinase cascade. *Journal of Neuroscience Research, 70*, 274–282.

Killiany, R. J., Gomez-Isla, T., Moss, M., Kikinis, R., Sandor, T., Jolesz, F., et al. (2000). Use of structural magnetic resonance imaging to predict who will get Alzheimer's disease. *Annals of Neurology, 47*, 430–439.

Kilts, C. (2003). In vivo neuroimaging correlates of the efficacy of paroxetine in the treatment of mood and anxiety disorders. *Psychopharmacology Bulletin, 37*, 19–28.

Kilts, C. D., Gross, R. E., Ely, T. D., & Drexler, K. P. (2004). The neural correlates of cue-induced craving in cocaine-dependent women. *American Journal of Psychiatry, 161*, 233–241.

Kim, B. N., Lee, J. S., Shin, M. S., Cho, S. C., & Lee, D. S. (2002). Regional cerebral perfusion abnormalities in attention deficit/hyperactivity disorder. Statistical parametric mapping analysis. *European Archives of Psychiatry and Clinical Neuroscience, 252*, 219–225.

Kim, C. H., Koo, M. S., Cheon, K. A., Ryu, Y. H., Lee, J. D., & Lee, H. S. (2003). Dopamine transporter density of basal ganglia assessed with [123I]IPT SPET in obsessive-compulsive disorder. *European Journal of Nuclear Medicine and Molecular Imaging, 30*, 1637–1643.

Kim, C. K., & Rivier, C. L. (2000). Nitric oxide and carbon monoxide have a stimulatory role in the hypothalamic-pituitary-adrenal response to physico-emotional stressors in rats. *Endocrinology, 141*, 2244–2253.

Kim, J. J., Kwon, J. S., Park, H. J., Youn, T., Kang, D. H., Kim, M. S., et al. (2003). Functional disconnection between the prefrontal and parietal cortices during working memory processing in schizophrenia: A [150]H20 PET study. *American Journal of Psychiatry, 160*, 919–923.

Kim, J. J., Lee, M. C., Kim, J., Kim, I. Y., Kim, S. I., Han, M. H., et al. (2001). Grey matter abnormalities in obsessive-compulsive disorder: Statistical parametric mapping of segmented magnetic resonance images. *British Journal of Psychiatry, 179*, 330–334.

Kim, J. W., Kim, D. H., Kim, S. H., & Cha, J. K. (2000). Association of the dopamine transporter gene with Parkinson's disease in Korean patients. *Journal of Korean Medical Science, 15*, 449–451.

Kim, K. J., & Peterson, B. S. (2003). Cavum septi pellucidi in Tourette syndrome. *Biological Psychiatry, 54*, 76–85.

Kim, K. W., Jhoo, J. H., Lee, K. U., Lee, D. Y., Lee, J. H., Youn, J. Y., et al. (1999). Association between apolipoprotein E polymorphism and Alzheimer's disease in Koreans. *Neuroscience Letters, 277*, 145–148.

Kim, M. C., Lee, T. K., & Choi, C. R. (2002). Review of long-term results of stereotactic psychosurgery. *Neurologia Medico-Chirurgica, 42*, 365–371.

Kim, M. C., Lee, T. K., Son, B. C., Choi, C. R., & Lee, C. (2001). Regional cerebral blood flow changes in patients with intractable obsessive compulsive disorders treated by limbic leucotomy. *Stereotactic and Functional Neurosurgery, 76*, 249–255.

Kim, S. S. (2003). Role of fluoxetine in anorexia nervosa. *Annals of Pharmacotherapy, 37*, 890–892.

Kimbrell, T. A., Ketter, T. A., George, M. S., Little, J. T., Benson, B. F., Willis, M. W., et al. (2002). Regional cerebral glucose utilization in patients with a range of severities of unipolar depression. *Biological Psychiatry, 51,* 237–252.

Kimura, H. (2002). Hydrogen sulfide as a neuromodulator. *Molecular Neurobiology, 26,* 13–19.

King, M. R., Heaton, M. B., & Walker, D. W. (2002). The effects of ethanol consumption on neurotrophins and their receptors in the rat hippocampus and basal forebrain. *Brain Research, 950,* 137–147.

Kinnear, C., Niehaus, D. J., Seedat, S., Moolman-Smook, J. C., Corfield, V. A., Malherbe, G., et al. (2001). Obsessive-compulsive disorder and a novel polymorphism adjacent to the oestrogen response element (ERE 6) upstream from the COMT gene. *Psychiatric Genetics, 11,* 85–87.

Kinney, H. C., Brody, B. A., Kloman, A. S., & Gilles, F. H. (1988). Sequence of central nervous system myelination in human infancy. II. Patterns of myelination in autopsied infants. *Journal of Neuropathology and Experimental Neurology, 47,* 217–234.

Kirino, E., & Inoue, R. (1999). The relationship mismatch negativity to quantitative EEG and morphological findings in schizophrenia. *Journal of Psychiatric Research, 33,* 445–456.

Kirley, A., Hawi, Z., Daly, G., McCarron, M., Mullins, C., Millar, N., et al. (2002). Dopaminergic system genes in ADHD: Toward a biological hypothesis. *Neuropsychopharmacology, 27,* 607–619.

Kirley, A., Lowe, N., Hawi, Z., Mullins, C., Daly, G., Waldman, I., et al. (2003). Association of the 480 bp DAT1 allele with methylphenidate response in a sample of Irish children with ADHD. *American Journal of Medical Genetics, 121B,* 50–54.

Kirov, G., Murphy, K. C., Arranz, M. J., Jones, I., McCandles, F., Kunugi, H., et al. (1998). Low activity allele of catechol-o-methyltransferase gene associated with rapid cycling bipolar disorder. *Molecular Psychiatry, 3,* 342–345.

Kirsch, I. (2003). St John's wort, conventional medicine, and placebo: An egregious double standard. *Complementary Therapies in Medicine, 11,* 193–195.

Klaassen, T., Klumperbeek, J., Deutz, N. E., Van Praag, H. M., & Griez, E. (1998). Effects of tryptophan depletion on anxiety and on panic provoked by carbon dioxide challenge. *Psychiatry Research, 77,* 167–174.

Kleiner-Fisman, G., Fisman, D. N., Sime, E., Saint-Cyr, J. A., Lozano, A. M., & Lang, A. E. (2003). Long-term follow up of bilateral deep brain stimulation of the subthalamic nucleus in patients with advanced Parkinson's disease. *Journal of Neurosurgery, 99,* 489–495.

Klimek, V., Roberson, G., Stockmeier, C. A., & Ordway, G. A. (2003). Serotonin transporter and MAO-B levels in monoamine nuclei of the human brainstem are normal in major depression. *Journal of Psychiatry Research, 37,* 387–397.

Klimesch, W. (1999). EEG alpha and theta oscillations reflect cognitive and memory performance: A review and analysis. *Brain Research Review, 29,* 169–195.

Klinberg, T., Vaidya, C. J., Gabrieli, J. D., Moseley, M. E., & Hedehus, M. (1999). Myelination and organization of the frontal white matter in children: A diffusion tensor MRI study. *Neuroreport, 10,* 2817–2821.

Klinger, M., Apelt, J., Kumar, A., Sorger, D., Sabri, O., Steinbach, J., et al. (2003). Alterations in cholinergic and non-cholinergic neurotransmitter receptor densities in transgenic Tg2576 mouse brain receptor with β-amyloid plaque pathology. *International Journal of Developmental Neuroscience, 21,* 357–369.

Kluger, A., Ferris, S. H., Golomb, J., Mittleman, M. S., & Reisberg, B. (1999). Neuropsychological prediction of decline to dementia in nondemented elderly. *Journal of Geriatric Psychiatry and Neurology, 12,* 168–179.

Klünemann, H. H., Fronhöfer, W., Wurster, H., Fischer, W., Ibach, B., & Klein, H. E. (2002). Alzheimer's second patient: Johann F. and his family. *Annals of Neurology, 52,* 520–523.

Knable, M. B., Barci, B. M., Webster, M. J., Meador-Woodruff, J., & Torrey, E. F. (2004). Molecular abnormalities of the hippocampus in severe psychiatric illness: Postmortem findings from the Stanley Neuropathology Consortium. *Molecular Psychiatry, 9,* 609–620.

Knivsberg, A. M., Reichelt, K. L., Høien, T., & Nødland, M. (2002). A randomised, controlled study of dietary intervention in autistic syndromes. *Nutritional Neuroscience, 5,* 251–261.

Knoll, J. (1992). The pharmacological profile of (-)deprenyl (selegiline) and its relevance for humans: A personal view. *Pharmacology & Toxicology, 70,* 317–321.

Koch, T., Kroslak, T., Averbeck, M., Mayer, P., Schroder, H., Raulf, E., et al. (2000). Allelic variation S268P of the human mu-opioid receptor affects both desensitization and G protein coupling. *Molecular Pharmacology, 58,* 328–334.

Kodl, M. M., & Wakschlag, L. S. (2004). Does a childhood history of externalizing problems predict smoking during pregnancy? *Addictive Behavior, 29,* 273–279.

Koenig, J. A., & Edwardson, J. M. (1997). Endocytosis and recycling of G protein-coupled receptors. *Trends in Pharmacolgical Science, 18,* 276–287.

Koenig, J. H., & Ikeda, K. (1996). Synaptic vesicles have two distinct recycling pathways. *Journal of Cell Biology, 135,* 797–808.

Kogure, D., Matsuda, H., Ohnishi, T., Asada, T., Uno, M., Kunihiro, T., et al. (2000). Longitudinal evaluation of early Alzheimer's disease using brain perfusion SPECT. *Journal of Nuclear Medicine, 41*, 1155–1162.

Kolata, G. (1984). Studying learning in the womb. *Science, 225*, 302–303.

Kolb, B. (1989). Brain development, plasticity, and behavior. *American Psychologist, 44*, 1203–1212.

Kolb, B., & Elliott, W. (1987). Recovery from early cortical lesions in rats: II. Effects of experience on anatomy and behavior following frontal lesions at 1 or 5 days of age. *Behavioural Brain Research, 26*, 119–137.

Kolb, B., & Whishaw, I. Q. (1996). *Fundamentals of human neuropsychology.* New York: Freeman.

Kolb, B., & Whishaw, I. Q. (2001). *An introduction to brain and behavior.* New York: Worth.

Konorski, J. (1948). *Conditioned reflexes and neuron organization.* Cambridge, England: Cambridge University Press.

Konrad, K., Gunther, T., Hanisch, C., & Herpertz-Dahlmann, B. (2004). Differential effects of methylphenidate on attentional functions in children with attention-deficit/hyperactivity disorder. *Journal of the American Academy of Child and Adolescent Psychiatry, 43*, 191–198.

Koob, G. F., & Nestler, E. J. (1997). The neurobiology of drug addiction. In S. Salloway, P. Malloy, & J. L. Cummings (Eds.), *The neuropsychiatry of limbic and subcortical disorders* (pp. 179–194). Washington, DC: American Psychiatric Press.

Kopala, L. C., Good, K. P., Morrison, K., Bassett, A. S., Alda, M., & Honer, W. G. (2001). Impaired olfactory identification in relatives of patients with familial schizophrenia. *American Journal of Psychiatry, 158*, 1286–1290.

Kopala, L. C., Good, K. P., Torrey, E. F., & Honer, W. G. (1998). Olfactory function in monozygotic twins discordant for schizophrenia. *American Journal of Psychiatry, 155*, 134–136.

Koran, L. M., Pallanti, S., & Quercioli, L. (2001). Sumatriptan, 5-HT(1D) receptors and obsessive-compulsive disorder. *European Neuropsychopharmacology, 11*, 169–172.

Kordower, J. H., Emborg, M. E., Bloch, J., Ma, S. Y., Chu, Y., Leventhal, L., et al. (2000). Neurodegeneration prevented by lentiviral vector delivery of GDNF in primate models of Parkinson's disease. *Science, 290*, 767–773.

Kosel, M., Rudolph, U., Wielepp, P., Luginbuhl, M., Schmitt, W., Fisch, H. U., et al. (2004). Diminished GABA(A) receptor-binding capacity and a DNA base substitution in a patient with treatment-resistant depression and anxiety. *Neuropsychopharmacology, 29*, 347–350.

Kosel, M., & Schlaepfer, T. E. (2003). Beyond the treatment of epilepsy: New applications of vagus nerve stimulation in psychiatry. *CNS Spectrums, 8*, 515–521.

Kosslyn, S. M. (1999). If neuroimaging is the answer, what is the question? *Philosophical Transactions of the Royal Society of London, Biological Sciences, 354*, 1283–1294.

Kossoff, E. H., & Singer, H. S. (2001). Tourette syndrome: Clinical characteristics and current management strategies. *Paediatric Drugs, 3*, 355–363.

Kostovic, I., Lukinovic, N., Judas, M., Bogdanovic, N., Mrzljak, L., Zecevic, N., et al. (1989). Structural basis of the developmental plasticity in the human cerebral cortex: The role of the transient subplate zone. *Metabolic Brain Diseases, 4*, 17–23.

Kotler, M., Barak, P., Cohen, H., Averbuch, I. E., Grinshpoon, A., Gritsenko, I., et al. (1999). Homicidal behavior in schizophrenia associated with a genetic polymorphism determining low catechol O-methyltransferase (COMT) activity. *American Journal of Medical Genetics, 88*, 628–633.

Kotzbauer, P. T., Trojanowsk, J. Q., & Lee, V. M. (2001). Lewy body pathology in Alzheimer's disease. *Journal of Molecular Neuroscience, 17*, 225–232.

Kovelman, J. A., & Scheibel, A. B. (1984). A neurohistologic correlate of schizophrenia. *Biological Psychiatry, 19*, 1601–1621.

Kowalska, A. (2003). Amyloid precursor protein gene mutations responsible for early-onset autosomal dominant Alzheimer's disease. *Folia Neuropathologica, 41*, 35–40.

Kowalska, A., Pruchnik-Wolinska, D., Florczak, J., Szczech, J., Kozubski, W., Rossa, G., et al. (2004). Amyloid precursor protein gene analysis in familial Alzheimer's disease cases: A lack of mutations in exons 16 and 17. *Folia Neuropathologica, 42*, 1–7.

Krack, P., Poepping, M., Weinert, D., Schrader, B., & Deuschl, G. (2000). Thalamic, pallidal, or subthalamic surgery for Parkinson's disease? *Journal of Neurology, 247*, 122–134.

Kramer, P. (1997). *Listening to Prozac.* New York: Penguin.

Krause, K. H., Dresel, S. H., Krause, J., Kung, H. F., & Tatsch, K. (2000). Increased striatal dopamine transporter in adult patients with attention deficit hyperactivity disorder: Effects of methylphenidate as measured by single photon emission computed tomography. *Neuroscience Letters, 285*, 107–110.

Krause, K.-H., Dresel, S. H., Krause, J., la Fougere, C., & Ackenheil, M. (2003). The dopamine transporter and neuroimaging in attention deficit hyperactivity disorder. *Neuroscience Behavioral Review, 27*, 605–613.

Krebs, M. O., Betancur, C., Leroy, S., Bourdel, M. C., Gillberg, C., & Leboyer, M. (2002). Absence of association between a polymorphic GGC repeat in the 5′ untranslated region of the reelin gene and autism. *Molecular Psychiatry, 7*, 801–804.

Krieg, J. C., Backmund, H., & Pirke, K. M. (1987). Cranial computed tomography findings in bulimia. *Acta Psychiatrica Scandinavica, 75*, 144–149.

Krieg, J. C., Lauer, C., & Pierke, K. M. (1987). Hormonal and metabolic mechanisms in the development of cerebral pseudoatrophy in eating disorders. *Psychotherapy and Psychosomatics, 48*, 176–180.

Krieg, J. C., Pirke, K. M., Lauer, C., & Backmund, H. (1988). Endocrine, metabolic, and cranial computed tomographic findings in anorexia nervosa. *Biological Psychiatry, 23*, 377–387.

Kroisel, P. M., Petek, E., Emberger, W., Windpassinger, C., Wladika, W., & Wagner, K. (2001). Candidate region for Gilles de la Tourette syndrome at 7q31. *American Journal of Medical Genetics, 101*, 259–261.

Kromkamp, M., Uylings, H. B. M., Smidt, M. P., Hellemons, A. J., Burback, P. H., & Kahn, R. S. (2003). Decreased thalamic expression of the homeobox gene DLX1 in psychosis. *Archives of General Psychiatry, 60*, 869–874.

Kronenberger, W. G., & Dunn, D. W. (2003). Learning disorders. *Neurologic Clinics, 21*, 941–952.

Kronofol, Z., Hamdan-Allen, G., Goel, K., & Hill, E. M. (1991). Effects of single and repeated electroconvulsive therapy sessions on plasma ACTH, prolactin, growth hormone and cortisol concentrations. *Psychoneuroendocrinology, 16*, 345–352.

Kruger, S., Seminowicz, D., Goldapple, K., Kennedy, S. H., & Mayberg, H. S. (2003). State and trait influences on mood regulation in bipolar disorder: Blood flow differences with an acute mood challenge. *Biological Psychiatry, 54*, 1274–1283.

Krystal, J. H., Cramer, J. A., Krol, W. F., Kirk, G. F., & Rosenheck, R. A. (2001). Naltrexone in the treatment of alcohol dependence. *New England Journal of Medicine, 345*, 1734–1739.

Kugaya, A., Epperson, C. N., Zoghbi, S., van Dyck, C. H., Hou, Y., Fujita, M., et al. (2003). Increase in prefrontal cortex serotonin 2A receptors following estrogen treatment in postmenopausal women. *American Journal of Psychiatry, 160*, 1522–1524.

Kuhar, M. J. (1998). Recent biochemical studies of the dopamine transporter—A CNS drug target. *Life Sciences, 62*, 1573–1575.

Kuhl, D. E., Minoshima, S., Fessler, J. A., Frey, K. A., Foster, N. L., Ficaro, E. P., et al. (1996). In vivo mapping of cholinergic terminals in normal aging, Alzheimer's disease, and Parkinson's disease. *Annals of Neurology, 40*, 399–410.

Kuikka, J. T., Pitkänen, A., Lepola, U., Partanen, K., Vainio, P., Bergström, K. A., et al. (1995). Abnormal regional benzodiazepine receptor uptake in the prefrontal cortex in patients with panic disorder. *Nuclear Medicine Communications, 16*, 273–280.

Kukull, W. A., Larson, E. B., Bowen, J. D., McCormick, W. C., Teri, L., Pfanschmidt, M. L., et al. (1995). Solvent exposure as a risk factor for Alzheimer's disease: A case-control study. *American Journal of Epidemiology, 141*, 1059–1079.

Kultas-Ilinsky, K., & Ilinsky, I. A. (2001). *Basal ganglia and thalamus in health and movement disorders.* New York: Kluwer Academic/Plenum.

Kumar, A., Schapiro, M. B., Grady, C., Haxby, J. V., Wagner, E., Salerno, J. A., et al. (1991). High-resolution PET studies in Alzheimer's disease. *Neuropsychopharmacology, 4*, 35–46.

Kumar, S., Kralic, J. E., O'Buckley, T. K., Grobin, A. C., & Morrow, L. (2003). Chronic ethanol consumption enhances internalization of alpha1 subunit-containing GABAA receptors in cerebral cortex. *Journal of Neurochemistry, 86*, 700–708.

Kunkel, A., Kopp, B., Muller, G., Villringer, K. Taub, E., & Flor, H. (1999). Constraint-induced movement therapy for motor recovery in chronic stroke patients. *Archives of Physical and Medical Rehabilitation, 80*, 624–628.

Kuopio, A. M., Marttila, R. J., Helenius, H., & Rinne, U. K. (1999). Environmental risk factors in Parkinson's disease. *Movement Disorders, 14*, 928–939.

Kupfer, D. J., Frank, E., Grochocinski, V. J., Cluss, P. A., Houck, P. R., & Stapf, D. A. (2002). Demographic and clinical characteristics of individuals in a bipolar disorder case registry. *Journal of Clinical Psychiatry, 63*, 120–125.

Kupur, R. K., & Kupur, P. A. (2003). Schizoid neurochemical pathology-induced membrane Na+-K+ atpase inhibition in relation to neurological disorders. *International Journal of Neuroscience, 113*, 1705–1717.

Kurlan, R. (1994). Hypothesis II: Tourette's syndrome is part of a clinical spectrum that includes normal brain development. *Archives of Neurology, 51*, 1145–1150.

Kurlan, R. (2004). Disabling repetitive behaviors in Parkinson's disease. *Movement Disorders, 19*, 433–437.

Kurlan, R., Kersun, J., Ballantine, H. T. Jr., & Caine, E. D. (1990). Neurosurgical treatment of severe obsessive-compulsive disorder associated with Tourette's syndrome. *Movement Disorders, 5*, 152–155.

Kurup, R. K., & Kurup, P. A. (2002). Hypothalamic digoxin deficiency in obsessive compulsive disorder and la Tourette's syndrome. *International Journal of Neuroscience, 112*, 797–816.

Kustanovich, V., Ishii, J., Crawford, L., Yang, M., McGough, J. J., McCracken, J. T., et al. (2004). Transmission disequilibrium testing of dopamine-related candidate gene polymorphisms in ADHD: Confirmation of association of ADHD with DRD4 and DRD5. *Molecular Psychiatry, 9*, 711–7117.

Kutcher, S., Aman, M., Brooks, S. J., Buitelaar, J., van Daalen, E., et al. (2004). International consensus statement on attention-deficit/hyperactivity disorder (ADHD) and disruptive behavior disorders (DBDs): Clinical implications and treatment practice suggestions. *European Neuropsychopharmacology, 14*, 11–28.

Kwak, C. H., Hanna, P. A., & Jankovic, J. (2000). Botulinum toxin in the treatment of tics. *Archives of Neurology, 57*, 1190–1193.

Kwak, C. H., & Jankovic, J. (2002). Tourettism and dystonia after subcortical stroke. *Movement Disorders, 17*, 821–825.

Kwak, C., Vuong, K. D., & Jankovic, J. (2003). Migraine headache in patients with Tourette syndrome. *Archives of Neurology, 60*, 1595–1598.

Kwon, J. S., Kim, J. J., Lee, D. W., Lee, J. S., Lee, D. S., Kim, M. S., et al. (2003a). Neural correlates of clinical symptoms and cognitive dysfunctions in obsessive-compulsive disorder. *Psychiatry Research, 122*, 37–47.

Kwon, J. S., McCarley, R. W., Hirayasu, Y., Anderson, J. E., Fischer, I. A., Kikinis, R., et al. (1999). Left planum temporale volume reduction in schizophrenia. *Archives of General Psychiatry, 56*, 142–148.

Kwon, J. S., Shin, Y. W., Kim, C. W., Kim, Y. I., Youn, T., Han, M. H., et al. (2003b). Similarity and disparity of obsessive-compulsive disorder and schizophrenia in MR volumetric abnormalities of the hippocampus-amygdala complex. *Journal of Neurology, Neurosurgery, and Psychiatry, 74*, 962–964.

La Malfa, G., Lassi, S., Bertelli, M., Salvini, R., & Placidi, G. F. (2004). Autism and intellectual diability: A study of prevalence on a sample of the Italian population. *Journal of Intellectual Disabilities Research, 48*, 262–267.

Laakso, M. P., Frisoni, G. B., Könönen, M., Mikkonen, M., Beltramello, A., Geroldi, C., et al. (2000). Hippocampus and entorhinal cortex in frontotemporal dementia and Alzheimer's disease: A morphometric MRI study. *Biological Psychiatry, 47*, 1056–1063.

Laakso, M. P., Partanen, K., Riekkinen, P., Lehtovirta, M., Helkala, E. L., Hallikainen, M., et al. (1996). Hippocampal volumes in Alzheimer's disease, Parkinson's disease with and without dementia, and in vascular dementia: An MRI study. *Neurology, 46*, 678–681.

Laburn, H. P. (1996). How does the fetus cope with thermal challenges? *News in Physiological Sciences, 11*, 96–100.

Lacerda, A. L., Dalgalarrondo, P., Caetano, D., Camargo, E. E., Etchebehere, E. C., & Soares, J. C. (2003b). Elevated thalamic and prefrontal regional cerebral blood flow in obsessive-compulsive disorder: A SPECT study. *Psychiatry Research, 123*, 125–134.

Lacerda, A. L., Dalgalarrondo, P., Caetano, D., Haas, G. L., Camargo, E. E., & Keshavan, M. S. (2003a). Neuropsychological performance and regional cerebral blood flow in obsessive-compulsive disorder. *Progress in Neuro-Psychopharmacology & Biological Psychiatry, 27*, 657–665.

Lachman, H. M., Morrow, B., Shprintzen, R., Veit, S., Parisa, S. S., Faedda, G., et al. (1996a). Association of codon 108–158 catechol-o-methyltransferase gene polymorphism with the psychiatric manifestations of velo-cardio-facial syndrome. *American Journal of Medical Genetics, 67*, 468–472.

Lachman, H. M., Papolos, D. F., Saito, T., Yu, Y. M., Szumlanski, C. L., & Weinshilboum, R. M. (1996b). Human catechol-o-methyltransferase pharmacogenetics: Description of a functional polymorphism and its potential application to neuropsychiatric disorders. *Pharmacogenetics, 6*, 243–250.

Lagace, D. C., Kutcher, S. P., & Robertson, H. A. (2003). Mathematics deficits in adolescents with bipolar I disorder. *American Journal of Psychiatry, 160*, 100–104.

Lagnaoui, R., Moore, N., Moride, Y., Miremont-Salamé, G., & Bégaud, B. (2003). Benzodiazepine utilization patterns in Alzheimer's disease patients. *Pharmacoepidemiology and Drug Safety, 12*, 511–515.

LaHoste, G. J., Swanson, J. M., Wigal, S. B., Glabe, C., Wigal, T., King, N., et al. (1996). Dopamine D4 receptor gene polymorphism is associated with attention deficit hyperactivity disorder. *Molecular Psychiatry, 1*, 121–124.

Lai, I. C., Hong, C. J., & Tsai, S. J. (2001). Association study of nicotinic-receptor variants and major depressive disorder. *Journal of Affective Disorders, 66*, 79–82.

Lai, Y. Y., & Siegel, J. M. (2003). Physiological and anatomical link between Parkinson-like disease and REM sleep behavior disorder. *Molecular Neurobiology, 27*, 137–152.

Laifenfeld, D., Klein, E., & Ben-Shachar, D. (2002). Norepinephrine alters the expression of genes involved in neuronal sprouting and differentiation: Relevance for major depression and antidepressant mechanisms. *Journal of Neurochemistry, 83*, 1054–1064.

Laihinen, A., Ruottinen, H., Rinne, J. O., Haaparanta, M., Bergman, J., Solin, O., et al. (2000). Risk for Parkinson's disease: Twin studies for the detection of asymptomatic subjects using [18F]6–fluorodopa PET. *Journal of Neurology, 247*, 110–113.

Lambon R., M. A., Patterson, K., Graham, N., Dawson, K., & Hodges, J. R. (2003). Homogeneity and heterogeneity in mild cognitive impairment and Alzheimer's disease: A cross-sectional and longitudinal study of 55 cases. *Brain, 126*, 2350–2362.

Langleben, D. D., Acton, P. D., Austin, G., Elman, I., Krikorian, G., Monterosso, J. R., et al. (2002). Effects of methylphenidate discontinuation on cerebral blood flow in prepubescent boys with attention deficit hyperactivity disorder. *Journal of Nuclear Medicine, 43*, 1624–1629.

Langley, K., Marshall, L., van den Bree, M., Thomas, H., Owen, M., O'Donovan, M., & Thapar, A. (2004). Association of the dopamine D4 receptor gene 7-repeat allele with neuropsychological test performance of children with ADHD. *American Journal of Psychiatry, 161*, 133–138.

Langreth, R. (2002). Viagra for the brain. *Forbes,* Feb. 4, 46–52.

Langston, J. W., & Ballard, P. (1984). Parkinsonism induced by 1-methyl-4-phenyl-1, 2, 3, 6-tetrahydropyridine (MPTP): Implications for treatment and the pathogenesis of Parkinson's disease. *Canadian Journal of Neurological Sciences, 11*, 160–165.

Lanius, R. A., Hopper, J. W., & Menon, R. S. (2003). Individual differences in a husband and wife who developed PTSD after a motor vehicle accident: A functional MRI case study. *American Journal of Psychiatry, 160*, 667–669.

Lannfelt, L., Axelman, K., Lilius, L., & Basun, H. (1995). Genetic counseling in a Swedish Alzheimer family with amyloid precursor protein mutation. *American Journal of Human Genetics, 56*, 332–335.

Lappalainen, J., Dranzler, H. R., Malison, R., Price, L. H., Van Dyck, C., Rosenheck, R. A., et al. (2002). A functional neuropeptide Y leu7Pro polymorphism associated with alcohol dependence in a large population sample from the United States. *Archives of General Psychiatry, 59*, 825–831.

Larisch, R., Klimke, A., Mayoral, F., Hamacher, K., Herzog, H. R., Vosberg, H., et al. (2001). Disturbance of serotonin 5HT2 receptors in remitted patients suffering from hereditary depressive disorder. *Nuklearmedizin, 40*, 129–134.

Larsen, J. P., Hoien, T., Lundberg, I., & Odeggard, H. (1990). MRI evaluation of the size and symmetry of the planum temporale in adolescents with developmental dyslexia. *Brain and Language, 39*, 289–301.

Larsen, J. P., Hoien, T., Lundberg, I., & Odeggard, H. (1992). Magnetic resonance imaging of the corpus callosum in developmental dyslexia. *Cognitive Neuropsychology, 9*, 123–134.

Larsson, J. O., Larsson, H., & Lichtenstein, P. (2004). Genetic and environmental contributions to stability and change of ADHD symptoms between 8 and 13 years of age: A longitudinal twin study. *Journal of the American Academy of Child and Adolescent Psychiatry, 43*, 1267–1275.

Laruelle, M. (1998). Imagine dopamine transmission in schizophrenia – A review and meta-analysis. *Quarterly Journal of Nuclear Medicine, 42*, 211–221.

Laruelle, M., & Abi-Dargham, A. (1999). Dopamine as the wind of psychotic fire: New evidence from brain imaging studies. *Journal of Psychopharmacology, 13*, 358–371.

Laruelle, M., Abi-Dargham, A., van Dyck, C., Gil, R., D'Souza, C. D., Erdos, J., et al. (1996). Single photon emission computerized tomography imaging of amphetamine-induced dopamine release in drug-free schizophrenic subjects. *Proceedings of the National Academy of Science, 93*, 9235–9240.

Laruelle, M., Abi-Dargham, A., van Dyck, C., Gil, R., D'Souza, C. D., Krystal, J., et al. (2000). Dopamine and serotonin transporters in patients with schizophrenia: An imaging study with [123I]B-CIT. *Biological Psychiatry, 47*, 371–379.

Laruelle, M., Abi-Dargham, A., van Dyck, C. H., Rosenblatt, W., Zea-Ponce, Y., Zoghbi, S. S., et al. (1995). SPECT imaging of striatal dopamine release after amphetamine challenge. *Journal of Nuclear Medicine, 36*, 1182–1190.

Lauderback, C. M., Kanski, J., Hackett, J. M., Maeda, N., Kindy, M. S., & Butterfield, D. A. (2002). Apolipoprotein E modulates Alzheimer's Abeta (1-42)-induced oxidative damage to synaptosomes in an allele-specific manner. *Brain Research, 924*, 90–97.

Laurin, D., Masaki, K. H., Foley, D. J., White, L. R., & Launer, L. J. (2004). Midlife dietary intake of antioxidants and risk of late-life incident dementia: The Honolulu-Asia Aging Study. *American Journal of Epidemiology, 159*, 959–967.

Laurin, D., Verreault, R., Lindsay, J., Dewailly, E., & Holub, B. J. (2003). Omega-3 fatty acids and risk of cognitive impairment and dementia. *Journal of Alzheimer's Disease, 5*, 315–322.

Lauterbach, E. C., Freeman, A., & Vogel, R. L. (2003). Correlates of generalized anxiety and panic attacks in dystonia and Parkinson disease. *Cognitive and Behavioral Neurology, 16*, 225–233.

Lauzurica, N., Hurtado, A., Escarti, A., Delgado, M., Barrios, V., Morande, G., et al. (2003). Polymorphism within the promoter and the intron 2 of the serotonin transporter gene in a population of bulimic patients. *Neuroscience Letters, 352*, 226–230.

Lavalaye, J., Linszen, D. H., Booij, J., Dingemans, P. M. A. J., Reneman, L., Habraken, J. B. A., et al. (2001). Dopamine transporter density in young patients with schizophrenia assessed with [123]FP-CIT SPECT. *Schizophrenia Research, 47*, 59–67.

Law, A. J., & Deakin, J. F. W. (2001). Asymmetrical reductions of hippocampal NMDARI glutamate receptor mRNA in the psychoses. *Neurochemistry, 12*, 2971–2974.

Law, A. J., Weickert, C. S., Hyde, T. M., Kleinman, J. E., & Harrison, P. J. (2004). Reduced spinophilin but not microtubule-associated protein 2 expression in the hippocampal formation in schizophrenia and mood disorders: Molecular evidence for a pathology of dendritic spines. *American Journal of Psychiatry, 161*, 1848–1855.

Lawrence, A. D., Evans, A. H., & Lees, A. J. (2003). Compulsive use of dopamine replacement therapy in Parkinson's disease: Reward systems gone awry? *Lancet Neurology, 2*, 595–604.

Lawrie, S. M., & Abukmeil, S. S. (1998). Brain abnormality in schizophrenia. A systematic and quantitative review of volumetric magnetic resonance imaging studies. *British Journal of Psychiatry, 172*, 110–120.

Lawson, J. S., Galin, H., Adams, S. J., Brunet, D. G., Criollo, M., & MacCrimmon, D. J. (2003). Artefacting reliability in QEEG topographic maps. *Clinical Neurophysiology, 114*, 883–888.

Laxer, K. D., Sourkes, T. L., Fang, T. Y., Young, S. N., Gauthier, S. G., & Missala, K. (1979). Monoamine metabolites in the CSF of epileptic patients. *Neurology, 29*, 1157–1161.

Le Couteur, D. G., Leighteon, P. W., McCann, S. J., & Pond, S. (1997). Association of a polymorphism in the dopamine-transporter gene with Parkinson's disease. *Movement Disorders, 12*, 760–763.

Leake, A., Fairbairn, A. F., McKeith, I. G., & Ferrier, I. N. (1991). Studies on the serotonin uptake binding site in major depressive disorder and control post-mortem brain: Neurochemical and clinical correlates. *Psychiatry Reseach, 39*, 155–165.

Learned-Coughlin, S. M., Bergstrom, M., Savitcheva, I., Ascher, J., Schmith, V. D., & Langstrom, B. (2003). In vivo activity of bupropion at the human dopamine transporter as measured by positron emission tomography. *Biological Psychiatry, 54*, 800–805.

Leckman, J. F., Cohen, D. J., Detlor, J., Young, J. G., Harcherik, D., & Shaywitz, B. A. (1982). Clonidine in the treatment of Tourette syndrome: A review of data. *Advances in Neurology, 35*, 391–401.

Leckman, J. F., Cohen, D. J., Shaywitz, B. A., Caparulo, B. K., Heninger, G. R., & Bowers, M. B. Jr. (1980). CSF monoamine metabolites in child and adult psychiatric patients. *Archives of General Psychiatry, 37*, 677–681.

Leckman, J. F., Grice, D. E., Boardman, J., Zhang, H., Vitale, A., Bondi, C., et al. (1997). Symptoms of obsessive-compulsive disorder. *American Journal of Psychiatry, 154*, 911–917.

Leckman, J. F., Hardin, M. T., Riddle, M. A., Stevenson, J., Ort, S. I., & Cohen, D. J. (1991). Clonidine treatment of Gilles de la Tourette's syndrome. *Archives of General Psychiatry, 48*, 324–328.

Leckman, J. F., Mayes, L. C., Feldman, R., Evans, D. W., King, R. A., & Cohen, D. J. (1999). Early parental preoccupations and behaviors and their possible relationship to the symptoms of obsessive-compulsive disorder. *Acta Psychiatrica Scandinavica, 396*, Supplement, 1–26.

Lecrubier, Y. (2001). The burden of depression and anxiety in general medicine. *Journal of Clinical Psychiatry, 62*, 4–9.

LeDoux, J. (2002). *Synaptic self: How our brains become who we are.* New York: Viking.

Lee, M., Martin-Ruiz, C., Graham, A., Court, J., Jaros, E., Perry, R., et al. (2002). Nicotinic receptor abnormalities in the cerebellar cortex in autism. *Brain, 125*, 1483–1495.

Lee, M. S., Kim, H. S., Cho, E. K., Lim, J. H., & Rinne, J. O. (2002). COMT genotype and effectiveness of entacapone in patients with fluctuating Parkinson's disease. *Neurology, 58*, 564–567.

Leekam, S. R., Libby, S. J., Wing, L., Gould, J., & Taylor, C. (2002). The diagnostic interview for social and communication disorders: Algorithms for ICD-10 childhood autism and Wing and Gould autistic spectrum disorder. *Journal of Child Psychology and Psychiatry, 43*, 327–342.

Lehrmann, E., Hyde, T. M., Vawter, M. P., Becker, K. G., Kleinman, J. E., & Freed, W. J. (2003). The use of microarrays to characterize neuropsychiatric disorders: Postmortem studies of substance abuse and schizophrenia. *Current Molecular Medicine, 3*, 437–446.

Leino, K., Mildh, L., Lertola, K., Seppala, T., & Kirvela, O. (1999). Time course of changes in breathing pattern in morphine- and oxycodone-induced respiratory depression. *Anaesthesia, 54*, 835–840.

Leite-Morris, K. A., Fukudome, E. Y., Shoeb, M. H., & Kaplan, G. B. (2004). GABAB receptor activation in the ventral tegmental area inhibits the acquisition and expression of opiate-induced motor sensitization. *Journal of Pharmacology and Experimental Therapy, 308*, 667–678.

Lemelson, R. (2003). Obsessive-compulsive disorder in Bali: The cultural shaping of a neuropsychiatric disorder. *Transcultural Psychiatry, 40*, 377–408.

Lemke, M. R. (2002). Effect of reboxetine on depression in Parkinson's disease patients. *Journal of Clinical Psychiatry, 63*, 300–304.

Lenn, N. J., & Freinkel, A. J. (1989). Facial sparing as a feature of prenatal-onset hemiparesis. *Pediatric Neurology, 5*, 291–295.

Lenox, R. H., & Hahn, C. G. (2000). Overview of the mechanism of action of lithium in the brain: Fifty year update. *Journal of Clinical Psychiatry, 61*, 5–15.

Leon, J., Cheng, C. K., & Neumann, P. J. (1998). Alzheimer's disease care: Costs and potential savings. *Health Affairs, 17*, 206–216.

Leon, M. R. (2000). Effects of caffeine on cognitive, psychomotor, and affective performance of children with attention-deficit/hyperactivity disorder. *Journal of Attention Disorders, 4*, 27–47.

Leonard, B. (2000). Stress, depression and the activation of the immune system. *World Journal of Biological Psychiatry, 1*, 17–25.

Leonard, H. L., Topol, D., Bukstein, O., Hindmarsh, D., Allen, A. J., & Swedo, S. E. (1994). Clonazepam as an augmenting agent in the treatment of childhood-onset obsessive-compulsive disorder. *Journal of the American Academy of Child and Adolescent Psychiatry, 33*, 792–794.

Lepine, J. P. (2002). The epidemiology of anxiety disorders: Prevalence and societal costs. *Journal of Clinical Psychiatry, 63*, 4–8.

Leppamaki, S., Partonen, T., & Lonnqvist, J. (2002). Bright-light exposure combined with physical exercise elevates mood. *Journal of Affective Disorders, 72*, 139–144.

Leroi, I., Brandt, J., Reich, S. G., Lyketsos, C. G., Grill, S., Thompson, R., et al. (2004). Randomized placebo-controlled trial of donepezil in cognitive impairment in Parkinson's disease. *International Journal of Geriatric Psychiatry, 19*, 1–8.

Leroi, I., O'Hearn, E., Marsh, L., Lyketsos, C. G., Rosenblatt, A., Ross, C. A., et al. (2002). Psychopathology in patients with degenerative cerebellar diseases: A comparison to Huntington's disease. *American Journal of Psychiatry, 159*, 1306–1314.

Leuchter, A. F., Cook, I. A., Witte, E. A., Morgan, M., & Abrams, M. (2002). Changes in brain function of depressed subjects during treatment with placebo. *American Journal of Psychiatry, 159*, 122–129.

Levant, B. (1997). The D3 dopamine receptor: Neurobiology and potential clinical relevance. *Pharmacological Reviews, 49*, 231–252.

Levecque, C., Elbaz, A., Clavel, J., Vidal, J. S., Amouyel, P., Alperovitch, A., et al. (2004). Association of polymorphisms in the tau and saitohin genes with Parkinson's disease. *Journal of Neurology, Neurosurgery, and Psychiatry, 75*, 478–480.

Levine, J. (1997). Controlled trials of inositol in psychiatry. *European Neuropsychopharmacology, 7*, 147–155.

Levine, J., Panchalingam, K., Rapaport, A., Gershon, S., McClure, R., & Pettegrew, J. W. (2000). Increased cerebrospinal fluid glutamine levels in depressed patients. *Biological Psychiatry, 47*, 586–593.

Levine, J., Stahl, Z., Sela, A. B., Gavendo, S., Ruderman, V., & Belmaker, R. H. (2002). Elevated homocysteine levels in young male patients with schizophrenia. *American Journal of Psychiatry, 159*, 1790–1792.

Levinson, D. F., Holmans, P., Laurent, C., Riley, B., Pulver, A. E., Gejman, P. V., et al. (2002). No major schizophrenia locus detected on chromosome 1q in a large multicenter sample. *Science, 296*, 793–741.

Levitan, I. B., & Kaczmarek, L. K. (1997). *The neuron* (2nd ed.). New York: Oxford University Press.

Levitan, I. B., and Kaczmarek, L. K. (1997). *The neuron: Cell and molecular biology.* New York: Oxford University Press.

Levy, L. A., Savit, J. M., & Hodes, M. (1983). Parkinsonism: Improvement by electroconvulsive therapy. *Archives of Physical Medical Rehabilitation, 64*, 432–433.

Levy, R. M., Steffens, D. C., McQuoid, D. R., Provenzale, J. M., MacFall, J. R., & Krishnan, K. R. (2003). MRI lesion severity and mortality in geriatric depression. *American Journal of Geriatric Psychiatry, 11*, 678–682.

Levy, S. E., Mandell, D. S., Merhar, S., Ittenbach, R. F., & Pinto-Martin, J. A. (2003). Use of complementary and alternative medicine among children recently diagnosed with autistic spectrum disorder. *Journal of Developmental and Behavioral Pediatrics, 24*, 418–423.

Lewis, D. A. (2000). GABAergic local circuit neurons and prefrontal dysfunction in schizophrenia. *Brain Research Reviews, 31*, 270–276.

LeWitt, P. A., & Nyholm, D. (2004). New developments in levodopa therapy. *Neurology, 62*, 9–16.

Leyton, M., Boileau, I., Benkelfat, C., Diksic, M., Baker, G., & Dagher, A. (2002). Amphetamine-induced increases in extracellular dopamine, drug wanting, and novelty seeking: A PET/[11C]Raclopride study in healthy men. *Neuropsychopharmacology, 27*, 1027–1035.

Li, C. Y., Sung, F. C., & Wu, S. C. (2002). Risk of cognitive impairment in relation to elevated exposure to electromagnetic fields. *Journal of Occupational and Environmental Medicine, 44*, 66–72.

Li, C. Y., Wu, S. C., & Sung, F. C. (2002). Lifetime principal occupation and risk of cognitive impairment among the elderly. *Industrial Health, 40*, 7–13.

Li, J., Nguyen, L., Gleason, C., Lotspeich, L., Spiker, D., Risch, N., et al. (2004). Lack of evidence for an association between WNT2 and RELN polymorphisms and autism. *American Journal of Medical Genetics, 126*, 51–57.

Li, T., Liu, X., Zhao, J., Hu, X., Ball, D. M., Loh, E. W., et al. (2002). Allelic association analysis of the dopamine D2, D3, 5-HT2A, and GABA(A)gamma2 receptors and serotonin transporter genes with heroin abuse in Chinese subjects. *American Journal of Medical Genetics, 114*, 329–335.

Li, T., Vallada, H., Curtis, D., Arranz, M., Xu, K., Cai, G., et al. (1997). Catechol-O-methyltransferase Va1158Met polymorphism: Frequency analysis in Han Chinese subjects and allelic association of the low activity allele with bipolar affective disorder. *Pharmacogenetics, 7*, 349–353.

Li, T., Xu, K., Deng, H., Cai, G., Liu, J., Liu, X., et al. (1997). Association analysis of the dopamine D4 gene exon III VNTR and heroin abuse in Chinese subjects. *Molecular Psychiatry, 2*, 413–416.

Li, T., Zhu, Z. H., Liu, X., Hu, X., Zhao, J., Sham, P. C., et al. (2000). Association analysis of polymorphisms in the DRD4 gene and heroin abuse in Chinese subjects. *American Journal of Medical Genetics, 96*, 616–621.

Liddle, P. F., Friston, K. J., Frith, C. D., Hirsch, S. R., Jones, T., & Frackowiak, R. S. J. (1992). Patterns of cerebral blood flow in schizophrenia. *British Journal of Psychiatry, 160*, 179–186.

Lieb, R., Isensee, B., Hoefler, M., Pfister, H., & Wittchen, H. U. (2002). Parental major depression and the risk of depression and other mental disorders in offspring. *Archives of General Psychiatry, 59*, 365–374.

Lieberman, J. A., Tollefson, G., Tohen, M., Green, A., Gur, R. E., Kahn, R., et al. (2003). Comparative efficacy and safety of atypical and conventional antipsychotic drugs in first-episode psychosis: A randomized double-blind trial of olanzapine versus haloperidol. *American Journal of Psychiatry, 160*, 1396–1404.

Lile, J. A., Stoops, W. W., Allen, T. S., Glaser, P. E., Hays, L. R., & Rush, C. R. (2004). Baclofen does not alter the reinforcing, subject-rated or cardiovascular effects of intranasal cocaine in humans. *Psychopharmacology, 171*, 441–449.

Lim, K., Tew, W., Kushner, M., Chow. K., Matsumoto, B., & DeLisi, L. E. (1996). Cortical gray matter volume deficits in patients with first-episode schizophrenia. *American Journal of Psychiatry, 153*, 1548–1553.

Lim, K. O., Choi, S. J., Pomara, N., Wolkin, A., & Rotrosen, J. P. (2002). Reduced frontal white matter integrity in cocaine dependence: A controlled diffusion tensor imaging study. *Bilogical Psychiatry, 51*, 890–895.

Lim, K. O., Rosenbloom, M. J., Faustman, W. O., Sullivan, E. V., & Pfefferbaum, A. (1999). Cortical gray matter deficit in patients with bipolar disorder. *Schizophrenia Research, 40*, 219–227.

Lima, L., Obregón, F., Urbina, M., Carreira, I., Baccichet, E., & Peña, S. (2003). Taurine concentration in human blood peripheral lymphocytes: Major depression and treatment with the antidepressant mirtazapine. *Advances in Experimental Medicine and Biology, 526*, 297–304.

Limousin, P., Greene, J., Pollak, P., Rothwell, J., Benabid, A. L., & Frackowiak, R. (1997). Changes in cerebral activity pattern due to subthalamic nucleus or internal pallidum stimulation in Parkinson's disease. *Annals of Neurology, 42*, 283–291.

Lin, J. J., Yueh, K. C., Chang, D. C., Chang, C. Y., Yeh, Y. H., & Lin, S. Z. (2003). The homozygote 10-copy genotype of variable number tandem repeat dopamine transporter gene may confer protection against Parkinson's disease for male, but not for female patients. *Journal of Neurological Science, 209*, 87–92.

Lin, J. J., Yueh, K. C., Chang, D. C., & Lin, S. Z. (2002). Association between genetic polymorphism of angiotensin-converting enzyme gene and Parkinson's disease. *Journal of Neurological Science, 199*, 25–29.

Linazasoro, G., Antonini, A., Maguire, R. P., & Leenders, K. L. (2004). Pharmacological and PET studies in patients with Parkinson's disease and a short duration motor response: Implications in the pathophysiology of motor complications. *Journal of Neural Transmission, 111*, 497–509.

Linazasoro, G., Obeso, J. A., Gomez, J. C., Martinez, M., Antonini, A., & Leenders, K. L. (1999). Modification of dopamine D2 receptor activity by pergolide in Parkinson's disease: An in vivo study by PET. *Clinical Neuropharmacology, 22*, 277–280.

Lindsay, R. L., & Aman, M. G. (2003). Pharmacologic therapies aid treatment for autism. *Pediatric Annals, 32*, 671–676.

Lindstrom L. H., Gefvert, O., Hagberg, G., Lundberg, T., Bergstrom, M., Hartvi, P. et al. (1999). Increased dopamine synthesis rate in medial prefrontal cortex and striatum in schizophrenia indicated by L-(B-11C) DOPA and PET. *Biological Psychiatry, 46*, 681–688.

Lindvall, O., Brundin, P., Widner, H., Rehncrona, S., Gustavii, B., Frackowiak, R., et al. (1990). Grafts of fetal dopamine neurons survive and improve motor function in Parkinson's disease. *Science, 247*, 574–577.

Lindvall, O., Sawle, G., Widner, H., Rothwell, J. C., Björklund, A., Brooks, D., et al. (1994). Evidence for long-term survival and function of dopaminergic grafts in progressive Parkinson's disease. *Annals of Neurology, 35*, 172–180.

Linnarsson, S., Bjorklund, A., & Ernfors, P. (1997). Learning deficits in BDNF mutant mice. *Journal of Neuroscience, 9*, 2581–2587.

Linterman, I., & Weyandt, L. (2001). Divided attention skills in college students with ADHD: Is it advantageous to have ADHD? *ADHD Report, 9*, 1–6.

Liotti, M., Mayberg, H. S., McGinnis, S., Brannan, S. L., & Jerabek, P. (2002). Unmasking disease-specific cerebral blood flow abnormalities: Mood challenge in patients with remitted unipolar depression. *American Journal of Psychiatry, 159*, 1830–1840.

Liou, H. H., Tsai, M. C., Chen, C. J., Jeng, J. S., Chang, Y. C., Chen, S. Y., et al. (1997). Environmental risk factors and Parkinson's disease: A case-control study in Taiwan. *Neurology, 48*, 1583–1588.

Lipinski, J. F., Sallee, F. R., Jackson, C., & Sethuraman, G. (1997). Dopamine agonist treatment of Tourette disorder in children: Results of an open-label trial of pergolide. *Movement Disorders, 12*, 402–407.

Lisanby, S. H., Luber, B., Schlaepfer, T. E., & Sackeim, H. A. (2003). Safety and feasibility of magnetic seizure therapy (MST) in major depression: Randomized within-subject comparison with electroconvulsive therapy. *Neuropsychopharmacology, 28*, 1852–1865.

Lishman, W. A. (1990). Alcohol and the brain. *British Journal of Psychiatry, 156*, 635–644.

Little, J. T., Ketter, T. A., Kimbrell, T. A., Danielson, A., Benson, B., Willis, M. W., et al. (1996). Venlafaxine or bupropion responders but not nonresponders show baseline prefrontal and paralimbic hypometabolism compared with controls. *Psychopharmacology Bulletin, 32*, 629–635.

Little, K. Y., McLaughlin, D. P., Ranc, J., Gilmore, J., Lopez, J. F., Watson, S. J., et al. (1997). Serotonin transporter binding sites and mRNA levels in depressed persons committing suicide. *Biological Psychiatry, 41*, 1156–1164.

Liu, J. G., & Anand, K. J. (2001). Protein kinases modulate cellular adaptations associated with opioid tolerance and dependence. *Brain Research Review, 38*, 1–19.

Livingstone, M. S., Rosen, G. D., Drislane, F. W., & Galaburda, A. M. (1991). Physiological and anatomical evidence for a magnocellular defect in developmental dyslexia. *Proceedings of the National Academy of Sciences, 88*, 7943–7947.

Llerena, A., Berecz, R., Dorado, P., Gonzalez, A. P., Penas-Lledo, E. M., & De La Rubia, A. (2003). CYP2C9 gene and susceptibility to major depressive disorder. *Pharmacogenomics, 3*, 300–302.

Lochner, C., Hemmings, S. M., Kinnear, C. J., Moolman-Smook, J. C., Corfield, V. A., Knowles, J. A., et al. (2004). Gender in obsessive-compulsive disorder: Clinical and genetic findings. *European Neuropsychopharmacology, 14*, 105–113.

Lockwood, A. H. (2000). Pesticides and Parkinsonism: Is there an etiological link? *Current Opinions in Neurology, 13*, 687–690.

Logan, A. C. (2003). Neurobehavioral aspects of omega-3 fatty acids: Possible mechanisms and therapeutic value in major depression. *Alternative Medicine Review, 8*, 410–425.

Lohr, J. B., & Braff, D. L. (2003). The value of referring to recently introduced antipsychotics as "second generation". *American Journal of Psychiatry, 160*, 1371–1372.

Loiselle, C. R., Wendlandt, J. T., Rohde, C. A., & Singer, H. S. (2003). Antistreptococcal, neuronal, and nuclear antibodies in Tourette syndrome. *Pediatric Neurology, 28*, 119–125.

Lombroso, C. T. (1999). Lamotrigine-induced tourettism. *Neurology, 52*, 1191–1194.

Loo, C., Sachdev, P., Elsayed, H., McDarmont, B., Mitchell, P., Wilkinson, M., et al. (2001). Effects of a 2- to 4-week course of repetitive transcranial magnetic stimulation (rTMS) on neuropsychologic functioning, electroencephalogram, and auditory threshold in depressed patients. *Biological Psychiatry, 49*, 615–623.

Loo, S. K. (2003). EEG and neurofeedback findings in ADHD. *ADHD Report, 11*, 1–9.

Loo, S. K., Teale, P. D., & Reite, M. L. (1999). EEG correlated of methylphenidate response among children with ADHD: A preliminary report. *Biological Psychiatry, 45*, 1657–1660.

Looney, S. W., & El-Mallakh, R. S. (1997). Meta-analysis of erythrocyte, Na, K-ATPase activity in bipolar illness. *Depression and Anxiety, 5*, 53–65.

Lopez, O. L., Becker, J. T., Sweet, R. A., Klunk, W., Kaufer, D. I., Saxton, J., et al. (2003). Psychiatric symptoms vary with the severity of dementia in probable Alzheimer's disease. *Journal of Neuropsychiatry and Clinical Neurosciences, 15*, 346–353.

Lopez, O. L., Becker, J. T., Wisniewski, S., Saxton, J., Kaufer, D. I., & DeKosky, S. T. (2002). Cholinesterase inhibitor treatment alters the natural history of Alzheimer's disease. *Journal of Neurology, Neurosurgery, and Psychiatry, 72*, 310–314.

Lorberboym, M., Watemberg, N., Nissenkorn, A., Nir, B., & Lerman-Sagie, T. (2004). Technetium 99m ethylcys- teinate dimmer single-photon emission computed tomography (SPECT) during intellectual stress test in children and adolescents with pure versus comorbid attention-deficit hyperactivity disorder (ADHD). *Journal of Child Neurology, 19*, 91–96.

Lorenzo, A., Yuan, M., Zhang, Z., Paganetti, P. A., Sturchler-Pierrat, C., Staufenbiel, M., et al. (2000). Amyloid β interacts with the amyloid precursor protein: A poltential toxic mechanism in Alzheimer's disease. *Nature Neuroscience, 3*, 460–464.

Lotsch, J., Skarke, C., Grosch, S., Darimont, J., Schmidt, H., & Geisslinger, G. (2002). The polymorphism A118G of the human opioid receptor gene decreases the pupil constrictory effect of morphine-6-glucuronide but not that of morphine. *Pharmacogenetics, 12*, 3–9.

Lou, H. C., Henriksen, L., & Bruhn, P. (1984). Focal cerebral hypoperfusion in children with dysphasia and/or attention deficit disorder. *Archives of Neurology, 41*, 825–829.

Lou, H. C., Henriksen, L., Bruhn, P., Borner, H., & Nielsen, J. B. (1989). Striatal dysfunction in attention deficit and hyperkinetic disorder. *Archives of Neurology, 46*, 48–52.

Lou, H. C., Rosa, P., Pryds, O., Karrebaek, H., Lunding, J., Cumming, P., et al. (2004). ADHD: Increased dopamine receptor availability linked to attention deficit and low neonatal cerebral blood flow. *Development in Medicine and Child Neurology, 46*, 179–183.

Louie, A. K., Lannon, R. A., Rutzick, E. A., Browne, D., Lewis, T. B., & Jones, R. (1996). Clinical features of cocaine-induced panic. *Biological Psychiatry, 40*, 938–940.

Lowe, N., Kirley, A., Hawi, Z., Sham, P., Wickham, H., Kratochvil, C. J., et al. (2004). Joint analysis of the DRD5 marker concludes association with attention-deficit/hyperactivity disorder confined to the predominantly inattentive and combined subtypes. *American Journal of Human Genetics, 74*, 348–356.

Lozza, C., Marié, R. M., & Baron, J. C. (2002). The metabolic substrates of bradykinesia and tremor in uncomplicated Parkinson's disease. *NeuroImage, 17*, 688–699.

Lucey, J. V., Costa, D. C., Adshead, G., Deahl, M., Busatto, G., Gacinovic, S., et al. (1997). Brain blood flow in anxiety disorders. OCD, panic disorder with agoraphobia, and post-traumatic stress disorder on 99mTcHMPAO single photon emission tomography (SPET). *British Journal of Psychiatry, 171*, 346–350.

Lucey, J. V., Costa, D. C., Busatto, G., Pilowsky, L. S., Marks, I. M., Ell, P. J., et al. (1997). Caudate regional cerebral blood flow in obsessive-compulsive disorder, panic disorder and healthy controls on single photon emission computerised tomography. *Psychiatry Research, 74*, 25–33.

Luchsinger, J. A., Tang, M. X., Shea, S., & Mayeux, R. (2002). Caloric intake and the risk of Alzheimer disease. *Archives of Neurology, 59*, 1258–1263.

Luchsinger, J. A., Tang, M. X., Shea, S., & Mayeux, R. (2003). Antioxidant vitamin intake and risk of Alzheimer disease. *Archives of Neurology, 60*, 203–208.

Luchsinger, J. A., Tang, M. X., Siddiqui, M., Shea, S., & Mayeux, R. (2004). Alcohol intake and risk of dementia. *Journal of the American Geriatrics Society, 52*, 540–546.

Lucki, I., & O'Leary, O. F. (2004). Distinguishing roles for norepinephrine and serotonin in the behavioral effects of antidepressant drugs. *Journal of Clinical Psychiatry, 65, Supplement 4*, 11–24.

Luk, S. L., Leung, P. W., & Lee, P. L. (1988). Conners' Teacher Rating Scale in Chinese children in Hong Kong. *Journal of Child Psychology and Psychiatry, 29*, 165–174.

Lundh, L. G., Thulin, U., Czyzykow, S., & Ost, L. G. (1998). Recognition bias for safe faces in panic disorder with agoraphobia. *Behaviour Research and Therapy, 36*, 323–337.

Luria, A. R. (1970). Functional organization of the brain. *Scientific American, 222*, 66–78.

Luria, A. R. (1980). *Higher cortical functions in man.* New York: Basic Books.

Lustman, P. J., Clouse, R. E., & Freedland, K. E. (1998). Management of major depression in adults with diabetes: Implications of recent clinical trials. *Seminars in Clinical Neuropsychiatry, 3*, 102–114.

Lyoo, I. K., Lee, D. W., Kim, Y. S., Kong, S. W., & Kwon, J. S. (2001). Patterns of temperament and character in subjects with obsessive-compulsive disorder. *Journal of Clinical Psychiatry, 62*, 637–641.

Lyoo, I. K., Noam, G. G., Lee, C. K., Lee, H. K., Kennedy, B. P., & Renshaw, P. F. (1996). The corpus callosum and lateral ventricles in children with attention-deficit hyperactivity disorder: A brain magnetic resonance imaging study. *Biological Psychiatry, 40*, 1060–1063.

Ma, Y., Feigin, A., Dhawan, V., Fukunda, M., Shi, Q., Greene, P., et al. (2002). Dyskinesia after fetal cell transplantation for Parkinsonism: A PET study. *Annals of Neurology, 52*, 628–634.

Mac Master, F. P., Keshavan, M. S., Dick, E. L., & Rosenberg, D. R. (1999). Corpus callosal signal intensity in treatment-naive pediatric obsessive compulsive disorders. *Progress in Neuro-Psychopharmacology & Biological Psychiatry, 23*, 601–612.

Macdonald, S., Halliday, J., MacEwan, T., Sharkery, V., Farrington, S., Wall, S., et al. (2003). Nithsdale schizophrenia surveys 24: Sexual dysfunction. *British Journal of Psychiatry, 182*, 50–56.

Machado, C. J., & Bachevalier, J. (2003). Non-human primate models of childhood psychopathology: The promise and the limitations. *Journal of Child Psychology and Psychiatry, 44*, 64–87.

MacKinnon, D. F., Zandi, P. P., Cooper, J., Potash, J. B., Simpson, S. G., Gershon, E., et al. (2002). Comorbid bipolar disorder and panic disorder in families with a high prevalence of bipolar disorder. *American Journal of Psychiatry, 159*, 30–35.

Maddock, R. J, Buonocore, M. H., Kile, S. J., & Garrett, A. S. (2003). Brain regions showing increased activation by threat-related words in panic disorder. *Neuroreport, 14*, 325–328.

Maddux, J. F., & Desmond, D. P. (2000). Addiction or dependence? *Addiction, 95*, 661–665.

Madsen, T. M., Treschow, A., Bengzon, J., Bolwig, T. G., Lindvall, O., & Tingström, A. (2000). Increased neurogenesis in a model of electroconvulsive therapy. *Biological Psychiatry, 47*, 1043–1049.

Maes, M., Scharpé, S., Van Grootel, L., Uyttenbroeck, W., Cooreman, W., Cosyns, P., et al. (1992). Higher alpha 1-antitrypsin, haptoglobin, ceruloplasmin and lower retinol binding protein plasma levels during depression: Further evidence for the existence of an inflammatory response during that illness. *Journal of Affective Disorders, 24*, 183–192.

Maes, M., & Smith, R. S. (1998). Fatty acids, cytokines, and major depression. *Biological Psychiatry, 43*, 313–314.

Maestrini, E., Lai, C., Marlow, A., Matthews, N., Wallace, S., Bailey, A., et al. (1999). Serotonin transporter (5-HTT) and gamma-aminobutyric acid receptor subunit beta3 (GABRB3) gene polymorphisms are not associated with autism in the IMGSA families. International Molecular Genetic Study of Autism Consortium. *American Journal of Medical Genetics, 88*, 492–496.

Maestro, S., Muratori, F., Cavallaro, M. C., Pei, F., Stern, D., Golse, B., et al. (2002). Attentional skills during the first 6 months of age in autism spectrum disorders. *Journal of the American Academy of Child and Adolescent Psychiatry, 41*, 1239–1245.

Maestu, F., Quesney, M. F., Ortiz, A. T., Fernandez, L. A., Amo, C., Campo, P., et al. (2003). Cognition and neural networks, a new perspective based on functional neuroimaging. *Revista de neurologia, 37*, 962–966.

Maggini, C., Ampollini, P., Gariboldi, S., Cella, P. L., Peqlizza, L., & Marchesi, C. (2001). The Parma High School Epidemiological Survey: Obsessive-compulsive symptoms. *Acta Psychiatrica Scandinavica, 103*, 441–446.

Magnusson, P., Smari, J., Gretarsdottir, H., & Pranadardottir, H. (1999). Attention-deficit/hyperactivity symptoms in Icelandic school children: Assessment with the Attention Deficit/hyperactivity Rating Scale-IV. *Scandinavian Journal of Psychology, 40*, 301–306.

Mahendra, N., & Arkin, S. (2003). Effects of four years of exercise, language, and social interventions on Alzheimer discourse. *Journal of Communication Disorders, 36*, 395–422.

Maher, B. S., Marazita, M. L., Zubenko, W. N., Spiker, D. G., Giles, D. E., Kaplan, B. B., et al. (2002). Genetic segregation analysis of recurrent early-onset major depression: Evidence for single major locus transmission. *American Journal of Medical Genetics, 114*, 214–221.

Mahmood, T., & Silverstone, T. (2001). Serotonin and bipolar disorder. *Journal of Affective Disorders, 66*, 1–11.

Maia, A. F., Pinto, A. S., Barbosa, E. R., Menezes, P. R., & Miguel, E. C. (2003). Obsessive-compulsive symptoms, obsessive-compulsive disorder, and related disorders in Parkinson's disease. *Journal of Neuropsychiatry and Clinical Neurosciences, 15*, 371–374.

Maj, M. (2003). The effect of lithium in bipolar disorder: A review of recent research evidence. *Bipolar Disorder, 5*, 180–188.

Maki, P. M., & Resnick, S. M. (2000). Longitudinal effects of estrogen replacement therapy on PET cerebral blood flow and cognition. *Neurobiology of Aging, 21*, 373–383.

Maki, P. M., Zonderman, A. B., & Resnick, S. M. (2001). Enhanced verbal memory in nondemented elderly women receiving hormone-replacement therapy. *American Journal of Psychiatry, 158*, 227–233.

Malaspina, D., Harkavy-Friedman, J., Corcoran, C., Mujica-Parodi, L., Printz, D., Gorman, J. M., & van Heertum, R. (2004). Resting neural activity distinguishes subgroups of schizophrenia patients. *Biological Psychiatry, 56*, 931–937.

Malaspina, D., Harlap, S., Fennig, S., Heiman, D., Hahon, D., Feldman, D., et al. (2001). Advancing paternal age and the risk of schizophrenia. *Archives of General Psychiatry, 58*, 361–367.

Maldonado, R. (2003). The neurobiology of addiction. *Journal of Neurotransmission, 66*, 1–14.

Maletzky, B., McFarland, B., & Burt, A. (1994). Refractory obsessive compulsive disorder and ECT. *Convulsive Therapy, 10*, 34–42.

Malison, R. T., McDougle, C. J., van Dyck, C. H., Scahill, L., Baldwin, R. M., Seibyl, J. P., et al. (1995). [123I]beta-CIT SPECT imaging of striatal dopamine transporter binding in Tourette's disorder. *American Journal of Psychiatry, 152*, 1359–1361.

Malison, R. T., Price, L. H., Berman, R., van Dyck, C. H., Pelton, G. H., Carpenter, L., et al. (1998). Reduced brain serotonin transporter availability in major depression as measured by [123I]-2 beta-carbomethoxy-3 beta-(4-iodophenyl)tropane and single photon emission computed tomography. *Biological Psychiatry, 44*, 1090–1098.

Malizia, A. L. (1999). What do brain imaging studies tell us about anxiety disorders? *Journal of Psychopharmacology, 13*, 372–378.

Malizia, A. L., Cunningham, V. J., Bell, C. J., Liddle, P. F., Jones, T., & Nutt, D. J. (1998). Decreased brain GABA(A)-benzodiazepine receptor binding in panic disorder: Preliminary results from a quantitative PET study. *Archives of General Psychiatry, 55*, 715–720.

Malla, A. K., Norman, R. M. G., Manchanda, R. M., Ahmed, R., Scholten, D., Harricharan, R., et al. (2002). One year outcome in first episode psychosis: Influence of DUP and other predictors. *Schizophrenia Research, 54*, 231–242.

Mallet, L., Mesnage, V., Houeto, J. L., Pelissolo, A., Yelnik, J., Behar, C., et al. (2002). Compulsions, Parkinson's disease, and stimulation. *Lancet, 360*, 1302–1304.

Maltête, D., Navarro, S., Welter, M. L., Roche, S., Bonnet, A. M., Houeto, J. L., et al. (2004). Subthalamic stimulation in Parkinson disease: With or without anesthesia? *Archives of Neurology, 61*, 390–392.

Mamo, D. C., Sweet, R. A., Chengappa, K. N. R., Reddy, R. R., & Jeste, D. V. (2002). The effect of age on the pharmacological management of ambulatory patients treated with depot neuroleptic medications for schizophrenia and related psychotic disorders. *International Journal of Geriatric Psychiatry, 17*, 1012–1017.

Mandel, S., Grunblatt, E., Riederer, P., Gerlach, M., Levites, Y., & Youdim, M. B. (2003). Neuroprotective strategies in Parkinson's disease: An update on progress. *CNS Drugs, 17*, 729–762.

Mandzia, J., & Black, S. E. (2001). Neuroimaging and behavior: Probing brain behavior relationships in the 21st century. *Current Neurological and Neuroscience Reports, 1*, 553–561.

Manes, F., Piven, J., Vrancic, D., Nanclares, V., Plebst, C., & Starkstein, S. E. (1999). An MRI study of the corpus callosum and cerebellum in mentally retarded autistic individuals. *Journal of Neuropsychiatry and Clinical Neurosciences, 11*, 470–474.

Mangone, C. A., Gorelick, P. B., Hier, D. B., & Ganellen, R. J. (1990). MRI in the elderly. *Neurology, 40*, 1011–1012.

Manjaly, Z. M., Marshall, J. C., Stephan, K. E., Gurd, J. M., Zilles, K., & Fink, G. R. (2003). In search of the hidden: An fMRI study with implications for the study of patients with autism and with acquired brain injury. *Neuroimage, 19*, 674–683.

Manji, H. (2003). Depression, III. *American Journal of Psychiatry, 160*, 24.

Manji, H. K., & Chen, G. (2000). Post-receptor signaling pathways in the pathophysiology and treatment of mood disorders. *Current Psychiatry Report, 2*, 479–489.

Manji, H. K., & Lenox, R. H. (2000). The nature of bipolar disorder. *Journal of Clinical Psychiatry, 61*, 42–57.

Manji, H. K., Quiroz, J. A., Sporn, J., Payne, J. L., Denicoff, K., Gray, N. A., et al. (2003). Enhancing neuronal plasticity and cellular resilience to develop novel, improved therapeutics for difficult-to-treat depression. *Biological Psychiatry, 53*, 707–742.

Mann, D. M., Takeuchi, A., Sato, S., Cairns, N. J., Lantos, P. L., Rossor, M. N., et al. (2001). Cases of Alzheimer's disease due to deletion of exon 9 of the presenilin-1 gene show an unusual but characteristic beta-amyloid pathology known as "cotton wool" plaques. *Neuropathology and Applied Neurobiology, 27*, 189–196.

Mao, J. (1999). NMDA and opioid receptors: Their interactions and antinociception, tolerance, and neuroplasticity. *Brain Research Reviews, 30*, 289–304.

Maraganore, D. M., O'Connor, M. K., Bower, J. H., Kuntz, K. M., McDonnell, S. K., Schaid, D. J., et al. (1999). Detection of preclinical Parkinson disease in at-risk family members with use of [123I]beta-CIT and SPECT: An exploratory study. *Mayo Clinic Proclamations, 74*, 681–685.

Marangell, L. B., Martinez, J. M., Zboyan, H. A., Kertz, B., Seung Kim, H. F., & Puyear, L. J. (2003). A double-blind, placebo-controlled study of omega-3 fatty acid docosahexaenoic acid in the treatment of major depression. *American Journal of Psychiatry, 160*, 996–998.

Marangell, L. B., Rush, A. J., George, M. S., Sackeim, H. A., Johnson, C. R., Hussain, M. M., et al. (2002). Vagus nerve stimulation (VNS) for major depressive episodes: One year outcomes. *Biological Psychiatry, 51*, 280–287.

March, J. S, Mulle, K., & Herbel, B. (1994). Behavioral psychotherapy for children and adolescents with obsessive-compulsive disorder: An open trial of a new protocol-driven treatment package. *Journal of the American Academy of Child and Adolescent Psychiatry, 33*, 333–341.

Marder, K., Tang, M. X., Alfaro, B., Mejia, H., Cote, L., Louis, E., et al. (1999). Risk of Alzheimer's disease in relatives of Parkinson's disease patients with and without dementia. *Neurology, 52*, 719–724.

Marder, S. R., McQuade, R. D., Stock, E., Kaplita, S., Marcus, R., Safferman, A., et al. (2003). Aripiprazole in the treatment of schizophrenia: Safety and tolerability in short-term, placebo-controlled trials. *Schizophrenia Research, 61*, 123–136.

Marek, G. J. (2002). Preclinical pharmacology of mGlu2/3 receptor agonists: novel agents for schizophrenia? *Current Drug Targets—CNS and Neurological Disorders, 1*, 215–225.

Marek, K. L., Seibyl, J. P., Zoghbi, S. S., Zea-Ponce, Y., Baldwin, R. M., Fussell, B., et al. (1996). [123I] beta-CIT/SPECT imaging demonstrated bilateral loss of dopamine transporters in hemi-Parkinson's disease. *Neurology, 46*, 231–237.

Margolis, E. B., Hjelmstad, G. O., Bonci, A., & Fields, H. L. (2003). Kappa-opioid agonists directly inhibit midbrain dopaminergic neurons. *Journal of Neuroscience, 23*, 9981–9986.

Marks, I. (1997). Behaviour therapy for obsessive-compulsive disorder: A decade of progress. *Canadian Journal of Psychiatry, 42*, 1021–1027.

Marrazzi, M. A., Bacon, J. P., Kinzie, J., & Luby, E. D. (1995). Naltrexone use in the treatment of anorexia nervosa and bulimia nervosa. *International Clinical Psychopharmacology, 10*, 163–172.

Marriott, L. K., Hauss-Wegrzyniak, B., Benton, R. S., Vraniak, P. D., & Wenk, G. L. (2002). Long-term estrogen therapy worsens the behavioral and neuropathological consequences of chronic brain inflammation. *Behavioral Neuroscience, 116*, 902–911.

Martin, A., Scahill, L., Klin, A., & Volkmar, F. R. (1999). Higher-functioning pervasive developmental disorders: Rates and patterns of psychotropic drug use. *Journal of the American Academy of Child and Adolescent Psychiatry, 38*, 923–931.

Martin, J. H. (1991). The collective electrical behavior of cortical neurons: The electroencephalogram and the mechanisms of epilepsy. In E. R. Kandel, J. H. Schwartz, & T. M. Jessell (Eds.), *Principles of neural science* (3rd ed., pp. 778–791). Norwalk, CT: Appleton & Lange.

Martin, J. L., Barbanoj, M. J., Schlaepfer, T. E., Thompson, E., Perez, V., & Kulisevsky, J. (2003). Repetitive transcranial magnetic stimulation for the treatment of depresssion. Systematic review and meta-analysis. *British Journal of Psychiatry, 182,* 480–491.

Martin, K. C., & Kandel, E. R. (1996). *Neuron, 17,* 567–570.

Martin, P., & Albers, M. (1995). Cerebellum and schizophrenia: A selective review. *Schizophrenia Bulletin, 21,* 241–250.

Martini, C., Trincavelli, M. L., Tuscano, D., Carmassi, C., Ciapparelli, A., Lucacchini, A., et al. (2004). Serotonin-mediated phosphorylation of extracellular regulated kinases in platelets of patients with panic disorder versus controls. *Neurochemistry International, 44,* 627–639.

Martini, F. H. (1998). *Fundamentals of anatomy and physiology* (4th ed.). Upper Saddle River, NJ: Prentice-Hall.

Martinsen, E. W., Hoffart, A., & Solberg, O. (1989). Comparing aerobic with nonaerobic forms of exercise in the treatment of clinical depression: A randomized trial. *Comparative Psychiatry, 30,* 324–331.

Martis, B., Alam, D., Dowd, S. M., Hill, S. K., Sharma, R. P., Rosen, C., et al. (2003). Neurocognitive effects of repetitive transcranial magnetic stimulation in severe major depression. *Clinical Neurophysiology, 114,* 1125–1132.

Marx, D. (2000). Drug shows promise for advanced disease. *Science, 289,* 375–376.

Maschke, M., Gomez, C. M., Tuite, P. J., & Konczak, J. (2003). Dysfunction of the basal ganglia, but not the cerebellum, impairs kinaesthesia. *Brain, 126,* 2312–2322.

Masi, G., Cosenza, A., Mucci, M., & Brovedani, P. (2003). A 3-year naturalistic study of 53 preschool children with pervasive developmental disorders treated with risperidone. *Journal of Clinical Psychiatry, 64,* 1039–1047.

Masi, G., Perugi, G., Toni, C., Millepiedi, S., Mucci, M., Bertini, N., et al. (2004). Obsessive-compulsive bipolar comorbidity: Focus on children and adolescents. *Journal of Affective Disorders, 78,* 175–183.

Mason, B. J., Goodman, A. M., Dixon, R. M., Abdel Hameed, M. H., Hulot, T., Wesnes, K., et al. (2002). A pharmacokinetic and pharmacodynamic drug interaction study of acamprosate and naltrexone. *Neuropsychopharmacology, 27,* 596–606.

Massagli, T. L., Fann, J. R., Burington, B. E., Jaffe, K. M., Katon, W. J., & Thompson, R. S. (2004). Psychiatric illness after mild traumatic brain injury in children. *Archives of Physical Medicine and Rehabilitation, 85,* 1428–1434.

Massana, G., Gastó, C., Junqué, C., Mercader, J. M., Gómez, B., Massana, J., et al. (2002). Reduced levels of creatine in the right medial temporal lobe region of panic disorder patients detected with (1)H magnetic resonance spectroscopy. *NeuroImage, 16,* Part 1, 836–842.

Massana, G., Serra-Grabulosa, J. M., Salgado-Pineda, P., Gastó, C., Junqué, C., Massana, J., et al. (2003a). Amygdalar atrophy in panic disorder patients detected by volumetric magnetic resonance imaging. *NeuroImage, 19,* 80–90.

Massana, G., Serra-Grabulosa, J. M., Salgado-Pineda, P., Gastó, C., Junqué, C., Massana, J., et al. (2003b). Parahippocampal gray matter density in panic disorder: A voxel-based morphometric study. *American Journal of Psychiatry, 160,* 566–568.

Massou, J. M., Trichard, C., Attar-Levy, D., Feline, A., Corruble, E., Beaufils, B., et al. (1997). Frontal 5-HT2A receptors studied in depressive patients during chronic treatment by selective serotonin reuptake inhibitors. *Psychopharmacology, 133,* 99–101.

Mathalon, D. H., Sullivan, E. V., O., Lim, K., & Pfefferbaum, A. (2001). Progressive brain volume changes and the clinical course of schizophrenia in men: A longitudinal magnetic resonance imaging study. *Archives of General Psychiatry, 58,* 148–157.

Mathews, C. A., Herrera Amighetti, L. D., Lowe, T. L., vam de Wetering, B. J., Freimer, N. B., & Reus, V. I. (2001). Cultural influences on diagnosis and perception of Tourette syndrome in Costa Rica. *Journal of the American Academy of Child and Adolescent Psychiatry, 40,* 456–463.

Mathews, C. A., & Reus, V. I. (2003). Genetic linkage in bipolar disorder. *CNS Spectrum, 8,* 891–904.

Matochik, J. A., Liebenauer, L. L., King, A. C., Szymanski, H. V., Cohen, R. M., & Zmetkin, A. J. (1994). Cerebral glucose metabolism in adults with attention deficit hyperactivity disorder after chronic stimulant treatment. *American Journal of Psychiatry, 151,* 658–664.

Matochik, J. A., London, E. D., Eldreth, D. A., Cadet, J. L., & Bolla, K. I. (2003). Frontal cortical tissue composition in abstinent cocaine abusers: A magnetic resonance imaging study. *Neuroimage, 19,* 1095–1102.

Matsumoto, N., David, D. E., Johnson, E. W., Konecki, D., Burmester, J. K., Ledbetter, D. H., et al. (2000). Breakpoint sequences of an 1;8 translocation in a family with Gilles de la Tourette syndrome. *European Journal of Human Genetics, 8,* 875–883.

Matsunaga, H., Kiriike, N., Iwasaki, Y., Miyata, A., Yamagami, S., & Kaye, W. H. (1999). Clinical characteristics in patients with anorexia nervosa and obsessive-compulsive disorder. *Psychological Medicine, 29,* 407–414.

Matsuo, K., Kato, N., & Kato, T. (2002). Decreased cerebral haemodynamic response to cognitive and physiological tasks in mood disorders as shown by near-infrared spectroscopy. *Psychological Medicine, 32,* 1029–1037.

Mattes, J. A., & Gittelman, R. (1981). Effects of artificial food colorings in children with hyperactive symptoms. A critical review and results of a controlled study. *Archives of General Psychiatry, 38,* 714–718.

Matthews, K., Bell, J. S., & Fowlie, D. G. (1996). Panic symptoms and cerebral electrical disturbance: Restoration of function with carbamazepine. *Behavioral Neurology, 9,* 37–40.

Mattila, P. M., Röyttä, M., Lönnberg, P., Marjamäki, P., Helenius, H., & Rinne, J. O. (2001). Choline acetytransferase activity and striatal dopamine receptors in Parkinson's disease in relation to cognitive impairment. *Acta Neuropathologica, 102,* 160–166.

Matur, Z., & Ucok, A. (2003). Quetiapine treatment in a patient with Tourette's syndrome, obsessive-compulsive disorder and drug-induced mania. *Israeli Journal of Psychiatry Related Sciences, 40,* 150–152.

Matus, A. (2000). Actin-based plasticity in dendritic spines. *Science, 290,* 754–758.

Maubach, K. (2003). GABA(A) receptor subtype selective cognitive enhancers. *Current Drug Targets—CNS and Neurological Disorders, 2,* 233–239.

Max, J. E., Fox, P. T., Lancaster, J. L., Kochunov, P., Mathews, K., Manes, F. F., Robertson, B. A. M., et al. (2002). Putamen lesions and the development of attention-deficit/hyperactivity symptomatology. *Journal of the American Academy of Child and Adolescent Psychology, 41,* 563–571.

Mayberg, H. S., Brannan, S. K., Tekell, J. L., Silva, J. A., Mahurin, R. K., McGinnis, S., et al. (2000). Regional metabolic effects of fluoxetine in major depression: Serial changes and relationship to clinical response. *Biological Psychiatry, 48,* 830–843.

Mayberg, H. S., Silva, J. A., Brannan, S. K., Mahurin, R. K., McGinnis, S., & Jerabek, P. A. (2002). The functional neuroanatomy of the placebo effect. *American Journal of Psychiatry, 159,* 728–735.

Mayer, P., & Hollt, V. (2001). Allelic and somatic variations in the endogenous opioid system of humans. *Pharmacological Therapy, 91,* 167–177.

Mayeux, R., Stern, Y., Cote, L., & Williams, J. B. (1984). Altered serotonin metabolism in depressed patients with Parkinson's disease. *Neurology, 34,* 642–646.

Maynard, C. J., Cappai, R., Volitakis, I., Cherny, R. A., White, A. R., Beyreuther, K., et al. (2002). Overexpression of Alzheimer's disease amyloid-beta opposes the age-dependent elevations of brain copper and iron. *Journal of Biological Chemistry, 277,* 44670–44676.

Maziade, M., Morette, C., Cayer, M., Roy, M. A., Szatmari, P., et al. (2000). Prolongation of brainstem auditory-evoked responses in autistic probands and theit unaffected relatives. *Archives of General Psychiatry, 57,* 1077–1083.

Mazzone, P. (2003). Deep brain stimulation in Parkinson's disease: Bilateral implantation of globus pallidus and subthalamic nucleus. *Journal of Neurosurgical Science, 47,* 47–51.

McCabe, S. (2000). Rapid detox: Understanding new treatment approaches for the addicted patient. *Perspectives in Psychiatric Care, 36,* 113–120.

McCarley, R. W., Wible, C. G., Frumin, M., Hirayasu, Y., Levitt, J. J., Fischer, I. A., & Shenton, M. E. (1999). MRI anatomy of schizophrenia. *Biological Psychiatry, 45,* 1099–1119.

McClung, C. A., & Nestler, E. J. (2003). Regulation of gene expression and cocaine reward by CREB and DeltaFosB. *Nature Neuroscience, 6,* 1208–1215.

McConnell, S. R. (2002). Interventions to facilitate social interaction for young children with autism: Review of available research and recommendations for educational intervention and future research. *Journal of Autism and Developmental Disorders, 32,* 351–372.

McConville, B. J., Fogelson, M. H., Norman, A. B., Klykylo, W. M., Manderscheid, P. Z., Parker, K. W., et al. (1991). Nicotine potentiation of haloperidol in reducing tic frequency in Tourette's disorder. *American Journal of Psychiatry, 148,* 793–794.

McCoy, P. A., Shao, Y., Wolpert, C. M., Donnelly, S. L., Ashley-Koch, A., Abel, H. L., et al. (2002). No association between the WNT2 gene and autistic disorder. *American Journal of Medical Genetics, 114,* 106–109.

McCracken, J. T., McGough, J., Shah, B., Cronin, P., Hong, D., Aman, M. G., et al. (2002). Risperidone in children with autism and serious behavioral problems. *New England Journal of Medicine, 347,* 314–321.

McCracken, J. T., Smalley, S. L., McGough, J. J., Crawford, L., Del'Homme, M., Cantor, R. M., et al. (2000). Evidence for linkage of a tandem duplication polymorphism upstream of the dopamine D4 receptor gene (DRD4) with attention deficit hyperactivity disorder (ADHD). *Molecular Psychiatry, 5,* 531–536.

McCurry, S. M., Gibbons, L. E., Logsdon, R. G., & Teri, L. (2004). Anxiety and nighttime behavioral disturbances. Awakenings in patients with Alzheimer's disease. *Journal of Gerontological Nursing, 30,* 12–20.

McDougle, C., & Posey, D. (2002). Genetics of childhood disorders: XLIV. Autism, Part 3: Psychopharmacology of autism. *Journal of the American Academy of Child and Adolescent Psychiatry, 41,* 1380–1383.

McDougle, C. J., Epperson, C. N., Pelton, G. H., Wasylink, S., & Price, L. H. (2000). A double-blind, placebo-controlled study of risperidone addition in serotonin reuptake inhibitor-refractory obsessive-compulsive disorder. *Archives of General Psychiatry, 57*, 794–801.

McDougle, C. J., Kresch, L. E., Goodman, W. K., Naylor, S. T., Volkmar, F. R., Cohen, D. J., et al. (1995). A case-controlled study of repetitive thoughts and behavior in adults with autistic disorder and obsessive-compulsive disorder. *American Journal of Psychiatry, 152*, 772–777.

McEachern, J. C., & Shaw, C. A. (2001). Revisiting the LTP orthodoxy: Plasticity versus pathology. In C. Holscher (Ed.), *Neural mechanisms of memory formation: Concepts of long-term potentiation and beyond* (pp. 26–293). Cambridge, England: Cambridge University Press.

McEvoy, J. P., & Allen, T. B. (2002). The importance of nicotinic acetylcholine receptors in bipolar disorder and Tourette's syndrome. *Current Drug Targets—CNS and Neurological Disorders, 1*, 433–442.

McEwen, B. S., & Sapolsky, R. M. (1995). Stress and cognitive function. *Current Opinion in Neurobiology, 5*, 205–216.

McFie, J., & Zanwill, O. L. (1960). Visual-constructive disabilities associated with lesions of the left cerebral hemisphere. *Brain, 83*, 243–260.

McGlashan, T. H., & Hoffman, R. E. (2000). Schizophrenia as a disorder of developmentally reduced synaptic connectivity. *Archives of General Psychiatry, 57*, 637–648.

McGorry, P. D., Yung, A. R., Phillips, L. J., Yuen, H. P., Francey, S., Cosgrave, E. M., et al. (2002). Randomized controlled trial of interventions designed to reduce the risk of progression to first-episode psychosis in a clinical sample with subthreshold symptoms. *Archives of General Psychiatry, 59*, 921–928.

McGrath, M. J., Campbell, K. M., Parks, C. R., & Burton, F. H. (2000). Glutamatergic drugs exacerbate symptomatic behavior in a transgenic model of comorbid Tourette's syndrome and obsessive-compulsive disorder. *Brain Research, 877*, 23–30.

McGuffin, P., & Mawson, D. (1980). Obsessive-compulsive neurosis: Two identical twin pairs. *British Journal of Psychiatry, 137*, 285–287.

McGuffin, P., Rijsdijk, F., Andrew, M., Sham, P., Katz, R., & Cardno, A. (2003). The heritability of bipolar affective disorder and the genetic relationship to unipolar disorder. *Archives of General Psychiatry, 60*, 497–502.

McGuire, P. K., Paulesu, E., Frackowiak, R. S. J., & Frith, C. D. (1996). Brain activity during stimulus independent thought. *Neuroreport, 7*, 2095–2099.

McGuire, P. K., Silbersweig, D. A., Murray, R. M., David, A. S., Frackowiak, R. S. J., & Frith, C. D. (1996). The functional anatomy of inner speech and auditory imagery. *Psychological Medicine, 26*, 29–38.

McIntire, S. L., Reimer, R. J., Schuske, K., Edwards, R. H., & Jorgensen, E. M. (1997). Identification and characterization of the vesicular GABA transporter. *Nature, 389*, 870–876.

McIntyre, C. C., Mori, S., Sherman, D. L., Thakor, N. V., & Vitek, J. L. (2004). Electric field and stimulating influence generated by deep brain stimulation of the subthalamic nucleus. *Clinical Neurophysiology, 115*, 589–595.

McKnight Investigators. (2003). Risk factors for the onset of eating disorders in adolescent girls: Result of the McKnight longitudinal risk factor study. *American Journal of Psychiatry, 160*, 248–254.

McLaughlin, T., Geissler, E. C., & Wan, G. J. (2003). Comorbidities and associated treatment charges in patients with anxiety disorders. *Pharmacotherapy, 23*, 1251–1256.

McMahon, F. J., Simpson, S. G., McInnis, M. G., Badner, J. A., MacKinnon, D. F., & DePaulo, R. (2001). Linkage of bipolar disorder to chromosome 18q and the validity of bipolar II disorder. *Archives of General Psychiatry, 58*, 1025–1031.

McMahon, W. M., Carter, A. S., Fredine, N., & Pauls, D. L. (2003). Children at familial risk for Tourette's disorder: Child and parent diagnoses. *American Journal of Medical Genetics, 121B*, 105–111.

McNamara, B., Ray, J. L., Arthurs, O. J., & Boniface, S. (2001). Transcranial magnetic stimulation for depression and other psychiatric disorders. *Psychological Medicine, 31*, 1141–1146.

Meador-Woodruff, J. H., Hogg, A. J. Jr., & Smith, R. E. (2001). Striatal ionotropic glutamate receptor expression in schizophrenia, bipolar disorder, and major depressive disorder. *Brain Research Bulletin, 55*, 631–640.

Meana, J. J., Gonzalez-Maeso, J., Garcia-Sevilla, J. A., & Guimon. J. (2000). Mu-opioid receptor and alpha2-adrenoceptor agonist stimulation of [35S]GTPgammaS binding to G-proteins in postmortem brains of opioid addicts. *Molecular Psychiatry, 5*, 308–315.

Mednick, S. A., Machon, R. A., & Huttunen, M. O. (1990). An update on Helsinki influenza project. *Archives of General Psychiatry, 47*, 292.

Mega, M. S., Cummings, J. L., O'Connor, S. M., Dinov, I. D., Reback, E., Felix, J., et al. (2001). Cognitive and metabolic responses to metrifonate therapy in Alzheimer's disease. *Journal of Geriatric Psychiatry and Neurology, 14*, 101–108.

Meguro, K., Ishii, H., Yamaguchi, S., Ishizaki, J., Schimada, M., Sato, M., et al. (2002). Prevalence of dementia and dementing diseases in Japan: The Tajiri project. *Archives of Neurology, 59*, 1109–1114.

Mellick, G. D., Buchman, D. D., Silburn, P. A., Chan, D. K., Le Couteur, D. G., Law, L. K., et al. (2000). The monoamine oxidase B gene GT repeat polymorphism and Parkinson's disease in a Chinese population. *Journal of Neurology, 247*, 52–55.

Mellman, L. A., & Gorman, J. M. (1984). Successful treatment of obsessive-compulsive disorder with ECT. *American Journal of Psychiatry, 141*, 596–597.

Meltzer, H. Y., Alphs, L., Green, A. I., Altamura, A. C., Anand, R., Bertoldi, A., et al. (2003). Clozapine treatment for suicidality in schizophrenia: International suicide prevention trial (InterSePT). *Archives of General Psychiatry, 60*, 82–91.

Mendez, I., Dagher, A., Hong, M., Gaudet, P., Weerasinghe, S., McAlister, V., et al. (2002). Simultaneous intrastriatal and intranigral fetal dopaminergic grafts in patients with Parkinson disease: Report of three cases. *Journal of Neurosurgery, 96*, 589–596.

Mendez, I., Dagher, A., Hong, M., Hebb, A., Gaudet, P., Law, A., et al. (2000). Enhancement of survival of stored dopaminergic cells and promotion of graft survival by exposure of human fetal nigral tissue to glial cell line-derived neurotrophic factor in patients with Parkinson's disease. Report of two cases and technical considerations. *Journal of Neurosurgery, 92*, 863–869.

Mendez, M. F., O'Connor, S. M., & Lim, G. T. H. (2004). Hypersexuality after right pallidotomy for Parkinson's disease. *Journal of Neuropsychiatry and Clinical Neuroscience, 16*, 37–40.

Mendis, T., Suchwersky, O., Lang, A., & Gauthier, S. (1999). Management of Parkinson's disease: A review of current and new therapies. *Canadian Journal of Neurological Science, 26*, 89–103.

Menegon, A., Board, P. G., Blackburn, A. C., Mellick, G. D., & Le Couteur, D. G. (1998). Parkinson's disease, pesticides, and glutathione transferase polymorphisms. *Lancet, 352*, 1344–1346.

Menon, V., Anagnoson, R. T., Glover, G. H., & Pfefferbaum, A. (2001). Functional magnetic resonance imaging evidence for disrupted basal ganglia function in schizophrenia. *American Journal of Psychiatry, 158*, 646–649.

Menza, M. A. (2000). The personality associated with Parkinson's disease. *Current Psychiatry Reports, 2*, 421–426.

Menza, M. A., Robertson-Hoffman, D. E., & Bonapace, A. S. (1993). Parkinson's disease and anxiety: Comorbidity with depression. *Biological Psychiatry, 34*, 465–470.

Merali, Z., Du, L., Hrdina, P., Palkovits, M., Faludi, G., Poulter, M. O., et al. (2004). Dysregulation in the suicide brain: mRNA expression of corticotrophin-releasing hormone receptors and GABA(A) receptor subunits in frontal cortical brain region. *Journal of Neuroscience, 24*, 1478–1485.

Merlo, M. C. G., Hofer, H., Gekle, W., Berger, G., Ventura, J., Panhuber, I., et al. (2002). Risperdone, 2mg/day vs. 4 mg/day, in first-episode acutely psychotic patients: Treatment efficacy and effects on fine motor functioning. *Journal of Clinical Psychiatry, 63*, 885–891.

Merrick, J., Kandel, I., & Morad, M. (2004). Trends in autism. *International Journal of Adolescent Medicine and Health, 16*, 75–78.

Merzenich, M. M, Jenkins, W. M., Johnston, P., Schreiner, C., Miller, S. L., & Tallal, P. (1996). Temporal processing deficits of language-learning impaired children ameliorated by training. *Science, 271*, 77–81.

Messaoudi, E., Bardsen, K., Srebro, B., & Bramham, C. R. (1998). Acute intrahippocampal infusion of BDNF induces lasting potentiation of synaptic transmission in the rat dentate gyrus. *Journal of Neurophysiology, 79*, 496–499.

Metin, O., Yazici, K., Tot, S., & Yazici, A. E. (2003). Amisulpiride augmentation in treatment resistant obsessive-compulsive disorder: An open trial. *Human Psychopharmacology, 18*, 463–467.

Meuret, A. E., Wilhelm, F. H., & Roth, W. T. (2004). Respiratory feedback for treating panic disorder. *Journal of Clinical Psychology, 60*, 197–207.

Meyer, J. H., Kapur, S., Houle, S., DaSilva, J., Owczarek, B., Brown, G. M., et al. (1999). Prefrontal cortex 5-HT2 receptors in depression: An [18F]setoperone PET imaging study. *American Journal of Psychiatry, 156*, 1029–1034.

Meyer, J. H., McMain, S., Kennedy, S. H., Korman, L., Brown, G. M., et al. (2003). Dysfunctional attitudes and 5-HT2 receptors during depression and self-harm. *American Journal of Psychiatry, 160*, 90–99.

Meyer, J. H., Swinson, R., Kennedy, S. H., Houle, S., & Brown, G. M. (2000). Increased left posterior parietal-temporal cortex activation after D-fenfluramine in women with panic disorder. *Psychiatry Research, 98*, 133–143.

Meyer, P., Bohnen, N. I., Minoshima, S., Koeppe, R. A., Wernette, K., Kilbourn, M. R., et al. (1999). Striatal presynaptic monoaminergic vesicles are not increased in Tourette's syndrome. *Neurology, 53*, 371–374.

Micallef, J., & Blin, O. (2001). Neurobiology and clinical pharmacology of obsessive-compulsive disorder. *Clinical Neuropharmacology, 24*, 191–207.

Michael, N., Erfurth, A., Ohrmann, P., Gossling, M., Arolt, V., Heindel, W., et al. (2003). Acute mania is accompanied by elevated glutamate/glutamine levels within the left dorsolateral prefrontal cortex. *Psychopharmacology, 168*, 344–346.

Michalak, E. E., & Lam, R. W. (2002). Breaking the myths: New treatment approaches for chronic depression. *Canadian Journal of Psychiatry, 47*, 635–643.

Michalski, B., & Fahnestock, M. (2003). Pro-brain-derived neurotrophic factor is decreased in parietal cortex in Alzheimer's disease. *Molecular Brain Research, 111*, 148–154.

Michelini, S., Cassano, G. B., Frare, F., & Perugi, G. (1996). Long-term use of benzodiazepines: Tolerance, dependence and chemical problems in anxiety and mood disorders. *Pharmacopsychiatry, 29*, 127–134.

Mielke, R., Zerres, K., Uhlhaas, S., Kessler, J., & Heiss, W. D. (1998). Apolipoprotein E polymorphism influences the cerebral metabolic pattern in Alzheimer's disease. *Neuroscience Letters, 254*, 49–52.

Miguel, E. C., Shavitt, R. G., Ferrao, Y. A., Brotto, S. A., & Diniz, J. B. (2003). How to treat OCD in patients with Tourette syndrome. *Journal of Psychosomatic Research, 55*, 49–57.

Miguel-Hidalgo, J. J., & Rajkowska, G. (2003). Comparison of prefrontal cell pathology between depression and alcohol dependence. *Journal of Psychiatric Research, 37*, 411–420.

Mihailescu, S., & Drucker-Colin, R. (2000). Nicotine, brain nicotinic receptors, and neuropsychiatric disorders. *Archives of Medical Research, 31*, 131–144.

Milev, P., Ho, B. C., Arndt, S., Nopoulos, P., & Andreasen, N. C. (2003). Initial magnetic resonance imaging volumetric brain measurements and outcome in schizophrenia: A prospective longitudinal study with 5–year follow-up. *Biological Psychiatry, 54*, 608–615.

Mill, J., Curran, S., Kent, L., Gould, A., Huckett, L., Richards, S., et al. (2002). Association study of a SNAP-25 microsatellite and attention deficit hyperactivity disorder. *American Journal of Medical Genetics, 114*, 269–271.

Miller, E. (2003). Measles-mumps-rubella vaccine and the development of autism. *Seminars in Pediatric Infectious Diseases, 14*, 199–206.

Miller, H. L., Delgado, P. L., Salomon, R. M., Berman R., Krystal, J. H., Heninger, G. R., et al. (1996). Clinical and biochemical effects of catecholamine depletion on antidepressant-induced remission of depression. *Archives of General Psychiatry, 53*, 117–128.

Miller, L. K. (1999). The savant syndrome: Intellectual impairment and exceptional skill. *Psychological Bulletin, 125*, 31–46.

Miller, N. S., & Greenfeld, A. (2004). Patient characteristics and risk factors for development of dependence on hydrocodone and oxycodone. *American Journal of Therapy, 11*, 26–32.

Miller, N. S., Ninonuevo, F. G., Klamen, D. L., Hoffman, N. G., & Smith, D. E. (1997). Integration and posttreatment variables in predicting results of abstinence-based outpatient treatment after one year. *Journal of Psychoactive Drugs, 29*, 239–248.

Millet, B., Chabane, N., Delorme, R., Leboyer, M., Leroy, S., Poirier, M. F., et al. (2003). Association between the dopamine receptor D4 (DRD4) gene and obsessive-compulsive disorder. *American Journal of Medical Genetics, 116B*, 55–59.

Mills, D. L., Coffey-Corina, S. A., & Neville, H. J. (1993). Language acquisition and cerebral specialization in 20-month old infants. *Journal of Cognitive Neuroscience, 5*, 317–334.

Mills, I. H., Park, G. R., Manara, A. R., & Merssiman, R. J. (1998). Treatment of compulsive behavior in eating disorders with intermittent ketamine infusions. *Quarterly Journal of Medicine, 91*, 493–503.

Millward, C., Ferriter, M., Calver, S., & Connell-Jones, G. (2004). Gluten- and casein-free diets for autistic spectrum disorder. *Cochrane Database of Systematic Reviews*, CD003498.

Milo, T. J., Kaufman, G. E., Barnes, W. E., Konopka, L. M., Crayton, J. W. Ringelstein, J. G., et al. (2001). Changes in regional cerebral blood flow after electroconvulsive therapy for depression. *Journal of ECT, 17*, 15–21.

Mimmack, M. L., Ryan, M., Baba, H., Navarro-Ruiz, J., Iritani, S., Faull, R. L. M., et al. (2002). Gene expression analysis in schizophrenia: Reproducible up-regulation of several members of the apolipoprotein L family located in a high-susceptibility locus for schizophrenia on chromosome 22. *Proceedings of the National Academy of the Sciences, 99*, 4680–4685.

Minami, Y., Yamamoto, R., Nishikouri, M., Fukao, A., & Hisamichi, S. (2000). Mortality and cancer incidence in patients with Parkinson's disease. *Journal of Neurology, 247*, 429–434.

Minett, T. S., Thomas, A., Wilkinson, L. M., Daniel, S. L., Sanders, J., Richardson, J., et al. (2003). What happens when donepezil is suddenly withdrawn? An open label trial in dementia with Lewy bodies and Parkinson's disease with dementia. *International Journal of Geriatric Psychiatry, 18*, 988–993.

Minzer, K., Lee, O., Hong, J. J., & Singer, H. S. (2004). Increased prefrontal D2 protein in Tourette syndrome: A postmortem analysis of frontal cortex and striatum. *Journal of Neurological Science, 219*, 55–61.

Mishizen-Eberz, A. J., Rissman, R. A., Carter, T. L., Ikonomovic, M. D., Wolfe, B. B., & Armstrong, D. M. (2004). Biochemical and molecular studies of NMDA receptor subunits NR1/2A/2B in hippocampal subregions throughout progression of Alzheimer's disease pathology. *Neurobiology of Disease, 15*, 80–92.

Misri, S., & Kostaras, X. (2002). Benefits and risks to mother and infant of drug treatment for postnatal depression. *Drug Safety, 25*, 903–911.

Moceri, V. M., Kukull, W. A., Emanuel, I., van Belle, G., & Larson, E. B. (2000). Early-life risk factors and the development of Alzheimer's disease. *Neurology, 54*, 415–420.

Moellentine, C., Rummans, T., Ahiskog, J. E., Harmsen, W. S., Suman, V. J., O'Connor, M. K., et al. (1998). Effectiveness of ECT in patients with Parkinsonism. *Journal of Neuropsychiatry and Clinical Neuroscience, 10,* 187–193.

Mogi, M., Togari, A., Kondo, T., Mizuno, Y., Komure, O., Kuno, S., et al. (1999). Brain-derived growth factor and nerve growth factor concentrations are decreased in the substantia nigra in Parkinson's disease. *Neuroscience Letters, 270,* 45–48.

Mohler-Kuo, M., Lee, J. E., & Wechsler, H. (2003). Trends in marijuana and other illicit drug use among college students: Results from 4 Harvard School of Public Health College Alcohol Study surveys: 1993–2001. *Journal of American College Health, 52,* 17–24.

Molfese, D. (1984). Auditory evoked responses recorded from 16–month-old human infants to words they did and did not know. *Brain and Language, 22,* 109–127.

Molfese, D. L. (2000). Predicting dyslexia at 8 years of age using neonatal brain responses. *Brain and Language, 72,* 238–245.

Molfese, D. L., Molfese, U. J., Key, A. F., & Kelly, S. D. (2003). Influence of environment on speech-sound discrimination: Findings from a longitudinal study. *Developmental Nuropsychology, 24,* 541–558.

Molina, J. A., Jiménez-Jiménez, F. J., Gomez, P., Vargas, C., Navarro, J. A., Ortí-Pareja, M., et al. (1997). Decreased cerebrospinal fluid levels of neutral and basic amino acids in patients with Parkinson's disease. *Journal of the Neurological Sciences, 150,* 123–127.

Molina, V., Montz, R., Perez-Castejon, M. J., Carreras, J. L., Calcedo, A., & Rubia, F. J. (1995). Cerebral perfusion, electrical activity and effects of serotonergic treatment in obsessive-compulsive disorder. A preliminary study. *Neuropsychobiology, 32,* 423–430.

Moll, G. H., Heinrich, H., Trott, G., Wirth, S., & Rothenberger, A. (2000). Deficient intracortical inhibition in drug-naïve children with attention-deficit hyperactivity disorder is enhanced by methylphenidate. *Neuroscience Letters, 284,* 121–125.

Moller, H. J. (2003). Bipolar disorder and schizophrenia: Distinct illnesses or a continuum? *Journal of Clinical Psychiatry, 64,* 23–27.

Momose, Y., Murata, M., Kobayashi, K., Tachikawa, M., Nakabayashi, Y., Kanazawa, I., et al. (2002). Association studies of multiple candidate genes for Parkinson's disease using single nucleotide polymorphisms. *Annals of Neurology, 51,* 133–136.

Monastra, V. J., Monastra, D. M., & George, S. (2002). The effects of stimulant therapy, EEG, biofeedback, and parenting style on the primary symptoms of attention-deficit/hyperactivity disorder. *Applied Psychophysiological Biofeedback, 27,* 231–249.

Moniz, E. (1994). Prefrontal leucotomy in the treatment of mental disorders. 1937. *American Journal of Psychiatry, 151, Supplement,* 236–239.

Monteggia, L. M., & Nesterl, E. J. (2003). Opiate addiction. In R. Maldonado (Ed.), *Molecular biology of drug addiction* (pp. 37–44). Totowa, NJ: Humana.

Monteleone, P., Brambilla, F., Bortolotti, F., LaRocca, M., & Maj, M. (1998). Prolactin response to d-fenfluramine is blunted in people with anorexia nervosa. *British Journal of Psychiatry, 172,* 438–442.

Montgomery, S. A. (1995). Safety of mirtazapine: A review. *International Clinical Psychopharmacology, Supplement 4,* 37–45.

Montoya, A., Weiss, A. P., Price, B. H., Cassem, E. H., Dougherty, D. D., Nierenberg, A. A., Rauch, S. L., & Cosgrove, G. R. (2002). Magnetic resonance imaging-guided limbic leucotomy for treatment of intractable psychiatric disease. *Neurosurgery, 50,* 1049–1052.

Moore, G. J., Bebchuk, J. M., Wilds, I. B., Chen, G., & Manji, H. K. (2000). Lithium-induced increase in human brain gray matter. *Lancet, 365,* 1241–1242.

Moore, P. B., El-Badri, S. M., Cousins, D., Shepherd, D. J., Young, A. H., McAllister, V. L., et al. (2001). White matter lesions and season of birth of patients with bipolar affective disorder. *American Journal of Psychiatry, 158,* 1521–1524.

Morcuende, S., Gadd, C. A., Peters, M., Moss, A., Harris, E. A., Sheasby, A., et al. (2003). Increased neurogenesis and brain-derived neurotrophic factor in neurokinin-1 receptor gene knockout mice. *European Journal of Neuroscience, 18,* 1828–1836.

Morens, D. M., Davis, J. W., Grandinetti, A., Ross, G. W., Popper, J. S., & White, L. R. (1996). Epidemiologic observations on Parkinson's disease: Incidence and mortality in a prospective study of middle-aged men. *Neurology, 46,* 1044–1050.

Morgan, B., Maybery, M., & Durkin, K. (2003). Weak central coherence, poor joint attention, and low verbal ability: Independent deficits in early autism. *Developmental Psychology, 39,* 646–656.

Morgan, C. M., Mefeez, A., Brandner, B., Bromley, L., & Curran, H. V. (2003). Acute effects of ketamine on memory systems and psychotic symptoms in healthy volunteers. *Neuropsychopharmacology, 29,* 208–218.

Moriarty, J., Eapen, V., Coasta, D. C., Gacinovic, S., Trimble, M., Ell, P. J., & Robertson, M. M. (1997). HMPAO SPET does not distinguish obsessive-compulsive and tic syndromes in families multiply affected with Gilles de la Tourette's syndrome. *Psychological Medicine, 27*, 737–740.

Morris, J. S., Smith, K. A., Cowen, P. J., Friston, K. J., & Dolan, R. J. (1999). Covariation of activity in habenula and dorsal raphé nuclei following tryptophan depletion. *Neuroimage, 10*, 163–172.

Morris, M. C., Evans, D. A., Bienias, J. L., Tangney, C. C., Bennett, D. A., Aggarwal, N., et al. (2002). Dietary intake of antioxidant nutrients and the risk of incident Alzheimer disease in a biracial community study. *Journal of the American Medical Association, 287*, 3230–3237.

Morris, M. C., Evans, D. A., Bienias, J. L., Tangney, C. C., Bennett, D. A., Wilson, R. S., et al. (2003). Consumption of fish and n-3 fatty acids and risk of incident Alzheimer disease. *Archives of Neurology, 60*, 940–946.

Morris, R. L., & Hollenbeck, P. J. (1995). Axonal transport of mitochondria along microtubules and F-actin in living vertebrate neurons. *Journal of Cell Biology, 131*, 1315–1326.

Morrison, J. R., & Stewart, M. A. (1973). The psychiatric status of the legal families of adopted hyperactive children. *Archives of General Psychiatry, 28*, 888–891.

Moscarillo, F. M., & Annunziata, C. M. (2000). ECT in a patient with a deep brain-stimulating electrode in place. *Journal of ECT, 16*, 287–290.

Moshe, K., Iulian, I., Seth, K., Eli, L., & Joseph, Z. (1994). Clomipramine-induced tourettism in obsessive-compulsive disorder: Clinical and theoretical implications. *Clinical Neuropharmacology, 17*, 338–343.

Moskovitz, C., Moses, H. III, & Klawans, H. L. (1978). Levodopa-induced psychosis: A kindling phenomenon. *American Journal of Psychiatry, 135*, 669–675.

Mostofsky, S. H., Cooper, K. L., Kates, W. R., Denckla, M. B., & Kaufmann, W. E. (2002). Smaller prefrontal and premotor volumes in boys with attention-deficit/hyperactivity disorder. *Biological Psychiatry, 52*, 785–794.

Mostofsky, S. H., Reiss, A. L., Lockhart, P., & Denckla, M. B. (1998). Evaluation of cerebellar size in attention-deficit hyperactivity disorder. *Journal of Child Neurology, 13*, 434–439.

Mostofsky, S. H., Wendlandt, J., Cutting, L., Denckla, M. B., & Singer, H. S. (1999). Corpus callosum measurements in girls with Tourette syndrome. *Neurology, 53*, 1345–1347.

Mozley, L. H., Gur, R. C., Mozley, P. D., & Gur, R. E. (2001). Striatal dopamine transporters and cognitive functioning in healthy men and women. *American Journal of Psychiatry, 158*, 1492–1499.

Mueller, B. K. (1999). Growth cone guidance: First steps towards a deeper understanding. *Annual Reviews of Neuroscience, 22*, 351–388.

Mueller, N., Kroll, B., Scharz, M. J., Riedel, M., Straube, A., Luetticken, R., et al. (2001). Increased titers of antibodies against streptococcal M12 and M19 proteins in patients with Tourette's syndrome. *Psychiatry Research, 101*, 187–193.

Mueller, N., Riedel, M., Straube, A., Guenther, W., & Wilske, B. (2000). Increased anti-streptococcal antibodies in patients with Tourette's syndrome. *Psychiatry Research, 94*, 43–49.

Mueller-Vahl, K. R., Koblenz, A., Joebges, M., Kolbe, H., Emrich, H. M., & Schneider, U. (2001). Influence of treatment of Tourette syndrome with Δ9-Tetrahydrocannabinol (Δ9-THC) on neuropsychological performance. *Pharmacopsychiatry, 34*, 19–24.

Mueller-Vahl, K. R., Schneider, U., Koblenz, A., Joebges, M., Kolbe, H., Daldrup, T., et al. (2002). Treatment of Tourette's syndrome with Δ9-tetrahydrocannabinol (THC): A randomized crossover trial. *Pharmacopsychiatry, 35*, 57–61.

Mueller-Vahl, K. R., Schneider, U., Prevedel, H., Theloe, K., Kolbe, H., Daldrup, T., et al. (2003). Δ9–tetrahydrocannabinol (THC) is effective in the treatment of tics in Tourette syndrome: A 6-week randomized trial. *Journal of Clinical Psychiatry, 64*, 459–465.

Muglia, P., Jain, U., Macciardi, F., & Kennedy, J. L. (2000). Adult attention deficit hyperactivity disorder and the dopamine D4 receptor gene. *American Journal of Medical Genetics, 96*, 273–277.

Muhle, R., Trentacoste, S. V., & Rapin, I. (2004). The genetics of autism. *Pediatrics, 113*, 472–486.

Muller, J. L., Deuticke, C., Putzhammer, A., Roder, C. H., Hajak, G., & Winkler, J. (2003). Schizophrenia and Parkinson's disease lead to equal motor-related changes in cortical and subcortical brain activation: An fMRI fingertapping study. *Psychiatry and Clinical Neuroscience, 57*, 562–568.

Muller, M. B., Lucassen, P. J., Yassaouridis, A., Hoogendijk, W. J., Holsboer, F., & Swaab, D. F. (2001). Neither major depression nor glucocorticoid treatment affects the cellular integrity of the hippocampus. *European Journal of Neuroscience, 14*, 1603–1612.

Müller, N., Putz, A., Kathmann, N., Lehle, R., Günther, W., & Straube, A. (1997). Characteristics of obsessive-compulsive symptoms in Tourette's syndrome, obsessive-compulsive disorder, and Parkinson's disease. *Psychiatry Research, 70*, 105–114.

Muller, T., Farahati, J., Kuhn, W., Eising, E. G., Przuntek, H., Reiners, C., et al. (1998). [123I]beta-CIT SPECT visualizes dopamine transporter loss in de novo Parkinsonian patients. *European Neurology, 39*, 44–48.

Muller-Vahl, K. R., Schneider, U., Koblenz, A., Jobges, M., Kolbe, H., Daldrup, T., et al. (2002). Treatment of Tourette's syndrome with Delta 9-tetrahydrocannabinol (THC): A randomized crossover trial. *Pharmacopsychiatry, 35,* 57–61.

Mulnard, R. A., Cotman, C. W., Kawas, C., van Dyck, C. H., Sano, M., Doody, R., et al. (2000). Estrogen replacement therapy or treatment of mild to moderate Alzheimer's disease. *Journal of the American Medical Association, 283,* 1007–1015.

Mundo, E., Richter, M. A., Sam, F., Macciardi, F., & Kennedy, J. L. (2000). Is the 5-HT(1Dbeta) receptor gene implicated in the pathogenesis of obsessive-compulsive disorder? *American Journal of Psychiatry, 157,* 1160–1161.

Mundo, E., Tharmalingham, S., Neves-Pereia, M., Dalton, E. J., Macciardi, F., Parikh, S. V., ct al. (2003). Evidence that the N-methyl-D-aspartate subunit 1 receptor gene (GRIN1) confers susceptibility to bipolar disorder. *Molecular Psychiatry, 8,* 241–245.

Mundo, E., Walker, M., Cate, T., Macciardi, F., & Kennedy, J. L. (2001). The role of serotonin transporter protein gene in antidepressant-induced mania in bipolar disorder. *Archives of General Psychiatry, 58,* 539–544.

Mundo, E., Walker, M., Tims, H., Macciardi, F., & Kennedy, J. L. (2000). Lack of linkage disequilibrium between serotonin transporter protein gene (*SCL6A4*) and bipolar disorder. *American Journal of Medical Genetics, 96,* 379–383.

Mundy, P. (2003). Annotation: The neural basis of social impairments in autism: The role of the dorsal medial-frontal cortex and anterior cingulate system. *Journal of Child Psychology and Psychiatry, and Allied Disciplines, 44,* 793–809.

Murakami, J. W., Courchesne, E., Press, G. A., Yeung-Courchesne, R., & Hesselink, J. R. (1989). Reduced cerebellar hemisphere size and its relationship to vermal hypoplasia in autism. *Archives of Neurology, 46,* 689–694.

Murata, T., Suziki, R., Higuchi, T., & Oshima, A. (2000). Regional cerebral blood flow in the patients with depressive disorders. *Keio Journal of Medicine, 49,* 112–113.

Murck, H., Song, C., Horrobin, D. F., & Uhr, M. (2004). Ethyl-eicosapentaenoate and dexamethasone resistance in therapy-refractory depression. *International Journal of Neuropsychopharmacology, 7,* 341–349.

Murer, M. G., Yan, Q., & Raisman-Vozari, R. (2001). Brain-derived neurotrophic factor in the control human brain, and in Alzheimer's disease and Parkinson's disease. *Progress in Neurology, 63,* 71–124.

Muris, P., Schmidt, H., Engelbrecht, P., & Perold, M. (2002). DSM-IV-defined anxiety disorder symptoms in South African children. *Journal of the American Academy of Child and Adolescent Psychiatry, 41,* 1360–1368.

Murphy, D. D., Rueter, S. M., Trojanowski, J. Q., & Lee, V. M. Y. (2000). Synucleins are developmentally expressed, and alpha-synuclein regulates the size of the presynaptic vesicular pool in primary hippocampal neurons. *Journal of Neuroscience, 20,* 3214–3200.

Murphy, K. C., Jones, L. A., & Owen, M. J. (1999). High rates of schizophrenia in adults with velo-cardio-facial syndrome. *Archives of General Psychiatry, 56,* 940–945.

Murphy, M. L., & Pichichero, M. E. (2002). Prospective identification and treatment of children with pediatric autoimmune neuropsychiatric disorder associated with group A streptococcal infection (PANDAS). *Archives of Pediatrics & Adolescent Medicine, 156,* 356–361.

Murphy, V. E., Mynett-Johnson, L. A., Claffey, E., Begin, P., McAuliffe, M., Kealey, C., et al. (2000). Search for bipolar disorder susceptibility loci: The application of a modified genome scan concentrating on gene-rich regions. *American Journal of Medical Genetics, 96,* 728–732.

Murrell, J. R., Hake, A. M., Quaid, K. A., Farlow, M. R., & Ghetti, B. (2000). Early-onset Alzheimer disease caused by a new mutation (V717L) in the amyloid precursor protein gene. *Archives of Neurology, 57,* 885–887.

Musalek, M., Podreka, H., Walter, E., Suess, V., Passweg, D., Nutzinger, R., et al. (1989). Regional brain function in hallucinations: A study of regional cerebral blood flow with Tc-HMPAO-SPECT in patients with auditory hallucinations, tactile hallucinations and normal controls. *Comprehensive Psychiatry, 30,* 99–108.

Nahas, Z., Molloy, M., Risch, S. C., & George, M. S. (2000). TMS in schizophrenia. In M. S. George & R. H. Belmaker (Eds.), *Transcranial magnetic stimulation in neuropsychiatry* (pp. 237–252). Washington, DC: American Psychiatric Press.

Nahas, Z., Speer, A., Molloy, M., Arana, G. W., Risch, S. C., & George, M. S. (1998). Frequency and intensity in the antidepressant effect of left prefrontal rTMS. *Biological Psychiatry, 43,* 94–95.

Nakamura, T., Dhawan, V., Chaly, T., Fukunda, M., Ma, Y., Breezem R., et al. (2001). Blinded positron emission tomography study of dopamine cell implantation for Parkinson's disease. *Annals of Neurology, 50,* 181–187.

Nakano, S., Asada, T., Matsuda, H., Uno, M., & Takasaki, M. (2001). Donepezil hydrochloride preserves regional cerebral blood flow in patients with Alzheimer's disease. *Journal of Nuclear Medicine, 42,* 1441–1445.

Nakatani, E., Nakgawa, A., Ohara, Y., Goto, S., Uozumi, N., Iwakiri, M., et al. (2003). Effects of behavior therapy on regional cerebral blood flow in obsessive-compulsive disorder. *Psychiatry Research, 124,* 113–120.

Narushima, K., Kosier, J. T., & Robinson, R. G. (2003). A reappraisal of poststroke depression, intra- and inter-hemispheric lesion location using meta-analysis. *Journal of Neuropsychiatry and Clinical Neuroscience, 15,* 422–430.

Näslund, J., Haroutunian, V., Mohs, R., Davis, K. L., Davies, P., Greengard, P., et al. (2000). Correlation between elevated levels of amyloid β-peptide in the brain and cognitive decline. *Journal of the American Medical Association, 283*, 1571–1577.

Nazemi, H., & Dager, S. R. (2003). Coping strategies of panic and control subjects undergoing lactate infusion during magnetic resonance imaging confinement. *Comprehensive Psychiatry, 44*, 190–197.

Nee, L. E., Caine, E. D., Polinsky, R. J., Eldridge, R., & Ebert, M. H. (1980). Gilles de la Tourette syndrome: Clinical and family study of 50 cases. *Annals of Neurology, 7*, 41–49.

Neerakal, I., & Srinivasan, K. (2003). A study of the phenomenology of panic attacks in patients from India. *Psychopathology, 36*, 92–97.

Nelson, J. C., Mazure, C. M., Jatlow, P. I., Bowers, M. B., & Price, L. H. (2004). Combining norepinephrine and serotonin reuptake inhibition mechanisms for treatment of depression: A double-blind, randomized study. *Biological Psychiatry, 55*, 296–300.

Nelson, K. B., Greether, J. K., Croen, L. A., Dambrosia, J. M., Dickens, B. F., Jelliffe, L. L., et al. (2001). Neuropeptides and neurotrophins in neonatal blood of children with autism or mental retardation. *Annals of Neurology, 49*, 597–606.

Nemeroff, C. B. (1998). Psychopharmacology of affective disorders in the 21st century. *Biological Psychiatry, 44*, 517–525.

Nestadt, G., Samuels, J., Riddle, M. A., Liang, K. Y., Bienvenu, O. J., Hoehn-Saric, R., et al. (2001). The relationship between obsessive-compulsive disorder and anxiety and affective disorders: Results from the Johns Hopkins OCD Family Study. *Psychological Medicine, 31*, 481–487.

Nestler, E. J. (2002). Common molecular and cellular substrates of addiction and memory. *Neurobiology of Learning and Memory, 78*, 637–647.

Nestler, E. J. (2004). Cellular and molecular mechanisms of drug addiction. In D. S. Charney & E. J. Nestler (Eds.), *Neurobiology of mental illness* (2nd ed., pp. 698–709). New York: Oxford University Press.

Nestler, E. J., Alreja, M., & Aghajanian, G. K. (1999). Molecular control of locus coeruleus neurotransmission. *Biological Psychiatry, 46*, 1131–1139.

Nestler, E. J., Barrot, M., & Self, D. W. (2001). ΔFosB: A sustained molecular switch for addiction. *Proceedings for the National Academy of Science, 98*, 11042–11046.

Netrakom, P., Krasuski, J. S., Miller, N. S., & O'Tuama, L. A. (1999). Structural and functional neuroimaging findings in substance-related disorders. *Psychiatric Clinics in North America, 22*, 313–329.

Neu, P., Schlattmann, P., Schilling, A., & Hartmann, A. (2004). Cerebrovascular reactivity in major depression: A pilot study. *Psychosomatic Medicine, 66*, 6–8.

Neuman, R. J., Todd, R. D., Heath, A. C., Reich, W., Hudziak, J. J., Bucholz, K. K., et al. (1999). Evaluation of ADHD typology in three contrasting samples: A latent class approach. *Journal of the American Academy and Child and Adolescent Psychiatry, 38*, 25–33.

Neumeister, A., Bain, E., Nugent, A. C., Carson, R. E., Bonne, O., Luckenbaugh, D. A., et al. (2004). Reduced serotonin type 1A receptor binding in panic disorder. *Journal of Neuroscience, 24*, 589–591.

Neumeister, A., Pirker, W., Willeit, M., Praschak-Rieder, N., Asenbaum, S., Brucke, T., et al. (2000). Seasonal variation of availability of serotonin transporter binding sites in healthy female subjects as measured by [(123)I]-2 beta-carbomethoxy-3 beta-(4-iodophenyl)tropane and single photon emission computed tomography. *Biological Psychiatry, 47*, 158–160.

Neville, B. G. R., Spratt, H. C., & Birtwistle, J. (2001). Early onset epileptic auditory and visual agnosia with spontaneous recovery associated with Tourette's syndrome. *Journal of Neurology, Neurosurgery, and Psychiatry, 71*, 556–567.

Neville, H. J., Schmidt, A., & Kutas, M. (1983). Altered visual-evoked potentials in congenitally deaf adults. *Brain Research, 266*, 127–132.

Neziroglu, F., Yaryura-Tobias, J. A., Walz, J., & McKay, D. (2000). The effect of fluvoxamine and behavior therapy on children and adolescents with obsessive-compulsive disorder. *Journal of Child and Adolescent Psychopharmacology, 10*, 295–306.

Ngan, E. T., Yatham, L. N., Ruth, T. J., & Liddle, P. F. (2000). Decreased serotonin 2A receptor densities in neuroleptic-naive patients with schizophrenia: A PET study using [(18)F]setoperone. *American Journal of Psychiatry, 157*, 1016–1018.

Nibuya, M., Nestler, E. J., & Duman, R. S. (1996). Chronic antidepressant administration increases the expression of cAMP response element-binding protein (CREB) in rat hippocampus. *Journal of Neuroscience, 16*, 2356–2372.

Nicholson, L. F. B., & Faull, R. L. M. (2002). *The basal ganglia VII*. New York: Kluwer Academic/Plenum.

Nicoll, J. A. R., Mrak, R. E., Graham, D. I., Stewart, J., Wilcock, G., MacGowan, S., et al. (2000). Association of Interleukin-1 gene polymorphisms with Alzheimer's disease. *Annals of Neurology, 47*, 365–368.

Nicolson, R., & Rapport, J. L. (2000). Childhood-onset schizophrenia: What can it teach us? In J. L. Rapoport (Ed.), *Childhood onset of "adult" psychopathology.* Washington, DC: American Psychiatric Press.

Niranjan, A., Jawahar, A., Kondziolka, D., & Lunsford, L. D. (1999). A comparison of surgical approaches for the management of tremor: Radiofrequency thalamotomy, gamma knife thalamotomy and thalamic stimulation. *Stereotactic and Functional Neurosurgery, 72,* 178–184.

Nishi, R. (1994). Neurotropic factors: Two are better than one. *Science, 265,* 1052–1053.

Nishizawa, S., Benkelfat, C., Young, S. N., Leyton, M., Mzengeza, S., de Montigny, C., et al. (1997). Differences between males and females in rates of serotonin synthesis in human brain. *Proceedings of the National Academy of Sciences of the United States of America, 94,* 5308–5313.

Nobili, F., Vitali, P., Canfora, M., Girtler, N., De Leo, C., Mariani, G., et al. (2002). Effects of long-term Donepezil therapy on rCBF of Alzheimer's patients. *Clinical Neurophysiology, 113,* 1241–1248.

Noble, E. P. (2003). D2 receptor gene in psychiatric and neurologic disorders and its phenotypes. *American Journal of Medical Genetics, 116B,* 103–125.

Noble, F., Coric, P., Turcaud, S., Fournie-Zaluski, M. C., & Roques, B. P. (1994). Assessment of phyical dependence after continuous perfusion into the rat jugular vein of the mixed inhibitor of enkephalin-degrading enzymes, RB 101. *European Journal of Pharmacology, 253,* 283–287.

Noble, F., & Roques, B. P. (2003). The role of CCK(2) receptors in the homeostasis of the opioid system. *Drugs Today, 39,* 897–908.

Nobler, M. S., Olvet, K. R., & Sackeim, H. A. (2002). Effects of medication on cerebral blood flow in late-life depression. *Current Psychiatry Reports, 4,* 51–58.

Nobler, M. S., Oquendo, M. A., Kegeles, L. S., Malone, K. M., Campbell, C. C., Sackeim, H. A., et al. (2001). Decreased regional brain metabolism after ECT. *American Journal of Psychiatry, 158,* 305–308.

Nobler, M. S., Pelton, G. H., & Sackeim, H. A. (1999). Cerebral blood flow and metabolism in late-life depression and dementia. *Journal of Geriatric Psychiatry and Neurology, 12,* 118–127.

Nobler, M. S., Sackheim, H. A., Prohovnik, I., Moeller, J. R., Mukherjee, S., Schnur, D. B., et al. (1994). Regional cerebral blood flow in mood disorders, III. Treatment and clinical response. *Archives of General Psychiatry, 51,* 884–897.

Nomura, T., Inoue, Y., Mitani, H., Kawahara, R., Miyake, M., & Nakashima, K. (2003). Visual hallucinations as REM sleep behavior disorders in patients with Parkinson's disease. *Movement Disorders, 18,* 812–817.

Nomura, Y., Fukunda, H., Terao, Y., Hikosaka, O., & Segawa, M. (2003). Abnormalities of voluntary saccades in Gilles de la Tourette's syndrome: Pathophysiological consideration. *Brain Development, 25,* 48–54.

Nomura, Y., Sakuma, H., Taketa, K., Tugami, T., Okuda, Y., & Nakagawa, T. (1994). Diffusional anisotropy of the human brain assessed with diffusion-weighted MR: Relation with brain development and aging. *American Journal of Neuroradiology, 15,* 231–238.

Nomura, Y., & Segawa, M. (2003). Neurology of Tourette's syndrome (TS) TS as a developmental dopamine disorder: A hypothesis. *Brain Development, 25,* 37–42.

Nonacs, R., & Cohen, L. S. (2003). Assessment and treatment of depression during pregnancy: An update. *Psychiatric Clinics of North America, 26,* 547–562.

Nordahl, T. E., Semple, W. E., Gross, M., Mellman, T. A., Stein, M. B., Goyer, P., et al. (1990). Cerebral glucose metabolic differences in patients with panic disorder. *Neuropsychopharmacology, 3,* 261–272.

Nordahl, T. E., Stein, M. B., Benkelfat, C., Semple, W. E., Andreason, P., Zametkin, A., et al. (1998). Regional cerebral metabolic asymmetries replicated in an independent group of patients with panic disorders. *Biological Psychiatry, 44,* 998–1006.

Nordstrom, E. J., & Burton, F. H. (2002). A transgenic model of comorbid Tourette's syndrome and obsessive-compulsive disorder circuitry. *Molecular Psychiatry, 7,* 617–625.

Novak, G., Kim, D., Seeman, P., & Tallerico, T. (2002). Schizophrenia and Nogo: Elevated mRNA in cortex, and high prevalence of a homozygous CAA insert. *Molecular Brain Research, 107,* 183–189.

Nurmi, E. L., Dowd, M., Tadevosyan-Leyfer, O., Haines, J. L., Folstein, S. E., & Sutcliffe, J. S. (2003). Exploratory subsetting of autism families based on savant skills improves evidence of genetic linkage to 15q11-q13. *Journal of the American Academy of Child and Adolescent Psychiatry, 42,* 856–863.

Nutt, D., Lingford-Hughes, A., & Daglish, M. (2003). Future directions in substance dependence research. *Journal of Neural Transmission, 64,* 95–103.

Nutt, D. J., & Malizia, A. L. (2004). Structural and functional brain changes in posttraumatic stress disorder. *Journal of Clinical Psychiatry, 65,* 11–17.

Nuttin, B., Cosyns, P., Demeulemeester, H., Gybels, J., & Meyerson, B. (1999). Electrical stimulation in anterior limbs of internal capsules in patients with obsessive-compulsive disorder. *Lancet, 354,* 1526.

Nuttin, B. J., Gabriëls, L. A., Cosyns, P. R., Meyerson, B. A., Andréewitch, S., Sunaert, S. G., et al. (2003). Long-term electrical capsular stimulation in patients with obsessive-compulsive disorder. *Neurosurgery, 52,* 1263–1274.

Nuwer, M. R., Lehmann, D., Lopes Da Silva, F., Matsuoka, S., Sutherling, W., & Vibert, J. F. (1994). IFCN guidelines for topographic and frequency analysis of EEGs and EPs. Report of an IFCN committee. *Electroencephalography and Clinical Neurophysiology, 91*, 1–5.

Nyegaard, M., Børglum, A. D., Brunn, T. G., Collier, D. A., Russ, C., Mors, O., et al. (2002). Novel polymorphisms in the somatostatin receptor 5 (SSTR5) gene associated with bipolar affective disorder. *Molecular Psychiatry, 7*, 745–754.

Nygaard, T. G., Raymond, D., Chen, C., Nishino, I., Greene, P. E., Jennings, D., et al. (1999). Localization of a gene for myoclonus-dystonia to chromosome 7q21-q31. *Annals of Neurology, 46*, 794–798.

Nystrom, C., Matousek, M., & Hallstrom, T. (1986). Relationships between EEG and clinical characteristics in major depressive disorder. *Acta Psychiatrica Scandinavica, 73*, 390–394.

Obadia, Y., Rotily, M., Degrand-Guillaud, A., Guelain, J., Ceccaldi, M., Severo, C., et al. (1997). The PREMAP Study: Prevalence and risk factors of dementia and clinically diagnosed Alzheimer's disease in Provence, France. Prevalence of Alzheimer's disease in Provence. *European Journal of Epidemiology, 13*, 247–253.

Obarzanek, E., Lesem, M. D., Goldstein, D. S., & Jimerson, D. C. (1991). Reduced resting metabolic rate in patients with bulimia nervosa. *Archives of General Psychiatry, 48*, 456–462.

Oberlander, T. F., Grunau, R. E., Fitzgerald, C., Papsdorf, M., Rurak, D., & Riggs, W. (2005). Pain Reactivity in 2-month-old infants after prenatal & postnatal serotonin reuptake inhibitor medication exposure. *Pediatrics, 115*, 411–425.

Obeso, J. A., Rodriguez, M. C., Guridi, J., Alvarez, L., Alvarez, E., Macias, R., et al. (2001). Lesion of the basal ganglia and surgery for Parkinson disease. *Archives of Neurology, 58*, 1165–1166.

O'Brien, C. P., Childress, A. R., McLellan, A. T., & Ehrman, R. (1992). Classical conditioning in drug-dependent humans. *Annals of the New York Academy of Science, 654*, 400–415.

O'Brien, J. T., Metcalfe, S., Swann, A., Hobson, J., Jobst, K., Ballard, C., et al. (2000). Medial temporal lobe width on CT scanning in Alzheimer's disease: Comparison with vascular dementia, depression, and dementia with Lewy bodies. *Dementia Geriatric Cognitive Disorders, 11*, 114–118.

O'Brien, K. M., & Vincent, N. K. (2003). Psychiatric comorbidity in anorexia and bulimia nervosa: Nature, prevalence, and causal relationships. *Clinical Psycholical Review, 23*, 57–74.

O'Connell, R. A., Van Heertum, R. L., Luck, D., Yudd, A. P., Cueva, J. E., Billick, S. B., et al. (1995). Single-photon emission computed tomography of the brain in acute mania and schizophrenia. *Journal of Neuroimaging, 5*, 101–104.

O'Connor, N., & Hermelin, B. (1984). Idiot savant calendrical calculations: Maths or memory? *Psychological Medicine, 14*, 801–806.

O'Connor, N., & Hermelin, B. (1991). Talents and preoccupations in idiots-savants. *Psychological Medicine, 21*, 959–964.

O'Doherty, J. P., Deichmann, R., Critchley, H. D., & Dolan, R. J. (2002). Neural responses during anticipation of a primary taste reward. *Neuron, 33*, 668–671.

Ogawa, M., Fukuyama, H., Ouchi, Y., Yamauchi, H., & Kimura, J. (1996). Altered energy metabolism in Alzheimer's disease. *Journal of the Neurological Sciences, 139*, 78–82.

Ogden, J. A. (1996). Phological dyslexia and phonological dysgraphia following left and right hemispherectomy. *Neuropsychologia, 34*, 905–918.

Ohara, K., Nagai, M., Suzuki, Y., Ochiai, M., & Ohara, K. (1998). No association between anxiety disorders and catechol-O-methyltransferase polymorphism. *Psychiatry Research, 80*, 145–148.

Ohara, K., Nagai, M., Suzuki, Y., & Ohara, K. (1998). Low activity allele of catechol-o-methyltransferase gene and Japanese unipolar depression. *Neuroreport, 9*, 1305–1308.

Ohnishi, T., Matsuda, H., Hashimoto, T., Kunihiro, T., Nishikawa, M., Uema, T., et al. (2000). Abnormal regional cerebral blood flow in childhood autism. *Brain, 123*, 1838–1844.

Ohye, C., Shibazaki, T., Zhang, J., & Andou, Y. (2002). Thalamic lesions produced by gamma thalamotomy for movement disorders. *Journal of Neurosurgery, 97*, 600–606.

Ojemann, G. A., & Schoenfield-McNeill, J. (1999). Activity in neurons in human temporal cortex during identification and memory for names and words. *Journal of Neuroscience, 19*, 5674–5682.

Okasha, A., Saad, A., Khalil, A. H., el Dawla, A. S., & Yehia, N. (1994). Phenomenology of obsessive-compulsive disorder: A transcultural study. *Comprehensive Psychiatry, 35*, 191–197.

Okubo, Y., Suhara, T., Suzuki, K., Kobayashi, K., Inoue, O., Terasaki, O., et al. (1997). Decreased prefrontal dopamine D1 receptors in schizophrenia revealed by PET. *Nature, 385*, 634–636.

Okugawa, G., Sedvall, G. C., & Agartz, I. (2003). Smaller cerebellar vermis but not hemisphere volume in patients with chronic schizophrenia. *American Journal of Psychiatry, 160*, 1614–1617.

Okugawa, G., Sedvall, G., Nordstrom, M., Andreasen, N., Pierson, R., Magnotta, V., et al. (2002). Selective reduction of posterior superior vermis in men with chronic schizophrenia. *Schizophrenia Research, 55*, 61–67.

Olanow, C. W., Goetz, C. G., Kordower, J. H., Stoessl, A. J., Sossi, V., Brin, M. F., et al. (2003). A double-blind controlled trial of bilateral fetal nigral transplantation in Parkinson's disease. *Annals of Neurology, 54*, 403–414.

Olanow, C. W., & Stocchi, F. (2004). COMT inhibitors in Parkinson's disease: Can they prevent and/or reverse levodopa-induced motor complications? *Neurology, 62*, 72–81.

Oliveri, R. L., Annesi, G., Zappia, M., Civitelli, D., De Marco, E. V., Pasqua, A. A., et al. (2000). The dopamine D2 receptor gene is a susceptibility locus for Parkinson's disease. *Movement Disorders, 15*, 127–131.

Olney, J. W., & Farber, N. B. (1995). Glutamate receptor dysfunction and schizophrenia. *Archives of General Psychiatry, 52*, 998–1007.

Olson, L. (2000). Combating Parkinson's disease—step three. *Science, 290*, 721–772.

Olson, R., Wise, B., Conners, F., Rack, J., & Fulker, D. (1989). Specific deficits in component reading and language skills: Genetic and environmental influences. *Journal of Learning Disabilities, 22*, 339–348.

Oluboka, O. J., Stewart, S. L., Sharma, V., Mazmanian, D., & Persad, E. (2002). Preliminary assessment of intrahemispheric QEEG measures in bipolar mood disorders. *Canadian Journal of Psychiatry, 47*, 368–374.

Ongur, D., Drevets, W. C., & Price, J. L. (1998). Glial reduction in the subgenual prefrontal cortex in mood disorders. *Proclamations of the National Academy of Science, U.S.A., 95*, 13290–13295.

Onitsuka, T., Shenton, M. E., Salisbury, D. F., Dickey, C. C., Kasai, K., et al. (2004). Middle and inferior temporal gyrus gray matter volume abnormalities in chronic schizophrenia: An MRI study. *American Journal of Psychiatry, 161*, 1603–1611.

Ontiveros, A., Fontaine, R., Breton, G., Elie, R., Fontaine, S., & Déry, R. (1989). Correlation of severity of panic disorder and neuroanatomical changes on magnetic resonance imaging. *Journal of Neuropsychiatry and Clinical Neurosciences, 1*, 404–408.

Ophoff, R. A., Escamilla, M. A., Service, S. K., Spesny, M., Meshi, D. B., Poon, W., et al. (2002). Genomewide linkage disequilibrium mapping of severe bipolar disorder in a population isolate. *American Journal of Human Genetics, 71*, 565–574.

Oquendo, M. A., Ellis, S. P., Greenwald, S., Malone, K. M., Weissman, M. M., & Mannm, J. J. (2001). Ethnic and sex differences in suicide rates relative to major depression in the United States. *American Journal of Psychiatry, 158*, 1652–1658.

Orton, S. T. (1928). Specific reading disability-strephosymbolia. *Journal of the American Medical Association, 90*, 1095–1099.

Orvidas, L. J., & Slattery, M. J. (2001). Pediatric autoimmune neuropsychiatric disorders and streptococcal infections: Role of otolaryngologist. *Laryngoscope, 111*, 1515–1519.

Oswald, P., Souery, D., & Medlewicz, J., (2003). Molecular genetics of affective disorders. *International Journal of Neuropsychopharmacology, 6*, 155–169.

Otero, G. A., Pliego-Rivero, F. B., Fernandez, T., & Ricardo, J. (2003). EEG development in children with sociocultural disadvantages: A follow-up study. *Clinical Neurophysiology, 114*, 1918–1925.

Otten, U., März, P., Heese, K., Hock, C., Kunz, D., & Rose-John, S. (2001). Signals regulating neurotrophin expression in glial cells. In B. C. Lopez & M. Nieto-Sampedro (Eds.), *Progress in brain research, 132*, 545–565.

Ovbiagele, B., Kindwell, C. S., Starkman, S., & Saver, J. L. (2003). Potential role of neuroprotective agents in the treatment of patients with acute ischemic stroke. *Current Treatment Options in Cardiovascular Medicine, 5*, 441–449.

Overall, K. L., & Dunham, A. E. (2002). Clinical features and outcome in dogs and cats with obsessive-compulsive disorder: 126 cases (1989–2000). *Journal of the American Veterinary Medical Association, 221*, 1445–1452.

Overmeyer, S., Bullmore, E. T., Suckling, J., Simmons, A., Williams, S. C. R., Santosh, P. J., ct al. (2001). Distributed grey and white matter deficits in hyperkinetic disorder: MRI evidence for anatomical abnormality in an attentional network. *Psychological Medicine, 31*, 1425–1435.

Overmeyer, S., Simmons, A., Santosh, J., Andrew, C., Williams, S. C., Taylor, A., et al. (2000). Corpus callosum may be similar in children with ADHD and siblings of children with ADHD. *Developments in Medicine and Child Neurology, 42*, 8–13.

Owley, T., McMahon, W., Cook, E. H., Laulhere, T., South, M., Mays, L. Z., Shernoff, E. S., et al. (2001). Multisite, double-blind, placebo-controlled trial of porcine secretin in autism. *Journal of the American Academy of Child and Adolescent Psychiatry, 40*, 1293–1299.

Ozaki, N., Goldman, D., Kaye, W. H., Plotnicov, K., Greenberg, B. D., Lappalainen, J., et al. (2003). Serotonin transporter missense mutation associated with a complex neuropsychiatric phenotype. *Molecular Psychiatry, 8*, 933–936.

Ozer, O. A., Kutanis, R., Agargun, M. Y., Besiroglu, L., Bal, A. C., Selvi, Y., et al. (2004). Serum lipid levels, suicidality, and panic disorder. *Comprehensive Psychiatry, 45*, 95–98.

Pacchierotti, C., Bossini, L., Castrogiovanni, A., Pieraccini, F., Soreca, I., & Castrogiovanni, P. (2002). Attachment and panic disorder. *Psychopathology, 35*, 347–354.

Padberg, F., Zwanzger, P., Thoma, H., Kathmann, N., Haag, C., Greenberg, B. D., et al. (1999). Repetitive transcranial magnetic stimulation (rTMS) in pharmacotherapy-refractory major depression: Comparative study of fast, slow and sham rTMS. *Psychiatry Research, 88*, 163–171.

Pakkenberg, B. (1990). Pronounced reduction of nerve cell number in mediodorsal thalamic nucleus and nucleus accumbens in schizophrenics. *Archives of General Psychiatry, 47*, 1023–1028.

Pal, P. K., Thennarasu, K., Fleming, J., Schulzer, M., Brown, T., & Calne, S. M. (2004). Nocturnal sleep disturbances and daytime dysfunction in patients with Parkinson's disease and in their caregivers. *Parkinsonism & Related Disorders, 10*, 157–168.

Palatnik, A., Frolov, K., Fux, M., & Benjamin, J. (2001). Double-blind, controlled, crossover trial of inositol versus fluvoxamine for the treatment of panic disorder. *Journal of Clinical Psychopharmacology, 21*, 335–339.

Pallanti, S., & Mazzi, D. (1992). MDMA (Ecstasy) precipitation of panic disorder. *Biological Psychiatry, 32*, 91–95.

Pallier, C., Dehaene, S., Poline, J. B., & LeBihan, D. (2003). Brain imaging of language plasticity in adopted adults: Can a second language replace the first? *Cerebral Cortex, 2*, 155–161.

Palmer, K., Inskip, H., Martyn, C., & Coggon, D. (1998). Dementia and occupational exposure to organic solvents. *Occupational and Environmental Medicine, 55*, 712–715.

Pandey, S. C. (2003). Anxiety and alcohol abuse disorders: A common role for CREB and its target, the neuropeptide Y gene. *Trends in Pharmacological Science, 24*, 456–460.

Panerai, S., Ferrante, L., & Zingale, M. (2002). Benefits of the treatment and education of autistic and communication handicapped children (TEACCH) programme as compared with a non-specific approach. *Journal of Intellectual Disability Research, 46*, 318–327.

Panizzon, M. S., Hoff, A. L., Nordahl, T. E., Kremen, W. S., Reisman, B., Wieneke, M., et al. (2003). Sex differences in the corpus callosum of patients with schizophrenia. *Schizophrenia Research, 62*, 115–122.

Papakostas, G. I., Petersen, T., Mahal, Y., Mischoulon, D., Nierenberg, A. A., & Fava, M., (2004). Quality of life assessments in major depressive disorder: A review of the literature. *General Hospital Psychiatry, 26*, 13–17.

Papanicolaou, A. (1998). *Fundamentals of functional brain imaging*. Lisse, Netherlands: Swets & Zeitlinger.

Papapetropoulos, S., Ellul, J., Argyriou, A. A., Talelli, P., Chroni, E., & Papapetropoulos, T. (2004). The effect of vascular disease on late onset Parkinson's disease. *European Journal of Neurology, 11*, 231–235.

Papassotiropoulos, A., Hawellek, B., Frahnert, C., Rao, G. S., & Rao, M. L. (1999). The risk of acute suicidality in psychiatric inpatients increases with low plasma cholesterol. *Pharmacopsychiatry, 32*, 1–4.

Paquette, V., Levesque, J., Mensour, B., Leroux, J. M., Beaudoin, G., Bourgouin, P., et al. (2003). Change the mind and you change the brain: Effects of cognitive-behavioral therapy on the neural correlates of spider phobia. *Neuroimage, 18*, 401–409.

Paradiso, S., Andreasen, N. C., Crespo-Facorro, B., O'Leary, D. S., Watkins, G. L., Boles Ponto, L. L., et al. (2003). Emotions in unmedicated patients with schizophrenia during evaluation with positron emission tomography. *American Journal of Psychiatry, 160*, 1775–1783.

Parain, K., Murer, M. G., Yan, Q., Faucheux, B., Agid, Y., Hirsch, E., et al. (1999). Reduced expression of brain-derived neurotrophic factor protein in Parkinson's disease substantia nigra. *Neuroreport, 10*, 557–561.

Pardo, R., Andreolotti, A. G., Ramos, B., Picatoste, F., & Claro, E. (2003). Opposed effects of lithium on the MEK-ERK pathway in neural cells: Inhibition in astrocytes and stimulation in neurons by GSK3 independent mechanisms. *Journal of Neurochemistry, 87*, 417–426.

Park, T. W., Yoon, K. S., Kim, J. H., Park, W. Y., Hirvonen, A., & Kang, D. (2002). Functional catechol-O-methyltransferase gene polymorphism and susceptibility to schizophrenia. *European Neuropsychopharmacology, 12*, 299–303.

Park, Y. D. (2003). The effects of vagus nerve stimulation on patients with intractable seizures and either Landau-Kleffner syndrome or autism. *Epilepsy and Behavior, 4*, 286–290.

Parker, G. (2002). Differential effectiveness of newer and older antidepressants appears mediated by an age effect on the phenotypic expression of depression. *Acta Psychiatrica Scandinavica, 106*, 168–170.

Parkinson, J. (1871). *An essay on the shaking palsy*. London: Sherwood, Neely and Jones.

Pary, R., Matuschka, P. R., Lewis, S., Caso, W., & Lippmann, S. (2003). Generalized anxiety disorder. *Southern Medical Journal, 96*, 581–586.

Pascual-Leone, A., & Dhuna, A. (1990). Cocaine-associated multifocal tics. *Neurology, 40*, 999–1000.

Pascual-Leone, A., Tarazona, F., Keenan, J., Tormos, J. M., Hamilton, R., & Catala, M. D. (1999). Transcranial magnetic stimulation and neuroplasticity. *Neuropsychologia, 37*, 207–217.

Pastor, P., Ezquerra, M., Munoz, E., Marti, M. J., Blesa, R., Tolosa, E., & et al. (2000). Significant association between the tau gene A0/A0 genotype and Parkinson's disease. *Annals of Neurology, 47*, 242–245.

Patterson, P. H. (1978). Environmental determination of autonomic neurotransmitter functions. *Annual Review of Neuroscience, 1*, 1–17.

Paulesu, E., Frith, U., Snowling, M., Gallagher, A., Morton, J., Frackowiak, R. S. J., et al. (1996). Is developmental dyslexia a disconnection syndrome? Evidence from PET scanning. *Brain, 119*, 143–157.

Pauls, D. L., Towbin, K. E., Leckman, J. F., Zahner, G. E., & Cohen, D. J. (1986). Gilles de la Tourette's syndrome and obsessive-compulsive disorder. Evidence supporting a genetic relationship. *Archives of General Psychiatry, 43*, 1180–1182.

Paulsen, J. S., Salmon, D. P., Thal, L. J., Romero, R., Weisstein-Jenkins, C., Galasko, D., Hofstetter, C. R., Thomas, R., Grant, I., & Jeste, D. V. (2000). Incidence of and risk factors for hallucinations and delusions in patients with probable AD. *Neurology, 54*, 1965–1971.

Paulus, M. P., Hozack, N. E., Zauscher, B. E., Frank, L., Brown, G. G., Braff, D. L., et al. (2002). Behavioral and functional neuroimaging evidence for prefrontal dysfunction in methamphetamine-dependent subjects. *Neuropsychopharmacology, 26*, 53–63.

Paulus W., & Jellinger K. (1991). The neuropathologic basis of different clinical subgroups of Parkinson's disease. *Journal of Neuropathology and Experimental Neurology, 50*, 743–755.

Paus, T., Koski, L., Zograos, C., & Westbury, C. (1998). Regional differences in the effects of task difficulty and motor output on bloodflow response in the human anterior cingulate cortex: A review of 107 PET activation studies. *Neuroreport, 9*, 37–47.

Payton, A., Holmes, J., Barrett, J. H., Sham, P., Harrington, R., McGuffin, P., et al. (2001). Susceptibility genes for a trait measure of attention deficit hyperactivity disorder: A pilot study in a non-clinical sample of twins. *Psychiatry Research, 105*, 273–278.

Pearlson, G. D., Wong, D. F., Tune, L. E., Ross, C. A., Chase, G. A., Links, J. M., et al. (1995). In vivo D2 dopamine receptor density in psychotic and nonpsychotic patients with bipolar disorder. *Archives of General Psychiatry, 52*, 471–477.

Pedersen, C. B., & Mortensen, P. B. (2001). Evidence of a dose-response relationship between urbanicity during upbringing and schizophrenia risk. *Archives of General Psychiatry, 58*, 1039–1045.

Pedersen, N. L., Gatz, M., Berg, S., & Johansson, B. (2004). How heritable is Alzheimer's disease late in life? Findings from Swedish twins. *Annals of Neurology, 55*, 180–185.

Pedrosa-Sanchez, M., & Sola, R. G. (2003). Modern day psychosurgery: A new approach to neurosurgery in psychiatric disease. *Review of Neurology, 36*, 887–897.

Penn, D. L., Meuser, K. T., Tarrier, N., Gloege, A., Cather, C., Serrano, D., et al. (2004). Supportive therapy for schizophrenia: Possible mechanisms and implications for adjuctive psychosocial treatments. *Schizophrenia Bulletin, 30*, 101–112.

Pennington, B. F. (1999). Toward an integrated understanding of dyslexia: Genetic, neurological, and cognitive mechanisms. *Development and Psychopathology, 11*, 629–654.

Pennington, B. F., Filipek, P. A., Lefly, D., Churchwell, J., Kennedy, D. N., Simon, J. H., et al. (1999). Brain morphometry in reading-disabled twins. *Neurology, 53*, 723–729.

Pennington, B. F., & Lefly, D. L. (2001). Early reading development in children at family risk for dyslexia. *Child Development, 72*, 816–833.

Peplonska, B., Zekanowski, C., Religa, D., Czyzewski, K., Styczynska, M., Pfeffer, A., et al. (2003). Strong association between Saitohin gene polymorphism and tau haplotype in the Polish population. *Neuroscience Letters, 348*, 163–166.

Peralta, V., & Cuesta, M. J. (2001). How many and which are the psychopathological dimensions in schizophrenia? Issues influencing their ascertainment. *Schizophrenia Research, 49*, 269–285.

Perl, D. P., Olanow, C. W., & Calne, D. (1998). Alzheimer's disease and Parkinson's disease: Distinct entities or extremes of a spectrum of neurodegeneration? *Annals of Neurology, 44*, 19–31.

Perlis, R. H., Mischoulon, D., Smoller, J. W., Wan, Y. J., Lamon-Fava, S., Lin, K. M., et al. (2003). Serotonin transporter polymorphisms and adverse effects with fluoxetine treatment. *Biological Psychiatry, 54*, 879–883.

Perna, G., Bertani, A., Caldirola, D., Gabriele, A., Cocchi, S., & Bellodi, L. (2002). Antipanic drug modulation of 35% CO_2 hyperreactivity and short-term treatment outcome. *Journal of Clinical Psychopharmacology, 22*, 300–308.

Perner, J., Frith, U., Leslie, A. M., & Leekam, S. R. (1989). Exploration of the autistic child's theory of mind: Knowledge, belief, and communication. *Child Development, 60*, 688–700.

Perrine, D. M. (1996). *The chemistry of mind-altering drugs: History, pharmacology, and cultural context.* Washington, DC: American Chemical Society.

Perry, E. K., Kilford, L., Lees, A. J., Burn, D. J., & Perry, R. H. (2003). Increased Alzheimer pathology in Parkinson's disease related to antimuscarinic drugs. *Annals of Neurology, 54*, 235–238.

Persico, A. M., D'Agruma, L., Maiorano, N., Totaro, A., Militerni, R., Bravaccio, C., et al. (2001). Reelin gene alleles and haplotypes as a factor predisposing to autistic disorder. *Molecular Psychiatry, 6*, 150–159.

Persico, A. M., Reich, S., Henningfield, J. E., Kuhar, M. J., & Uhl, G. R. (1998). Parkinsonian patients report blunted subjective effects of methylphenidate. *Experimental and Clinical Psychopharmacology, 6*, 54–63.

Perugi, G., Toni, C., Frare, F., Travierso, M. C., Hantouche, E., & Akiskal, H. S. (2002). Obsessive-compulsive-bipolar comorbidity: A systematic exploration of clinical features and treatment outcome. *Journal of Clinical Psychiatry, 63*, 1129–1134.

Petanceska, S. S., DeRosa, S., Sharma, A., Diaz, N., Duff, K., & Tint, S. G. (2003). Changes in apolipoprotein E expression in response to dietary and pharmacological modulation of cholesterol. *Journal of Molecular Neuroscience, 20*, 395–406.

Petek, E., Windpassinger, C., Vincent, J. B., Cheung, J., Boright, A. P., Scherer, S. W., et al. (2001). Disruption of a novel gene (IMMP2L) by a breakpoint in 7q31 associated with Tourette syndrome. *American Journal of Human Genetics, 68*, 848–858.

Peter, H., Hand, I., Hohagen, F., Koenig, A., Mindermann, O., Oeder, F., et al. (2002). Serum cholesterol level comparison: Control subjects, anxiety disorder patients, and obsessive-compulsive disorder patients. *Canadian Journal of Psychiatry, 47*, 557–561.

Peterson, A. L., & Azrin, N. H. (1992). An evaluation of behavioral treatments for Tourette syndrome. *Behavioral Research and Therapy, 30*, 167–174.

Peterson, B., Riddle, M. A., Cohen, D. J., Katz, L. D., Smith, J. C., Hardin, M. T., et al. (1993). Reduced basal ganglia volumes in Tourette's syndrome using three-dimensional reconstruction techniques from magnetic resonance images. *Neurology, 43*, 941–949.

Peterson, B. S. (1995). Neuroimaging in child and adolescent neuropsychiatric disorders. *Journal of the American Academy of Child and Adolescent Psychiatry, 34*, 1560–1576.

Peterson, B. S., Leckman, J. F., Duncan, J. S., Wetzles, R., Riddle, M. A., Hardin, M. T., et al. (1994). Corpus callosum morphology from magnetic resonance images in Tourette's syndrome. *Psychiatry Research, 55*, 85–99.

Peterson, B. S., Leckman, J. F., Tucker, D., Scahill, L., Staib, L., Zhang, H., et al. (2000). Preliminary findings of antistreptococcal antibody titers and basal ganglia volumes in tic, obsessive-compulsive, and attention deficit/hyperactivity disorders. *Archives of General Psychiatry, 57*, 364–372.

Peterson, B. S., Skudlarski, P., Anderson, A. W., Zhang, H., Gatenby, J. C., Lacadie, C. M., et al. (1998). A functional magnetic resonance imaging study of tic suppression in Tourette syndrome. *Archives of General Psychiatry, 55*, 326–333.

Peterson, B. S., Staib, L., Scahill, L., Zhang, H., Anderson, C., Leckman, J. F., et al. (2001). Regional brain and ventricular volumes in Tourette syndrome. *Archives of General Psychiatry, 58*, 427–440.

Peterson, B. S., Thomas, P., Kane, M. J., Scahill, L., Zhang, H., Bronen, R., et al. (2003). Basal ganglia volumes in patients with Gilles de la Tourette syndrome. *Archives of General Psychiatry, 60*, 415–424.

Peterson, R. C., Jack, Jr., C. R., Xu, Y. C., Waring, S. C., O'Brien, P. C., Smith, G. E., et al. (2000). Memory and MRI-based hippocampal volumes in aging and AD. *Neurology, 54*, 581–587.

Petit, E., Hérault, J., Raynaud, M., Cherpi, C., Perrot, A., Barthélémy, C., et al. (1996). X chromosome and infantile autism. *Biological Psychiatry, 40*, 457–464.

Petrakis, I., Limoncelli, D., Gueorguievva, R., Jatlow, P., Boutros, N. N., Trevisan, L., et al. (2004). Altered NMDA Glutamate receptor antagonist response in individuals with a family vulnerability to alcoholism. *American Journal of Psychiatry, 161*, 1776–1782.

Petrovitch, H., Ross, G. W., Abbott, R. D., Sanderson, W. T., Sharp, D. S., Tanner, C. M., et al. (2002). Plantation work and risk of Parkinson disease in a population-based longitudinal study. *Archives of Neurology, 59*, 1787–1792.

Pettmann, B., & Henderson, C. E. (1998). Neuronal cell death. *Neuron, 20*, 633–647.

Petty, F., Davis, L. L., Kabel, D., & Kramer, G. L. (1996). Serotonin dysfunction disorders: A behavioral neurochemistry perspective. *Journal of Clinical Psychiatry, 57*, 11–16.

Petty, F., Kramer, G. L., Dunnam, D., & Rush, A. J. (1990). Plasma gaba in mood disorders. *Psychopharmacology Bulletin, 26*, 157–161.

Petty, R. G., Barta, P. W., Pearlson, G. D., McGilchrist, I. K., Lewis, R. W., Tien, A. Y., et al. (1995). Reversal of asymmetry of the planum temporale in schizophrenia. *American Journal of Psychiatry, 152*, 715–721.

Pfefferbaum, A., Desmond, J. E., Galloway, C., Menon, V., Glover, G. H., & Sullivan, E. V. (2001). Reorganization of frontal systems used by alcoholics for spatial working memory: An fMRI study. *Neuroimage, 14*, 7–20.

Pfefferbaum, A., & Sullivan, E. V. (2002). Microstructural but not macrostructural disruption of white matter in women with chronic alcoholism. *Neuroimage, 15*, 708–718.

Phelan, A. T. (2002). MMR and autism: An overview of the debate to date. *British Journal of Nursing, 11*, 621–625.

Phillips, M. L., Marks, I. M., Senior, C., Lythgoe, D., O'Dwyer, A. M., Meehan, O., et al. (2000). A differential neural response in obsessive-compulsive disorder patients with washing compared with checking symptoms to disgust. *Psychological Medicine, 30*, 1037–1050.

Physician's Desk Reference, 57th ed. (2003). Stanford, CT: Thomson.

Pian, K. L., Westenberg, H. G., van Megen, H. J., & den Boer, J. A. (1998). Sumatriptan (5-HT1D receptor agonist) does not exacerbate symptoms in obsessive compulsive disorder. *Psychopharmacology, 140*, 365–370.

Pickar, D., Breir, A., Hsiao, J. K., Doran, A. R., Wolkowitz, O. M., Pato, C. N., et al. (1990). Cerebrospinal fluid and monoamine metabolites and their relation to psychosis: Implications for regional brain dysfunction in schizophrenia. *Archives of General Psychiatry, 47*, 641–648.

Pieribone, V. A., Shupliakov, O., Brodin, L., Hilfiker-Rothenfluh, S., Czernik, A. J., & Greengard, P. (1995). Distinct pools of synaptic vesicles in neurotransmitter release. *Nature, 375*, 493–497.

Pierot, L., Desnos, C., Blin, J., Raisman, R., Scherman, D., Javoy-Agid, F., et al. (1988). D1 and D2–type dopamine receptors in patients with Parkinson's disease and progressive supranuclear palsy. *Journal of the Neurological Sciences, 86*, 291–306.

Pies, R. (1999). Individualized risperidone dosing. *American Journal of Psychiatry, 156*, 1123–1124.

Piet, R., Vargova, L., Sykova, E., Poulain, D. A., & Oliet, S. H. (2004). Physiological contribution of astrocytic environment of neurons to intersynaptic crosstalk. *Proceedings of the National Academy of Sciences USA, 101*, 2151–2155.

Piggott, M. A., Owens, J., O'Brien, J., Colloby, S., Fenwick, J., Wyper, D., et al. (2003). Muscarinic receptors in basal ganglia in dementia with Lewy bodies, Parkinson's disease, and Alzheimer's disease. *Journal of Chemistry and Neuroanatomy, 25*, 161–173.

Pigott, T. A., & Seay, S. M. (1999). A review of the efficiency of selective serotonin reuptake inhibitors in obsessive-compulsive disorder. *Journal of Clinical Psychiatry, 60*, 101–106.

Pilowsky, L. S., Costa, D. C., & Eli, P. J. (1992). Clozapine single photo emissiontomography and the D2 receptor blockade hypothesis of schizophrenia. *Lancet, 340*, 199–202.

Pimlott, S. L., Piggott, M., Owens, J., Greally, E., Court, J. A., Jaros, E., et al. (2004). Nicotinic acetylcholine receptor distribution in Alzheimer's disease, dementia with Lewy bodies, Parkinson's disease, and vascular dementia: In vitro binding study using 5–[(125)i]-a-85380. *Neuropsychopharmacology, 29*, 108–116.

Pinel, J. J. (2000). *Biological psychology* (4th ed.). Needham Heights, MA: Allyn & Bacon.

Pinto, S., Thobois, S., Costes, N., Le Bars, D., Benabid, A. L., Broussoulle, E., et al. (2004). Subthalamic nucleus stimulation and dysarthia in Parkinson's disease: A PET study. *Brain, 127*, 602–615.

Pitchot, W., Ansseau, M., Gonzalez Moreno, A., Hansenne, M., & von Frenckell, R. (1992). Dopaminergic function in panic disorder: Comparison with major and minor depression. *Biological Psychiatry, 32*, 1004–1011.

Piven, J., Arndt, S., Bailey, J., & Andreasen, N. (1996). Regional brain enlargement in autism: A magnetic resonance imaging study. *Journal of the American Academy of Child and Adolescent Psychiatry, 35*, 530–536.

Piven, J., Bailey, J., Ranson, B. J., & Arndt, S. (1997). An MRI study of the corpus callosum in autism. *American Journal of Psychiatry, 154*, 1051–1056.

Piven, J., Bailey, J., Ranson, B. J., & Arndt, S. (1998). No difference in hippocampus volume detected on magnetic resonance imaging in autistic individuals. *Journal of Autism and Developmental Disorders, 28*, 105–110.

Pizzagalli, D. A., Oakes, T. R., Fox, A. S., Chung, M. K., Larson, C. L., Larson, C. L., et al. (2003). Functional but not structural subgenual prefrontal cortex abnormalities in melancholia. *Molecular Psychiatry, 9*, 393–405.

Plaitakis, A. & Shashidharan, P. (2000). Glutamate transport and metabolism in dopaminergic neurons of substantia nigra: Implications for the pathogenesis of Parkinson's disease. *Journal of Neurology, 247*, 25–35.

Plassman, B. L., Havlik, R. J., Steffens, D. C., Helms, M. J., Newman, T. N., Drosdick, D., et al. (2000). Documented head injury in early adulthood and risk of Alzheimer's disease and other dementias. *Neurology, 55*, 1158–1166.

Playford, E. D., Jenkins, I. H., Passingham, R. E., Nutt, J., Frackowiak, R. S., & Brooks, D. J. (1992). Impaired mesial frontal and putamen activation in Parkinson's disease: A positron emission tomography study. *Annals of Neurology, 32*, 151–161.

Plessen, K. J., Wentzel-Larsen, T., Hugdahl, K., Feineigle, P., Klein, J., Staib, L. H., et al. (2004). Altered interhemispheric connectivity in individuals with Tourette's disorder. *American Journal of Psychiatry, 161*, 2028–2037.

Plioplys, A. V., Hemmens, S. E., & Regan, C. M. (1990). Expression of a neural cell adhesion molecule serum fragment is depressed in autism. *Journal of Neuropsychiatry and Clinical Neurosciences, 2*, 413–417.

Pliszka, S. R. (2003). *Neuroscience for the mental health clincian*. New York: Guilford.

Poewe, W. (2004). The role of COMT inhibition in the treatment of Parkinson's disease. *Neurology, 62*, 31–38.

Poewe, W., Deuschl, G., Gordin, A., Kultalahti, E. R., & Leinonen, M. (2002). Efficacy and safety of entacapone in Parkinson's disease patients with suboptimal levodopa response: A 6–month randomized placebo-controlled double-blind study in Germany and Austria (Celomen study). *Acta Neurologica Scandinavica, 105*, 245–255.

Pogarell, O., Hamann, C., Pöpperl, G., Juckel, G., Choukèr, M., Zaudig, M., et al. (2003). Elevated brain serotonin transporter availability in patients with obsessive-compulsive disorder. *Biological Psychiatry, 54*, 1406–1413.

Poldrack, R. A., Wagner, A. D., Prull, M. W., Desmond, J. E., Glover, G. H., & Gabrieli, J. D. E. (1999). Functional specialization for semantic and phonological processing in the left inferior prefrontal cortex. *NeuroImage, 10*, 15–35.

Pollack, M. H., Allgulander, C., Bandelow, B., Cassano, G. B., Greist, J. H., Hollander, E., et al. (2003). WCA recommendations for the long-term treatment of panic disorder. *CNS Spectrums, 8, Supplement 1*, 17–30.

Polluzi, E., Motola, D., Silvani, C., De Ponti, F., Vaccheri, A., & Montanaro, N. (2003). Prescriptions of antidepressants in primary care in Italy: Pattern of use after admission of selective serotonin reuptake inhibitors for reimbursement. *European Journal of Pharmacology, 59*, 825–31.

Pols, H. J., Hauzer, R. C., Meijer, J. A., Verburg, K., & Griez, E. J. (1996). Fluvoxamine attenuates panic induced by 35% CO2 challenge. *Journal of Clinical Psychiatry, 57*, 539–542.

Porta, M., Maggioni, G., Ottaviani, F., & Schindler, A. (2004). Treatment of phonic tics in patients with Tourette's syndrome using botulinum toxin type A. *Neurological Science, 24*, 420–423.

Posener, J. A., Wang, L., Price, J. L., Gado, M. H., Province, M. A., Miller, M. I., et al. (2003). High-dimensional mapping of the hippocampus in depression. *American Journal of Psychiatry, 160*, 83–89.

Posey, D. J., & McDougle, C. J. (2001). The pathophysiology and treatment of autism. *Current Psychiatry Reports, 3*, 101–108.

Posey, T. B., & Losch, M. E. (1983). Auditory hallucinations of hearing voices in 375 normal subjects. *Imagination, Cognition and Personality, 3*, 99–113.

Potash, J. B., Willour, V. L., Chiu, Y. F., Simpson, S. G., MacKinnon, D. F., Pearlson, G. D., et al. (2001). The familial aggregation of psychotic symptoms in bipolar disorder pedigrees. *American Journal of Psychiatry, 158*, 1258–1264.

Potash, J. B., Zandi, P. P., Willour, V. L., Lan, T. H., Huo, Y., Avramopoulos, D., et al. (2003). Suggestive linkage to chromosomal regions 13q31 and 22q12 in families with psychotic bipolar disorder. *American Journal of Psychiatry, 160*, 680–686.

Potter, W. Z., Hsiao, J. K., & Goldman, S. M. (1989). Effects of renal clearance on plasma concentrations of homovanillic acid. Methodological cautions. *Archives of General Psychiatry, 46*, 558–562.

Pralong, E., Magistretti, P., & Stoop, R. (2002). Cellular perspectives on the glutamate-monoamine interactions in limbic lobe structures and their relevance for some psychiatric disorders. *Progress in Neurobiology, 67*, 173–202.

Preston, J. D., O'Neal, J. H., & Talaga, M. C. (2002). Substance related disorders. In *Handbook of clinical psychopharmacology for therapists* (3rd ed., pp. 144–152). Oakland, CA: New Harbinger.

Preuss, U. W., Koller, G., Zill, P., Bondy, B., & Soyka, M. (2003). Alcoholism-related phenotypes and genetic variants of the CB1 receptor. *European Archives of Psychiatry and Clinical Neuroscience, 253*, 275–280.

Preux, P. M., Condet, A., Anglade, C., Druet-Cabanac, M., Debrock, M., Macharia, W., et al. (2000). Parkinson's disease and environmental factors. Matched case-control study in the Limousin region, France. *Neuroepidemiology, 19*, 333–337.

Price, R. A., Kidd, K. K., Cohen, D. J., Paulus, D. L., & Leckman, J. F. (1985). A twin study of Tourette syndrome. *Archives of General Psychiatry, 42*, 815–820.

Price, R. A., Leckman, J. F., Pauls, D. L., Cohen, D. J., Kidd, K. K. (1986). Gilles de la Tourette's syndrome: Tics and central nervous system stimulants in twins and nontwins. *Neurology, 36*, 232–237.

Priyadarshi, A., Khuder, S. A., Schaub, E. A., & Shrivastava, S. (2000). A meta-analysis of Parkinson's disease and exposure to pesticides. *Neurotoxicity, 21*, 435–440.

Przewlocki, R., & Przewlocka, B. (2001). Opioids in chronic pain. *European Journal of Pharmacology, 429*, 79–91.

Pu, L., Bao, G. B., Xu, M. J., Ma, L., & Pei, G. (2002). Hippocampal long-term potentiation is reduced by chronic opiate treatment and can be restored by re-exposure to opiates. *Journal of Neuroscience, 22*, 1914–1921.

Pueyo, R., Maneru, C., Junque, C., Vendrell, P., Pujol, J., Mataro, M., et al. (2003). Quantitative signal intensity measures on magnetic resonance imaging in attention-deficit hyperactivity disorder. *Cognitive Behavioral Neurology, 16*, 75–81.

Pulvar, A. E. (2000). Search for schizophrenia susceptibility genes. *Biological Psychiatry, 47*, 221–230.

Purcell, A. E., Rocco, M. M., Lenhart, J. A., Hyder, K., Zimmerman, A. W., & Pevsner, J. (2001). Assessment of neural cell adhesion molecule (NCAM) in autistic serum and postmortem brain. *Journal of Autism and Developmental Disorders, 31*, 183–194.

Puzantian, T., & Hart, L. L. (1993). Clonidine in panic disorder. *Annals of Pharmacotherapy, 27*, 1351–1353.

Quertemont, E., de Neuville, J., & De Witte, P. (1998). Changes in the amygdala amino acid microdialysate after conditioning with a cue associated with ethanol. *Psychopharmacology, 139*, 71–78.

Quintin, P., Benkelfat, C., Launay, J. M., Arnulf, I., Pointereau-Bellenger, A., Barbault, S., et al. (2001). Clinical and neurochemical effect of acute tryptophan depletion in unaffected relatives of patients with bipolar affective disorder. *Biological Psychiatry, 50*, 184–190.

Quirk, G. J., & Gehlert, D. R. (2003). Inhibition of the amygdala: Key to pathological states? *Annals of the New York Academy of Sciences, 985*, 263–272.

Quitkin, F. M., Petkova, E., McGrath, P. J., Taylor, B., Beasley, C., Stewart, J., et al. (2003). When should a trial of fluoxetine for major depression be declared failed? *American Journal of Psychiatry, 160*, 734–740.

Raboniwitz, J., Cohen, H., & Atias, S. (2002). Outcomes of naltrexone maintenance following ultra rapid opiate detoxification versus intensive inpatient detoxification. *American Journal of Addiction, 11*, 52–56.

Raedler, T. J., Knable, M. B., Jones, D. W., Urbina. R. A., Corey, J. G., Lee, K. S., et al. (2003). In vivo determination of muscarinic acetylcholine receptor availability in schizophrenia. *American Journal of Psychiatry, 160*, 118–127.

Ragonese, P., Salemi, G., Morgante, L., Aridon, P., Epifanio, A., Buffa, D., et al. (2003). A case-control study on cigarette, alcohol, and coffee consumption preceding Parkinson's disease. *Neuroepidemiology, 22*, 297–304.

Raichle, M. E. (2000). A brief history of human functional brain mapping. In A. W. Toga & J. C. Mazziotta (Eds.), *Brain mapping: The systems* (pp. 33–76). CA: Academic Press.

Raiha, I., Kaprio, J., Koskenvuo, M., Rajala, T., & Sourander, L. (1996). Alzheimer's disease in Finnish twins. *Lancet, 347*, 573–578.

Raine, A., Buchsbaum, M. S., Stanley, J., Lottenberg, S., Abel, L., & Stoddard, J. (1994). Selective reductions in prefrontal glucose metabolism in murderers. *Biological Psychiatry, 36*, 365–373.

Raison, C. L., & Miller, A. H. (2003). When not enough is too much: The role of insufficient glucocorticoid signaling in the pathophysiology of stress-related disorders. *American Journal of Psychiatry, 160*, 1554–1565.

Raiteri, M. (2001). Presynaptic autoreceptors. *Journal of Neurochemistry, 78*, 673–675.

Rajkowska, G. (2003). Depression: What we can learn from postmortem studies. *Neuroscientist, 9*, 273–284.

Rajkowska, G., Halaris, A., & Selemon, L. D. (2001). Reductions in neuronal and glial density characterize the dorsolateral prefrontal cortex in bipolar disorder. *Biological Psychiatry, 49*, 741–752.

Rakic, P. (1995) A small step for the cell, a giant leap for mankind—a hypothesis of neocortical expansion during evolution. *Trends in Neuroscience, 18*, 383–388.

Ramachandran, V. S. (1993). Behavioral and magnetoencephalographic correlates of plasticity in the adult human brain. *Proceedings of the National Academy of the Sciences, USA, 90*, 10413–10420.

Ramachandran, V. S., & Rogers-Ramachandran, D. (2000). Phantom limbs and neural plasticity. *Archives of Neurology, 57*, 317–320.

Ramoz, N., Reichert, J. G., Smith, C. J., Silverman, J. M., Bespalova, I. N., Davis, K. L., et al. (2004). Linkage and association of the mitochondrial aspartate/glutamate carrier SLC25A12 gene with autism. *American Journal of Psychiatry, 161*, 662–669.

Ranade, S. S., Mansour, H., Wood, J., Chowdari, L. K., Brar, L. K., Kupfer, D. J., et al. (2003). Linkage and association between serotonin 2A receptor gene polymorphism and bipolar I disorder. *American Journal of Medical Genetics, 121B*, 28–34.

Rao, M. L., Hawellek, B., Papassotiropoulos, A., Deister, A., & Frahnert, C. (1998). Upregulation of the platelet serotonin 2A receptor and low blood serotonin in suicidal psychiatric patients. *Neuropsychobiology, 38*, 84–98.

Rao, V. L., Dogan, A., Todd, K. G., Bowen, K. K., & Dempsey, R. J. (2001). Neuroprotection by memantine, a non-competitive NMDA receptor antagonist after traumatic brain injury in rats. *Brain Research, 911*, 96–100.

Rapoport, J., Giedd, J., Blumenthal, J., Hamburger, S., Jeffries, N., Fernandez, T., et al. (1999). Progressive cortical change during adolescence in childhood-onset schizophrenia. A longitudinal magnetic resonance imaging study. *Archives of General Psychiatry, 56*, 649–654.

Rapoport, J. L., Gield, J., Kumra, S., Jacobsen, L., Smith, A., Lee, P., et al. (1997). Childhood-onset schizophrenia: Progressive ventricular change during adolescence. *Archives of General Psychiatry, 54*, 897–903.

Rapoport, M., Feder, V., & Sandor, P. (1998). Response of major depression and Tourette's syndrome to ECT: A case report. *Psychosomatic Medicine, 60*, 528–529.

Rapoport, S. I. (2003). Coupled reductions in brain oxidative phosphorylation and synaptic function can be quantified and staged in the course of Alzheimer disease. *Neurotoxicity Research, 5*, 385–398.

Rapoport, S. I., Horwitz, B., Grady, C. L., Haxby, J. V., DeCarli, C., & Schapiro, M. B. (1991). Abnormal brain glucose metabolism in Alzheimer's disease, as measured by position emission tomography. *Advances in Experimental Medicine and Biology, 291*, 231–248.

Rapoport, S. I., Pettigrew, K. D., & Schapiro, M. B. (1991). Discordance and concordance of dementia of the Alzheimer type (DAT) in monozygotic twins indicate heritable and sporadic forms of Alzheimer's disease. *Neurology, 41*, 1549–1553.

Rasmussen, E. R., Neuman, R. J., Heath, A. C., Levy, F., Hay, D. A., & Todd, R. D. (2004). Familial clustering of latent class and DSM-IV defined attention-deficit/hyperactivity disorder (ADHD) subtypes. *Journal of Child Psychology and Psychiatry, 45*, 589–598.

Rasmussen, K., Almvik, R., & Levander, S. (2001). Attention deficit hyperactivity disorder, reading disability, and personality disorders in a prison population. *Journal of the American Academy of Psychiatry and Law, 29*, 186–193.

Ratzoni, G., Hermesh, H., Brandt, N., Lauffer, M., & Munitz, H. (1990). Clomipramine efficacy for tics, obsessions, and compulsions in Tourette's syndrome and obsessive-compulsive disorder: A case study. *Biological Psychiatry, 27*, 95–98.

Rauch, S. L., Shin, L. M., Dougherty, D. D., Alpert, N. M., Fischman, A. J., & Jenike, M. A. (2002). Predictors of fluvoxamine response in contamination-related obsessive compulsive disorder: PET symptom provocation study. *Neuropsychopharmacology, 27*, 782–791.

Rauch, S. L., Shin, L. M., & Wright, C. I. (2003). Neuroimaging studies of amygdala function in anxiety disorders. *Annals of the New York Academy of Sciences, 985*, 389–410.

Ravaglia, G., Forti, P., Maioli, F., Sacchetti, L., Mariani, E., Nativio, V., et al. (2002). Education, occupation, and prevalence of dementia: Findings from the Conselice study. *Dementia and Geriatric Cognitive Disorders, 14*, 90–100.

Ravnkilde, B., Videbech, P., Clemmensen, K., Egander, A., Rasmussen, N. A., Gjedde, A., et al. (2003). The Danish PET/depression project: Cognitive function and regional cerebral blood flow. *Acta Psychiatrica Scandinavica, 108*, 32–40.

Rayburn, N. R., & Otto, M. W. (2003). Cognitive-behavioral therapy for panic disorder: A review of treatment elements, strategies, and outcomes. *CNS Spectrums, 8*, 356–362.

Reba, R. C. (1993). PET and SPECT: Opportunities and challenges for psychiatry. *Journal of Clinical Psychiatry, 54, Supplement*, 26–32.

Rechlin, T., Weis, M., & Claus, D. (1994). Heart rate variability in depressed patients and differential effects of paroxetine and amitriptyline on cardiovascular autonomic functions. *Pharmacopsychiatry, 27*, 124–128.

Rees, T. M., & Brimijoin, S. (2003). The role of acetylcholinesterase in the pathogenesis of Alzheimer's disease. *Drugs of Today, 39*, 75–83.

Reid, I. C., & Stewart, C. A. (2001). How antidepressants work: New perspectives on the pathophysiology of depressive disorder. *British Journal of Psychiatry, 178*, 299–303.

Reiman, E. M., Caselli, R. J., Chen, K., Alexander, G. E., Bandy, D., & Frost, J. (2001). Declining brain activity in cognitively normal apolipoprotein E ε4 heterozygotes: A foundation for using positron emission tomography to efficiently test treatments to prevent Alzheimer's disease. *Proceedings of the National Academy of Sciences, 98*, 3334–3339.

Reimer, R. J., Fon, E. A., & Edwards, R. H. (1998). Vesicular neurotransmitter transport and the presynaptic regulation of quantal size. *Current Opinion in Neurobiology, 8*, 405–412.

Reimherr, F. W., Amsterdam, J. D., Quitkin, F. M., Rosenbaum, F., Fava, M., Zajecka, J., et al. (1998). Optimal length of continuation therapy in depression: A prospective assessment during long-term fluoxetine treatment. *American Journal of Psychiatry, 15*, 1247–1253.

Reisberg, B., Doody, R., Stöffler, A., Schmitt, F., Ferris, S., & Möbius, H. J. (2003). Memantine in moderate-to-severe Alzheimer's disease. *New England Journal of Medicine, 348*, 1333–1341.

Retz, W., Thome, J., Blocher, D., Baader, M., & Roesler, M. (2002). Association of attention deficit hyperactivity disorder-related psychopathology and personality traits with the serotonin transporter promoter region polymorphism. *Neuroscience Letters, 319*, 133–136.

Reynolds, C. F. (1992). Treatment of depression in special populations. *Journal of Clinical Psychiatry, 53*, 45–53.

Rice, J. A., & Weyandt, L. L. (2000). Performance in measures of executive function in adults with Tourette's syndrome. *ADHD Report, 8*, 1–7.

Richardson, A. J., & Puri, B. K. (2002). A randomized double-blind, placebo-controlled study of the effects of supplementation with highly unsaturated fatty acids on ADHD-related symptoms in children with specific learning difficulties. *Progress in Neuropsychopharmacology and Biological Psychiatry, 26*, 233–239.

Riddle, M. A., Hardin, M. T., King, R., Scahill, L., & Wollston, J. L. (1990). Fluoxetine treatment of children and adolescents with Tourette's and obsessive-compulsive disorders: Preliminary clinical experiences. *Journal of the American Academy of Child and Adolescent Psychiatry, 29*, 45–48.

Riedel, G., Platt, B., & Micheau, J. (2003). Glutamate receptor function in learning and memory. *Behavioural Brain Research, 140*, 1–47.

Rietveld, M. J., Hudziak, J. J., Bartels, M., van Beijsterveldt, C. E., & Boomsma, D. I. (2003). Heritability of attention problems in children: I. Cross-sectional results from a study of twins, age 3–12 years. *American Journal of Medical Genetics, 117B*, 102–113.

Rinne, J. O., Laihinen, A., Lönnberg, P., Marjamäki, P., & Rinne, U. K. (1991). A postmortem study on striatal dopamine receptors in Parkinson's disease. *Brain Research, 556*, 117–122.

Rioux, L., Nissanov, J., Lauber, K., Bilker, W. B., & Arnold, S. E. (2003). Distribution of microtubule-associated protein MAP2-immunoreactive interstitial neurons in the parahippocampal white matter in subjects with schizophrenia. *American Journal of Psychiatry, 160*, 149–155.

Ritvo, E. R., Freeman, B. J., Scheibel, A. B., Duong, T., Robinson, H., Guthrie D., et al. (1986). Lower Purkinje cell counts in the cerebella of four autistic subjects: Initial findings of the UCLA-NSAC Autopsy Research Report. *American Journal of Psychiatry, 143*, 862–866.

Ritz, M. C., Lamb, R. J., Goldberg, S. R., & Kuhar, M. J. (1987). Cocaine receptors on dopamine transporters are related to self-administration of cocaine. *Science, 237*, 1219–1223.

Rive, B., Vercelletto, M., Damier, F. D., Cochran, J., & François, C. (2004). Memantine enhances autonomy in moderate to severe Alzheimer's disease. *International Journal of Geriatric Psychiatry, 19*, 458–464.

Roane, H. S., Piazza, C. C., Cercone, J. J., & Grados, M. (2002). Assessment and treatment of vocal tics associated with Tourette's syndrome. *Behavior Modification, 26*, 482–498.

Roberts, A. J., McDonald, J. S., Heyser, C. J., Kieffer, B. L., Matthes, H. W., Koob, G. F., et al. (2000). Mu-opioid receptor knockout mice do not self-administer alcohol. *Journal of Pharmacology and Experimental Therapy, 293*, 1002–1008.

Roberts, R. E., Attkinsson, C. C., & Rosenblatt, A. (1998). Prevalence of psychopathology among children and adolescents. *American Journal of Psychiatry, 155*, 715–725.

Robertson, M. M. (2003). Diagnosing Tourette syndrome: Is it a common disorder? *Journal of Psychosomatic Research, 55*, 3–6.

Robinson, D., Wu, H., Munne, R. A., Ashtari, M., Alvir, J. M., Lerner, G., et al. (1995). Reduced caudate nucleus volume in obsessive-compulsive disorder. *Archives of General Psychiatry, 52*, 393–398.

Robinson, T. E., & Berridge, K. C. (2000). The psychology and neurobiology of addiction: An incentive-sensitization view. *Addiction, 95*, 91–117.

Robinson, T. E., Gorny, G., Mitton, E., & Kolb, B. (2001). Cocaine self-administration alters the morphology of dendrites and dendritic spines in the nucleus accumbens and neocortex. *Synapse, 39*, 257–266.

Robinson, T. E., & Kolb, B. (2004). Structural plasticity associated with exposure to drugs of abuse. *Neuropharmacology, 47*, 33–46.

Rocca, P., Beoni, A. M., Eva, C., Ferrero, P., Maina, G., Bogetto, F., et al. (2000). Lymphocyte peripheral benzodiazepine receptor mRNA decreases in obsessive-compulsive disorder. *European Neuropsychopharmacology, 10*, 337–340.

Rodriguez, G., Nobili, F., Rocca, G., De Carli, F., Gianelli, M. V., & Rosadini, G. (1998). Quantitative electroencephalography and regional cerebral blood flow: Discriminant analysis between Alzheimer's patients and healthy controls. *Dementia and Geriatric Cognitive Disorders, 9*, 274–283.

Rohan, M., Parow, A., Stoll, A. L., Demopulos, C., Friedman, S., Dager, S., et al. (2004). Low-field magnetic stimulation in bipolar depression using an MRI-based stimulator. *American Journal of Psychiatry, 161*, 93–98.

Rohde, L. A., Roman, T., Szobot, C., Cunha, R. D., Hutz, M. H., & Biederman, J. (2003). Dopamine transporter gene, response to methylphenidate and cerebral blood flow in attention-deficit/hyperactivity disorder: A pilot study. *Synapse, 48*, 87–89.

Roizen, N. J., Blondis, T. A., Irwin, M., Rubinoff, A., Kieffer, J., & Stein, M. A. (1996). Psychiatric and developmental disorders in families of children with attention-deficit hyperactivity disorder. *Archives of Pediatric and Adolescent Medicine, 150*, 203–208.

Rojas, D. C., Smith, J. A., Benkers, T. L., Camou, S. L., Reite, M. L., & Rogers, S. J. (2004). Hippocampus and amygdala volumes in parents of children with autistic disorder. *American Journal of Psychiatry, 161*, 2038–2044.

Roks, G., Dermaut, B., Heutink, P., Julliams, A., Backhovens, H., Van de Broeck, M., et al. (1999). Mutation screening of the tau gene in patients with early-onset Alzheimer's disease. *Neuroscience Letters, 277*, 137–139.

Roman, T., Schmitz, M., Polanczyk, G. V., Eizirik, M., Rohde, L. A., & Hutz, M. H. (2001). Attention-deficit hyperactivity disorder: A study of association with both the dopamine transporter gene and the dopamine D4 receptor gene. *American Journal of Medical Genetics, 105*, 471–478.

Roman, T., Schmitz, M., Polanczyk, G. V., Eizirik, M., Rohde, L. A., & Hutz, M. H. (2002). Further evidence for the association between attention-deficit/hyperactivity disorder and the dopamine-β-hydroxylase gene. *American Journal of Medical Genetics, 114*, 154–158.

Roman, T., Schmitz, M., Polanczyk, G. V., Eizirik, M., Rohde, L. A., & Hutz, M. H. (2003). Is the alpha-2A adrenergic receptor gene (ADRA2A) associated with attention-deficit/hyperactivity disorder? *American Journal of Human Genetics, 120B*, 116–120.

Romano, S. J., Halmi, K. A., Sarkar, N. P., Koke, S. C., & Lee, J. S. (2002). A placebo-controlled study of fluoxetine in continued treatment of bulimia nervosa after successful acute fluoxetine treatment. *American Journal of Psychiatry, 159*, 96–102.

Romstad, A., Dupont, E., Krag-Olsen, B., Ostergaard, K., Guldberg, P., & Guttler, F. (2003). Dopa-responsive dystonia and Tourette syndrome in a large Danish family. *Archives of Neurology, 60*, 618–622.

Rosenberg, D. R., Benazon, N. R., Gilbert, A., Sullivan, A., & Moore, G. J. (2000). Thalamic volume in pediatric obsessive-compulsive disorder patients before and after cognitive behavioral therapy. *Biological Psychiatry, 48*, 294–300.

Rosenberg, D. R., Keshavan, M. S., Dick, E. L., Bagwell, W. W., MacMaster, F. P., & Birmaher, B. (1997). Corpus callosal morphology in treatment-naive pediatric obsessive compulsive disorder. *Progress in Neuro-Psychopharmacology & Biological Psychiatry, 21*, 1269–1283.

Rosenberg, D. R., Keshavan, M. S., O'Hearn, K. M., Dick, E. L., Bagwell, W. W., Seymour, A. B., et al. (1997). Frontostriatal measurement in treatment-naive children with obsessive-compulsive disorder. *Archives of General Psychiatry, 54*, 824–830.

Rosenberg, D. R., MacMaster, F. P., Keshavan, M. S., Fitzgerald, K. D., Stewart, C. M., & Moore, G. J. (2000). Decrease in caudate glutamatergic concentrations in pediatric obsessive-compulsive disorder patients taking paroxetine. *Journal of the American Academy of Child and Adolescent Psychiatry, 39*, 1096–1103.

Rosenvinge, J. H., Matinussen, M., & Ostensen, E. (2000). The comorbidity of eating disorders and personality disorders: A meta-analytic review of studies published between 1983 and 1998. *Eating and Weight Disorders, 5*, 52–61.

Roskies, A. (2002). Neuroethics for a new millenium. *Neuron, 35*, 21–23.

Roslin, M., & Kurian, M. (2003). Vagus nerve stimulation in the treatment of morbid obesity. In S. C. Schachter & D. Schmidt (Eds.), *Vagus nerve stimulation* (2nd ed., pp. 113–121). New York: Martin Dunitz, Taylor & Francis Group.

Ross, G. W., Abbott, R. D., Petrovitch, H., Morens, D. M., Grandinetti, A., Tung, K. H., et al. (2000). Association of coffee and caffeine intake with the risk of Parkinson disease. *Journal of the American Medical Association, 283*, 2674–2679.

Rossi, A., Barraco, A., & Donda, P. (2004). Fluoxetine: A review on evidence based medicine. *Annals of General Hospital Psychiatry, 12*, 2.

Rotondo, A., Mazzanti, C., Dell'Osso, L., Rucci, P., Sullivan, P., Bouanani, S., et al. (2002). Catechol o-methyltransferase, serotonin transporter, and tryptophan hydroxylase gene polymorphism in bipolar disorder patiens with and without comorbid panic disorder. *American Journal of Psychiatry, 159*, 23–29.

Rowe, D. C., Stever, C., Giedinghagen, L. N., Gard, J. M. C., Cleveland, H. H., Terris, S. T., et al. (1998). Dopamine DRD4 receptor polymorphism and attention deficit hyperactivity disorder. *Molecular Psychiatry, 3*, 419–426.

Rowland, A. S., Lesesne, C. A., & Abramowitz, A. J. (2002). The epidemiology of attention-deficit/hyperactivity disorder (ADHD): A public health view. *Mental Retardation and Developmental Disabilities Research Reviews, 8*, 162–170.

Roy, A., Dejong, J., & Ferraro, T. (1991). CSF GABA in depressed patients and normal controls. *Psychological Medicine, 21*, 613–618.

Roy-Byrne, P., Russo, J., Pollack, M., Stewart, R., Bystrisky, A., Bell, J., et al. (2003). Personality and symptom sensitivity predictors of alprazolam withdrawal in panic disorder. *Psychological Medicine, 33*, 511–518.

Rubia, K., Overmeyer, S., Taylor, E., Brammer, M., Williams, S. C., Simmons, A., & Bullmore, E. T. (1999). Hypofrontality in attention deficit hyperactivity disorder during higher-order motor control: A study with functional MRI. *American Journal of Psychiatry, 156*, 891–896.

Rubin, E., Sackeim, H. A., Prohovnik, I., Moeller, J. R., Schnur, D. B., & Mukherjee, S. (1995). Regional cerebral blood flow in mood disorders: IV. Comparison of mania and depression. *Psychiatry Research, 61*, 1–10.

Rück, C., Andréewitch, S., Flyckt, K., Edman, G., Nyman, H., Meyerson, B. A., et al. (2003). Capsulotomy for refractory anxiety disorders: Long-term follow-up of 26 patients. *American Journal of Psychiatry, 160*, 513–521.

Ruitenberg, A., Ott, A., van Swieten, J. C., Hofman, A., & Breteler, M. M. (2001). Incidence of dementia: Does gender make a difference? *Neurobiology of Aging, 22*, 575–580.

Ruitenberg, A., van Swieten, J. C., Witteman, J. C., Mehta, K. M., van Duijn, C. M., Hofman, A., et al. (2002). Alcohol consumption and risk of dementia: The Rotterdam Study. *Lancet, 359*, 281–286.

Rumsey, J. M., Duara, R., Grady, C., Rapoport, J. L., Margolin, R. A., Rapoport, S. I., et al. (1985). Brain metabolism in autism. Resting cerebral glucose utilization rates as measured with positron emission tomography. *Archives of General Psychiatry, 42*, 448–455.

Runeson, B., & Åsberg, M. (2003). Family history of suicide among suicide victims. *American Journal of Psychiatry, 160*, 1525–1526.

Rupprecht, R., & Zwanzger, P. (2003). Significance of GABAA receptors for the pathophysiology and therapy of panic disorders. *Der Nervenarzt, 74*, 543–551.

Rush, J. A. (2003). Vagus nerve stimulation: Clinical results in depression. In S. C. Schachter & D. Schmidt (Eds.), *Vagus nerve stimulation* (2nd ed., pp. 85–112). New York: Martin Dunitz, Taylor & Francis Group.

Russ, C., Powell, J. F., Zhao, J., Baker, M., Hutton, M., Crawford, F., et al. (2001). The microtubule associated protein tau gene and Alzheimer's disease—An association study and meta-analysis. *Neuroscience Letters, 314*, 92–96.

Russell, J., & Hill, E. L. (2001). Action-monitoring and intention reporting in children with autism. *Journal of Child Psychology and Psychiatry, and Allied Disciplines, 42*, 317–328.

Russell, P. S., Tharyan, P., Arun Kumar, K., & Cherian, A. (2002). Electro convulsive therapy in a pre-pubertal child with severe depression. *Journal of Postgraduate Medicine, 48*, 290–291.

Rutter, M. (2000). Genetic studies of autism: From the 1970s into the millennium. *Journal of Abnormal Child Psychology, 28*, 3–15.

Rutter, M., Caspi, A., Fergusson, D., Horwood, L. J., Goodman, R., Maughan, B., et al. (2004). Sex differences in developmental reading disability: New findings from 4 epidemiological studies. *Journal of the American Medical Association, 291*, 2007–2012.

Ryan, J. M., Kidder, S. W., Daiello, L. A., & Tariot, P. N. (2002). Mental health services in nursing homes: Psychopharmacologic interventions in nursing homes: What do we know and where should we go? *Psychiatric Services, 53*, 1407–1413.

Ryan, N. D. (2003). Child and adolescent depression: Short-term treatment effectiveness and long-term opportunities. *International Journal of Methods in Psychiatric Research, 12*, 44–53.

Rybicki, B. A., Johnson, C. C., Peterson, E. L., Kortsha, G. X., & Gorell, J. M. (1999). A family history of Parkinson's disease and its effect on other PD risk factors. *Neuroepidemiology, 18*, 270–278.

Sánchez, J. L., Buriticá, O., Pineda, D., Uribe, C. S., & Palacio, L. G. (2004). Prevalence of Parkinson's disease and Parkinsonism in a Colombian population using the capture–recapture method. *International Journal of Neuroscience, 114*, 175–182.

Sánchez-Fernández, C., González, C., Mercer, L. D., Beart, P. M., Ruiz-Gayo, M., & Fernández-Alfonso, M. S. (2003). Cholecystokinin induces cerebral vasodilatation via presynaptic CCK2 receptors: New implications for the pathophysiology of panic. *Journal of Cerebral Blood Flow and Metabolism, 23*, 364–370.

Sachdev, P., Trollor, J., Walker, A., Wen, W., Fulham, M., Smith, J. S., et al. (2001). Bilateral orbitomedial leucotomy for obsessive-compulsive disorder: A single-case study using positron emission tomography. *Australian and New Zealand Journal of Psychiatry, 35*, 684–690.

Sachdev, P. S., McBride, R., Loo, C. K., Mitchell, P. B., Malhi, G. S., & Croker, V. M. (2001). Right versus left prefrontal transcranial magnetic stimulation for obsessive-compulsive disorder: A preliminary investigation. *Journal of Clinical Psychiatry, 62*, 981–984.

Sackeim, H. A., Prohovnik, I., Moeller, J. R., Mayeux, R., Stern, Y., & Devanand, D. P. (1993). Regional cerebral blood flow in mood disorders. II. Comparison of major depression and Alzheimer's disease. *Journal of Nuclear Medicine, 34*, 1090–1101.

Sackeim, H. A., Rush, A. J., George, M. S., Marangell, L. B., Husain, M. M., Nahas, Z., et al. (2001). Vagus nerve stimulation (TNS) for treatment-resistant depression: Efficacy, side effects, and predictors of outcome. *Neuropsychopharmacology, 25*, 713–728.

Sackheim, H. A. (1997). What's new with ECT. *American Society of Clinical Psychopharmacology Progress Notes, 8*, 27–33.

Sadato, N., Okada, T., Honda, M., & Yonekura, Y. (2002). Critical period for cross-modal plasticity in blind humans: A functional MRI study. *Neuroimage, 16*, 389–400.

Sadato, N., Pascual-Leone, A., Grafman, J., Deibe, M. P., Ibanez, V., & Hallett, M. (1998). Neural networks for Braille reading by the blind. *Brain, 121*, 1213–1229.

Saemundsen, E., Magnússon, P., Smári, J., & Sigurdardóttir, S. (2003). Autism diagnostic interview-revised and the childhood autism rating scale: Convergence and discrepancy in diagnosing autism. *Journal of Autism and Developmental Disorders, 33*, 319–328.

Safer, D. J. (1973). A familial factor in minimal brain dysfunction. *Behavioral Genetics, 3*, 175–186.

Safer, D. J., & Zito, J. M. (2000). Pharmacoepidemiology of methylphenidate and other stimulants for the treatment of attention deficit hyperactivity disorder. In L. L. Greenhill & B. B. Osman (Eds.), *Ritalin: Theory and practice* (2nd ed. pp. 7–26). New York: Mary Ann Liebert.

Safer, D. J., Zito, J. M., & dosReis, S. (2003). Concomitant psychotropic medication for youths. *American Journal of Psychiatry, 160*, 438–449.

Safren, S. A., Gershuny, B. S., Marzol, P., Otto, M. W., & Pollack, M. H. (2002). History of childhood abuse in panic disorder, social phobia, and generalized anxiety disorder. *Journal of Nervous and Mental Disease, 190*, 453–456.

Sallee, F. R., Gilbert, D. L., Vinks, A. A., Miceli, J. J., Robarge, L., & Wilner, K. (2003). Pharmacodynamics of ziprasidone in children and adolescents: Impact on dopamine transmission. *Journal of the American Academy of Child and Adolescent Psychiatry, 42*, 902–907.

Sallee, F. R., Nesbitt, L., Jackson, C., Sine, L., & Sethuraman, G. (1997). Relative efficiency of haloperidol and pimozide in children and adolescents with Tourette's disorder. *American Journal of Psychiatry, 154*, 1057–1062.

Sallee, F. R., Sethuraman, G., Sine, L., & Liu, H. (2000). Yohimbine challenge in children with anxiety disorders. *American Journal of Psychiatry, 157*, 1236–1242.

Sallet, P. C., Elkis, H., Alves, T. M., Oliveira, J. R., Sassi, E., de Castro, C. C., et al. (2003). Reduced cortical folding in schizophrenia: An MRI morphometric study. *American Journal of Psychiatry, 160*, 1606–1613.

Salloway, S., Malloy, P., Kohn, R., Gillard, E., Duffy, J., Rogg, J., et al. (1996). MRI and neuropsychological differences in early- and late-life-onset geriatric depression. *Neurology, 46*, 1567–1574.

Salokangas, R. K. R., Honkonen, T., Stengard, E., Koivisto, A. M., & Hietala, J. (2002). Negative symptoms and neuroleptics in catatonic schizophrenia. *Schizophrenia Research, 59*, 73–76.

Saloviita, T., Ruusila, L., & Ruusila, U. (2000). Incidence of savant syndrome in Finland. *Perception and Motor Skills, 91*, 120–122.

Salthouse, T. A., Atkinson, T. M., & Berish, D. E. (2003). Executive functioning as a potential mediator of age-related cognitive decline in normal adults. *Journal of Experimental Psychology: General, 132*, 566–594.

Samson, S., & Zatorre, R. J. (1988). Discrimination of melodic and harmonic stimuli after unilateral cerebral excisions. *Brain and Cognition, 7*, 348–360.

Samuels, S. C., Brickman, A. M., Burd, J. A., Purohit, D. P., Qureshi, P. Q., & Serby, M. (2004). Depression in autopsy-confirmed dementia with Lewy bodies and Alzheimer's disease. *Mount Sinai Journal of Medicine, 71*, 55–62.

Samuels, S. C., & Grossman, H. (2003). Emerging therapeutics for Alzheimer's disease: An avenue of hope. *CNS Spectrums, 8*, 834–845.

Sanberg, P. R., Shytle, D., & Silver, A. A. (1998). Treatment of Tourette's syndrome with mecamylamine. *Lancet, 352*, 705–706.

Sanberg, P. R., Silver, A. A., Shytle, R. D., Philipp, M. K., Cahill, D. W., Fogelson, H. M., et al. (1997). Nicotine for the treatment of Tourette's syndrome. *Pharmacological Therapy, 74*, 21–25.

Sand, P. G., Mori, T., Godau, C., Stöber, G., Flachenecker, P., Franke, P., et al. (2002). Norepinephrine transporter gene (NET) variants in patients with panic disorder. *Neuroscience Letters, 333*, 41–44.

Sanderson, W. C., Rapee, R. M., & Barlow, D. H. (1989). The influence of an illusion of control on panic attacks induced via inhalation of 5.5% carbon dioxide-enriched air. *Archives of General Psychiatry, 46*, 157–162.

Sandor, P. (2003). Pharmacological management of tics in patients with TS. *Journal of Psychosomatic Research, 55*, 41–48.

Sandoval, V., Riddle, E. L., Hanson, G. R., & Fleckenstein, A. E. (2003). Methylphenidate alters vesicular monoamine transport and prevents methamphetamine-induced dopaminergic deficits. *Journal of Pharmacology and Experimental Therapy, 304*, 1181–1187.

Sano, M., Ernesto, C., Thomas, R. G., Klauber, M. R., Schafer, K., Grundman M., et al. (1997). A controlled trial of selegiline, alpha-tocopherol, or both as treatment for Alzheimer's disease. The Alzheimer's Disease Cooperative Study. *New England Journal of Medicine, 336*, 1216–1222.

Sanz, E., De-las-Cuevas, C., Kiuru, A., Bate, A., & Edwards, R. (2005). Selective serotonin reuptake inhibitors in pregnant women & neonatal withdrawal syndrome: A database analysis. *Lancet, 365*, 482–487.

Sargent, P. A., Kjaer, K. H., Bench, C. J., Rabiner, E. A., Messa, C., Meyer, J., et al. (2000). Brain serotonin1A receptor binding measured by positron emission tomography with [11C]WAY-100635: Effects of depression and antidepressant treatment. *Archives of General Psychiatry, 57*, 174–180.

Sarup, A., Larsson, O. M., & Schousboe, A. (2003). GABA transporters and GABA-transaminase as drug targets. *Current Drug Targets—CNS and Neurological Disorders, 2*, 269–277.

Sassi, R. B., Nicoletti, M., Brambilla, P., Harenski, K., Mallinger, A. G., Frank, E., et al. (2001). Decreased pituitary volume in patients with bipolar disorder. *Biological Psychiatry, 50*, 271–280.

Sattler, J. M., & Weyandt, L. (2002). Specific learning disabilities. In J. M. Sattler (Ed.), *Assessment of children: Behavioral and clinical applications* (4th ed., pp. 281–335). San Diego: Sattler.

Saunders-Pullman, R., Shriberg, J., Heiman, G., Raymond, D., Wendt, K., Kramer, P., et al. (2002). Myoclonus dystonia: possible association with obsessive-compulsive disorder and alcohol dependence. *Neurology, 58*, 242–245.

Savas, H. A., Unal, B., Erbagci, H., Inaloz, S., Herken, H., Canan, S., et al. (2002). Hippocampal volume in schizophrenia and its relationship with risperdone treatment: A stereological study. *Neuropsychobiology, 46*, 61–66.

Sawle, G. V., Bloomfield, P. M., Bjorklund, A., Brooks, D. J., Brundin, P., Leenders, K. L., et al. (1992). Transplantation of fetal dopamine neurons in Parkinson's disease: PET [18F]6-L-fluorodopa studies in two patients with putaminal implants. *Annals of Neurology, 31*, 166–173.

Saxena, S., Brody, A. L., Ho, M. L., Alborzian, S., Ho, M. K., Maidment, K. M., et al. (2001). Cerebral metabolism in major depression and obsessive-compulsive disorder occurring separately and concurrently. *Biological Psychiatry, 50*, 159–170.

Saxena, S., Brody, A. L., Ho, M. L., Alborzian, S., Maidment, K. M., Zohrabi, N., et al. (2002). Differential cerebral metabolic changes with paroxetine treatment of obsessive-compulsive disorder vs major depression. *Archives of General Psychiatry, 59*, 250–261.

Saxena, S., Brody, A. L., Ho, M. L., Zohrabi, N., Maidment, K. M., & Baxter L. R. Jr. (2003). Differential brain metabolic predictors of response to paroxetine in obsessive-compulsive disorder versus major depression. *American Journal of Psychiatry, 160*, 522–532.

Saxena, S., Brody, A. L., Schwartz, J. M., & Baxter, L. R. (1998). Neuroimaging and frontal-subcortical circuitry in obsessive-compulsive disorder. *British Journal of Psychiatry, Supplement*, 26–37.

Saxena, S., Brody, A. L., Ho, M., Zohrabi, N., Maidment, K. M., & Baxter, L. R. (2003). Differential brain metabolic predictors of response to parozetine in obsessive-compulsive disorder versus major depression. *American Journal of Psychiatry, 160*, 522–532.

Saxena, S., Maidment, K. M., Vapnik, T., Golden, G., Rishwain, T., Rosen, R. M., et al. (2002). Obsessive-compulsive hoarding: Symptom severity and response to multimodal treatment. *Journal of Clinical Psychiatry, 63*, 21–27.

Scahill, L., Leckman, J. F., Schultz, R. T., Katsovich, L., & Peterson, B. S. (2003). A placebo-controlled trial of risperidone in Tourette syndrome. *Neurology, 60*, 1130–1135.

Scahill, L., Riddle, M. A., King, R. A., Hardin, M. T., Rasmusson, A., Makuch, R. W., et al. (1997). Fluoxetine has no market effect of tic symptoms in patients with Tourette's syndrome: A double-blind placebo-controlled study. *Journal of Child and Adolescent Psychopharmacology, 7*, 75–85.

Scarr, E., Pavey, G., Sundram, S., MacKinnon, A., & Dean, B. (2003). Decreased hippocampal NMDA, but not kainite or AMPA receptors in bipolar disorder. *Bipolar Disorders, 5*, 257–264.

Scherrer, J. F., True, W. R., Xian, H., Lyons, M. J., Eisen, S. A., Goldberg, J., et al. (2000). Evidence for genetic influences common and specific to symptoms of generalized anxiety and panic. *Journal of Affective Disorders, 57*, 25–35.

Schiffer, H. H. (2002). Glutamate receptor genes: Susceptibility factors in schizophrenia and depressive disorders? *Molecular Neurobiology, 25*, 191–212.

Schiffman, J., Edstrom, M., LaBrie, J., Schulsinger, F., Sorensen, H., & Mednick, S. (2002). Minor physical anomolies and schizophrenia spectrum disorders: A prospective investigation. *American Journal of Psychiatry, 159*, 238–243.

Schildkaut, J. J. (1965). The catecholamine hypothesis of affective disorders: A review of supporting evidence. *American Journal of Psychiatry, 122*, 509–522.

Schindler, K. M., Richter, M. A., Kennedy, J. L., Pato, M. T., & Pato, C. N. (2000). Association between homozygosity at the COMT gene locus and obsessive compulsive disorder. *American Journal of Medical Genetics, 96*, 721–724.

Schlaepfer, T. E., Harris, G. J., Tien, A. Y., Peng, L., Lee, S., & Pearlson, G. (1995). Structural differences in the cerebral cortex of healthy female and male subjects: A magnetic resonance imaging study. *Psychiatry Research: Neuroimaging, 61*, 129–135.

Schlaepfer, T. E., Pearlson, G. D., Wong, D. F., Marenco, S., & Dannals, R. F. (1997). PET study of competition between intravenous cocaine and [11C]-raclopride at dopamine receptors in human subjects. *American Journal of Psychiatry, 154*, 1209–1213.

Schlaggar, B. L., & O'Leary, D. D. (1991). Potential of visual cortex to develop an array of functional units unique to somatosensory cortex. *Science, 252*, 1556–1560.

Schlicker, E., & Gothert, M. (1998). Interactions between the presynaptic alpha2-autoreceptor and presynaptic inhibitory heteroreceptors on noradrenergic neurones. *Brain Research Bulletin, 15*, 129–132.

Schloss, P., & Williams, D. C. (1998). The serotonin transporter: A primary target for antidepressant drugs. *Journal of Psychopharmacology, 12*, 115–121.

Schmahl, C. G., Vermetten, E., Elzinga, B. M., & Bremner, D. J. (2003). Magnetic resonance imaging of hippocampal and amygdala volume in women with childhood abuse and borderline personality disorder. *Psychiatry Research, 122*, 193–198.

Schmauss, C., Haroutunian, V., Davis, K. L., & Davidson, M. (1993). Selective loss of dopamine D3-type receptor mRNA expression in parietal and motor cortices of patients with chronic schizophrenia. *Proceedings of the National Academy of Sciences of the United States of America, 90*, 8942–8946.

Schmitt, A., Weber, S., Jatzko, A., Braus, D. F., & Henn, F. A. (2004). Hippocampal volume and cell proliferation after acute and chronic clozapine or haloperidol treatment. *Journal of Neural Transmission, 111*, 91–100.

Schott, K., Schaefer, J. E., Richartz, E., Batra, A., Eusterschulte, B., Klein, R., et al. (2003). Autoantibodies to serotonin in serum of patients with psychiatric disorders. *Psychiatry Research, 121*, 51–57.

Schotte, A., Janssen, P. F., Gommeren, W. Luyten, W. H., Van Gompel, P., Lesage, A. S., et al. (1996). Risperidone compared with new and reference antipsychotic drugs: In vitro and in vivo receptor binding. *Psychopharmacology, 124*, 57–73.

Schrag, A., Ben-Shlomo, Y., & Quinn, N. (2002). How valid is the clinical diagnosis of Parkinson's disease in the community? *Journal of Neurology, Neurosurgery, and Psychiatry, 73*, 529–534.

Schrag, A., Jahanshahi, M., & Quinn, N. P. (2001). What contributes to depression in Parkinson's disease? *Psychological Medicine, 31*, 65–73.

Schröder, J., Buchsbaum, M. S., Shihabuddin, L., Tang, C., Wei, T. C., Spiegel-Cohen, J., et al. (2001). Patterns of cortical activity and memory performance in Alzheimer's disease. *Biological Psychiatry, 49*, 426–436.

Schroeder, U., Kuehler, A., Haslinger, B., Erhard, P., Fogel, W., Tronnier, V. M., et al. (2002). Subthalamic nucleus stimulation affects striato-anterior cingulate cortex circuit in a response conflict task: A PET study. *Brain, 125*, 1995–2004.

Schultz, R. T., Cho, N. K., Staib, L. H., Kier, L. E., Fletcher, J. M., Shaywitz, S. E., et al. (1994). Brain morphology in normal and dyslexic children: The influence of sex and age. *Annals of Neurology, 35*, 732–742.

Schultz, R. T., & Klin, A. (2002). Genetics of childhood disorder: XLIII. Autism, Part 2: Neural foundations. *Journal of the American Academy of Child and Adolescent Psychiatry, 41*, 1259–1262.

Schulz, K. P., Fan, J., Tang, C. Y., Newcorn, J. H., Buchsbaum, M., Cheung, A., et al. (2004). Response inhibition in adolescents diagnosed with attention deficit hyperactivity disorder during childhood: An event-related fMRI study. *American Journal of Psychiatry, 161*, 1650–1657.

Schumacher, J., Otte, A. C., Becker, T., Sun, Y., Wienker, T. F., Wirth, B., et al. (2003). No evidence for DUP25 in patients with panic disorder using a quantitative real-time PCR approach. *Human Genetics, 114*, 115–117.

Schuman, E. M. (1999). Neurotrophin regulation of synaptic transmission. *Current Opinion in Neurobiology, 9*, 105–109.

Schurhoff, F., Bellivier, F., Jouvent, R., Mouren-Simeoni, M., Bouvard, M., Allilaire, J. F., et al. (2000). Early and late onset bipolar disorders: Two different forms of manic-depressive illness? *Journal of Affective Disorders, 58*, 215–221.

Schwab, S. G., Hallmayer, J., Hanses, C., Albus, M., Lerer, B., Kanyas, K., et al. (1998). Further evidence for a susceptibility locus on chromosome 10p14-p11 in 72 families with schizophrenia by nonparapmetric linkage analysis. *American Journal of Medical Genetics, 81*, 302–307.

Schwartz, G., Amor, L. B., Grizenko, N., Lageix, P., Baron, C., Boivin, D., et al. (2004). Actigraph monitoring during sleep of children with ADHD on methylphenidate and placebo. *Journal of the American Academy of Child and Adolescent Psychiatry, 43*, 1267–1282.

Schwartz, J. M., & Beyette, B. (1996). *Brain lock: Free yourself from obsessive-compulsive disorder.* New York: ReganBooks.

Schweinsburg, B. C., Taylor, M. J., Alhassoon, O. M., Videen, J. S., Brown, G. G., Patterson, T. L., et al. (2001). Chemical pathology in brain white matter of recently detoxified alcoholics: A 1H magnetic resonance spectroscopy investigation of alcohol-associated frontal lobe injury. *Alcoholism: Clinical and Experimental Research, 25*, 924–934.

Schweitzer, J. B., Lee, D. O., Hanford, R. B., Tagamets, M. A., Hoffman, J. M., Grafton, S. T., et al. (2003). A positron emission tomography study of methylphenidate in adults with ADHD: Alterations in resting blood flow and predicting treatment response. *Neuropsychopharmacology, 28*, 967–973.

Scott, F. J., Baron-Cohen, S., Bolton, P., & Brayne, C. (2002). The CAST (Childhood Asperger Syndrome Test): Preliminary development of a UK screen for mainstream primary-school-age children. *Autism, 6*, 9–31.

Scott, W. K., Grubber, J. M., Conneally, P. M., Small, G. W., Hulette, C. M., Rosenberg, C. K., et al. (2000). Fine mapping of the chromosome 12 late-onset Alzheimer's disease locus: Potential genetic and phenotypic heterogeneity. *American Journal of Human Genetics, 66*, 922–932.

Scott, W. K., Nance, M. A., Watts, R. L., Hubble, J. P., Koller, W. C., Lyons, K., et al. (2001). Complete genomic screen in Parkinson disease: Evidence for multiple genes. *Journal of the American Medical Association, 286*, 2239–2244.

Scoville, W. B., & Miller, B. (1957). Loss of recent memory after bilateral hippocampal lesions. *Journal of Neurology, Neurosurgery, and Psychiatry, 20*, 11–21.

Sedvall, G., Farde, L., Persson, A., & Wiesel, F. A. (1986). Imaging of neurotransmitter receptors in the living human brain. *Archives of General Psychiatry, 43*, 995–1005.

Seeman, P., Guan, H. C., & Van Tol, H. H. (1995). Schizophrenia: Elevation of dopamine D4-like sites, using [3H]nemonapride and [125I]epidepride. *European Journal of Pharmacology, 286*, 3–5.

Seeman, P., & Tallerico, T. (1999). Rapid release of antipsychotic drugs from dopamine D2 receptors: An explanation for low receptor occupancy and early clinical relapse upon withdrawal of clozapine or quetiapine. *American Journal of Psychiatry, 156*, 876–884.

Segawa, M. (2003). Neurophysiology of Tourette's syndrome: Pathophysiological considerations. *Brain Development, 25*, supplement, 62–69.

Seibyl, J. P., Marek, K. L., Quinlan, D., Sheff, K., Zoghbi, S., Zea-Ponce, Y., et al. (1995). Decreased single-photon emission computed tomographic [123I]beta-CIT striatal uptake correlates with symptom severity in Parkinson's disease. *Annals of Neurology, 38*, 589–598.

Seidman, L. J., Faraone, S. V., Goldstein, J. M., Goodman, J. M., Kremen, W. S., Matsuda, G., et al. (1997). Reduced subcortical brain volumes in nonpsychotic siblings of schizophrenic patients: A pilot MRI study. *American Journal of Medical Genetics, Neuropsychiatric Genetics, 74*, 507–514.

Seidman, L. J., Faraone, S. V., Goldstein, J. M., Kremen, W. S., Horton, N. J., Makris, N., et al. (2002). Left hippocampal volume as a vulnerability indicator for schizophrenia: A magnetic resonance imaging morphometric sudy of nonpsychotic first-degree relatives. *Archives of General Psychiatry, 9*, 839–849.

Selemon, L. D. (2004). Increased cortical neuronal density in schizophrenia. *American Journal of Psychiatry, 161*, 1564.

Selemon, L. D., & Goldman-Rakic, P. S. (1999). The reduced neuropil hypothesis: A circuit based model of schizophrenia. *Biological Psychiatry, 45*, 17–25.

Selemon, L. D., Kleinman, J. E., Herman, M. M., & Goldman-Rakic, P. S. (2002). Smaller frontal gray matter volume in postmortem schizophrenic brains. *American Journal of Psychiatry, 159*, 1983–1991.

Selemon, L. D., & Rajkowska, G. (2003). Cellular pathology in the dorsolateral prefrontal cortex distinguishes schizophrenia from bipolar disorder. *Current Molecular Medicine, 3*, 427–436.

Selemon, L. D., Rajkowska, G., & Goldman-Rakic, P. S. (1995). Abnormally high neuronal density in the schizophrenic cortex. *Archives of General Psychiatry, 52*, 805–818.

Self, D. (2004). Drug dependence and addiction. *American Journal of Psychiatry, 161*, 223.

Sell, L. A., Morris, J., Bearn, J., Frackowiak, R. S. J., Friston, K. J., & Dolan, R. J. (1999). Activation of reward circuitry in human opiate addicts. *European Journal of Neuroscience, 11*, 1042–1048.

Semla, T. P., Cohen, D., Freels, S., Paveza, G. J., Ashford, J. W., Gorelick, P., et al. (1995). Psychotropic drug use in relation to psychiatric symptoms in community-living persons with Alzheimer's disease. *Pharmacotherapy, 15*, 495–501.

Semrud-Clikeman, M. (1997). Evidence from imaging on the relationship between brain structure and developmental language disorders. *Seminars in Pediatric Neurology, 4*, 117–124.

Semrud-Clikeman, M., Filipek, P. A., Biederman, J., Steingard, R., Kennedy, D., Renshaw, P., et al. (1994). Attention-deficit hyperactivity disorder: Magnetic resonance imaging morphometric analysis of the corpus callosum. *Journal of the American Academy of Child and Adolescent Psychology, 33*, 875–881.

Senanarong, V., Harnphadungkit, K., Lertrit, P., Mitrpant, C., Udompunthurak, S., Limwong, C., et al. (2001). Experience of ApoE study in Thai elderly. *Journal of the Medical Association of Thailand, 84*, 182–187.

Sepkuty, J. P., Cohen, A. S., Eccles, C., Rafiq, A., Behar, K., Ganel, R., et al. (2002). A neuronal glutamate transporter contributes to neurotransmitter GABA synthesis and epilepsy. *Journal of Neuroscience, 22*, 6372–6379.

Serby, M. (2003). Methylphenidate-induced obsessive-compulsive symptoms in an elderly man. *CNS Spectrums, 8*, 612–613.

Sestini, S., Scotto di Luzio, A., Ammannati, F., De Cristofaro, M. T., Passeri, A., Martini, S., et al. (2002). Changes in regional cerebral blood flow caused by deep-brain stimulation of the subthalamic nucleus in Parkinson's disease. *Journal of Nuclear Medicine, 43*, 725–732.

Shafran, R., Ralph, J., & Tallis, F. (1995). Obsessive-compulsive symptoms and the family. *Bulletin of the Menninger Clinic, 59*, 472–492.

Shafritz, K. M., Marchione, K. E, Gore, J. C., Shaywitz, S. E., & Shaywitz, B. A. (2004). The effects of methylphenidate on neural systems of attention in attention deficit hyperactivity disorder. *American Journal of Psychiatry, 161*, 1990–1997.

Shagass, C., Roemer, R. A., Straumanis, J. J., & Josiassen, R. C. (1984). Psychiatric diagnostic discriminations with combinations of quantitative EEG variables. *British Journal of Psychiatry, 144*, 581–592.

Shah, A., & Frith, U. (1983). An islet of ability in autistic children: A research note. *Journal of Child Psychology and Psychiatry, 24*, 613–620.

Shah, A., & Frith, U. (1993). Why do autistic individuals show superior performance on the block design task? *Journal of Child Psychology and Psychiatry, 34*, 1351–1364.

Shalev, U., Grimm, J. W., & Shaham, Y. (2002). Neurobiology of relapse to heroine and cocaine seeking: A review. *Pharmacological Reviews, 54*, 1–42.

Shao, Y., Cuccaro, M. L., Hauser, E. R., Raiford, K. L., Menold, M. M., Wolpert, C. M., Ravan, S. A., et al. (2003). Fina mapping of autistic disorder to chromosome 15q11-q13 by use of phenotypic subtypes. *American Journal of Human Genetics, 72*, 539–548.

Shao, Y., Wolpert, C. M., Raiford, K. L., Menold, M. M., Donnelly, S. L., Ravan, S. A., et al. (2002). Genomic screen and follow-up analysis for autistic disorder. *American Journal of Medical Genetics, 114*, 99–105.

Shapira, N. A., Liu, Y., He, A. G., Bradley, M. M., Lessig, M. C., James, G. A., et al. (2003). Brain activation by disgust-inducing pictures in obsessive-compulsive disorder. *Biological Psychiatry, 54*, 751–756.

Shapleske, J., Rossell, S. L., Woodruff, P. W., & David, A. S. (1999). The planum temporale: A systematic, quantitative review of its structural, functional and clinical significance. *Brain Research, 29*, 26–49.

Sharma, S. K., Yashpal, K., Fundytus, M. E., Sauriol, F., Henry, J. L., & Coderre, T. J. (2003). Alterations in brain metabolism induced by chronic morphine treatment: NMR studies in rat CNS. *Neurochemistry Research, 28*, 1369–1373.

Sharp, W. S., Gottesman, R. F., Greenstein, D. K., Ebens, C. L., Rapoport, J. L., & Castellanos, F. X. (2003). Monozygotic twins discordant for attention-deficit/hyperactivity disorder: Ascertainment and clinical characteristics. *Journal of the American Academy of Child and Adolescent Psychiatry, 42*, 93–97.

Shaw, P., Lawrence, E. J., Radbourne, C., Bramham, J., Polkey, C. E., & David, A. S. (2004). The impact of early and late damage to the human amygdala on "theory of mind" reasoning. *Brain, 127*, 1535–1748.

Shaywitz, B. A., Shaywitz, S. E., Pugh, K. R., Constable, R. T., Skudlarski, P., Fulbright, R. K., et al. (1995). Sex differences in the functional organization of the brain for language. *Nature, 373*, 607–609.

Sheehan, D. V. (2002). The management of panic disorder. *Journal of Clinical Psychiatry, 63, Supplement 14*, 17–21.

Sheinkopf, S. J., Mundy, P., Oller, D. K., & Steffens, M. (2000). Vocal atypicalities of preverbal autistic children. *Journal of Autism and Developmental Disorders, 30*, 345–354.

Shekhar, A., Sajdyk, T. J., Gehlert, D. R., & Rainnie, D. G. (2003). The amygdala, panic disorder, and cardiovascular responses. *Annals of the New York Academy of Sciences, 985*, 308–325.

Sheline, Y., Bardgett, M. E., & Csernansky, J. G. (1997). Correlated reductions in cerebrospinal fluid 5-HIAA and MHPG concentrations after treatment with selective serotonin reuptake inhibitors. *Journal of Clinical Psychopharmacology, 17*, 11–14.

Sheline, Y. I., Gado, M. H., & Kraemer, H. C. (2003). Untreated depression and hippocampal volume loss. *American Journal of Psychiatry, 160*, 1516–1518.

Sheline, Y. I., Mintun, M. A., Moerlein, S. M., & Snyder, A. Z. (2002). Greater loss of 5-HT(2A) receptors in midlife than in late life. *American Journal of Psychiatry, 159*, 430–435.

Sheline, Y. I., Mokhtar, H. G., & Price, J. L. (1998). Amygdala core nuclei volumes are decreased in recurrent major depression. *NeuroReport, 9*, 2023–2028.

Sheline, Y. I., Wang, P. W., Gado, M. H., Csernansky, J. G., & Vannier, M. W. (1996). Hippocampal atrophy in recurrent major depression. *Proceedings of the National Academy of Sciences of the United States of America, 93*, 3908–3913.

Shelter, D. (1985). Prenatal music experiences. *Music Education Journal, 71*, 26–27.

Shen, K., & Bargmann, C. I. (2003). The immunoglobulin superfamily protein SYG-1 determines the location of specific synapses in C. elegans. *Cell, 112*, 619–630.

Sheng, M. H. T. (2001). The postsynaptic specialization. In M. W. Cowan, T. C. Sudhof, & C. F. Stevens (Eds.), *Synapses* (pp. 315–356). Baltimore: Johns Hopkins University Press.

Shenton, M. E., Dickey, C. C., Frumin, M., & McCarley, R. W. (2001). A review of MRI findings in schizophrenia. *Schizophrenia Research, 49*, 1–52.

Sherer, T. B., Betarbet, R., & Greenamyre, J. T. (2002). Environment, mitochondria, and Parkinson's disease. *Neuroscientist, 8*, 192–197.

Sherman, D. K., Iacono, W. G., & McGue, M. K. (1997). Attention-deficit hyperactivity disorder dimensions: A twin study of attention and impulsivity-hyperactivity. *Journal of the American Academy of Childhood and Adolescent Psychiatry, 36*, 745–753.

Sherman, D. K., McGue, M. K., & Iacono, W. G. (1997). Twin concordance for attention deficit hyperactivity disorder: A comparison of teachers' and mothers' response. *American Journal of Psychiatry, 154*, 532–535.

Sherrington, C. S. (1897). The central nervous system. In M. Foster (Ed.), *A textbook of physiology* (7th ed., Part III, p. 929). London: Macmillan.

Shimamoto, H., Takasaki, K., Shigemori, M., Imaizumi, T., Aybe, M., & Shoji, H. (2001). Therapeutic effect and mechanism of repetitive transcranial magnetic stimulation in Parkinson's disease. *Journal of Neurology, 248*, 48–52.

Shimizu, E., Hashimoto, K., Okamura, N., Koike, K., Komatsu, N., Kumakiri, C., et al. (2003). Alterations of serum levels of brain-derived neurotrophic factor (BDNF) in depressed patients with or without antidepressants. *Biological Psychiatry, 54*, 70–75.

Shinahara, K., Saijo, T., Mori, K., & Kuroda, Y. (2004). Single-strand conformation polymorphism analysis of the FMR1 gene in autistic and mentally retarded children in Japan. *Journal of Medical Investigation, 51*, 52–58.

Shioe, K., Ichimiya, T., Suhara, T., Takano, A., Sudo, Y., Yasuno, F., et al. (2003). No association between genotype of the promoter region of serotonin transporter gene and serotonin transporter binding in human brain measured by PET. *Synapse, 48*, 184–188.

Shioiri, T., Oshitani, Y., Kato, T., Murashita, J., Hamakawa, H., Inubushi, T., et al. (1996). Prevalence of cavum septum pellucidum detected by MRI patients with bipolar disorder, major depression, and schizophrenia. *Psychological Medicine, 26*, 431–434.

Shippenberg, T. S., & Elmer, G. I. (1998). The neurobiology of opiate reinforcement. *Critical Reviews in Neurobiology, 12*, 267–303.

Shoptaw, S., Yang, X., Rotheram-Fuller, E. J., Hsieh, Y. C., Kintaudi, P. C., Charuvastra, V. C., et al. (2003). Randomized placebo-controlled trial of baclofen for cocaine dependence: Preliminary effects for individuals with chronic patterns of cocaine use. *Journal of Clinical Psychiatry, 64*, 1440–1448.

Short, E. J., Manos, M. J., Findling, R. L., & Schubel, E. A. (2004). A prospective study of stimulant response in preschool children: Insights from ROC analyses. *Journal of the American Academy of Child and Adolescent Psychiatry, 43*, 251–259.

Shulman, R. B. (2003). Maintenance ECT in the treatment of PD. Therapy improves psychotic symptoms, physical function. *Geriatrics, 58*, 43–45.

Sichel, D. A., Cohen, L. S., Dimmock, J. A., & Rosenbaum, J. F. (1993). Postpartum obsessive compulsive disorder: A case series. *Journal of Clinical Psychiatry, 54*, 156–159.

Sichel, D. A., Cohen, L. S., Robertson, L. M., Ruttenberg, A., & Rosenbaum, J. F. (1995). Prophylactic estrogen in recurrent postpartum affective disorder. *Biological Psychiatry, 38*, 814–818.

Siegel, B. V. Jr., Nuechterlein, K. H., Abel, L., Wu, J. C., & Buchsbaum, M. S. (1995). Glucose metabolic correlates of continuous performance test performance in adults with a history of infantile autism, schizophrenics, and controls. *Schizophrenia Research, 17*, 85–94.

Siegle, G. J., Steinhauer, S. R., Thase, M. E., Stenger, V. A., & Carter, C. S. (2002). Can't shake that feeling: Event-related fMRI assessment of sustained amygdala activity in response to emotional information in depressed individuals. *Biological Psychiatry, 51*, 693–707.

Sigurdsson, E., Fombonne, E., Sayal, K., & Chekley, S. (1999). Neurodevelopmental antecedents of early-onset bipolar affective disorder. *British Journal of Psychiatry, 174*, 121–127.

Sigurdsson, E. M., Permanne, B., Soto, C., Wisniewski, T., & Frangione, B. (2000). In vivo reversal of amyloid-β lesions in rat brain. *Journal of Neuropathology and Experimental Neurology, 59*, 11–17.

Silbersweig, D. A., Stern, E., Frith, C., Cahill, C., Holmes, A., Grootoonk, S., et al. (1995). A functional neuroanatomy of hallucinations in schizophrenia. *Nature, 378*, 176–179.

Silbert, L. C., Quinn, J. F., Moore, M. M., Corbridge, E., Ball, M. J., Murdoch, G., et al. (2003). Changes in premorbid brain volume predict Alzheimer's disease pathology. *Neurology, 61*, 487–492.

Silfverskiold, P., & Risberg, J. (1989). Regional cerebral blood flow in depression and mania. *Archives of General Psychiatry, 46*, 253–259.

Silver, A. A., Shytle, R. D., Philipp, M. K., Wilkinson, B. J., McConville, B., & Sanberg, P. R. (2001). Transdermal nicotine and haloperidol in Tourette's disorder: A double-blind placebo-controlled study. *Journal of Clinical Psychiatry, 62*, 707–714.

Silver, H. (2003). Selective serotonin reuptake inhibitor augmentation in the treatment of negative symptoms of schizophrenia. *International Clinical Psychopharmacology, 18*, 305–313.

Silverman, J. M., Smith, C. J., Marin, D. B., Birstein, S., Mare, M., Mohs, R. C., et al. (1999). Identifying families with likely genetic protective factors against Alzheimer's disease. *American Journal of Human Genetics, 64*, 832–838.

Silverman, J. M., Smith, C. J., Marin, D. B., Mohs, R. C., & Propper, C. B. (2003). Familial patterns of risk in very late-onset Alzheimer disease. *Archives of General Psychiatry, 60*, 190–197.

Simon, G. E., Fleck, M., Lucas, R., Bushnell, D. M., & LIDO Group. (2004). Prevalence and predictors of depression treatment in an international primary care study. *American Journal of Psychiatry, 161*, 1626–1634.

Simpson, D., & Plosker, G. L. (2004). Spotlight on atomoxetine in adults with attention-deficit hyperactivity disorder. *CNS Drugs, 18*, 397–401.

Simpson, H. B., Gorfinkle, K. S., & Liebowitz, M. R. (1999). Cognitive-behavioral therapy as an adjunct to serotonin reuptake inhibitors in obsessive-compulsive disorder: An open trial. *Journal of Clinical Psychiatry, 60*, 584–590.

Simpson, H. B., Lombardo, I., Slifstein, M., Huang, H. Y., Hwang, D. R., Abi-Dargham, A., et al. (2003). Serotonin transporters in obsessive-compulsive disorder: A positron emission tomography study with [(11)C]McN 5652. *Biological Psychiatry, 54*, 1414–1421.

Singer, H. S., Hahn, I. H., Krowiak, E., Nelson, E., & Moran, T. (1990). Tourette's syndrome: A neurochemical analysis of postmortem cortical brain tissue. *Annals of Neurology, 27*, 443–446.

Singer, H. S., Hahn, I. H., & Moran, T. H. (1991). Abnormal dopamine uptake sites in postmortem striatum from patients with Tourette's syndrome. *Annals of Neurology, 30*, 558–562.

Singer, H. S., Reiss, A. L., Brown, J. E., Aylward, E. H., Shih, B., Chee, E., et al. (1993). Volumetric MRI changes in basal ganglia of children with Tourette's syndrome. *Neurology, 43*, 950–956.

Singer, H. S., Szymanski, S., Giuliano, J., Yokoi, F., Dogan, A. S., Brasic, J. R., et al. (2002). Elevated intrasynaptic dopamine release in Tourette's syndrome measured by PET. *American Journal of Psychiatry, 159*, 1329–1336.

Singh, A., & Kulkarni, S. K. (2002). Role of adenosine in drug-induced catatonia in mice. *Indian Journal of Experimental Biology, 40*, 882–888.

Singhal, A. B., Caviness, V. S., Begleiter, A. F., Mark, E. J., Rordorf, G., & Koroshetz, W. J. (2002). Cerebral vasoconstriction and stroke after use of serotonergic drugs. *Neurology, 58*, 130–133.

Sjogren, M., Minthon, L., Passant, U., Blennow, K., & Wallin, A. (1998). Decreased monoamine metabolites in frontotemporal dementia and Alzheimer's disease. *Neurobiology of Aging, 19*, 379–384.

Sjøholt, G., Gulbrandsen, A. K., Løvlie, R., Berle, J., Molven, A., & Steen, V. M. (2000). A human *myo*-inositol monophosphatase gene (*IMPA2*) localized in a putative susceptibility region for bipolar disorder on chromosome 18p11.2: Genomic structure and polymorphism screening in manic-depressive patients. *Molecular Psychiatry, 5*, 172–180.

Skalabrin, E. J., Laws, E. R. Jr., & Bennett, J. P. Jr. (1998). Pallidotomy improves motor responses and widens the levodopa therapeutic window in Parkinson's disease. *Movement Disorders, 13*, 775–781.

Skinner, J. E., Molnar, M., & Kowalik, Z. J. (2000). The role of the thalamic reticular neurons in alpha-andgamma-oscillations in neocortex: A mechanism for selective perception and stimulus binding. *Acta Neurobilogiae Experimentalis, 60*, 123–142.

Sklair-Tavron, L., Shi, W. X., Lane, S. B., Harris, H. W., Bunney, B. S., & Nestler, E. J. (1996). Chronic morphine induces visible changes in the morphology of mesolimbic dopamine neurons. *Proceedings of the National Academy of Sciences, 93*, 11202–11207.

Skre, I., Onstad, S., Torgersen, S., Lygren, S., & Kringlen, E. (1993). A twin study of DSM-III-R anxiety disorders. *Acta Psychiatrica Scandinavica, 88*, 85–92.

Slaughter, J. R., Slaughter, K. A., Nichols, D., Holmes, S. E., & Martens, M. P. (2001). Prevalence, clinical manifestations, etiology, and treatment of depression in Parkinson's disease. *Journal of Neuropsychiatry and Clinical Neuroscience, 13*, 187–196.

Small, D. M., Zatorre, R. J., Dagher, A., Evans, A. C., & Jones-Gotman, M. (2001). Changes in brain activity related to eating chocolate: From pleasure to aversion. *Brain, 124*, 1720–1733.

Small, S. L., Flores, D. K., & Noll, D. C. (1998). Different neural circuits subserve reading before and after therapy for acquired dyslexia. *Brain and Language, 62*, 298–308.

Smalley, S. L. (1997). Genetic influences in childhood-onset psychiatric disorders: Autism and attention-deficit/ hyperactivity disorder. *American Journal of Human Genetics, 60*, 1276–1282.

Smart, D., Smith, G., & Lambert, D. G. (1994). Mu-opioid receptor stimulation of inositol (1,4,5) triphosphate formation via a pertussis toxin-sensitive G protein. *Journal of Neurochemistry, 62*, 1009–1014.

Smith, A., & Sugar, O. (1975). Development of above normal language and intelligence 21 years after left hemispherectomy. *Neurology, 25*, 813–818.

Smith, C. E., Leenerts, M. H., & Gajewski, B. J. (2003). A systematically tested intervention for managing reactive depression. *Nursing Research, 52*, 401–409.

Smith, K. A., Fairburn, C. G., & Cowen, P. J. (1999). Symptomoatic relapse in bulimia nervosa following acute tryptophan depletion. *Archives of General Psychiatry, 56*, 171–176.

Smith, K. M., Daly, M., Fischer, M., Yiannoutsos, C. T., Bauer, L., Barkley, R., & Navia, B. A. (2003). Association of the dopamine beta hydroxylase gene with attention deficit hyperactivity disorder: Genetic analysis of the Milwaukee longitudinal study. *American Journal of Medical Genetics, 119*, 77–85.

Smith, R. S. (1991). The macrophage theory of depression. *Medical Hypotheses, 35*, 298–306.

Smith, T. (1999). Outcome of early intervention for children with autism. *Clinical Psychology and Scientific Practice, 6*, 33–49.

Smoller, J. W., & Finn, C. T. (2003). Family, twin, and adoption studies of bipolar disorder. *American Journal of Medical Genetics, Part C, 123*, 48–58.

Smoller, J. W., Pollack, M. H., Wassertheil-Smoller, S., Barton, B., Hendrix, S. L., Jackson, R. D., et al. (2003). Prevalence and correlates of panic attacks in postmenopausal women: Results from an ancillary study to the Women's Health Initiative. *Archives of Internal Medicine, 163*, 2041–2050.

Snider, L. A., & Swedo, S. E. (2003). Post-streptococcal autoimmune disorders of the central nervous system. *Current Opinion in Neurology, 16*, 359–365.

Snow, D., & Anderson, C. (2000). Exploring the factors influencing relapse and recovery among drug and alcohol addicted women. *Journal of Psychosocial Nursing and Mental Health Service, 38*, 8–19.

Snowdon, J., & Lane, F. (2001). The prevalence and outcome of depression and dementia in Botany elderly population. *International Journal of Geriatric Psychiatry, 16*, 293–299.

Snyder, S. H., Jaffrey, S. R., & Zakhary, R. (1998). Nitric oxide and carbon monoxide: Parallel roles and neural messengers. *Brain Research Reviews, 26*, 167–175.

Soares, J. C., & Innis, R. B. (1999). Neurochemical brain imaging investigations of schizophrenia. *Biological Psychiatry, 46*, 600–615.

Soares, J. C., & Mann, J. J. (1997). The functional neuroanatomy of mood disorders. *Journal of Psychiatric Research, 31*, 393–432.

Sodersten, P., Bergh, C., & Ammar, A. (2003). Anorexia nervosa: Towards a neurobiology based therapy. *European Journal of Pharmacology, 480*, 67–74.

Sodhi, M. S., & Sanders-Bush, E. (2004). Serotonin and brain development. *International Review of Neurobiology, 59*, 111–174.

Sokol, D. K., Dunn, D. W., Edwards-Brown, M., & Feinberg, J. (2002). Hydrogen proton magnetic resonance spectroscopy in autism: Preliminary evidence of elevated choline/creatine ratio. *Journal of Child Neurology, 17*, 245–249.

Sokoloff, L. (1989). Circulation and energy metabolism of the brain. In G. J. Siegel (Ed.), *Basic neurochemistry: Molecular, cellular, and medical aspects* (4th edition, pp. 565–590). New York: Raven.

Soldin, O. P., Lai, S., Lamm, S. H., & Mosee, S. (2003). Lack of relation between human neonatal thyroxine and pediatric neurobehavioral disorders. *Thyroid, 13*, 193–198.

Soloff, P. H., Meltzer, C. C., Becker, C., Greer, P. J., Kelly, T. M., & Constantine, D. (2003). Impulsivity and prefrontal hypometabolism in borderline personality disorder. *Psychiatric Research, 123*, 153–163.

Solomon, R., Rich, C. L., & Darko, D. F. (1990). Antidepressant treatment and occurrence of mania in bipolar patients admitted for depression. *Journal of Affective Disorders, 18*, 253–257.

Someya, T., Kitamura, H., Uehara, T., Sakado, K., Kaiya, H., Tang, S. W., et al. (2000). Panic disorder and perceived parental rearing behavior investigated by the Japanese version of the EMBU scale. *Depression and Anxiety, 11*, 158–162.

Song, F., Freemantle, N., Sheldon, T. A., House, A., Watson, P., Long, A., et al. (1993). Selective serotonin reuptake inhibitors: Meta-analysis of efficacy and acceptability. *British Medical Journal, 306*, 683–687.

Sora, I., Elmer, G., Funada, M., Pieper, J., Li, X. F., Hall, F. S., et al. (2001). Mu opiate receptor gene dose effects on different morphine actions: evidence for differential in vivo mu receptor reserve. *Neuropsychopharmacology, 25*, 41–54.

Sowell, E., Thompson, P., Holmes, C., Batth, R., Jernigan, T., & Toga, A. (1999). Localizing age-related changes in brain structure between childhood and adolescence using statistical parametric mapping. *Neuroimage, 9,* 587–597.

Sowell, E. R., Thompson, P. M., Welcome, S. E., Henkenius, A. L., Toga. A. W., & Peterson, B. S. (2003). Cortical abnormalities in children and adolescents with attention-deficit hyperactivity disorder. *Lancet, 362,* 1699–1707.

Soyka, M., Preuss, U. W., Koller, G., Zill, P., & Bondy, B. (2004). Association of 5-HT1B receptor gene and antisocial behavior in alcoholism. *Journal of Neurotransmission, 111,* 101–109.

Spadafora, P., Annesi, G., Pasqua, A. A., Serra, P., Ciro Candiano, I. C., Carrideo, S., et al. (2003). NACP-REP1 polymorphism is not involved in Parkinson's disease: A case-control study in a population sample from southern Italy. *Neuroscience Letters, 35,* 75–78.

Spalletta, G., Pasini, A., Pau, F., Guido, G., Menghini, L., & Caltagirone, C. (2001). Prefrontal blood flow dysregulation in drug naïve ADHD children without structural abnormalities. *Journal of Neural Transmission, 108,* 1203–1216.

Spanagel, R. (2003). Behavioral and molecular aspects of alcohol craving and relapse. In R. Maldonado, (Ed.), *Molecular biology of drug addiction* (pp. 295–310). Totowa, NJ: Humana.

Sparks, B. F., Friedman, S. D., Shaw, D. W., Aylward, E. H., Echelard, D., Artru, A. A., et al. (2002). Brain structural abnormalities in young children with autism spectrum disorders. *Neurogy, 59,* 184–192.

Sparrevohn, R., & Howie, P. M. (1995). Theory of mind in children with autistic disorder: Evidence of developmental progression and the role of verbal ability. *Journal of Child Psychology and Psychiatry, and Allied Disciplines, 36,* 249–263.

Spence, D. W., Kayumov, L., Chen, A., Lowe, A., Jain, U., Katzman, M. A., et al. (2004). Acupuncture increases nocturnal melatonin secretion and reduces insomnia and anxiety: A preliminary report. *Journal of Neuropsychiatry and Clinical Neurosciences, 16,* 19–28.

Spencer, T., & Biederman, J. (2002). Non-stimulant treatment for Attention-Deficit/Hyperactivity Disorder. *Journal of Attention Disorders, 6,* 109–119.

Spencer, T., Biederman, J., Harding, M., O'Donnell, D., Wilens, T., Faraone, S., et al. (1998). Disentangling the overlap between Tourette's disorder and ADHD. *Journal of Child Psychology and Psychiatry, 39,* 1037–1044.

Spencer, T. J. (2004). ADHD treatment across the life cycle. *Journal of Clinical Psychiatry, 65,* 22–26.

Sperry, R. W. (1974). Lateral specialization in the surgically separated hemispheres. In F. Schmitt & F. Worden (Eds.), *The neurosciences: Third study program.* Cambridge, MA: MIT Press.

Spiegel, A. (1998). *G proteins, receptors, and disease.* Totowa, NJ: Humana.

Spiegel, D. A., & Bruce, T. J. (1997). Benzodiazepines and exposure-based cognitive behavior therapies for panic disorder: Conclusions from combined treatment trials. *American Journal of Psychiatry, 154,* 773–781.

Spielewoy, C., & Giros, B. (2002). Recent advances in the molecular mechanisms of psychostimulant abuse using knockout mice. In R. Maldonado (Ed.), *Molecular biology* (pp. 79–106). Totowa, NJ: Humana.

Spliethoff-Kamminga, N. G. A., Zwinderman, A. H., Springer, M. P., & Roos, R. A. C. (2003). Psychosocial problems in Parkinson's disease: Evaluation of a disease-specific questionnaire. *Movement Disorders, 18,* 503–509.

Sponheim, E., & Skjeldal, O. (1998). Autism and related disorders: Epidemiological findings in a Norwegian study using ICD-10 diagnostic criteria. *Journal of Autism and Developmental Disorders, 28,* 217–227.

Sponheim, S. R., Clementz, B. A., Iacono, W. G., & Beiser, M. (2000). Clinical and biological concomitants of resting state EEG power abnormalities in schizophrenia. *Biological Psychiatry, 48,* 1088–1097.

Springer, S. P., & Deutsch, G. (1993). *Left brain right brain* (4th ed.). New York: Freeman.

Srinivasagam, N. M., Kaye, W. H., Plotnicov, K. H., Greeno, C., Weltzin, T. E., & Rao, R. (1995). Persistent perfectionism, symmetry, and exactness after long-term recovery from anorexia nervosa. *American Journal of Psychiatry, 152,* 1630–1634.

St. James-Roberts, I. (1981). A reinterpretation of hemispherectomy data without functional plasticity of the brain. *Brain and Language, 13,* 31–53.

Staff, R. T., Gemmell, H. G., Shanks, M. F., Murray, A. D., & Venneri, A. (2000). Changes in the rCBF images of patients with Alzheimer's disease receiving Donepezil therapy. *Nuclear Medicine Communications, 21,* 37–41.

Stahl, S. M. (1998). Basic psychopharmacology of antidepressants: Antidepressants have seven distinct mechanisms of action. *Journal of Clinical Psychiatry, 59,* 5–14.

Stahl, S. M. (1998). Mechanism of action of serotonin selective reuptake inhibitors. Serotonin receptors and pathways mediate therapeutic effects and side effects. *Journal of Affective Disorders, 51,* 215–235.

Stahl, S. M. (2000). Blue genes and the mechanism of action of antidepressants. *Journal of Clinical Psychiatry, 6,* 164–165.

Stahl, S. M. (2000). Essential psychopharmacology of depression and bipolar disorder. New York: Cambridge University Press.

Stamatakis, E. A., & Hetherington, M. M. (2003). Neuroimaging in eating disorders. *Nutritional Neuroscience, 6,* 325–334.

Stamenkovic, M., Schindler, S. D., Asenbaum, S., Neumeister, A., Willeit, M., Willinger, U., et al. (2000). No change in striatal dopamine re-uptake site density in psychotropic drug naïve and in current treated Tourette's disorder patients: A [123I]-β-CIT SPECT study. *European Neuropsychopharmacology, 11*, 69–74.

Stanford, S. C. (2001a). Anxiety. In R. A. Webster (Ed.), *Neurotransmitters, drugs, and brain function* (pp. 395–423). New York: Wiley.

Stanford, S. C. (2001b). 5-Hydroxytryptamine. In R. A. Webster (Ed.), *Neurotransmitters, drugs, and brain function* (pp. 187–209). New York: Wiley.

Stanford, S. C. (2001c). Depression. In R. A. Webster (Ed.), *Neurotransmitters, drugs, and brain function* (pp. 425–452). New York: Wiley.

Starcevic, V., Kellner, R., Uhlenhuth, E. H., & Pathak, D. (1993). The phenomenology of panic attacks in panic disorder with and without agoraphobia. *Comprehensive Psychiatry, 34*, 36–41.

State, M. W., Pauls, D. L., & Leckman, J. F. (2001). Tourette's syndrome and related disorders. *Child and Adolescent Psychiatric Clinics of North America, 10*, 317–331.

Steffenburg, S., Gillberg, C., Hellgren, L., Andersson, L., Gillberg, I. C., Jakobsson, G., et al. (1989). A twin study of autism in Denmark, Finland, Iceland, Norway and Sweden. *Journal of Child Psychology and Psychiatry, and Allied Disciplines, 30*, 405–416.

Steiger, H. (2004). Eating disorders and the serotonin connection: State, trait, and developmental effects. *Journal of Psychiatry and Neuroscience, 29*, 20–29.

Steiger, H., Gauvin, L., Israel, M., Koerner, N., Ng Ying Kin, N. M. K., Paris, J., et al. (2001). Association of serotonin and cortisol indices with childhood abuse in bulimia nervosa. *Archives of General Psychiatry, 58*, 837–843.

Steiger, H., Leonard, S., Ng Ying Kin, N. M., Ladouceur, C., Ramdoyal, D., & Young, C. N. (2000). Childhood abuse and platelet tritiated paroxetine binding n bulimia nervosa: Implications of borderline personality disorder. *Journal of Clinical Psychiatry, 61*, 428–435.

Stein, D., Kaye, W. H., Matsunaga, H., Orbach, I., Har-Even, D., Frank, G., McConaha, C. W., et al. (2002). Eating-related concerns, mood, and personality traits in recovered bulimia nervosa subjects: A replication study. *International Journal of Eating Disorders, 32*, 225–229.

Stein, D. G., Brailowsky, S., & Will, B. (1995). *Brain repair* (pp. 41–45). New York: Oxford University Press.

Stein, D. J., Van Heerden, B., Wessels, C. J., Van Kradenburg, J., Warwick, J., & Wasserman, H. J. (1999). Single photon emission computed tomography of the brain with Tc-99m HMPAO during sumatriptan challenge in obsessive-compulsive disorder: Investigating the functional role of the serotonin auto-receptor. *Progress in Neuro-Psychopharmacology & Biological Psychiatry, 23*, 1079–1099.

Stein, L. (1962). Effects and interactions of imipramine, chlorpromazine, resperine and amphetamine on self-stimulation: Possible neurophysiological basis of depression. In J. Wortis (Ed.), *Recent advances in biological psychiatry* (pp. 288–308). New York: Plenum.

Stein, M. B., & Uhde, T. W. (1989). Infrequent occurrence of EEG abnormalities in panic disorder. *American Journal of Psychiatry, 146*, 517–520.

Steiner, M., Dunn, E., & Born, L. (2003). Hormones and mood: From menarche to menopause and beyond. *Journal of Affective Disorders, 74*, 67–83.

Steinlein, O. K., Stoodt, J., de Vos, R. A., Steur, E. N., Wevers, A., Schütz, U., et al. (1999). Mutation screening of the CHRNA4 and CHRNB2 nicotinic cholinergic receptor genes in Alzheimer's disease. *Neuroreport, 10*, 2919–2922.

Stern, E., Silbersweig, D. A., Chee, K. Y., Holmes, A., Robertson, M. M., Trimble, M., et al. (2000). A functional neuroanatomy of tics in Tourette syndrome. *Archives of General Psychiatry, 57*, 741–748.

Stern, M., Dulaney, E., Gruber, S. B., Golbe, L., Bergen, M., Hurtig, H., et al. (1991). The epidemiology of Parkinson's disease. A case-control study of young-onset and old-onset patients. *Archives of Neurology, 48*, 903–907.

Sternbach, H. (2003). Are antidepressants carcinogenic? A review of preclinical and clinical studies. *Journal of Clinical Psychiatry, 64*, 1153–1162.

Sterr, A., Elbert, T., & Rockstroh, B. (2002). Functional reorganization of human cerebral cortex and its perceptual concomitants. In M. Fahle & T. Poggio (Eds.), *Perceptual learning* (pp. 125–144). Cambridge, MA: MIT Press.

Stevenson, J. (1992). Evidence for a genetic etiology in hyperactivity in children. *Behavioral Genetics, 22*, 337–344.

Stewart, R. J., Chen, B., Dowlatshahi, D., MacQueen, G. M., & Young, T. (2001). Abonormalities in the camp signaling pathway in post-mortem brain tissue from the Stanley Neuropathology Consortium. *Brain Research Bulletin, 55*, 625–629.

Stiles, J. (2000). Neural plasticity and cognitive development. *Developmental Neuropsychology, 18*, 237–272.

Stimpson, N., Agrawal, N., & Lewis, G. (2002). Randomised controlled trials investigating pharmacological and psychological interventions for treatment-refractory depression. *British Journal of Psychiatry, 181*, 284–294.

Stocchi, F. (2003). Prevention and treatment of motor fluctuations. *Parkinsonism Related Disorders, 9*, 73–81.

Stockmeier, C. A. (2003). Involvement of serotonin in depression: Evidence from postmortem and imaging studies of serotonin receptors and the serotonin transporter. *Journal of Psychiatric Research, 37*, 357–373.

Stoll, A. L., Severus, W. E., Freeman, M. P., Reuter, S., Zboyan, H. A., Diamond, E., et al. (1999). Omega 3 fatty acids in bipolar disorder. *Archives of General Psychiatry, 56*, 407–412.

Strafella, A. P., Paus, T., Barrett, J., & Dagher, A. (2001). Repetitive transcranial magnetic stimulation o the human prefrontal cortex induces dopamine release in the caudate nucleus. *Journal of Neuoscience, 21*, 1–4.

Strafella, A. P., Paus, T., Fraraccio, M., & Dagher, A. (2003). Striatal dopamine release induced by repetitive transcranial magnetic stimulation of the human cortex. *Brain, 12*, 2609–2615.

Strakowski, S. M., DelBello, M. P., Zimmerman, M. E., Getz, G. E., Mills, N. P., Ret, J., et al. (2002). Ventricular and periventricular structural volumes in first-versus multiple-episode bipolar disorder. *American Journal of Psychiatry, 159*, 1841–1847.

Strange, P. G. (2001). Antipsychotic drugs: Importance of dopamine receptors for mechanisms of therapeutic actions and side effects. *Pharmacological Reviews, 45*, 119–134.

Straub, R. E., MacLean, C. J., Martin, R. B., Ma, Y., Myakishev, M. V., Harris-Kerr, C., et al. (1998). A schizophrenia locus may be located in region 10p15–p11. *American Journal of Medical Genetics, 81*, 296–301.

Strauss, W. L., Unis, A. S., Cowan, C., Dawson, G., & Dager, S. R. (2002). Fluorine magnetic resonance spectroscopy measurement of brain fluvoxamine and fluoxetine in pediatric patients treated for pervasive developmental disorders. *The American Journal of Psychiatry, 159*, 755–760.

Strickland, D., & Bertoni, J. M. (2004). Parkinson's prevalence estimated by a state registry. *Movement Disorders, 19*, 318–323.

Strober, M., Freeman, R., Lampert, C., Diamond, J., & Kaye, W. (2001). Males with anorexia nervosa: A controlled study of eating disorders in first-degree relatives. *International Journal of Eating Disorders, 29*, 263–269.

Ströhle, A., & Holsboer, F. (2003). Stress responsive neurohormones in depression and anxiety. *Pharmacopsychiatry, 36, Supplement 3*, S207–214.

Ströhle, A., Romeo, E., di Michele, F., Pasini, A., Yassouridis, A., Holsboer, F., et al. (2002). GABA(A) receptor-modulating neuroactive steroid composition in patients with panic disorder before and during paroxetine treatment. *American Journal of Psychiatry, 159*, 145–147.

Stubberfield, T., & Parry, T. (1999). Utilization of alternative therapies in attention-deficit hyperactivity disorder. *Journal of Pediatrics and Child Health, 35*, 450–453.

Sturm, V., Lenartz, D., Koulousakis, A., Treuer, H., Herholz, K., Klein, J. C., et al. (2003). The nucleus accumbens: A target for deep brain stimulation in obsessive-compulsive and anxiety disorders. *Journal of Chemical Neuroanatomy, 26*, 293–299.

Südof, T. C. (2001). The synaptic cleft and synaptic cell adhesion. In M. W. Cowan, T. C. Sudhof, & C. F. Stevens (Eds.), *Synapses* (pp. 1–88). Baltimore: Johns Hopkins University Press.

Sukhodolsky, D. G., Scahill, L., Zhang, H., Peterson, B. S., King, R. A., Lombroso, P. J., et al. (2003). Disruptive behavior in children with Tourette's syndrome: Association with ADHD comorbidity, tic severity, and functional impairment. *Journal of the American Academy of Child and Adolescent Psychiatry, 42*, 98–105.

Sullivan, P. F., Neale, M. C., & Kendler, K. S. (2000). Genetic epidemiology of major depression: Review and meta-analysis. *American Journal of Psychiatry, 157*, 1552–1562.

Sultzer, D. L. (2004). Psychosis and antipsychotic medications in Alzheimer's disease: Clinical management and research perspectives. *Dementia and Geriatric Cognitive Disorders, 17*, 78–90.

Sultzer, D. L., Brown, C. V., Mandelkern, M. A., Mahler, M. E., Mendez, M. F., Chen, S. T., et al. (2003). Delusional thoughts and regional frontal/temporal cortex metabolism in Alzheimer's disease. *American Journal of Psychiatry, 160*, 341–349.

Sumiyoshi, T., Stockmeier, C. A., Overholser, J. C., Dilley, G. E., & Meltzer, H. Y. (1996). Serotonin1A receptors are increased in postmortem prefrontal cortex in schizophrenia. *Brain Research, 708*, 209–214.

Sun, Y., Nadal-Vicens, M., Misono, S., Lin, M. Z., Zubiaga, A., Hua, X., et al. (2001). Neurogenin promotes neurogenesis and inhibits glial differentiation by independent mechanisms. *Cell, 104*, 365–376.

Sundaramurthy, D., Pieri, L. F., Gape, H., Markham, A. F., & Campbell, D. A. (2000). Analysis of the serotonin transporter gene linked polymorphism (5-HTTLPR) in anorexia nervosa. *American Journal of Medical Genetics, 96*, 53–55.

Sung, S., Yao, Y., Uryu, K., Yang, H., Lee, V. M., Trojanowski, J. Q., & Pratico, D. (2004). Early vitamin E supplementation in young but not aged mice reduces Abeta levels and amyloid deposition in a transgenic model of Alzheimer's disease. *Federation of the American Societies Experimental Biology Journal, 18*, 323–325.

Suri, R., Stowe, Z. N., Hendrick, V., Hostetter, A., Widawski, M., & Altshuler, L. L. (2002). Estimates of nursing infant daily dose of fluoxetine through breast milk. *Biological Psychiatry, 52*, 446–451.

Swanberg, M. M., Tractenberg, R. E., Mohs, R., Thal, L. J., & Cummings, J. L. (2004). Executive dysfunction in Alzheimer disease. *Archives of Neurology, 61*, 556–560.

Swann, A. C., Bowden, C. L., Morris, D., Calabrese, J. R., Petty, F., Small, J., et al. (1997). Depression during mania: Treatment response to lithium or divalproex. *Archives of General Psychiatry, 54*, 37–42.

Swann, A. C., Secunda, S., Davis, J. M., Robbins, E., Hanin, I., Koslow, S. H., et al. (1983). CSF monoamine metabolites in mania. *American Journal of Psychiatry, 140*, 396–400.

Swanson, J. M., Flodman, P., Kennedy, J., Spence, M. A., Moyzis, R., Schuck, S., et al. (2000). Dopamine genes and ADHD. *Neuroscience and Biobehavior Reviews, 24*, 21–25.

Swanson, J. M., Sunohara, G. A., Kennedy, J. L., Regino, R., Fineberg, E., Wigal, T., et al. (1998). Association of the dopamine receptor D4 (DRD4) gene with a refined phenotype of attention deficit hyperactivity disorder (ADHD): A family-based approach. *Molecular Psychiatry, 3*, 38–41.

Swanson, L. W. (2003). *Brain architecture: Understanding the basic plan.* New York: Oxford University Press.

Swayze, V. W., Andersen, A. E., Andreasen, N. C., Arndt, S., Sato, Y., & Ziebell, S. (2003). Brain tissue volume segmentation in patients with anorexia nervosa before and after weight normalization. *International Journal of Eating Disorders, 33*, 33–44.

Swedo, S. E., Leonard, H. L., Garvey, M., Mittleman, B., Allen, A. J., Perlmutter, S., et al. (1998). Pediatric autoimmune neuropsychiatric disorders associated with streptococcal infections: Clinical description of the first 50 cases. *American Journal of Psychiatry, 155*, 264–271.

Sweet, R. A., Nimgaonkar, V. L., Devlin, B., & Jeste, D. V. (2003). Psychotic symptoms in Alzheimer disease: Evidence for a distinct phenotype. *Molecular Psychiatry, 8*, 383–392.

Synder, S. H., & Ferris, C. D. (2001). Novel neurotransmitters and their neuropsychiatric relevance. In M. W. Cowan, T. C. Sudhof, & C. F. Stevens (Eds.), *Synapses* (pp. 651–680). Baltimore: Johns Hopkins University Press.

Szatmari, P., Bryson, S. E., Streiner, D. L., Wilson, F., Archer, L., & Ryerse, C. (2000). Two-year outcome of preschool schildren with autism or Asperger's syndrome. *American Journal of Psychiatry, 157*, 1980–1987.

Szatmari, P., Jones, M. B., Zwaigenbaum, L., & MacLean, J. E. (1998). Genetics of autism: Overview and new directions. *Journal of Autism and Developmental Disorders, 28*, 351–368.

Szeszko, P. R., Robinson, D., Alvir, J. M., Bilder, R. M., Lencz, T., Ashtari, M., et al. (1999). Orbital frontal and amygdala volume reductions in obsessive-compulsive disorder. *Archives of General Psychiatry, 56*, 913–919.

Szuster-Ciesielska, A., Tustanowska-Stachura, A., Slotwinska, M., Marmurowska-Michalowska, H., & Kandefer-Szerszen, M. (2003). In vitro immunoregulatory effects of antidepressants in healthy volunteers. *Polish Journal of Pharmacology, 55*, 353–362.

Tabet, N., Birks, J., & Grimley Evans, J. (2000). Vitamin E for Alzheimer's disease. *Cochrane Database of Systematic Reviews*, CD002854.

Tabiner, M., Youings, S., Dennis, N., Baldwin, D., Buis, C., Mayers, A., et al. (2003). Failure to find DUP25 in patients with anxiety disorders, in control individuals, or in previously reported positive control cell lines. *American Journal of Human Genetics, 72*, 535–538.

Tafet, G. E., Idoyaga-Vargas, V. P., Abulafia, D. P., Calandria, J. M., Roffman, S. S., Chiovetta, A., et al. (2001). Correlation between cortisol level and serotonin uptake in patients with chronic stress and depression. *Cognitive, Affective, and Behavioral Neuroscience, 1*, 388–393.

Tahir, E., Yazgan, Y., Cirakoglu, B., Ozbay, F., Waldman, I., & Asherson, P. J. (2000). Association and linkage of DRD4 and DRD5 with attention deficit hyperactivity disorder (ADHD) in a sample of Turkish children. *Molecular Psychiatry, 5*, 396–404.

Takahashi, H., Suzumura, S., Shirakizawa, F., Wada, N., Tanaka-Taya, K., Arai, S., et al. (2003). An epidemiological study on Japanese autism concerning routine childhood immunization history. *Japanese Journal of Infectious Disorders, 56*, 114–117.

Takahashi, N., Miner, L. L., Sora, I., Ujike, H., Reva, R. S., Kostic, V., et al. (1997). VMAT2 knockout mice: Heterozygotes display reduced amphetamine-conditioned reward, enhanced amphetamine locomotion, and enhanced MPTP toxicity. *Proceedings of the National Academy of Science USA, 94*, 9938–9943.

Tamas, L. B., Shibasaki, T., Horikoshi, S., & Ohye, C. (1993). General activation of cerebral metabolism with speech: A PET study. *International Journal of Psychophysiology, 14*, 199–208.

Tan, E. K., Tan, C., Fook-Chong, S. M., Lum, S. Y., Chai, A., Chung, H., et al. (2003). Dose-dependent protective effect of coffee, tea, and smoking in Parkinson's disease: A study in ethnic Chinese. *Journal of Neurological Science, 216*, 163–167.

Tan, E. K., Tan, C., Shen, H., Chai, A., Lum, S. Y., Teoh, M. L., et al. (2003). Alpha sinuclein promoter and risk of Parkinson's disease: Microsatellite and allelic size variability. *Neuroscience Letters, 336*, 70–72.

Tan, Z. S., Seshadri, S., Beiser, A., Wilson, P. W., Kiel, D. P., Tocco, M., et al. (2003). Plasma total cholesterol level as a risk factor for Alzheimer disease: The Framingham Study. *Archives of Internal Medicine, 163*, 1053–1057.

Tanahashi, H., Asada, T., & Tabira, T. (2004). Association between tau polymorphism and male early-onset Alzheimer's disease. *Neuroreport, 15*, 175–179.

Tanaka, S., Matsunaga, H., Kimura, M., Tatsumi, K., Hidaka, Y., Takano, T., et al. (2003). Autoantibodies against four kinds of neurotransmitter receptors in psychiatric disorders. *Journal of Neuroimmunology, 141*, 155–164.

Tandon, R., DeQuardo, J. R., Goodson, J., Mann, N. A., & Greden, J. F. (1992). Effect of anticholinergics on positive and negative symptoms in schizophrenia. *Psychopharmacology Bulletin, 28,* 297–302.

Tang, M. X., Cross, P., Andrews, H., Jacobs, D. M., Small, S., Bell, K., et al. (2001). Incidence of AD in African-Americans, Caribbean Hispanics, and Caucasians in northern Manhattan. *Neurology, 56,* 49–56.

Tang, M. X., Stern, Y., Marder, K., Bell, K., Gurland, B., Lantigua, R., et al. (1998). The *APOE-ε*4 allele and the risk of Alzheimer's disease among African Americans, whites, and Hispanics. *Journal of the American Medical Association, 279,* 751–755.

Tanner, C. M., Goldman, S. M., Aston, D. A., Ottman, R., Ellenberg, J., Mayeux, R., et al. (2002). Smoking and Parkinson's disease in twins. *Neurology, 58,* 581–588.

Tariot, P. N., Farlow, M. R., Grossberg, G. T., Graham, S. M., McDonald, S., & Gergel, I. (2004). Memantine treatment in patients with moderate to severe Alzheimer disease already receiving donepezil: A randomized controlled trial. *Journal of the American Medical Association, 291,* 317–324.

Tarumi, S., & Tashiiro, N. (2004). Stress situations of daily living in patients with obsessive-compulsive disorder: A retrospective case note study. *Psychological Reports, 94,* 139–150.

Tass, P. A., Klosterdotter, J., Schneider, F., Lenartz, D., Koulousakis, A., & Sturm, V. (2003). Obsessive-compulsive disorder: Development of demand-controlled deep brain stimulation with methods from stochastic phase resetting. *Neuropsychopharmacology, 28,* 27–34.

Taub, E., Miller, N. E., Novack, T. A., Cook, E. W., III, Fleming, W. C., Nepomuncen, C. S., et al. (1993). Technique to improve chronic motor deficit after stroke. *Archives of Physical and Medical Rehabilitation, 74,* 347–354.

Taub, E., Uswatte, G., & Elbert, T. (2002). New treatments in neurorehabilitation founded on basic research. *Nature Reviews in Neuroscience, 3,* 228–236.

Tauscher, J., Bagby, R. M., Javanmard, M., Christensen, B. K., Kasper, S., & Kapur, S. (2001). Inverse relationship between serotonin 5-HT(1A) receptor binding and anxiety: A [(11)C]WAY-100635 PET investigation in healthy volunteers. *American Journal of Psychiatry, 158,* 1326–1328.

Tauscher, J., Hussain, T., Agid, O., Verhoeff, P., Wilson, A. A., Houle, S., et al. (2004). Equivalent occupancy of dopamine D1 and D2 receptors with clozapine: Differentiation from other atypical antipsychotics. *American Journal of Psychiatry, 161,* 1620–1625.

Tauscher, J., Kapur, S., Verhoeff, P. L. G., Hussey, D. F., Daskalakis, Z. J., Tauscher-Wisniewski, S., et al. (2002). Brain serotonin 5-HT1A receptor binding in schizophrenia measured by positron emission tomography and [11C]WAY-100635. *Archives of General Psychiatry, 59,* 514–520.

Tauscher, J., Pirker, W., Willeit, M., de Zwaan, M., Bailer, U., Neumeister, A., et al. (2001). [123I]beta-CIT and single photon emission computed tomography reveal reduced brain serotonin transporter availability in bulimia nervosa. *Biological Psychiatry, 49,* 326–332.

Tauscher-Wisniewski, S., Kapur, A., Tauscher, J., Jones, C., Daskalakis, J., Paptheodorou, G., et al. (2002). Quetiapine: An effective antipsychotic in first-episode schizophrenia despite only transiently high dopamine-2 receptor blockade. *Journal of Clinical Psychiatry, 63,* 992–997.

Taylor, H. G., Wade, S. L., Stancin, T., Yeates, K. O., Drotar, D., & Minich, N. (2002). A prospective study of short and long term outcomes after traumatic brain injury in children: Behavior and achievement. *Neuropsychology, 16,* 15–27.

Taylor, M. C., Le Couteur, D. G., Mellick, G. D., & Board, P. G. (107). Paraoxonase polymorphisms, pesticide exposure and Parkinson's disease in a Caucasian population. *Journal of Neural Transmission, 107,* 979–983.

Taylor, S. F. (1996). Cerebral blood flow activation and functional lesions in schizophrenia. *Schizophrenia Research, 19,* 129–140.

Taylor, S. F., Tandon, R., Shipley, J. E., Eiser, A. S., & Goodson, J. (1991). Sleep onset REM periods in schizophrenic patients. *Society of Biological Psychiatry, 30,* 205–209.

Tedroff, J., Ekesbo, A., Rydin, E., Långström, B., & Hagberg, G. (1999). Regulation of dopaminergic activity in early Parkinson's disease. *Annals of Neurology, 46,* 359–365.

Teicher, M. H., Anderson, C. M., Polcari, A., Glod, C. A., Maas, L. C., & Renshaw, P. F. (2000). Functional deficits in basal ganglia of children with attention-deficit/hyperactivity disorder shown with functional magnetic resonance imaging relaxometry. *Nature Medicine, 6,* 470–473.

Teicher, M. H., Glod, C. A., & Cole, J. O. (1993). Antidepressant drugs and the emergence of suicidal tendencies. *Drug Safety, 8,* 186–212.

Tek, C., & Ulug, B. (2001). Religiosity and religious obsessions in obsessive-compulsive disorder. *Psychiatry Research, 104,* 99–108.

Temel, Y., & Visser-Vandewalle, V. (2004). Surgery in Tourette syndrome. *Movement Disorders, 19,* 3–14.

Temple, E., Deutsche, G. K., Poldrack, R. A., Miller, S. L., Tallal, P., Merzenich, M. M., & Gabrieli, J. D. E. (2003). Neural deficits in children with dyslexia ameliorated by behavioral remediation: Evidence from functional MRI. *Proceedings of the National Academy of Sciences, 100*, 2860–2865.

Temple, E., Poldrack, R. A., Salidis, J., Deutsch, G. K., Tallal, P., Merzenich, M. M., et al. (2001). Disrupted neural responses to phonological and orthographic processing in dyslexic children: An fMRI study. *Neuroreport, 12*, 299–307.

Teri, L., Gibbons, L. E., McCurry, S. M., Logsdon, R. G., Buchner, D. M., Barlow, W. E., et al. (2003). Exercise plus behavioral management in patients with Alzheimer disease: A randomized controlled trial. *Journal of the American Medical Association, 290*, 2015–2022.

Terman, J. R., & Kolodkin, A. L. (1999). Attracted or repelled? Look within. *Neuron, 23*, 193–195.

Thaker, U., McDonagh, A. M., Iwatsubo, T., Lendon, C. L., Pickering-Brown, S. M., & Mann, D. M. (2003). Tau load is associated with apolipoprotein E genotype and the amount of amyloid beta protein, Abeta40, in sporadic and familial Alzheimer's disease. *Neuropathology and Applied Neurobiology, 29*, 35–44.

Thaut, M. H. (1988). Measuring musical responsiveness in autistic children: A comparative analysis of improvised musical tone sequences of autistic, normal, and mentally retarded individuals. *Journal of Autism and Developmental Disorders, 18*, 561–571.

Thirumala, P., Hier, D. B., & Patel, P. (2002). Motor recovery after stroke: Lessons from functional brain imaging. *Neurological Research, 24*, 453–458.

Thobois, S., Dominey, P., Fraix, V., Mertens, P., Guenot, M., Zimmer, L., et al. (2002). Effects of subthalamic nucleus stimulation on actual and imagined movement in Parkinson's disease: A PET study. *Journal of Neurology, 249*, 1689–1698.

Thoenen, H., Zafra, F., Hengerer, B., & Lindholm, D. (1991). The synthesis of nerve growth factor and brain-derived neurotrophic factor in hippocampal and cortical neurons is regulated by specific transmitter systems. *Annual of the New York Academy Science, 640*, 86–90.

Thomas, A. J., Davis, S., Ferrier, I. N., Kalaria, R. N., & O'Brien, J. T. (2004). Elevation of cell adhesion molecule immunoreactivity in the anterior cingulated cortex in bipolar disorder. *Biological Psychiatry, 55*, 652–655.

Thomas, A. J., Ferrier, I. N., Kalaria, R. N., Perry, R. H., Brown, A., & O'Brien, J. T. (2001). A neuropathological study of vascular factors in late-life depression. *Journal of Neurology, Neurosurgery, and Psychiatry, 70*, 83–87.

Thomas, K. M., Drevets, W. C., Dahl, R. E, Ryan, N. D., Birmaher, B., Eccard, C. H., et al. (2001). Amygdala response to fearful faces in anxious and depressed children. *Archives of General Psychiatry, 58*, 1057–1063.

Thomas, S. G., & Kellner, C. H. (2003). Remission of major depression and obsessive-compulsive disorder after a single unilateral ECT. *Journal of ECT, 19*, 50–51.

Thompson, P. M., Vidal, C., Giedd, J., Gochman, P., Blumenthal, J., Nicolson, R., et al. (2001). Mapping adolescent brain changes reveals dynamic wave of accelerated gray matter loss in very early-onset schizophrenia. *Proceedings of the National Academy of Sciences, 98*, 11650–11655.

Thompson, R. F. (2000). *The brain: A neuroscience primer* (3rd ed.). New York: Worth.

Thompson, R. J., & Bolton, P. F. (2003). Case report: Angleman syndrome in an individual with a small SMC(15) and paternal uniparental disomy: A case report with reference to the assessment of cognitive functioning and autistic symptomatology. *Journal of Autism and Developmental Disorders, 33*, 171–176.

Thorén, P., Asberg, M., Bertilsson, L., Mellström, B., Sjöqvist, F., & Träskman, L. (1980). Clomipramine treatment of obsessive-compulsive disorder. II. Biochemical aspects. *Archives of General Psychiatry, 37*, 1289–1294.

Thurman, D., Alverson, C., Dunn, K., Guerreor, J., & Sniezek, J. (1999). Traumatic brain injury in the United States: A public health perspective. *Journal of Head Trauma and Rehabilitation, 14*, 602–605.

Tiemeier, H. (2003). Biological risk factors for late life depression. *European Journal of Epidemiology, 18*, 745–750.

Tiemeier, H., Bakker, S. L., Hofman, A., Koudstaal, P. J., & Breteler, M. M. (2002). Cerebral haemodynamics and depression in the elderly. *Journal of Neurology, Neurosurgery, and Psychiatry, 73*, 34–39.

Tien, A. Y. (1991). Distributions of hallucinations in the population. *Social Psychiatry and Psychiatric Epidemiology, 26*, 287–292.

Tiihomem, J., Kuikka, J., Bergstrom, K., Hakola, P., Karhu, J., Ryynanen, O. P., et al. (1995). Altered striatal dopamine re-uptake site densities in habitually violent and non-violent alcoholics. *National Medicine, 1*, 654–657.

Tiihonen, J., Vilkman, H., Rasanen, P., Ryynanen, O. P., Hakko, H., Bergman, J., et al. (1998). Striatal presynaptic dopamine function in type 1 alcoholics measured with positron emission tomography. *Molecular Psychiatry, 3*, 156–161.

Tiraboschi, P., Hansen, L. A., Alford, M., Merdes, A., Masliah, E., Thal, L. J., et al. (2002). Early and widespread cholinergic losses differentiate dementia with Lewy bodies from Alzheimer disease. *Archives General Psychiatry, 59*, 946–951.

Tizabi, Y., Louis, V. A., Taylor, C. T., Waxman, D., Culver, K. E., & Szechtman, H. (2002). Effect of nicotine on quinpirole-induced checking behavior in rats: Implications for obsessive-compulsive disorder. *Biological Psychiatry, 51*, 164–171.

Todd, R. D., Sitdhiraksa, N., Reich, W., Ji, T. H., Joyner, C. A., Heath, A. C., & et al. (2002). Discrimination of DSM-IV and latent class attention-deficit/hyperactivity disorder subtypes by educational and cognitive performance in a population-based sample of child and adolescent twins. *Journal of the American Academy of Child and Adolescent Psychiatry, 41*, 820–828.

Toft, M., & Aasly, J. (2004). The genetics of Parkinson disease. *Tidsskrift For Den Norske Iaegeforening, 124*, 922–924.

Tohda, C., Tamura, T., & Komatsu, K. (2003). Repair of amyloid β(25–35)-induced memory impairment and synaptic loss by a Kampo formula, Zokumei-to. *Brain Research, 990*, 141–147.

Tohgi, H., Abe, T., Takahashi, S., Takahashi, J., Nozaki, Y., Ueno, M., et al. (1993). Monoamine metabolism in the cerebrospinal fluid in Parkinson's disease: Relationship to clinical symptoms and subsequent therapeutic outcomes. *Journal of Neural Transmission, 5*, 17–26.

Tokumaru, A. M., Barkovich, A. J., O'ichi, T., Matsuo, T., & Kusano, S. (1999). The evolution of cerebral blood flow in the developing brain. Evaluation with iodine-123 iodoamphetamine SPECT and correlation with MR imagin. *American Journal of Neuroradiology, 20*, 845–852.

Tokunaga, H., Nishikawa, T., Ikejiri, Y., Nakagawa, Y., Yasuno, F., Hashikawa, K., et al. M. (1999). Different neural substrates for Kanji and Kana writing: A PET study. *NeuroReport, 10*, 3315–3319.

Tolar, M., Keller, J. N., Chan, S., Mattson, M. P., Marques, M. A., & Crutcher, K. A. (1999). Truncated apolipoprotein E (ApoE) causes increased intracellular calcium and may mediate ApoE neurotoxicity. *Journal of Neuroscience, 19*, 7100–7110.

Tolin, D. F., Abramowitz, J. S., Brigidi, B. D., & Foa, E. B. (2003). Intolerance of uncertainty in obsessive-compulsive disorder. *Journal of Anxiety Disorders, 17*, 233–242.

Tolosa, E. (2003). Advances in the pharmacological management of Parkinson disease. *Journal of Neural Transmission, Supplementum*, 65–78.

Tomizawa, K., Ohta, J., Matsushita, M., Moriwaki, A., Li, S. T., Takel, K., & et al. (2002). Cdk5/p35 regulates neurotransmitter release through phosphorylation and downregulation of P/Q-type voltage-dependent calcium channel activity. *Journal of Neuroscience, 22*, 2590–2597.

Toni, N., Buchs, P. A., Nikonenko, I., Bron, C. R., & Muller, D. (1999). LTP promotes formation of multiple spine synapses between a single axon terminal and a dendrite. *Nature, 402*, 421–425.

Tonini, G., Shanks, M. F., & Venneri, A. (2003). Short-term longitudinal evaluation of cerebral blood flow in mild Alzheimer's disease. *Neurological Sciences, 24*, 24–30.

Tordjman, S., Gutknecht, L., Carlier, M., Spitz, E., Antoine, C., Slama, F., et al. (2001). Role of the serotonin transporter gene in the behavioral expression of autism. *Molecular Psychiatry, 6*, 434–439.

Torgesen, J. K., Wagner, R. K., & Rashotte, C. A. (1994). Longitudinal studies of phonological processing and reading. *Journal of Learning Disabilities, 27*, 276–286.

Torres, A. R. (2003). Is fever suppression involved in the etiology of autism and neurodevelopmental disorders? *BMC Pediatrics, 3*, 9.

Torrey, E. F., Miller, J., Rawlings, R., & Yoken, R. H. (1997). Seasonality of births in schizophrenia and bipolar disorder: A review of the literature. *Schizophrenia Research, 28*, 1–38.

Tot, S., Ozge, A., Comelekoglu, U., Yazici, K., & Bal, N. (2002). Association of QEEG findings with clinical characteristics of OCD: Evidence of left frontotemporal dysfunction. *Canadian Journal of Psychiatry, 47*, 538–545.

Tran, M., Bédard, M., Molloy, D. W., Dubois, S., & Lever, J. A. (2003). Associations between psychotic symptoms and dependence in activities of daily living among older adults with Alzheimer's disease. *International Psychogeriatrics, 15*, 171–179.

Trenton, A., Currier, G., & Zwemer, F. (2003). Fatalities associated with therapeutic use and overdose of atypical antipsychotics. *CNS Drugs, 17*, 307–324.

Trevarthen, C., & Aitken, K. J. (2001). Infant intersubjectivity: Research, theory, and clinical applications. *Journal of Child Psychology and Psychiatry, and Allied Disciplines, 42*, 3–48.

Trivedi, H. K., Mendelowitz, A. J., & Fink, M. (2003). Gilles de la Tourette form of catatonia: Response to ECT. *Journal of ECT, 19*, 115–117.

Trivedi, M. H. (1996). Functional neuroanatomy of obsessive-compulsive disorder. *Journal of Clinical Psychiatry, 57 Supplement 8*, 26–35.

Trivedi, M. H. (2003). Treatment-resistant depression: New therapies on the horizon. *Annals of Clinical Psychiatry, 15*, 59–70.

Trixler, M., Tenyi, T., Csabi, G., & Szabo, R. (2001). Minor physical anomalies in schizophrenia and bipolar affective disorder. *Schizophrenia Research, 52*, 195–201.

Trott, C. T., Fahn, S., Greene, P., Dillon, S., Winfield, H., Winfield, L., et al. (2003). Cognition following bilateral implants of embryonic dopamine neurons in PD: A double blind study. *Neurology, 60*, 1938–1943.

Trottier, G., Srivastava, L., & Walker, C. D. (1999). Etiology of infantile autism: A review of recent advances in genetic and neurobiological research. *Journal of Psychiatry and Neuroscience, 24*, 103–115.

Trzonkowski, P., Mysliwska, J., Godlewska, B., Szmit, E., Lukaszuk, K., Wieckiewicz, J., et al. (2004). Immune consequences of the spontaneous pro-inflammatory status in depressed elderly patients. *Brain, Behavior, and Immunity, 18*, 135–148.

Tsai, G. E., & Coyle, J. T. (1998). The role of glutamatergic neurotransmission in the pathophysiology of alcoholism. *Annual Reviews of Medicine, 49*, 173–184.

Tsatsanis, K. D., Rourke, B. P., Klin, A., Volkmar, F. R., Cicchetti, D., & Schultz, R. T. (2003). Reduced thalamic volume in high-functioning individuals with autism. *Biological Psychiatry, 53*, 121–129.

Tsuang, M. T., Lyons, M. J., Eisen, S. A., Golberg, J., True, W., Lin, W., et al. (1996). Genetic influences on DSM-III-R drug abuse and dependence: A study of 3, 372 twin pairs. *American Journal of Medical Genetics, 67*, 473–477.

Tully, L. A., Arseneault, L., Caspi, A., Moffitt, T. E., & Morgan, J. (2004). Does maternal warmth moderate the effects of birth weight on twins' attention-deficit/hyperactivity disorder (ADHD) symptoms and low IQ? *Journal of Consultation in Clinical Psychology, 72*, 218–226.

Tunbridge, E., Burnet, P. W., Sodhi, M. S., & Harrison, P. J. (2004). Catechol-o-methyltransferase (COMT) and praline dehydrogenase (PRODH) mRNAs in the dorsolateral prefrontal cortex in schizophrenia, bipolar disorder, and major depression. *Synapse, 51*, 112–118.

Tupala, E., Hall, H., Bergstrom, K., Mantere, T., Rasanen, P., Sarkioja, T., et al. (2003a). Different effect of age on dopamine transporters in the dorsal and ventrical striatum of controls and alcoholics. *Synapse, 48*, 205–211.

Tupala, E., Hall, H., Bergstrom, K., Mantere, T., Rasanen, P., Sarkioja, T., et al. (2003b). Dopamine D2 receptors and transporters in type 1 and 2 alcoholics measured with human whole hemisphere autoradiography. *Human Brain Mapping, 20*, 91–102.

Turetsky, B. I., Moberg, P. J., Arnold, S. E., Doty, R. L., & Gur, R. E. (2003). Low olfactory bulb volume in first-degree relatives of patients with schizophrenia. *American Journal of Psychiatry, 160*, 703–708.

Turgeon, L., O'Connor, K. P., Marchand, A., & Freeston, M. H. (2002). Recollections of parent-child relationships in patients with obsessive-compulsive disorder and panic disorder with agoraphobia. *Acta Psychiatrica Scandinavica, 105*, 310–316.

Turic, D., Langley, K., Kirov, G., Owen, M. J., Thapar, A., & O'Donovan, M. C. (2004). Direct analysis of the genes encoding G proteins GalphaT2, Galphao, GalpaZ in ADHD. *American Journal of Medical Genetics, 127B*, 68–72.

Turjanski, N., Sawle, G. V., Playford, E. D., Weeks, R., Lammerstma, A. A., Lees, A. J., et al. (1994). PET studies of the presynaptic and ppostsynaptic dopaminergic system in Tourette's syndrome. *Journal of Neurology, Neurosurgery, and Psychiatry, 57*, 688–692.

Turner, R. S., Grafton, S. T., McIntosh, A. R., DeLong, M. R, & Hoffman, J. M. (2003). The functional anatomy of Parkinsonian bradykinesia. *NeuroImage, 19*, 163–179.

Tutus, A., Simek, A., Sofuoglu, S., Nardali, M., Kugu, N., Karaaslan, F., & Gonul, A. S. (1998). Changes in regional cerebral blood flow demonstrated by single photon emission computed tomography in depressive disorders: Comparison of unipolar vs. bipolar subtypes. *Psychiatry Research, 83*, 169–177.

Twelves, D., Perkins, K. S., & Counsell, C. (2003). Systematic review of incidence studies of Parkinson's disease. *Movement Disorders, 18*, 19–31.

Tyas, S. L., Manfreda, J., Strain, L. A., & Montgomery, P. R. (2001). Risk factors for Alzheimer's disease: A population-based, longitudinal study in Manitoba, Canada. *International Journal of Epidemiology, 30*, 590–597.

Uboga, N. V., & Price, J. L. (2000). Formation of diffuse and fibrillar tangles in aging and early Alzheimer's disease. *Neurobiology of Aging, 21*, 1–10.

Uchida, R. R., Del-Ben, C. M., Santos, A. C., Araújo, D., Crippa, J. A., Guimarães, F. S., et al. (2003). Decreased left temporal lobe volume of panic patients measured by magnetic resonance imaging. *Brazilian Journal of Medical and Biological Research, 36*, 925–929.

Uesugi, H., Toyoda, J., & Iio, M. (1995). Positron emission tomography and plasma biochemistry findings in schizophrenic patients before and after electroconvulsive therapy. *Psychiatry Clinical Neuroscience, 49*, 131–135.

Uitti, R. J. (1998). Medical treatment of essential tremor and Parkinson's disease. *Geriatrics, 53*, 53–57.

Ulmann, R. K., & Sleator, E. K. (1986). Responders, nonresponders, and placebo responders among children with attention deficit disorder: Importance of a blinded placebo evaluation. *Clinical Pediatrics, 25*, 594–599.

US Surgeon General (1999). Mental health: A report of the US Surgeon General. Retrieved September 19, 2003, from http://www.surgeongeneral.gov/library/mentalhealth/chapter2/sec2_1.

Vaccarino, F. J., Bloom F. E., & Koob, G. F. (1985). Blockade of nucleus accumbens opiate receptors attenuates heroin reward in the rat. *Psychopharmacology, 86*, 37–42.

Vaidya, C. J., Austin, G., Kirkorian, G., Ridlehuber, H. W., Desmond, J. E., Glover, G. H., et al. (1998). Selective effects of methylphenidate in attention deficit hyperactivity disorder: A functional magnetic resonance study. *Proclamations of the National Academy of Sciences, U.S.A., 95*, 14494–14499.

Vaidya, V. A., & Duman, R. S. (2001). Depression—emerging insights from neurobiology. *British Medical Bulletin, 57*, 61–79.

Vakili, K., Pillay, S. S., Lafer, B., Fava, M., Renshaw, P. F., Bonello-Cintron, C. M., et al. (2000). Hippocampal volume in primary unipolar major depression: A magnetic resonance imaging study. *Biological Psychiatry, 47*, 1087–1090.

Valdes, R. M., Huff, M. O., El-Masri, M. A., & El-Mallakh, R. S. (2003). Effect of ethacrynic acid on sodium pump isoforms in SH-SY5Y cells. *Bipolar Disorders, 5*, 123–128.

Valenstein, M., Taylor, K. K., Austin, K., Kales, H. C., McCarthy, J. F., & Blow, F. C. (2004). Benzodiazepine use among depressed patients treated in mental health settings. *American Journal of Psychiatry, 161*, 654–661.

Valente, E. M., Abou-Sleiman, P. M., Caputo, V., Muqit, M. M., Harvey, K., Gispert, S., et al. (2004). Hereditary early-onset Parkinson's disease caused by mutations in PINK1. *Science, 304*, 1158–1160.

van Balkom, A. J., de Haan, E., van Oppen, P., Spinhoven, P., Hoogduin, K. A., & van Dyck, R. (1998). Cognitive and behavioral therapies alone versus in combination with fluvoxamine in the treatment of obsessive compulsive disorder. *Journal of Nervous and Mental Disease, 186*, 492–499.

van der Stelt, M., & Di Marzo, V. (2003). The endocannabinoid system in the basal ganglia and in the mesolimbic reward system: Implications for neurological and psychiatric disorders. *European Journal of Pharmacology, 480*, 133–150.

van Dongen, Y. C., & Groenewegen, H. J. (2002). Core and shell of the nucleus accumbens are interconnected via intrastriatal projections. In L. F. B. Nicholson, & R. L. M. Faull (Eds.), *The basal ganglia VII* (pp. 191–200). New York: Kluwer Academic/Plenum.

van Duijn, C. M., Farrer, L. A., Cupples, L. A., & Hofman, A. (1993). Genetic transmission of Alzheimer's disease among families in a Dutch population based study. *Journal of Medical Genetics, 30*, 640–646.

Van Dyck, C. H., Malison, R. T., Seibyl, J. P., Laruelle, M., Klumpp, H., Zoghbi, S. S., et al. (2000). Age-related decline in central serotonin transporter availability with [(123)I]beta-CIT SPECT. *Neurobiology of Aging, 21*, 497–501.

Van Dyck, C. H., Quinlan, D. M., Cretella, L. M., Staley, J. K., Malison, R. T., Baldwin, R. M., et al. (2002). Unaltered dopamine transporter availability in adult attention deficit hyperactivity disorder. *American Journal of Psychiatry, 159*, 309–312.

Van Heeringen, K. (2003). The neurobiology of suicide and suicidality. *Canadian Journal of Psychiatry, 48*, 292–300.

Van Heertum, R. L., & Tikofsky, R. S. (2003). Positron emission tomography and single-photon emission computed tomography brain imaging in the evaluation of dementia. *Seminars in Nuclear Medicine, 33*, 77–85.

van Os, J., Hanssen, M., Bijl, R. V., & Vollebergh, W. (2001). Prevalence of psychotic disorder and community level of psychotic symptoms. *Archives of General Psychiatry, 58*, 663–668.

van Praag, H., Kempermann, G., & Gage, F. H. (1999). Running increases cell proliferation and neurogenesis in the adult mouse dentate gyrus. *Nature Neuroscience, 2*, 266–270.

Vanacore, N., Nappo, A., Gentile, M., Brustolin, A., Palange, S., Liberati, A., et al. (2002). Evaluation of risk of Parkinson's disease in a cohort of licensed pesticide users. *Neurological Science, 23*, 119–120.

Varrone, A., Marek, K. L, Jennings, D., Innis, R. B., & Seibyl, J. P. (2001). [123I]beta-CIT SPECT imaging demonstrates reduced density of striatal dopamine transporters in Parkinson's disease and multiple system atrophy. *Movement Disorders, 16*, 1023–1032.

Varrone, A., Salvatore, E., De Michele, G., Barone, P., Sansone, V., Pellecchia, M. T., et al. (2004). Reduced striatal [123 I]FP-CIT binding in SCA2 patients without Parkinsonism. *Annals of Neurology, 55*, 426–430.

Vega, W. A., Sribney, W. M., Aguilar-Gaxiola, S., & Kolody, B. (2004). 12-month prevalence of DSM-III-R psychiatric disorders among Mexican-Americans: Nativity, social assimilation, and age determinants. *Journal of Nervous and Mental Disease, 192*, 532–541.

Verburg, K., Griez, E., Meijer, J., & Pols, H. (1995). Discrimination between panic disorder and generalized anxiety disorder by 35% carbon dioxide challenge. *American Journal of Psychiatry, 152*, 1081–1083.

Verhulst, F. C., Achenbach, T. M., van der Ende, J., Erol, N., Lambert, M. C., Leung, P. W. L., et al. (2003). Comparison of problems reported by youths from seven countries. *American Journal of Psychiatry, 160*, 1479–1485.

Verkerk, A. J., Mathews, C. A., Joosse, M., Eussen, B. H., Heutink, P., & Oostra, B. A. (2003). CNTNAP2 is disrupted in a family with Gilles de la Tourette syndrome and obsessive compulsive disorder. *Genomics, 82*, 1–9.

Vermeulen, T. (1998). Distribution of paroxetine in three postmortem cases. *Journal of Analytical Toxicology, 22*, 541–544.

Videbech, P. (2000). PET measures of brain glucose metabolism and blood flow in major depressive disorder: A critical review. *Acta Psychiatrica Scandinavica, 101*, 11–20.

Videbech, P., & Ravnkilde, B. (2004). Hippocampal volume and depression: A meta-analysis of MRI studies. *American Journal of Psychiatry, 161*, 1957–1966.

Vingerhoets, F. J., Villemure, J. G., Temperli, P., Pollo, C., Pralong, E., & Ghika, J. (2002). Subthalamic DBS replaces levodopa in Parkinson's disease: Two-year follow-up. *Neurology, 58*, 396–401.

Visser-Vandewalle, V., Temel, Y., Boon, P., Vreeling, F., Colle, H., Hoogland, G., et al. (2003). Chronic bilateral thalamic stimulation: A new therapeutic approach in intractable Tourette syndrome. Report of three cases. *Journal of Neurosurgery, 99*, 1094–1100.

Vitousek, K., & Manke, F. (1994). Personality variable and disorders in anorexia nervosa and bulimia nervosa. *Journal of Abnormal Psychology, 103*, 137–147.

Vles, J. S., Feron, F. J., Hendriksen, J. G., Jolles, J., van Kroonenburgh, M. J., & Weber, W. E. (2003). Methylphenidate down-regulates the dopamine receptor and transporter system in children with attention deficit hyperkinetic disorder (ADHD). *Neuropediatrics, 34*, 77–80.

Voigt, R. G., Llorente, A. M., Jensen, C. L., Fraley, J. K., Berretta, M. C., & Heird, W. C. (2001). A randomized, double-blind, placebo-controlled trial of docosahexaenoic acid supplementation in children with attention-deficit/hyperactivity disorder. *Journal of Pediatrics, 139*, 189–196.

Vokaer, M., Bier, J. C., Elincx, S., Claes, T., Paquier, P., Goldman, S., et al. (2002). The cerebellum may be directly involved in cognitive functions. *Neurology, 58*, 967–970.

Volkow, N. D., Chang, L., Wang, G. J., Fowler, J. S., Ding, Y. S. Sedler, M., et al. (2001). Low level of brain dopamine D2 receptors in methamphetamine abusers: Association with metabolism in the orbitofrontal cortex. *American Journal of Psychiatry, 158*, 2015–2021.

Volkow, N. D., Fowler, J. S., & Wang, G. J. (2002). Roles of dopamine in drug reinforcement and addiction in humans: Results from imaging studies. *Behavioral Pharmacology, 13*, 355–366.

Volkow, N. D., Fowler, J. S., & Wang, G. J. (2003). Positron emission tomography and single-photon emission computed tomography in substance abuse. *Seminars in Nuclear Medicine, 33*, 114–128.

Volkow, N. D., Fowler, J. S., Wang, G., Ding, Y., & Gatley, S. J. (2002). Mechanism of action of methylphenidate: Insights from PET imaging studies. *Journal of Attention Disorders, 6*, S31–43.

Volkow, N. D., Fowler, J. S., Wolf, A. P., & Gillespi, H. (1991). Metabolic studies of drugs of abuse. *NIDA Research Monograph, 105*, 47–53.

Volkow, N. D., Wang, G. J., Fischman, M. W., Foltin, R. W., Fowler, J. S., Abumrad, N. N., et al. (1997). Relationship between subjective effects of cocaine and dopamine transporter occupancy. *Nature, 386*, 827–830.

Volkow, N. D., Wang, G. J., Fowler, J. S., Fischman, M., Foltin, R., Abumrad, N. N., et al. (1999). Methylphenidate and cocaine have a similar in vivo potency to block dopamine transporters in the human brain. *Life Science, 65*, 7–12.

Volkow, N. D., Wang, G. J., Fowler, J. S., Logan, J., Francheschi, D., Maynard, L., et al. (2002). Relationship between blockade of dopamine transporters by oral methylphenidate and the increase in extracellular dopamine: Therapeutic implications. *Synapse, 43*, 181–187.

Volkow, N. D., Wang, G. J., Fowler, J. S., Logan, J., Gerasimov, M., Maynard, L., et al. (2001). Therapeutic doses of oral methylphenidate significantly increase extracellular dopamine in human brain. *Journal of Neuoscience, 21*, 1–5.

Volkow, N. D., Wang, G. J., Fowler, J. S., Logan, J., Hitzemann, R., Ding, Y. S., et al. (1996). Decreases in dopamine receptors but not in dopamine transporters in alcoholics. *Alcoholism: Clinical and Experimental Research, 20*, 1594–1598.

Volkow, N. D., Wang, G. J., Maynard, L., Fowler, J. S., Jayne, B., Telang, F., et al. (2002). Effects of alcohol detoxification on dopamine D2 receptors in alcoholics: A preliminary study. *Psychiatry Research, 116*, 163–172.

Vollenweider, F. X., Vontobel, P., Hell, D., & Leenders, K. L. (1999). 5-HT modulation of dopamine release in basal ganglia in psilocybin-induced psyhosis in man—a PET study with [11C]raclopride. *Neuropsychopharmacology, 20*, 424–433.

Volpato Cordioli, A., Heldt, E., Braga Bochi, D., Margis, R., Basso de Sousa, M., Fonseca Tonello, J., et al. (2003). Cognitive-behavioral group therapy in obsessive-compulsive disorder: A randomized clinical trial. *Psychotherapy and Psychosomatics, 72*, 211–216.

von Bohlen und Halbach, O., & Dermietzel, R. (2002). *Neurotransmitters and neuromodulators: Handbook of receptors and biological effects*. Wenheim, Germany: Wiley-VCH.

Vrontakis, M. E. (2002). Galanin: A biologically active peptide. *Current Drug Targets–CNS and Neurological Disorders, 1*, 531–541.

Vythilingam, M., Anderson, E. R., Goddard, A., Woods, S. W., Staib, L. H., Charney, D. S., et al. (2000). Temporal lobe volume in panic disorder: A quantitative magnetic resonance imaging study. *Psychiatry Research, 99*, 75–82.

Vythilingam, M., Charles, H. C., Tupler, L. A., Blitchington, T., Kelly, L., & Krishnan, K. R. (2003). Focal and lateralized subcortical abnormalities in unipolar major depressive disorder: An automated multivoxel proton magnetic resonance spectroscopy study. *Biological Psychiatry, 54*, 744–750.

Wadsworth, S. J., Olson, R. K., Pennington, B. F., & DeFries, J. C. (2000). Differential genetic etiology of reading disability as a function of IQ. *Journal of Learning Disabilities, 33*, 192–199.

Wagner, J. P., Black, I. B., & DiCicco-Bloom, E. (1999). Stimulation of neonatal and adult brain neurogenesis by subcutaneous injection of basic fibroblast growth factor. *Journal of Neuroscience, 19*, 6006–6016.

Wahlbeck, K., Forsen, T., Osmond, C., Barker, D. J. P., & Eriksson, J. G. (2001). Association of schizophrenia with low maternal body mass index, small size at birth, and thinness during childhood. *Archives of General Psychiatry, 58*, 48–53.

Waldman, I. D., Rowe, D. C., Abramowitz, A., Kozel, S. T., Mohr, J. H., Sherman, S. L., et al. (1998). Association and linkage of the dopamine transporter gene and attention-deficir hyperactivity disorder in children: Heterogeneity owing to diagnostic subtype and severity. *American Journal of Human Genetics, 63*, 1767–1776.

Walkup, J. T., LaBuda, M. C., Singer, H. S., Brown, J., Riddle, M. A., & Hurko, O. (1996). Family study and segregation analysis of Tourette syndrome: Evidence for a mixed model of inheritance. *American Journal of Human Genetics, 59*, 684–693.

Walsh, B. T., Hadigan, C. M., Devlin, M. J., Gladis, M., & Roose, S. P. (1991). Long-term outcome of antidepressant treatment for bulimia nervosa. *American Journal of Psychiatry, 148*, 1206–1212.

Walsh, E., Buchanan, A., & Fahy, T. (2001). Violence and schizophrenia: Examining the evidence. *British Journal of Psychiatry, 180*, 490–495.

Walsh, L. E., & Garg, B. P. (1997). Ischemic strokes in children. *Indian Journal of Pediatrics, 64*, 613–623.

Walters, C. L., Kuo, Y. C., & Blendy, J. A. (2003). Differential distribution of CREB in the mesolimbic dopamine reward pathway. *Journal of Neurochemistry, 87*, 1237–1244.

Wang, C. T., Grishanin, R., Earles, C. A., Chang, P. Y., Martin, T. F., Chapman, E. R., et al. (2001). Synaptotagmin modulation of fusion pore kinetics in regulated exocytosis of dense-core vesicles. *Science, 294*, 1111–1115.

Wang, G. J., Volkow, N. D., Chang, L., Miller, E., Sedler, M., Hitzemann, R., et al. (2004). Partial recovery of brain metabolism in methamphetamine abusers after protracted abstinence. *American Journal of Psychiatry, 161*, 242–248.

Wang, H. S., & Kuo, M. F. (2003). Tourette's syndrome in Taiwan: An epidemiological study of tic disorder in an elementary school at Taipei County. *Brain Development, 25*, S29–31.

Wang, L., Swank, J. S., Glick, I. E., Gado, M. H., Miller, M. I., Morris, J. C., et al. (2003). Changes in hippocampal volume and shape across time distinguish dementia of the Alzheimer type from healthy aging. *NeuroImage, 20*, 667–682.

Wang, P. N., Liao, S. Q., Liu, R. S., Liu, C. Y., Chao, H. T., Lu, S. R., et al. (2000). Effects of estrogen on cognition, mood, and recebral blood flow in AD. *Neurology, 54*, 2061–2066.

Wang, R. (2002). Two's company, three's a crowd: Can H2S be the third endogenous gaseous transmitter? *Federation of American Societies of Experimental Biology Journal, 16*, 1792–1798.

Warkentin, S., Ohlsson, M., Wollmer, P., Edenbrandt, L., & Minthon, L. (2004). Regional cerebral blood flow in Alzheimer's disease: Classification and analysis of heterogeneity. *Dementia and Geriatric Cognitive Disorders, 17*, 207–214.

Warner, T. T., & Schapira, A. H. (2003). Genetic and environmental factors in the cause of Parkinson's disease. *Annals of Neurology, 53*, 16–25.

Warsh, J. J., Young, L. T., & Li, P. P. (2000). Guanine nucleotide binding (G) protein disturbances in bipolar affective disorder. In R. H. Belmker (Ed.), *Bipolar medications: Mechanisms of action* (pp. 299–329). Washington, DC: American Psychiatric Press.

Wassink, T. H., Piven, J., Vieland, V. J., Huang, J., Swiderski, R. E., Pietila, J., et al. (2001). Evidence supporting WNT2 as an autism susceptibility gene. *American Journal of Medical Genetics, 105*, 406–413.

Watanabe, T. K., Miller, M. A., & McElligott, J. M. (2003). Congenital and acquired brain injury: Outcomes after acquired brain injury. *Archives of Physical and Medical Rehabilitation, 84*, 23–31.

Waters, T. L., Barrett, P. M., & March, J. S. (2001). Cognitive-behavioral family treatment of childhood obsessive-compulsive disorder: Preliminary findings. *American Journal of Psychotherapy, 55*, 372–387.

Watkins, K. E., Paus, T., Lerch, J. P., Zijdenbos, A., Collins, D. L., Neelin, P., et al. (2001). Structural asymmetries in the human brain: A voxel-based statistical analysis of 142 MRI scans. *Cerebral Cortex, 9*, 868–877.

Watkins, P. B., Zimmerman, H. J., Knapp, M. J., Gracon, S. I., & Lewis, K. W. (1994). Hepatotoxic effects of tacrine administration in patients with Alzheimer's disease. *Journal of the American Medical Association, 271*, 992–998.

Webb, S. J., Monk, C. S., & Nelson, C. A. (2001). Mechanisms of postnatal neurobiological development: Implications for human development. *Developmental Neuropsychology, 19*, 147–171.

Weber, A. M., Egelhoff, J. C., McKellop, J. M., & Franz, D. N. (2000). Autism and the cerebellum: Evidence from tuberous sclerosis. *Journal of Autism and Developmental Disorders, 30*, 511–517.

Webster, R. A. (2001). Diseases of the basal ganglia. In R. A. Webster (Ed.), *Neurotransmitters, drugs and brain function* (pp. 299–323). New York: John Wiley & Sons.

Webster, R. A. (2001a). Dopamine (DA). In R. A. Webster (Ed.), *Neurotransmitters, drugs, and brain function* (pp. 137–161). New York: Wiley.

Webster, R. A. (2001b). Neurotransmitter systems and function: Overview. In R. A. Webster (Ed.), *Neurotransmitters, drugs, and brain function* (pp. 3–32). New York: Wiley.

Webster, R. A. (2001c). Schizophrenia. In R. A. Webster (Ed.), *Neurotransmitters, drugs, and brain function* (pp. 351–373). New York: Wiley.

Webster, S. D., Yang, A. J., Margol, L., Garzon-Rodriquez, W., Glabe, C. G., & Tenner, A. J. (2000). Complement component C1q modulates the phagocytosis of Aβ by microglia. *Experimental Neurology, 161*, 127–138.

Wehr, T. A., Muscettola, G., & Goodwin, F. K. (1980). Urinary 3-methoxy-4-hydroxyphenylglycol circadian rhythm. Early timing (phase-advance) in manic-depressives compared with normal subjects. *Archives of General Psychiatry, 37*, 257–263.

Weinberger, D. R. (1987). Implications of normal brain development for the pathogenesis of schizophrenia. *Archives of General Psychiatry, 44*, 600–669.

Weinberger, D. R. (1995). From neuropathology to neurodevelopment. *Lancet, 346*, 552–557.

Weinberger, D. R. (1996). On the plausibility of "the neurodevelopmental hypothesis" of schizophrenia. *Neuropsychopharmacology, 14*, 1–11.

Weinberger, D. R., & Lipska, B. K. (1995). Cortical maldevelopment, antipsychotic drugs and schizophrenia: A search for common ground. *Schizophrenia Research, 16*, 87–110.

Weiner, H. L., Lemere, C. A., Maron, R., Spooner, E. T., Grenfell, T. J., Mori, C., et al. (2000). Nasal administration of amyloid-peptide decreases cerebral amyloid burden in a mouse model of Alzheimer's disease. *Annals of Neurology, 48*, 567–579.

Weiner, M. F., Edland, S. D., & Luszcyzynska, H. (1994). Prevalence and incidence of major depression in Alzheimer's disease. *American Journal of Psychiatry, 151*, 1006–1009.

Weiner, M. F., Hynan, L. S., Parikh, B., Zaki, N., White, C. L. III, Bigio, E. H., et al. (2003). Can Alzheimer's disease and dementias with Lewy bodies be distinguished clinically? *Journal of Geriatric Psychiatry and Neurology, 16*, 245–250.

Weingarten, H. L. (1988). 1-Methyl-4-phenyl-1, 2, 3, 6-tetrahydropyridine (MPTP): One designer drug and serendipity. *Journal of Forensic Sciences, 33*, 588–595.

Weintraub, D., Moberg, P. J., Duda, J. E., Katz, I. R., & Stern, M. B. (2003). Recognition and treatment of depression in Parkinson's disease. *Journal of Geriatric Psychiatry and Neurology, 16*, 178–183.

Weisskopf, M. G., Chen, H., Schwarzschild, M. A., Kawachi, I., & Ascherio, A. (2003). Prospective study of phobic anxiety and risk of Parkinson's disease. *Movement Disorders, 18*, 646–651.

Weissman, M. M. (1993). Family genetic studies of panic disorder. *Journal of Psychiatric Research, 27, Supplement 1*, 69–78.

Weist, M. D. (1997). Expanded school mental health services: A national movement in progress. In T. H. Ollendick & R. J. Prinz (Eds.), *Advances in clinical and child psychology* (Vol. 19) 319–352. New York: Plenum.

Wender, E. H. (1986). The food additive-free diet in the treatment of behavior disorders: A review. *Journal of Development and Behavioral Pediatrics, 7*, 35–42.

Werman, R. (1966). Criteria for identification of a central nervous system transmitter. *Comparative Biochemistry and Physiology, 18*, 745–766.

West, A. B., & Maidment, N. T. (2004). Genetics of parkin-linked disease. *Human Genetics, 114*, 327–336.

West, P., Sweeting, H., Der, G., Barton, J., & Lucas, C. (2003). Voice-DISC identified DSM-IV disorders among 15-year-olds in the west of Scotland. *Journal of the American Academy of Child and Adolescent Psychiatry, 42*, 941–949.

Weyandt, L. L. (2001). *An ADHD primer.* Boston: Allyn & Bacon.

Weyandt, L. L. (2004). Alternative interventions: Nontraditional treatments for attention disorders. In *Helping children at home and school: Handouts from your school psychologist*. Bethesda, MD: National Association of School Psychologists.

Weyandt, L. L. (2005). Executive function in children, adolescents, and adults with attention-deficit/hyperactivity disorder: Introduction to the special issue. *Developmental Neuropsychology, 27*, 1–10.

Weyandt, L. L. (2005). Neuropsychological performance in adults with ADHD. In D. Gozal & D. Molfese (Eds.), *Attention deficit hyperactivity disorder: From genes to animal models to patients.* Totowa, NJ: Humana.

Weyandt, L. L., Iwaszuk, W., Fulton, K., Ollerton, M., Beatty, N., Fouts. H., et al. (2003). The Internal Restlessness Scale: Performance of college students with and without ADHD. *Journal of Learning Disabilities, 36*, 382–389.

Weyandt, L. L., Mitzlaff, L., & Thomas, L. (2002). The relationship between intelligence and performance on the Test of Variables of Attention (TOVA). *Journal of Learning Disabilities, 35*, 114–120.

Whalen, C., & Schreibman, L. (2003). Joint attention training for children with autism using behavior modification procedures. *Journal of Child Psychology and Psychiatry, 44*, 456–468.

Whalen, P. J., Shin, L. M., McInerney, S. C., Fischer, H., Wright, C. I., & Rauch, S. L. (2001). A functional MRI study of human amygdala responses to facial expressions of fear versus anger. *Emotion, 1*, 70–83.

Whitall, J., McCombe-Waller, S., Silver, K. H. C., & Macko, R. F. (2000). Repetitive bilateral arm training with rhythmic auditory cueing improves motor function in chronic hemiparetic stroke. *Stroke, 31*, 2390–2397.

White, B. L., & Held, R. (1966). Plasticity of sensorimotor development. In J. F. Rosenblith & W. Allinsmith (Eds.), *The causes of behavior*. Boston: Allyn & Bacon.

White, F. J., & Kalivas, P. W. (1998). Neuroadaptations involved in amphetamine and cocaine addiction. *Drug and Alcohol Dependence, 51*, 141–153.

White, H. S. (2003). Mechanism of action of newer anticonvulsants. *Journal of Clinical Psychiatry, 64*, 5–8.

Whitehouse, P. J., Martino, A. M., Marcus, K. A., Zweig, R. M., Singer, H. S., Price, D. L., et al. (1988). Reductions in acetylcholine and nicotine binding in several degenerative diseases. *Archives of Neurology, 45*, 722–724.

Wiedemann, G., Pauli, P., Dengler, W., Lutzenberger, W., Birbaumer, N., & Buchkremer, G. (1999). Frontal brain asymmetry as a biological substrate of emotions in patients with panic disorders. *Archives of General Psychiatry, 56*, 78–84.

Wiesel, F. A. (1992). Glucose metabolism in psychiatric disorders: How can we facilitate comparisons among studies? *Journal of Neural Transmission, 37, Supplement*, 1–18.

Wilcock, G. K., Birks, J., Whitehead, A., & Evans, S. J. (2002). The effect of selegiline in the treatment of people with Alzheimer's disease: A meta-analysis of published trials. *International Journal of Geriatric Psychiatry, 17*, 175–183.

Wilcox, J., Tsuang, M. T., Ledger, E., Algeo, J., & Schnurr, T. (2002). Brain perfusion in autism varies with age. *Biological Psychiatry, 46*, 13–16.

Wilens, T. E. (2004). Impact of ADHD and its treatment on substance abuse in adults. *Journal of Clinical Psychiatry, 65*, 38–45.

Wilhelm, S., Deckersbach, T., Coffey, B. J., Bohne, A., Peterson, A. L., & Baer, L. (2003). Habit reversal versus supportive psychotherapy for Tourette's disorder: A randomized controlled trial. *American Journal of Psychiatry, 160*, 1175–1177.

Wilkinson, B. J., Newman, M. B., Shytle, R. D., Silver, A. A., Sanberg, P. R., & Sheehan, D. (2002). Family impact of Tourette's syndrome. *Journal of Child and Family Studies, 10*, 477–483.

Willcutt, E. (2005). The etiology of ADHD: Behavioral and molecular genetic approaches. In D. Barch (Ed.), *Cognitive and affective neuroscience of psychopathology*. NY: Oxford University Press.

Willcutt, E. G., Pennington, B. F., & DeFries, J. C. (2000). Twin study of the etiology of comorbidity between reading disability and attention-deficit/hyperactivity disorder. *American Journal of Medical Genetics, 96*, 293–301.

Willencutt, E. G., Pennington, B. F., & DeFries, J. C. (1999). Etiology of inattention and hyperactivity/impulsivity in a community sample of twins with learning difficulties. *Journal of Abnormal Child Psychology, 28*, 149–159.

Williams, J., Spurlock, G., Holmans, P., Mant, R., Murphy, K., Jones, L., et al. (1998). A meta-analysis and transmission disequilibrium study of association between the dopamine D3 receptor gene and schizophrenia. *Molecular Psychiatry, 3*, 141–149.

Williams, R. S., Hauser, S. L., Purpura, D. P., DeLong, G. R., & Swisher, C. N. (1980). Autism and mental retardation: Neuropathologic studies performed in four retarded persons with autistic behavior. *Archives of Neurology, 37*, 749–753.

Williams, S. E., Ris, M. D., & Ayangar, R. (1998). Recovery in pediatric brain injury: Is psychostimulant medication beneficial? *Journal of Head Trauma, 13*, 73–81.

Willis, W. G., & Weiler, M. D. (2005). Neural substrates of childhood attention-deficit/hyperactivity disorder: Electroencephalographic and magnetic resonance imaging evidence. *Developmental Neuropsychology, 27*, 135–187.

Wilson, R. S., Evans, D. A., Bienias, J. L., Mendes de Leon, C. F., Schneider, J. A., & Bennett, D. A. (2003). Proneness to psychological distress is associated with risk of Alzheimer's disease. *Neurology, 61*, 1479–1485.

Wilson, R. S., Mendes de Leon, C. F., Barnes, L. L., Schneider, J. A., Bienias, J. L., Evans, D. A., et al. (2002). Participation in cognitively stimulating activities and risk of incident Alzheimer's disease. *Journal of the American Medical Association, 287*, 742–748.

Wilson, R. S., Schneider, J. A., Bienias, J. L., Arnold, S. E., Evans, D. A., & Bennett, D. A. (2003). Depressive symptoms, clinical AD, and cortical plaques and tangles in older persons. *Neurology, 61*, 1102–1107.

Wimpory, D. (2002). Social timing, clock genes and autism: A new hypothesis. *Journal of Intellectual Disability Research, 46*, 352–358.

Wise, R. A., & Gardner, E. L. (2004). Animal models of addiction. In D. S. Charney & E. J. Nestler (Eds.), *Neurobiology of mental illness* (2nd ed., pp. 683–697). New York: Oxford University Press.

Wise, R. A., Newton, P. L., Leeb, K., Burnette, B., Pocock, D., & Justice, J. (1995). Fluctuations in nucleus accumbens dopamine concentration during intravenous cocaine self-administration in rats. *Psychopharmacology, 120*, 10–20.

Wisner, K. L., Perel, J. M., Peindl, K. S., & Hanusa, B. H. (2004). Timing of depression recurrence in the first year after birth. *Journal of Affective Disorders, 78*, 249–252.

Witelson, S. F. (1989). Hand and sex differences in the isthmus and genu of the human corpus callosum. *Brain, 112*, 799–835.

Wittchen, H. U. (2002). Generalized anxiety disorder: Prevalence, burden, and cost to society. *Depression and Anxiety, 16*, 162–171.

Woerner, M. G., Robinson, D. G., Alvir, J. J., Sheitman, B. B., Lieberman, J. A., & Kane, J. M. (2003). Clozapine as a first treatment for schizophrenia. *American Journal of Psychiatry, 160*, 1514–1516.

Wolf, S. S., Jones, D. W., Knable, M. B., Gorey, J. G., Lee, K. S., Hyde, T. M., et al. (1996). Tourette syndrome: Prediction of phenotypic variation in monozygotiz twins by caudate nucleus D2 receptor. *Science, 273*, 1225–1227.

Wolfe, B. E., Metzger, E. D., Levine, J. M., Finkeltein, D. M., Cooper, T. B., & Jimerson, D. C. (2000). Serotonin function following remission from bulimia nervosa. *Neuropsychopharmacology, 22*, 257–263.

Wolfe, P. (2001). *Brain matters: Translating research into classroom practice.* Alexandria, VA: Association for Supervision and Curriculum Development.

Wonderlich, S. A., Crosby, R. D., Mitchell, J. E., Thompson, K. M., Redlin, J., Demuth, G., et al. (2001). Eating disturbance and sexual trauma in childhood and adulthood. *International Journal of Eating Disorders, 30*, 401–412.

Wong, D. F., Wanger, H. N., Tune, L. E., Dannals, R. F., Pearlson, G. D., Links, J. M., et al. (1986). Positron emission tomography reveals elevated D2 dopamine receptors in drug-naive schizophrenics. *Science, 234*, 1558–1563.

Woo, J., Lau, E., Ziea, E., & Chan, D. K. (2004). Prevalence of Parkinson's disease in a Chinese population. *Acta Neurologica Scandinavica, 109*, 228–231.

Woo, J. M., Yoon, K. S., & Yu, B. H. (2002). Catechol O-methyltransferase genetic polymorphism in panic disorder. *American Journal of Psychiatry, 159*, 1785–1787.

Wood, B. L., Klebba, K., Gbadebo, O., Lichter, D., Kurlan, R., & Miller, B. (2003). Pilot study of effect of emotional stimuli on tic severity in children with Tourette's syndrome. *Movement Disorders, 18*, 1392–1395.

Woodruff, P., McManus, I., & David, A. (1995). A meta-analysis of corpus callosum size in schizophrenia. *Journal of Neurology, Neurosurgery, and Psychiatry, 58*, 457–461.

Woods, D. W., Twohig, M. P., Flessner, C. A., & Roloff, T. J. (2003). Treatment of vocal tics in children with Tourette syndrome: Investigating the efficacy of habit reversal. *Journal of Applied Behavior Analysis, 36*, 109–112.

Wooten, G. F., Currie, L. J., Bovbjerg, V. E., Lee, J. K., & Patrie, J. (2004). Are men at greater risk for Parkinson's disease than women? *Journal of Neurology, Neurosurgery, and Psychiatry, 75*, 637–639.

Wu, L. T., Kouzis, A. C., & Schlenger, W. E. (2003). Substance use, dependence, and service utilization among US uninsured nonelderly population. *American Journal of Public Health, 93*, 2079–2085.

Xian, H., Scherrer, J. F., Madden, P. A., Lyons, M. J., Tsuang, M., True, W. R., et al. (2003). The heritability of failed smoking cessation and nicotine withdrawal in twins who smoked and attempted to quit. *Nicotine and Tobacco Research, 5*, 245–254.

Xu, P. Y., Liang, R., Jankovic, J., Hunter, C., Zeng, Y. X., Ashizawa, T., et al. (2002). Association of homozygous 7048G7049 variant in the intron six of *Nurr1* gene with Parkinson's disease. *Neurology, 58*, 881–884.

Xu, X., Ozbay, F., Wigg, K., Shulman, R., Tahir, E., Yazgan, Y., et al. (2003). Evaluation of the genes for the adrenergic receptors alpha 2A and alpha 1C and Gilles de la Tourette syndrome. *American Journal of Medical Genetics, 119B*, 54–59.

Yamada, K., Watanabe, A., Iwayama-Shigeno, Y., & Yoshikawa, T. (2003). Evidence of association between gamma-aminobutyric acid type A receptor genes located on 5q34 and female patients with mood disorders. *Neuroscience Letters, 349*, 9–12.

Yamamoto, M., Kondo, I., Ogawa, N., Asanuma, M., Yamashita, Y., & Mizuno, Y. (1997). Genetic association between susceptibility to Parkinson's disease and alpha1-antichymotrypsin polymorphism. *Brain Research, 759*, 153–155.

Yamashita, Y., Fujimoto, C., Nakajima, E., Isagai, T., & Matsuishi, T. (2003). Possible association between congenital cytomegalovirus infection and autistic disorder. *Journal of Autism and Developmental Disorders, 33*, 455–459.

Yao, W. D., Gainetdinov, R. R., Arbuckle, M. I., Sotnikova, T. D., Cyr, M., Beaulieu, J. M., et al. (2004). Identification of PSD-95 as a regulator of dopamine-mediated synaptic and behavioral plasticity. *Neuron, 41*, 625–638.

Yaryura-Tobias, J. A., Mancebo, M., & Bubrick, J. (2001). Basal ganglia pathology in children and adolescents with obsessive-compulsive disorder, Tourette's syndrome, and attention-deficit hyperactivity disorder. *Psychiatric Annals, 31*, 565–572.

Yatham, L. N., Clark, C. C., & Zis, A. P. (2000). A preliminary study of the effects of electroconvulsive therapy on regional brain glucose metabolism in patients with major depression. *Journal of ECT, 16*, 171–176.

Yatham, L. N., Liddle, P. F., Dennie, J., Shiah, I. S., Adam, M. J., Lane, C. J., et al. (1999). Decrease in brain serotonin 2 receptor binding in patients with major depression following desipramine treatment: A positron emission tomography study with fluorine-18-labeled setoperone. *Archives of General Psychiatry, 56*, 705–711.

Yatham, L. N., Liddle, P. F., Shiah, I. S., Scarrow, G., Lam, R. W., Adam, M. J., et al. (2000). Brain serotonin 2 receptors in major depression: A positron emission tomography study. *Archives of General Psychiatry, 57*, 850–858.

Yeragani, V. K., Tancer, M., & Uhde, T. (2003). Heart rate and QT interval variability: Abnormal alpha-2 adrenergic function in patients with panic disorder. *Psychiatry Research, 121,* 185–196.

Yerevanian, B. I., Koek, R. J., & Mintz, J. (2003). Lithium, anticonvulsants and suicidal behavior in bipolar disorder. *Journal of Affective Disorders, 73,* 223–228.

Yildiz, A., & Sachs, G. S. (2003). Age of onset of psychotic versus non-psychotic bipolar illness in men & in women. *Journal of Affective Disorders, 74,* 197–201.

Yildiz, A., Sachs, G. S., Dorer, D. J., & Renshaw, P. F. (2001). 31P nuclear magnetic resonance spectroscopy findings in bipolar illness: A meta-analysis. *Psychiatry Research: Neuroimaging Section, 106,* 181–191.

Yirmiya, N., Pilowsky, T., Nemanov, L., Arbelle, S., Feinsilver, T., Fried I., et al. (2001). Evidence for an association with the serotonin transporter promoter region polymorphism and autism. *American Journal of Medical Genetics, 105,* 381–386.

Yoo, A. S., Cheng, I., Chung, S., Grenfell, T. Z., Lee, H., Pack-Chung, E., et al. (2000). Presenilin-mediated modulation of capacitative calcium entry. *Neuron, 27,* 561–572.

Yoon, I. S., Li, P. P., Siu, K. P., Kennedy, J. L., Macciardi, F., Cooke, R. G., et al. (2001). Altered TRPC7 gene expression in bipolar-I disorder. *Biological Psychiatry, 50,* 620–626.

Yoshida, K. Y., Takahashi, H., Higuchi, H., Kamata, M., Ito, K., Sato, K., et al. (2004). Prediction of antidepressant response to milnacipran by norepinephrine transporter gene polymorphisms. *American Journal of Psychiatry, 161,* 1575–1580.

Yoshizumi, T., Murase, S., Honjo, S., Kaneko, H., & Murakami, T. (2004). Hallucinatory experiences in a community sample of Japanese children. *Journal of the American Academy of Child and Adolescent Psychiatry, 43,* 1030–1036.

Young, L. T. (2001). Postreceptor pathways for signaling transduction in depression and bipolar disorder. *Journal of Psychiatry and Neuroscience, 26,* 17–22.

Young, L. T., Li, P. P., Kish, S. J., Siu, K. P., Kamble, A., Hornykiewicz, O., et al. (1993). Cerebral cortex Gs alpha protein levels and forskolin-stimulated cyclic AMP formation are increased in bipolar affective disorder. *Journal of Neurochemistry, 61,* 890–898.

Young, L. T., Warsh, J. J., Kish, S. J., Shannak, K., & Hornykeiwicz, O. (1994). Reduced brain 5-HT and elevated NE turnover and metabolites in bipolar affective disorder. *Biological Psychiatry, 35,* 121–127.

Young, R. F., Jacques, S., Mark, R., Kopyov, O., Copcutt, B., Posewitz, A., et al. (2000). Gamma knife thalamotomy for treatment of tremor: Long-term results. *Journal of Neurosurgery, 93,* 128–135.

Young, R. L., Brewer, N., & Pattison, C. (2003). Parental identification of early behavioral abnormalities in children with autistic disorder. *Autism, 7,* 125–143.

Yu, C., Li, Y., Chen, W., & Yue, M. (2002). Genotype of ethanol metabolizing enzyme genes by oligonucleotide microarray in alcoholic liver disease in Chinese people. *Chinese Medical Journal, 115,* 1085–1087.

Yu-Feng, L., Li, J., & Faraone, S. (2004). Association of norepinephrine transporter gene with methylphenidate response. *Journal of the American Academy of Child and Adolescent Psychiatry, 43,* 1154–1158.

Zaffanello, M., Zamboni, G., Fontana, E., Zoccante, L., & Tato, L. (2003). A case of partial biotinidase deficiency associated with autism. *Child Neuropsychology, 9,* 184–188.

Zaldy, S. T., Seshadri, S., Beiser, A., Wilson, P. W. F., Kiel, D. P., Tocco, M., et al. (2003). Plasma total cholesterol level as a risk factor for Alzheimer's disease. *Archives of Internal Medicine, 163,* 1053–1057.

Zametkin, A. J., Liebenauer, L. L., Fitzgerald, G. A., King, A. C., Minkunas, D. V., Herscovitch, P., et al. (1993). Brain metabolism in teenagers with attention-deficit hyperactivity disorder. *Archives of General Psychiatry, 50,* 333–340.

Zametkin, A. J., Nordahl, T. E., Gross, M., King, A. C., Semple, W. E., Rumsey, J., et al. (1990). Cerebral glucose metabolism in adults with hyperactivity of childhood onset. *New England Journal of Medicine, 323,* 1361–1366.

Zandi, P. P., Anthony, J. C., Khachaturian, A. S., Stone, S. V., Gustafson, D., Tschanz, J. T., et al. (2004). Reduced risk of Alzheimer disease in users of antioxidant vitamin supplements: The Cache County Study. *Archives of Neurology, 61,* 82–88.

Zandi, P. P., Carlson, M. C., Plassman, B. L., Welsh-Bohmer, K. A., Mayer, L. S., Steffens, D. C., et al. (2002). Hormone replacement therapy and incidence of Alzheimer disease in older women: The Cache County Study. *Journal of the American Medical Association, 288,* 2123–2129.

Zappia, M., Annesi, G., Nicoletti, G., Serra, P., Arabia, G., Pugliese, P., et al. (2003). Association of tau gene polymorphism with Parkinson's disease. *Neurological Science, 24,* 223–224.

Zarate, C. A. Jr., Du, J., Quiroz, J., Gray, N. A., Denicoff, K. D., Singh, J., et al. (2003). Regulation of cellular plasticity cascades in the pathophysiology and treatment of mood disorders: Role of the glutamatergic system. *Annals of the New York Academy of Sciences, 1003,* 273–291.

Zarranz, J. J., Alegre, J., Gomez-Esteban, J. C., Lezcano, E., Ros, R., Ampuero, I., et al. (2004). The new mutation, E46K, of alpha-synuclein causes Parkinson and Lewy body dementia. *Annals of Neurology, 55,* 164–173.

Zelnik, N., Newfield, R. S., Silman-Stolar, Z., & Goikhman, I. (2002). Height distribution in children with Tourette syndrome. *Journal of Child Neurology, 17,* 200–204.

Z'Graggen, W. J., Metz, G. A., Kartje, L., Thallmair, M., & Schwab, M. E. (1998). Functional recovery and enhanced corticofugal plasticity after unilateral pyramidal tract lesion and blockade of myelin-associated neurite growth inhibitor in adult rats. *Journal of Neuroscience, 18*, 4744–4757.

Zhang, R., Wang, Y., Zhang, L., Zhang, Z., Tsang, W., Lu, M., et al. (2002). Sildenafil (Viagra) induces neurogenesis and promotes functional recovery after stroke in rats. *Stroke, 33*, 2675–2680.

Zhou, F. M., Wilson, C., & Dani, J. A. (2003). Muscarinic and nicotinic cholinergic mechanisms in the mesostriatal dopamine systems. *The Neuroscientist, 9*, 23–36.

Zhu, G., Bartsch, O., Skrynyk, C., Rotonodo, A., Akhtar, L. A., Harris, C., et al. (2004). Failure to detect DUP25 in lymphoblastoid cells derived from patients with panic disorder and control individuals representing European and American populations. *European Journal of Human Genetics, 18*, 140–143.

Zhu, H., Guo, Q., & Mattson, M. P. (1999). Dietary restriction protects hippocampal neurons against the death-promoting action of a presenilin-1 mutation. *Brain Research, 842*, 224–229.

Ziemann, U., Corwell, B., & Cohen, L. G. (1998). Modulation of plasticity in human motor cortex after forearm ischemic nerve block. *Journal of Neuroscience, 18*, 1115–1123.

Zilberman, T., Tavares, H., & el-Guebaly, N. (2003). Gender similarities and differences: The prevalence and course of alcohol and other substance-related disorders. *Journal of Addiction Disorders, 22*, 61–74.

Zilbovicius, M., Boddaert, N., Belin, P., Poline, J. B., Remy, P., Mangin, J. F., et al. (2000). Temporal lobe dysfunction in childhood autism: A PET study. Positron emission tomography. *American Journal of Psychiatry, 157*, 1988–1993.

Zilbovicius, M., Garreau, B., Samson, Y., Remy, P., Barthélémy, C., Syrota, A., et al. (1995). Delayed maturation of the frontal cortex in childhood autism. *American Journal of Psychiatry, 152*, 248–252.

Zilbovicius, M., Garreau, B., Tzourio, N., Mazoyer, B., Bruck, B., Martinot, J. L., et al. (1992). Regional cerebral blood flow in childhood autism: A SPECT study. *American Journal of Psychiatry, 149*, 924–930.

Zimmerman, A. M., Abrams, M. T., Giuliano, J. D., Denckla, M. B., & Singer, H. S. (2000). Subcortical volumes in girls with Tourette syndrome: Support for a gender effect. *Neurology, 54*, 2224–2229.

Zimmerman, M., Chelminski, I., & McDermut, W. (2002). Major depressive disorder and axis I diagnostic comorbidity. *Journal of Clinical Psychiatry, 63*, 187–193.

Zink, M., Sartorius, A., Lederbogen, F., & Henn, F. A. (2002). Electroconvulsive therapy in patient receiving rivastigmine. *Journal of ECT, 18*, 162–164.

Zipursky, R. B., Seeman, M. V., Bury, A., Langevin, R., Wortzman, G., & Katz, R. (1997). Deficits in gray matter volume are present in schizophrenia but not bipolar disorder. *Schizophrenia Research, 26*, 85–92.

Zito, J. M., Safer, D. J., dosReis, S., Gardner, J. F., Boles, M., & Lynch, F. (2000). Trends in the prescribing of psychotropic medications to preschoolers. *Journal of the American Medical Association, 283*, 1025–1030.

Zito, J. M., Safer, D. J., dosReis, S., Gardner, J. F., Magder, L., Soeken, K., et al. (2003). Psychotropic practice patterns for youth. A ten year perspective. *Archives of Pediatrics and Adolescent Medicine, 157*, 17–25.

Zito, J. M., Safer, D. J., dosReis, S., Magder, L. S., Gardner, J. F., & Zarin, D. A. (1999). Psychotherapeutic medication patterns for youths with attention-deficit/hyperactivity disorder. *Archives of Pediatrics and Adolescent Medicine, 53*, 1257–1263.

Zohar, J., Insel, T. R., Zohar-Kadouch, R. C., Hill, J. L., & Murphy, D. L. (1988). Serotonergic responsivity in obsessive-compulsive disorder. Effects of chronic clomipramine treatment. *Archives of General Psychiatry, 45*, 167–172.

Zubieta, J. K., Dannals, R. F., & Frost, J. J. (1999). Gender and age influences in human brain mu-opioid receptor binding measured by PET. *American Journal of Psychiatry, 156*, 842–848.

Zubieta, J. K., Gorelick, D. A., Stauffer, R., Ravet, H. T., Dannals, R. F., & Frost, J. J. (1996). Increased mu opioid receptor binding detected by PET in cocaine-dependent men is associated with cocaine craving. *National Medicine, 2*, 1225–1229.

Zubieta, J. K., Greenwald, M. K., Lombardi, U., Woods, J. H., Kilbourn, M. R., Jewett, D. M., et al. (2000). Buprenorphrine-induced changes in mu-opioid receptor availability in male heroin-dependent volunteers: A preliminary study. *Neuropsychopharmacology, 23*, 326–334.

Zwanzger, P., Eser, D., Padberg, F., Baghai, T. C., Schule, C., Rötzer, F., et al. (2003). Effects of tiagabine on cholecystokinin-tetrapeptide (CCK-4)-induced anxiety in healthy volunteers. *Depression and Anxiety, 18*, 140–143.

Appendix: Website Information

General

American Medical Association
www.ama-assn.org

American Psychiatric Association
www.psych.org

American Psychological Association
www.apa.org

Blausen Medical Communications
www.blausen.com

Healthy Place
www.healthyplace.com

Internet Mental Health
www.mentalhealth.com

National Institute of Mental Health
www.nimh.nih.gov

WebMd
www.webmd.com

Alzheimer's Disease

Alzheimer's Association
www.alz.org

Alzheimer's Disease and Education
Referral Center
www.alzheimers.org

AlzheimerSupport.com
www.alzheimersupport.com

Anxiety Disorders

About, Inc.—"Panic/Anxiety Disorders"
www.panicdisorder.about.com

Anxiety Disorders Association of America
www.adaa.org

Anxietypanic.com—"Panic/Anxiety
Disorder"
www.anxietypanic.com

Attention-Deficit/Hyperactivity Disorder

About, Inc.* "Attention Deficit Disorder"
add.about.com

ADD Warehouse
www.addwarehouse.com

ADHD.com
www.adhd.com

ADHDnews.com
www.adhdnews.com

Children and Adults with Attention-Deficit/
Hyperactivity Disorder
www.chadd.org

Autistic Disorder

Autism—PDD Resources Network
www.autism-pdd.net

Autism Society of America
www.autism-society.org

Center for the Study of Autism
www.autism.org.

Cure Autism Now Foundation
www.canfoundation.org

Treatment and Education of Autistic and
Related Communication Handicapped
Children
www.teacch.com

Bipolar Disorder

About, Inc.* "Bipolar Disorder"
bipolar.about.com

Bipolar.com
www.bipolar.com

Bipolar Home
www.bipolarhome.org

Child and Adolescent Bipolar Foundation
www.bpkids.org

Depression and Bipolar Support Alliance
www.dbsalliance.org

Brain Anatomy

About, Inc.—"Anatomy of the Brain"
www.biology.about.com

Brain Connection—"Image gallery—Brain
Anatomy"
www.brainconnection.com

Harvard University—"The Whole
Brain Atlas"
www.med.harvard.edu

PBS—"The Secret Life of the Brain"
www.pbs.org/wnet/brain

Virtual Hospital—"The Human Brain:
Dissections of the Real Brain"
www.vh.org/adult/provider/anatomy/
BrainAnatomy/BrainAnatomy

Major Depression

About, Inc.—"About Depression"
www.depression.about.com

Depression.com
www.depression.com

Depression and Bipolar Support Alliance
www.dbsalliance.org

National Mental Health Association—
"Depression-Screening.org"
www.depression-screening.org

Psychology Online—"Depression—
Information and Treatment"
www.psychologyinfo.com/depression

Learning Disabilities

LDOnline
www.ldonline.org

LD Resources
www.ldresources.com

Learning Disabilities Association of America
www.ldanatl.org

National Center for Learning Disabilities
www.ld.org

Parkinson's Disease

American Parkinson Disease Association, Inc.
www.apdaparkinson.org

Parkinson's Disease Foundation
www.pdf.org

Parkinsons.org
www.parkinsons.org

Schizophrenia

National Alliance for Research on
Schizophrenia and Depression
www.narsad.org

Schizophrenia.com
www.schizophrenia.com

World Fellowship for Schizophrenia and
Allied Disorders
www.world-schizophrenia.org

Tourette's Disorder

Tourette's-Disorder.com
www.tourettes-disorder.com

Tourette Syndrome Association
www.tsa-usa.org

Tourette Syndrome "Plus"
www.tourettesyndrome.net

Index